Maternal and Newborn **Success**

A Q&A Review Applying Critical Thinking to Test Taking

D1511336

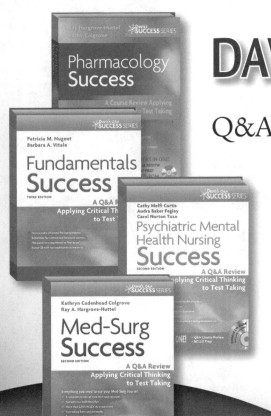
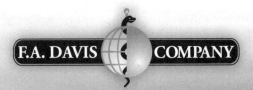
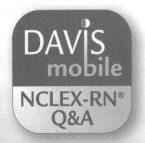
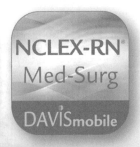
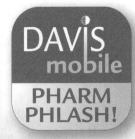
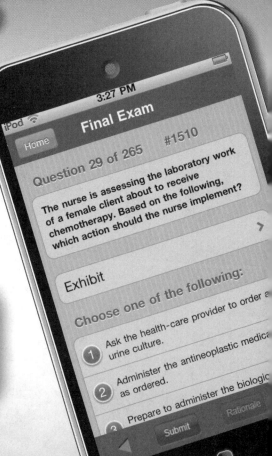

Maternal and Newborn **Success**

A Q&A Review Applying Critical Thinking to Test Taking

SECOND EDITION

Margot De Sevo, PhD, LCCE, IBCLC, RNC
Adelphi University School of Nursing
Garden City, New York

F.A. Davis Company • Philadelphia

F. A. Davis Company
1915 Arch Street
Philadelphia, PA 19103
www.fadavis.com

Copyright © 2013 by F. A. Davis Company

Printed in the United States of America

Last digit indicates print number: 10 9 8 7 6 5 4 3 2 1

Publisher, Nursing: Robert G. Martone
Director of Content Development: Darlene D. Pedersen
Project Editor: Jacalyn C. Clay
Electronic Project Editor: Sandra A. Glennie
Manager of Art and Design: Carolyn O'Brien

As new scientific information becomes available through basic and clinical research, recommended treatments and drug therapies undergo changes. The author(s) and publisher have done everything possible to make this book accurate, up to date, and in accord with accepted standards at the time of publication. The author(s), editors, and publisher are not responsible for errors or omissions or for consequences from application of the book, and make no warranty, expressed or implied, in regard to the contents of the book. Any practice described in this book should be applied by the reader in accordance with professional standards of care used in regard to the unique circumstances that may apply in each situation. The reader is advised always to check product information (package inserts) for changes and new information regarding dose and contraindications before administering any drug. Caution is especially urged when using new or infrequently ordered drugs.

I dedicate this book to my wonderful family. My husband, Richard, has loved me throughout our marriage and supported me at every point in my career. He is my best friend. My daughters Allison and Julia, my sons-in-law Craig and Adam, and my grandchildren Cameron and Abigail, give my life purpose and meaning, inspiring me each day to be the best person, mother, and grandmother that I can be. I cherish them all.

Reviewers

Marie Adorno, APRNC, MN
Associate Professor of Nursing
Our Lady of Holy Cross College
New Orleans, Louisiana

Rebecca L. Allen, RN, MNA
Assistant Professor
Clarkson College
Omaha, Nebraska

Anita Althans, RNC, BSN, MSN
Associate Professor of Nursing
Our Lady of Holy Cross College
New Orleans, Louisiana

Kimberly Attwood, PhD(c), CRNP,
APRN, BC, NP-C
Assistant Professor of Nursing
DeSales University
Center Valley, Pennsylvania

Bridgette Bailey, RN, MSN
Assistant Professor
Iowa Lakes Community College
Emmetsburg, Iowa

Laura Beyerle, MSN, RN
Director of Nursing Education
Indiana Business College
Indianapolis, Indiana

Kathleen Borge, MS, RNC, CNE
Department Chair, Nursing IV
School of Nursing
Samaritan Hospital
Troy, New York

Betty Carlson Bowles, PhD, RNC,
IBCLC, RLC, FACCE
Assistant Professor of Nursing
Midwestern State University
Wichita Falls, Texas

Jennifer B. Bradle, MSN, RN,
APN-CNS
Adjunct Faculty
Meridian Health School of Nursing
Georgian Court University
Red Bank, New Jersey

Tammy Bryant, RN, BSN
Program Director
Southwest Georgia Technical College
Thomasville, Georgia

Jackie Collins, RNC-OB, MSN,
IBCLC, CCM, CNE
Senior Level Coordinator
College of Nursing and Health
Professions
Central Maine Medical Center
Lewiston, Maine

Judith Drumm, DNS, RN, CPN
Associate Professor of Nursing
Palm Beach Atlantic University
West Palm Beach, Florida

Lisa Everhart, RN, MSN, WHNP-BC
Assistant Professor of Nursing—Health
of Women and Infants
Columbia State Community College
Franklin, Tennessee

Joyce A. Finch, MSN, MEd, RN, BA,
RNC, CNE
Assistant Professor, Nursing Education
Christ College of Nursing and Health
Sciences
Cincinnati, Ohio

Denise M. Fitzpatrick, RNC, MSN,
CNE
Course Coordinator
Dixon School of Nursing
Abington Memorial Hospital
Willow Grove, Pennsylvania

Sue Gabriel, MFS, MSN, RN, SANE,
EdD candidate
Assistant Professor
School of Nursing
BryanLGH College of Health Sciences
Lincoln, Nebraska

Marilyn Johnessee Greer, RN, MS
Associate Professor of Nursing
Rockford College
Rockford, Illinois

Mary E. Hancock, MSN/Ed, RNC
Nursing Faculty
Bon Secours Memorial School of Nursing
Richmond, Virginia

Paula Karnick, PhD, ANP-C, CPNP
Associate Professor
School of Nursing
North Park University
Chicago, Illinois

Kathy Jo Keever, RNC-OB, CNM, MS
Professor, Nursing/Health Professions
Anne Arundel Community College
Arnold, Maryland

Kathryn M.L. Konrad, MS, RNC-OB, LCCE, FACCE
Instructor
College of Nursing
The University of Oklahoma
Oklahoma City, Oklahoma

Barbara Lange, PhD, RN
Executive Director
Carolyn McKelvey Moore School of Nursing
University of Arkansas – Fort Smith
Fort Smith, Arkansas

Nancy Lugo-Baez, MSN, RN
Assistant Professor of Nursing
Bethel College
North Newton, Kansas

Jaclyn Mauldin, MSN, RN
Professor of Nursing
Florida State College at Jacksonville
Jacksonville, Florida

Barbara McClaskey, PhD, MN, RNC, ARNP
Professor
Department of Nursing
Pittsburg State University
Pittsburg, Kansas

Carrie Mines, RN, BScN, MSC(T), PhD student
Level 1 Coordinator and Faculty
Mohawk College
Hamilton, Ontario, Canada

Michelle R. Offutt, RN, MSN, ARNP
Associate Professor
St. Petersburg College
Pinellas Park, Florida

Robin L. Page, PhD, RN, CNM
Assistant Professor of Clinical Nursing
School of Nursing
University of Texas at Austin
Austin, Texas

Donna Paulsen, RN, MSN
Nursing Faculty
North Carolina A&T State University
Greensboro, North Carolina

Jacquelyn Reid, MSN, EdD, CNM, CNE
Associate Professor of Nursing
Indiana University, Southeast
New Albany, Indiana

Kellie Richardson, RN, MSN
MCH Lead Instructor
Kilgore College
Kilgore, Texas

Jean Smucker Rodgers, RN, MN
Nursing Faculty
Hesston College
Hesston, Kansas

Kathryn Rudd, RNC, MSN
Nurse Educator
Huron School of Nursing
Cuyahoga Community College
Cleveland, Ohio

Martha C. Ruder, RN, MSN
Coordinator, Associate Degree Nursing Program
Gulf Coast State College
Panama City, Florida

Teresa Salema, BSN
Nursing Educator
Camosun College
Victoria, British Columbia, Canada

Cordia A. Starling, RN, BSN, MS, EdD
Professor/Division Chair, Nursing
Dalton State College
Dalton, Georgia

Wendy Z. Thompson, EdD(c), MSN, BSBA, IBCLC
Assistant Professor/Technology
Coordinator
Nova Southeastern University
Fort Lauderdale, Florida

Leigh Anne Walker, RN, MSN
Nursing Instructor
Rowan-Cabarrus Community College
Kannapolis, North Carolina

Sherry Warner, MSN, RN
Nursing Instructor
Fulton-Montgomery Community College
Johnstown, New York

Acknowledgments

I want to thank Joan Arnold, RN, PhD, for persuading me to write this book. Without her words of encouragement, I would probably never have begun the project. Barbara Bruno, RN, deserves a special thanks for spending a full morning of her busy day at the hospital helping me with fetal monitor tracings. Virginia Moore, RN, IBCLC, must be thanked for her continued patience and frequent words of support. Robert Martone and Jacalyn Clay at F.A. Davis Company have been helpful, supportive, and instructive throughout the writing process. Thank you, all.

Contents

Introduction

This book is part of a series published by F. A. Davis designed to assist student nurses in reviewing essential information and in taking examinations, particularly the NCLEX-RN® and certification exams. The book focuses predominantly on childbearing—the antepartum, intrapartum, postpartum, and newborn periods—and, because of the childbearing focus, includes questions about fetal and neonatal development. In addition, because women are pregnant for such a short period of their lives, because childbearing occurs within the context of the family, and because embryonic and fetal development occur within the context of genetics, the text contains questions on those topics. Other subjects, including sexually transmitted illnesses, domestic violence, rape, and contraception, that affect women during the childbearing years—which make up about one third of a woman's life—are also included. As a result, this text is an excellent supplement for a number of nursing school courses, including parent-child nursing, fetal growth and development, basic genetics, family processes, and women's health.

To obtain the most from this book, the student is strongly encouraged to read the content related to the different topic areas and to study the material in a logical manner. Only if this is done will this book be valuable. Used as a supplement to foundational work, this book should be helpful in developing the skills needed to be successful on examinations in the relevant content areas.

A discussion of the types of questions asked on examinations, of techniques for approaching test questions to identify what is being asked, and of how to select correct responses follows.

USE THIS BOOK AS ONE EDUCATIONAL STRATEGY

This book contains 11 subsequent chapters and is accompanied online with two comprehensive examinations. This introductory chapter focuses on the types of questions included in the NCLEX-RN examination and on how to approach studying and preparing for an examination. Chapters 2 through 11 focus on topics related to maternity nursing, most specifically the antepartum, intrapartum, postpartum, and newborn periods. Each of these chapters contains practice questions that test a student's knowledge and answers and rationales with specific tips on how to approach answering the question. The reasons a particular answer is correct and the reasons other answer options are incorrect are given. This information serves as a valuable learning tool for the student and helps to reinforce knowledge. Chapter 12 consists of a 100-question Comprehensive Examination with questions, answers, and rationales. The two comprehensive online examinations include questions and answers that cover all topics included in the 10 content chapters. The online format will provide the test taker with practice in answering questions on the computer, a valuable help given that the NCLEX-RN examination is computer-based.

LEARN THE MATERIAL

The first step to take before attempting to answer questions in this text—or on an examination—is to study and learn the relevant material. Learning does not mean simply reading textbooks and/or attending class. Learning is an active process that requires a number of complex skills, including reading, discussing, and organizing information.

READ YOUR ASSIGNMENTS

Students must first read their assignments. By far the best time to read the assigned material is before the class in which the information will be discussed. Then, if students have any questions about what was read, they can ask the instructor during class and clarify anything that is confusing. In addition, students will find discussions much more meaningful when they have a basic understanding of the material.

DISCUSS THE INFORMATION

During class time, material should be discussed with students rather than fed to them. Teachers have an obligation to provide stimulating and thought-provoking classes, but students also have an obligation to be prepared to engage in discussions upon entering the classroom.

Although facts must be learned, nursing is not a fact-based profession. Nursing is an applied science. Nurses must use information. When a nurse enters a client's room, the client rarely asks the nurse to define a term or to recite a fact. Rather, the client presents the nurse with a set of data that the nurse must interpret and act on. In other words, the nurse must think critically. Students, therefore, must discuss client-based information by asking "why" questions rather than simply learning facts by asking "what" questions.

ORGANIZE THE INFORMATION

While reading and discussing information, nursing students must begin to organize their knowledge. Nursing knowledge cannot be memorized. There is too much information to be memorized and, more important, memorization negatively affects the ability to use information. Nurses must be able to analyze data critically to determine priorities and actions. To think critically, nurses develop connections between and among elements of information.

There are several steps for organizing basic information, including understanding the pathophysiology of a problem; determining its significance for a particular client; identifying signs and symptoms; and using the steps of the nursing process: assessment, formulation of a nursing diagnosis, development of a plan of care, implementation of that plan, and evaluation of the outcomes. An example—a woman with a diagnosis of placenta previa—is used in this chapter to illustrate the use of these interrelated steps to provide a pathway for organizing basic information. Whether studying for an examination or using skills in a specific clinical situation, it is often helpful to show graphically the relationships between and among various pieces of information, as is done below.

Example: A client has placenta previa.

The nurse must first understand the problem, determine its significance, and assess for signs and symptoms.

Understand the Problem

The first action is to understand (not memorize) the pathophysiology of the issue or problem. (Implicit is the prerequisite that the learner already fully understands the normal anatomy and physiology of pregnancy.)

The placenta usually attaches to a highly vascular site in the decidua on the posterior wall of the uterus. Women who have compromised uterine vascularity—women who are multiparous, are smokers, have diabetes, or are carrying multiple gestations, for example—are at high risk for placenta previa. In this condition, the placenta, rather than attaching to the posterior portion of the uterine wall, attaches to an area immediately above or adjacent to the internal os of the uterus.

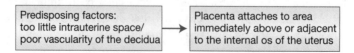

Determine the Significance of the Pathophysiology

The second phase of the process is to determine the significance of the pathophysiology. Often the nurse is able to deduce the significance based on knowledge of normal anatomy and physiology.

Because the placenta is the highly vascular organ that supplies oxygen and nutrients to the developing baby, it is essential to the well-being of the fetus. If the cervix were to dilate or be injured, the chorionic villi of the placenta would be disrupted. The mother would lose blood, and the baby's oxygenation and nutrition would be critically affected, resulting in a life-threatening situation for both mother and fetus.

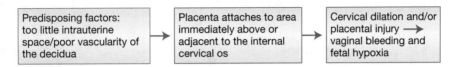

Identify Signs and Symptoms

Once the significance of the pathophysiology is deduced, it is essential to identify the signs and symptoms that are expected.

In the mother, the nurse would expect to see bleeding with its associated changes in hematological signs (hematocrit and hemoglobin) and vital signs, as well as anxiety. Because the placental bleeding will be unobstructed—that is, the blood will be able to escape easily via the vagina—the nurse would expect that the client would be in little to no pain and that the blood would be bright red. In addition, the nurse would expect the client's hematological signs to be affected and the vital signs to change. However, because women have significantly elevated blood volumes during pregnancy, the pulse rate will elevate first, and the blood pressure will stay relatively stable. A drop in blood pressure is a late, and ominous, sign. In addition, the nurse would expect the mother to be anxious regarding her own and her baby's well-being.

In the fetus, if there were significant maternal blood loss and placental disturbance, the nurse would expect to see adverse changes in heart rate patterns. Late decelerations result from poor uteroplacental blood flow.

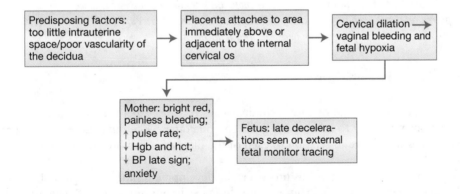

Once the problem and the data concerning it are understood, the significance determined, and expected signs and symptoms identified, it is time for the student (and nurse) to turn to the nursing process.

USE THE NURSING PROCESS

The nursing process is foundational to nursing practice. To provide comprehensive care to their clients, nurses must understand and use each part of the nursing process—assessment, formulation of a nursing diagnosis, development of a plan of care, implementation of that plan, and evaluation of the outcomes.

Assess

Nurses gather a variety of information during the assessment phase of the nursing process. Some of the information is objective, or fact-based. For example, a client's hematocrit level and other blood values in the chart are facts that the nurse can use to determine a client's needs. Nurses also must identify subjective data, or information as perceived through the eyes of the client. A client's rating of pain is an excellent example of subjective information. Nurses must be aware of which data must be assessed because each and every client situation is unique. In other words, nurses must be able to use the information taught in class and individualize it for each client interaction to determine which objective data must be accessed and which questions should be asked of the client. Once the information is obtained, the nurse analyzes it. (See example above.)

Formulate Nursing Diagnoses

After the nurse has analyzed the data, a diagnosis is made. Nurses are licensed to treat actual or potential health problems. Nursing diagnoses are statements of the health problems that the nurse, in collaboration with the client, has concluded are critical to the client's well-being.

The nurse now must develop the nursing diagnoses and prioritize them as they relate to the care of a client with placenta previa. Because a woman with placenta previa may begin to bleed, it is essential that the nurse develop two sets of diagnoses: one aimed at preventing complications—that is, "risk for" diagnoses—and one directed at the worst-case scenario—that is, if the client should start to bleed.

The "risk for" placenta previa nursing diagnoses are:

- *Risk for maternal imbalanced fluid volume related to (r/t) hypovolemia secondary to excessive blood loss*
- *Risk for impaired fetal gas exchange r/t decreased blood volume and maternal cardiovascular compromise*
- *Maternal anxiety r/t concern for personal and fetal health*

The worst-case scenario (active bleeding) nursing diagnoses are:

- *Imbalanced maternal fluid volume r/t hypovolemia secondary to excessive blood loss*
- *Impaired fetal gas exchange r/t decreased blood volume and maternal cardiovascular compromise*
- *Maternal anxiety r/t concern for personal and fetal health*

Develop a Plan of Care

The nurse develops a plan of care including goals of care, expected client outcomes, and interventions necessary to achieve the goals and outcomes. The nurse determines what he or she wishes to achieve in relation to each of the diagnoses and how to go about meeting those goals.

One very important part of this process is the development of the priorities of care. The nurse must determine which diagnoses are the most important and, consequently, which actions are the most important. For example, a client's physical well-being must take precedence over emotional well-being. It is essential that the nurse consider the client's priorities and the goals and orders of the client's primary health care provider.

The nurse caring for the client with placenta previa develops a plan of care based on the diagnoses listed above. Because the physical conditions must take precedence, the nurse prioritzes the plan with the physical needs first. The client's emotional needs will then be considered. The plan of care to meet the "at risk" nursing diagnoses is shown in Box 1-1, and a plan for the worst-case scenario—active bleeding—is shown in Box 1-2.

BOX 1-1 PLAN OF CARE FOR CLIENT WITH PLACENTA PREVIA AT RISK FOR BLEEDING

Nursing Diagnosis: Risk for imbalanced fluid volume (maternal) related to (r/t) hypovolemia secondary to excessive blood loss.
Goal: Client will not bleed throughout her pregnancy.
Proposed Actions: The nurse will:
- Assess for vaginal bleeding each shift.
- Assess for uterine contractions each shift.
- Assess vital signs each shift.
- Assess intake and output during each shift.
- Assess bowel function each shift.
- Insert nothing into the vagina.
- Maintain client on bed rest, as ordered.
- Monitor changes in laboratory data.

Nursing Diagnosis: Risk for impaired gas exchange (fetal) r/t decreased blood volume and maternal cardiovascular compromise.
Goal: The fetal heart rate will show average variability and no decelerations until delivery.
Proposed Actions: The nurse will:
- Monitor fetal heart rate every shift.
- Do nonstress testing, as ordered.

Nursing Diagnosis: Anxiety (maternal) r/t concern for personal and fetal health.
Goal: The mother will exhibit minimal anxiety throughout her pregnancy.
Proposed Actions: The nurse will:
- Provide emotional support.

BOX 1-2 PLAN OF CARE FOR PATIENT WITH PLACENTA PREVIA WHO IS BLEEDING

Nursing Diagnosis: Imbalanced fluid volume (maternal) r/t hypovolemia secondary to excessive blood loss.
Goal: Client will become hemodynamically stable.
Proposed Interventions: The nurse will:
- Measure vaginal bleeding.
  - Count number of saturated vaginal pads.
  - Weigh pads—1 g = 1 mL of blood.
- Monitor for uterine contraction pattern, if present.
- Assess vital signs every 15 minutes.
- Assess oxygen saturation levels continually.
- Assess intake and output every hour.
- Insert nothing into the vagina.
- Maintain client on bed rest.
- Monitor changes in laboratory data.
- Administer intravenous fluids, as ordered.
- Prepare for emergency cesarean section, as ordered.

Nursing Diagnosis: Risk for impaired gas exchange (fetal) r/t decreased blood volume and maternal cardiovascular compromise.
Goal: The fetal heart rate will show average variability and no late decelerations.
Proposed Interventions: The nurse will:
- Monitor fetal heart rate continually via external fetal monitor.

Nursing Diagnosis: Anxiety (maternal) r/t concern for personal and fetal health.
Goal: The mother will exhibit minimal anxiety.
Proposed Interventions: The nurse will:
- Provide clear, calm explanations of all assessments and actions.
- Provide emotional support.

Implement the Care

Once the plan is established, the nurse implements it. The plan may include direct client care by the nurse and/or care that is coordinated by the nurse but performed by other practitioners. If assessment data change during implementation, the nurse must reanalyze the data, change diagnoses, and reprioritize care.

One very important aspect of nursing care is that it be evidence-based. Nurses are independent practitioners. They are mandated to provide safe, therapeutic care that has a scientific basis. Nurses, therefore, must engage in lifelong learning. It is essential that nurses realize that much of the information in textbooks is outdated before the text was even published. To provide evidence-based care, nurses must keep their knowledge current by accessing information from reliable sources on the Internet, in professional journals, and at professional conferences.

Care of the placenta previa patient should be implemented as developed during the planning phase. If a situation should change, for example, should the woman begin to bleed spontaneously during a shift, the nurse would immediately revise his or her plan, as needed. In the example cited, the nurse would implement the active bleeding plan of care.

Evaluate the Care

The evaluation phase is usually identified as the last phase of the nursing process, but it also could be classified as another assessment phase. When nurses evaluate, they are reassessing clients to determine whether the actions taken during the implementation phase met the needs of the client. In other words, "Were the goals of the nursing care met?" If the goals were not met, the nurse is obligated to develop new actions to meet the goals. If some of the goals were met, priorities may need to be changed, and so on. As can be seen from this phase, the nursing process is ongoing and ever-changing.

Throughout the nursing care period, the nurse is assessing and reassessing the status of the client with placenta previa. If needed, the nurse may report significant changes to the health care provider or may determine independently that a change in nursing care is needed. For example, if the client begins to cry because she is concerned about her baby's health, and physiologically the client is stable, the nurse can concentrate on meeting the client's emotional needs. The nurse may sit quietly with the client while she communicates her concerns. Conversely, if the client begins to bleed profusely, the nurse would immediately report the change to the client's health care provider and implement the active bleeding plan.

TYPES OF QUESTIONS

There are four "integrative processes" upon which questions in the NCLEX-RN examination are based: "Nursing Process," "Caring," "Communication and Documentation," and "Teaching/Learning" (*2013 NCLEX-RN Detailed Test Plan, Candidate Version,* 2013, p. 10). The test taker must determine which process(es) is (are) being evaluated in each question. The test taker must realize that because nursing is an action profession, the NCLEX-RN questions simulate, in a written format, clinical situations. Critical reading is, therefore, essential.

Most of the questions on the NCLEX-RN exam are multiple-choice. Other types of questions, known as alternate-type questions, include "fill-in-the-blank" questions, "multiple-response" questions, "drag-and-drop" questions, and "hot spot" items. In addition, any one of the types of questions may include an item to interpret, including lab data, images, and/or audio or video files (*2013 NCLEX-RN Detailed Test Plan,* 2013, p. 46). The types of questions and examples of each are discussed below.

Multiple-Choice Questions

In these questions, a stem is provided (a situation), and the test taker must choose among four possible responses. Sometimes the test taker will be asked to choose the best response, sometimes to choose the first action that should be taken, and so on. There are numerous ways that multiple-choice questions may be asked. Below is one example related to a client with placenta previa.

A client, 36 weeks' gestation, has been diagnosed with a complete placenta previa. On nursing rounds, the client tells the nurse that she has a bad backache that comes and goes. Which of the following actions should the nurse perform first?

1. *Give the client a back rub.*
2. *Assess the client's vital signs.*
3. *Time the client's back pains.*
4. *Assess for vaginal bleeding.*

Answer: *4*

The nurse must realize that, because the backache comes and goes, this client may be in early labor. As dilation of the cervix can lead to bleeding, the nurse must first assess for placental injury—vaginal bleeding.

Fill-in-the-Blank Questions

These are calculation questions. The test taker may be asked to calculate a medication dosage, an intravenous (IV) drip rate, a minimum urinary output, or other factor. Included in the question will be the units that the test taker should have in the answer.

The nurse caring for a client with placenta previa must determine how much blood the client has lost. The nurse weighs a clean vaginal pad (5 g) and the client's saturated pad (25 g). How many milliliters of blood has the client lost? _____ mL

Answer: *20 mL*

The test taker must subtract 5 from 25 to determine that the client has lost 20 g of blood. Then, knowing that 1 g of blood is equal to 1 mL of blood, the test taker knows that the client has lost 20 mL of blood.

Drag-and-Drop Questions

In drag-and-drop questions, the test taker is asked to place four or five possible responses in chronological or rank order. The responses may be actions to be taken during a nursing procedure, steps in growth and development, and the like. The items are called drag-and-drop questions because the test taker will move the items with his or her computer mouse. Needless to say, in this book, the test taker will simply be asked to write the responses in the correct sequence.

The nurse must administer a blood transfusion to a client with placenta previa who has lost a significant amount of blood. Put the following nursing actions in the chronological order in which they should be performed.

1. *Stay with client for a full 5 minutes and take a full set of vital signs.*
2. *Compare the client's name and hospital identification number with the name and number on the blood product container.*
3. *Check the physician's order regarding the type of infusion that is to be administered.*
4. *Regulate the infusion rate as prescribed.*

Answer: *3, 2, 4, 1*

Of the four steps included in the answer options, the order should be 3, 2, 4, 1. First, the nurse must check the physician's order to determine exactly what blood product is being ordered. Second, the nurse must compare the information on the blood product bag with the client's name band. This must be done with another nurse or a doctor. Third, the nurse must begin the infusion and regulate the infusion. Finally, the nurse must closely monitor the client during the first 5 minutes of the infusion to assess for any transfusion reactions. At the end of the 5 minutes, a full set of vital signs must be taken.

Multiple-Response Questions

The sentence "Select all that apply" following a question means that the examiner has included more than one correct response to the question. Usually there will be five responses given, and the test taker must determine which of the five responses are correct. There may be two, three, four, or even five correct responses.

A nurse is caring for a client, 28 weeks' gestation, with placenta previa. Which of the following physician orders should the nurse question? **Select all that apply.**

1. *Encourage ambulation.*
2. *Weigh all vaginal pads.*
3. *Assess cervical dilation daily.*
4. *Perform a nonstress test every morning.*
5. *Administer Colace 100 mg PO three times a day*

Answer: *1 and 3 are correct.*

Because the placenta could be injured, no vaginal examinations should be performed; therefore, the nurse should question #3—assess cervical dilation daily. Also, because bleeding may occur, clients with placenta previa are allowed only minimal activity; therefore, ambulation would not be encouraged.

Hot Spot Items

These items require the test taker to identify the correct response to a question about a picture, graph, or other image. For example, a test taker may be asked to place an "X" on the location of a P wave on an electrocardiogram strip.

Below is a diagram of the uterus. Place an "X" where a complete placenta previa would be attached.

Answer: *The test taker should place an "X" on the internal os of the cervix.*

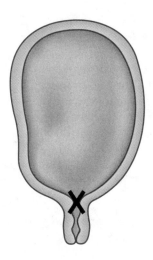

Items for Interpretation

Some questions may include an item to interpret. For example, the test taker is asked to interpret the sound on an audio file as inspiratory stridor, recognize that a client is becoming progressively more anemic by interpreting laboratory results, or perform a calculation based on information given on an intake and output sheet.

While caring for a client who had an emergency cesarean section because of active bleeding related to complete placenta previa, the nurse aide has emptied the Foley catheter three times during an 8-hour shift. See Output Record next page. How many mL of urine has the client voided during the shift?

Answer: *250 mL (60 + 90 + 100 = 250)*

Urine Output for 8-Hour Shift

7 a.m.	
8 a.m.	*60 mL*
9 a.m.	
10 a.m.	
11 a.m.	*90 mL*
12 p.m.	
1 p.m.	
2 p.m.	
3 p.m.	*100 mL*
TOTAL	

KNOW HOW TO APPROACH EXAM QUESTIONS

There are several techniques that a test taker should use when approaching examination questions.

- **Pretend that the examination is a clinical experience**—First and foremost, test takers must approach critical-thinking questions as if they were in a clinical setting and the situation were developing on the spot. If the test taker pretends he or she is in a clinical situation, the importance of the response becomes evident. In addition, the test taker is likely to prepare for the examination with more commitment. That is not to say that students are rarely committed to doing well on examinations, but rather that they often approach examinations differently than they approach clinical situations. It is a rare nurse who goes to clinical not having had sufficient sleep to care for his or her clients, and yet students often enter an examination room after only 2 or 3 hours of sleep. The student taking an exam and a nurse working on a clinical unit both need the same critical-thinking ability that sleep provides. It is essential that test takers be well rested before all exams.
- **Read the stem carefully before reading the responses**—As discussed above, there are a number of different types of questions on the NCLEX-RN examination, and most faculty are including alternate-format questions in their classroom examinations as well. Before answering any question, the test taker must be sure, therefore, what the questioner is asking. This is one enormous drawback to classroom examinations. A test taker standing in a client's room is much less likely to misinterpret the situation when he or she is facing a client than when reading a question on an examination.
- **Consider possible responses**—After clearly understanding the stem of the question, *but before reading the possible responses*, the test taker should consider possible correct answers to the question. It is important for the test taker to realize that test writers include only plausible answer options. A test writer's goal is to determine whether the test taker knows and understands the material. The test taker, therefore, must have an idea of what the correct answer might be before beginning to read the possible responses.
- **Read the responses**—Only after clearly understanding what is being asked and after developing an idea of what the correct answer might be should the test taker read the responses. The one response that is closest in content to the test taker's "guess" should be the answer that is chosen, and the test taker should not second-guess himself or herself. The first impression is almost always the correct response. Only if the test taker knows that he or she misread the question should the answer be changed.
- **Read the rationales for each question**—In this book, rationales are given for each answer option. The student should take full advantage of this feature. Read why the correct answer is correct. The rationale may be based on content, on interpretation of information, or on a number of other bases. Understanding why the answer to one

question is correct is likely to transfer over to other questions with similar rationales. Next, read why the wrong answers are wrong. Again, the rationales may be based on a number of different factors. Understanding why answers are wrong also may transfer over to other questions.

- **Finally, read all test-taking tips**—Some of the tips relate directly to test-taking skills, whereas others include invaluable information for the test taker.

If the test taker uses this text as recommended above, he or she should be well prepared to be successful when taking an examination in any or all of the content areas represented. As a result, the test taker should be fully prepared to function as a beginning registered professional nurse in the many areas of maternity and women's health.

Sexuality, Fertility, and Genetics

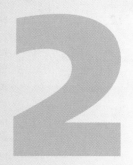

Before pregnancy can begin, a sperm and an ovum must unite. This usually occurs as a result of sexual intercourse but can be accomplished via artificial insemination, in vitro fertilization, and a number of other procedures used in attempts to overcome infertility. The nurse must be familiar with the male and female reproductive systems to understand why normal procreation occurs and why, in some instances, a woman fails to become pregnant. This chapter includes questions on three related issues surrounding the process of reproduction: sexuality, infertility, and genetics. Since genetics involves much more than simply parents and their offspring, additional concepts are included in the genetics section.

KEYWORDS

The following words include vocabulary, nursing/medical terminology, concepts, principles, or information relevant to content specifically addressed in the chapter or associated with topics presented in it. Dictionaries, your nursing textbooks, and medical dictionaries such as *Taber's Cyclopedic Medical Dictionary* are resources that can be used to expand your knowledge and understanding of these words and related information.

allele
amniocentesis
aneuploidy
autosomal dominant inheritance
autosomal recessive inheritance
autosome
basal body temperature
chorionic villus sampling (CVS)
chromosome
corpus cavernosum
corpus luteum
corpus spongiosum
deoxyribonucleic acid (DNA)
diploid
Down syndrome
Duchenne muscular dystrophy
ejaculatory duct
endometrial biopsy
epididymis
estrogen
expressivity
fallopian tubes
familial adenomatous polyposis (FAP)
ferning capacity
fertilization

fimbriae
follicle-stimulating hormone (FSH)
follicular phase
fragile X syndrome
gametes
gametogenesis
gene
genetics
genome
genotype
GIFT (gamete intrafallopian transfer)
glans
gonadotropin-releasing hormone
graafian follicle
haploid
hemophilia A
human chorionic gonadotropin
Huntington's disease
hysterosalpingogram
hysteroscopy
infertility
in vitro fertilization
ischemic phase
karyotype
laparoscopy

luteal phase

luteinizing hormone (LH)

meiosis

menses

menstrual cycle

menstrual phase

mitochondrial inheritance

mitosis

monosomy

oogenesis

ovary

ovulation

ovum

pedigree

penetrance

phenotype

phenylketonuria

polycystic kidney disease (PKD)

prepuce

progesterone

proliferative phase

prostate

ribonucleic acid (RNA)

scrotum

secretory phase

seminal vesicle

sex chromosome

spermatogenesis

spinnbarkeit

surrogate

testes

trisomy

urethra

uterus

vagina

vas deferens

X-linked recessive inheritance

Y-linked inheritance

ZIFT (zygote intrafallopian transfer)

QUESTIONS

Sexuality

1. A nurse is discussing sexual arousal during a preadolescent boys' sex education class. Which of the following should the nurse base her reply on when a boy asks, "What exactly happens when my body gets aroused, anyway?"
   1. The vas deferens thickens and expands.
   2. The sympathetic nerves of the penis are stimulated.
   3. The corpora of the penis become engorged.
   4. The prepuce of the penis elongates.

2. A woman, whose menstrual cycle is 35 days long, states that she often has a slight pain on one side of her lower abdomen on day 21 of her cycle. She wonders whether she has ovarian cancer. Which of the following is the nurse's best response?
   1. "Women often feel a slight twinge when ovulation occurs."
   2. "You should seek medical attention as soon as possible since ovarian cancer is definitely a possibility."
   3. "Ovarian cancer is unlikely because the pain is not a constant pain."
   4. "It is more likely that such pain indicates an ovarian cyst because pain is more common with that problem."

3. A nurse is explaining to a client about monthly hormonal changes. Starting with day 1 of the menstrual cycle, please place the following four hormones in the chronological order in which they elevate during the menstrual cycle.
   1. Follicle-stimulating hormone.
   2. Gonadotropin-releasing hormone.
   3. Luteinizing hormone.
   4. Progesterone.

4. A 54-year-old client calls her health care practitioner complaining of frequency and burning when she urinates. Which of the following factors that occurred within the preceding 3 days likely contributed to this client's problem?
   1. She had intercourse with her partner.
   2. She returned from a trip abroad.
   3. She stopped taking hormone replacement therapy.
   4. She started a weight-lifting exercise program.

5. A woman's temperature has just risen 0.4°F and will remain elevated during the remainder of her cycle. She expects to menstruate in about 2 weeks. Which of the following hormones is responsible for the change?
   1. Estrogen.
   2. Progesterone.
   3. Luteinizing hormone (LH).
   4. Follicle-stimulating hormone (FSH).

6. A woman is menstruating. If hormonal studies were to be done at this time, which of the following hormonal levels would the nurse expect to see?
   1. Both estrogen and progesterone are high.
   2. Estrogen is high and progesterone is low.
   3. Estrogen is low and progesterone is high.
   4. Both estrogen and progesterone are low.

7. A nurse teaches a woman who wishes to become pregnant that if she assesses for spinnbarkeit she will be able closely to predict her time of ovulation. Which technique should the client be taught to assess for spinnbarkeit?
   1. Take her temperature each morning before rising.
   2. Carefully feel her breasts for glandular development.
   3. Monitor her nipples for signs of tingling and sensitivity.
   4. Assess her vaginal discharge for elasticity and slipperiness.

8. In analyzing the need for teaching regarding sexual health in a client who is sexually active, which of the following questions is the most important for a nurse to ask?
   1. "How old are your children?"
   2. "Did you have intercourse last evening?"
   3. "With whom do you have intercourse?"
   4. "Do you use vaginal lubricant?"

9. When a nurse is teaching a woman about her menstrual cycle, which of the following is the most important change that happens during the follicular phase of the menstrual cycle?
   1. Maturation of the graafian follicle.
   2. Multiplication of the fimbriae.
   3. Secretion of human chorionic gonadotropin.
   4. Proliferation of the endometrium.

10. It is day 17 of a woman's menstrual cycle. She is complaining of breast tenderness and pain in her lower left quadrant. The woman states that her cycle is usually 31 days long. Which of the following is an appropriate reply by the nurse?
    1. "You are probably ovulating."
    2. "Your hormone levels should be checked."
    3. "You will probably menstruate early."
    4. "Your breast changes are a worrisome sign."

11. A man asks the nurse where his sperm are produced. On the diagram, please place an "X" on the site of spermatogenesis.

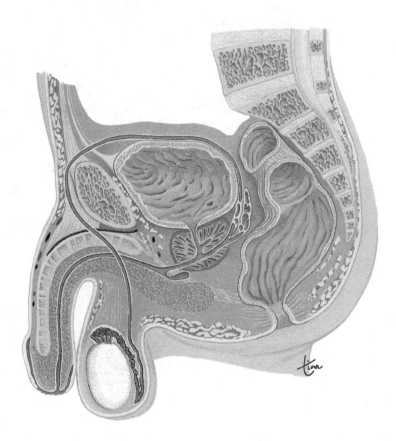

12. The nurse is teaching a class on reproduction. When asked about the development of the ova, the nurse would include which of the following?
    1. Meiotic divisions begin during puberty.
    2. At the end of meiosis, four ova are created.
    3. Each ovum contains the diploid number of chromosomes.
    4. Like sperm, ova have the ability to propel themselves.

13. A client complaining of secondary amenorrhea is seeking care from her gynecologist. Which of the following may have contributed to her problem?
    1. Athletic activities.
    2. Vaccination history.
    3. Pet ownership.
    4. History of asthma.

14. What is the function of the highlighted region on the drawing below?
    1. It produces a fluid that nourishes the sperm.
    2. It secretes a fluid that neutralizes the acidic environment of the vagina.
    3. It is the reservoir where sperm mature.
    4. It contracts during ejaculation, forcing the sperm and fluid out of the urethra.

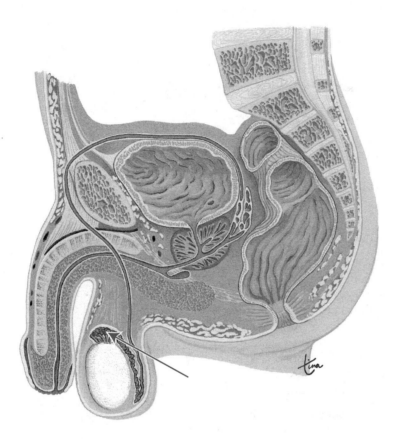

Infertility

15. A couple is seeking infertility counseling. During the history, it is noted that the man is a cancer survivor, drinks one beer every night with dinner, and takes a sauna every day after work. Which of the following is an appropriate response by the nurse?
    1. It is unlikely that any of these factors is affecting his fertility.
    2. Daily alcohol consumption could be causing his infertility problems.
    3. Sperm may be malformed when exposed to the heat of the sauna.
    4. Cancer survivors have the same fertility rates as healthy males.

16. A nurse is teaching an infertile couple about how the sperm travel through the man's body during ejaculation. Please put the following five major structures in order, beginning with the place where spermatogenesis occurs and continuing through the path that the sperm and semen travel until ejaculation.
    1. Epididymis.
    2. Prostate.
    3. Testes.
    4. Urethra.
    5. Vas deferens.

17. A client has been notified that endometriosis is covering her fimbriae. She asks the nurse why that is such a problem. The nurse advises the woman that fertilization is often impossible when the fimbriated ends are blocked. Please place an "X" on the diagram to show the woman where fertilization takes place.

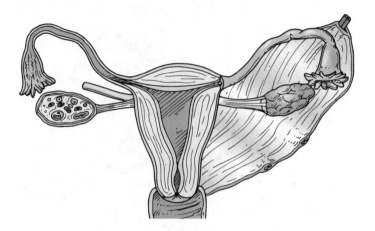

18. The nurse is providing counseling to a group of sexually active single women. Most of the women have expressed a desire to have children in the future, but not within the next few years. Which of the following actions should the nurse suggest the women take to protect their fertility for the future? **Select all that apply.**
    1. Use condoms during intercourse.
    2. Refrain from smoking cigarettes.
    3. Maintain an appropriate weight for height.
    4. Exercise in moderation.
    5. Refrain from drinking carbonated beverages.

19. A couple is seeking advice regarding actions that they can take to increase their potential of becoming pregnant. Which of the following recommendations should the nurse give to the couple?
    1. The couple should use vaginal lubricants during intercourse.
    2. The couple should delay having intercourse until the day of ovulation.
    3. The woman should refrain from douching.
    4. The man should be on top during intercourse.

20. A nurse working in an infertility clinic should include which of the following in her discussions with the couple?
    1. Adoption as an alternative to infertility treatments.
    2. The legal controversy surrounding artificial insemination.
    3. The need to seek marriage counseling before undergoing infertility treatments.
    4. Statistics regarding the number of couples who never learn why they are infertile.

21. An Orthodox Jewish couple is seeking infertility counseling. The woman states that her menstrual cycle is 21 days long. After testing, no physical explanation is found for the infertility. Which of the following may explain why the woman has been unable to conceive?
    1. Her kosher diet is lacking the essential nutrients needed for achieving optimal reproductive health.
    2. The positions allowed Orthodox Jewish couples during intercourse hinder the process of fertilization.
    3. Orthodox Jewish couples are known to have a high rate of infertility because of inborn genetic diseases.
    4. Orthodox Jewish couples refrain from intercourse during menses and for seven days after it ends.

22. An infertile woman has been diagnosed with endometriosis. She asks the nurse why that diagnosis has made her infertile. Which of the following explanations is appropriate for the nurse to make?
    1. "Scarring surrounds the ends of your tubes, preventing your eggs from being fertilized by your partner's sperm."
    2. "You are producing insufficient quantities of follicle-stimulating hormone that is needed to mature an egg every month."
    3. "Inside your uterus is a benign tumor that makes it impossible for the fertilized egg to implant."
    4. "You have a chronic infection of the vaginal tract that makes the secretions hostile to your partner's sperm."

23. A Roman Catholic couple is infertile. Their health care practitioner advises them that their best chance of getting pregnant is via in vitro fertilization with a mixture of the man's sperm and donor sperm. Which of the following issues, related to this procedure, should the nurse realize may be in conflict with the couple's religious beliefs? **Select all that apply.**
    1. The man will ejaculate by masturbation into a specially designed condom.
    2. The woman may become pregnant with donor sperm.
    3. Fertilization is occurring in the artificial environment of the laboratory.
    4. More embryos will be created than will be used to inseminate the woman.
    5. The woman will receive medications to facilitate the ripening of her ova.

24. Infertility increases a client's risk of which of the following diseases?
    1. Diabetes mellitus.
    2. Nystagmus.
    3. Cholecystitis.
    4. Ovarian cancer.

25. A client is to receive Pergonal (menotropins) injections for infertility prior to in vitro fertilization. Which of the following is the expected action of this medication?
    1. Prolongation of the luteal phase.
    2. Stimulation of ovulation.
    3. Suppression of menstruation.
    4. Promotion of cervical mucus production.

26. A 35-year-old client is being seen for her yearly gynecological examination. She states that she and her partner have been trying to become pregnant for a little over 6 months, and that a friend had recently advised her partner to take ginseng to improve the potency of his sperm. The woman states that they have decided to take their friend's advice. On which of the following information should the nurse base his or her reply?
    1. Based on their history, the client and her partner have made the appropriate decision regarding their fertility.
    2. Ginseng can cause permanent chromosomal mutations and should be stopped immediately.
    3. It is unnecessary to become concerned about this woman's fertility because she has tried to become pregnant for only a few months.
    4. Although ginseng may be helpful, it would be prudent to encourage the woman to seek fertility counseling.

27. A couple is seeking infertility counseling. The practitioner has identified the factors listed below in the woman's health history. Which of these findings may be contributing to the couple's infertility?
    1. The client is 36 years old.
    2. The client was 13 years old when she started to menstruate.
    3. The client works as a dental hygienist 3 days a week.
    4. The client jogs 2 miles every day.

28. A couple who has sought fertility counseling has been told that the man's sperm count is very low. The nurse advises the couple that spermatogenesis is impaired when which of the following occurs?
    1. The testes are overheated.
    2. The vas deferens is ligated.
    3. The prostate gland is enlarged.
    4. The flagella are segmented.

29. A nurse working with an infertile couple has made the following nursing diagnosis: Sexual dysfunction related to decreased libido. Which of the following assessments is the likely reason for this diagnosis?
    1. The couple has established a set schedule for their sexual encounters.
    2. The couple has been married for more than eight years.
    3. The couple lives with one set of parents.
    4. The couple has close friends who gave birth to a baby within the past year.

30. An infertile man is being treated with Viagra (sildenafil citrate) for erectile dysfunction (ED). Which of the following is a contraindication for this medication?
    1. Preexisting diagnosis of herpes simplex 2.
    2. Nitroglycerin ingestion for angina pectoris.
    3. Retinal damage from type I diabetes mellitus.
    4. Postsurgical care for resection of the prostate.

31. A client has been notified that because of fallopian tube obstruction, her best option for becoming pregnant is through in vitro fertilization. The client asks the nurse about the procedure. Which of the following responses is correct?
    1. "During the stimulation phase of the procedure, the physician will make sure that only one egg reaches maturation."
    2. "Preimplantation genetic diagnosis will be performed on your partner's sperm before they are mixed with your eggs."
    3. "After ovarian stimulation, you will be artificially inseminated with your partner's sperm."
    4. "Any extra embryos will be preserved for you if you wish to conceive again in the future."

32. A client asks the nurse about the gamete intrafallopian transfer (GIFT) procedure. Which of the following responses would be appropriate for the nurse to make?
    1. Fertilization takes place in the woman's body.
    2. Zygotes are placed in the fallopian tubes.
    3. Donor sperm are placed in a medium with donor eggs.
    4. A surrogate carries the infertile woman's fetus.

33. A client who is undergoing ovarian stimulation for infertility calls the infertility nurse and states, "My abdomen feels very bloated, my clothes are very tight, and my urine is very dark." Which of the following is the appropriate statement for the nurse to make at this time?
    1. "Please take a urine sample to the lab so they can check it for an infection."
    2. "Those changes indicate that you are likely already pregnant."
    3. "It is important for you to come into the office to be examined today."
    4. "Abdominal bloating is an expected response to the medications."

34. Nurses working in a midwifery office have attended a conference to learn about factors that increase a woman's risk of becoming infertile. To evaluate the nurses' learning, the conference coordinator tested the nurses' knowledge at the conclusion of the seminar. Which of the following problems should the nurses state increase a client's risk of developing infertility problems? **Select all that apply.**
    1. Women who have menstrual cycles that are up to 30 days long.
    2. Women who experience pain during intercourse.
    3. Women who have had pelvic inflammatory disease.
    4. Women who have excess facial hair.
    5. Women who have menstrual periods that are over 5 days long.

35. An infertility specialist is evaluating whether a woman's cervical mucus contains enough estrogen to support sperm motility. Which of the following tests is the physician conducting?
    1. Ferning capacity.
    2. Basal body temperature.
    3. Culposcopy.
    4. Hysterotomy.

36. A couple that has been attempting to become pregnant for 5 years is seeking assistance from an infertility clinic. The nurse assesses the clients' emotional responses to their infertility. Which of the following responses would the nurse expect to find? **Select all that apply.**
    1. Anger at others who have babies.
    2. Feelings of failure because they can't make a baby.
    3. Sexual excitement because they want so desperately to conceive a baby.
    4. Sadness because of the perceived loss of being a parent.
    5. Guilt on the part of one partner because he or she is not able to give the other a baby.

37. A client is to undergo a postcoital test for infertility. The nurse should include which of the following statements in the client's preprocedure counseling?
    1. "You will have the test the day after your menstruation ends."
    2. "You will have a dye put into your vein that will show up on x-ray."
    3. "You should refrain from having intercourse for the four days immediately prior to the test."
    4. "You should experience the same sensations you feel when your doctor does your Pap test."

38. A client is to have a hysterosalpingogram. In this procedure, the physician will be able to determine which of the following?
    1. Whether or not the ovaries are maturing properly.
    2. If the endometrium is fully vascularized.
    3. If the cervix is incompetent.
    4. Whether or not the fallopian tubes are obstructed.

39. A client's basal body temperature (BBT) chart for one full month is shown below. Based on the temperatures shown, what can the nurse conclude?
    1. It is likely that she has not ovulated.
    2. The client's fertile period is between 12 and 18 days.
    3. The client's period is abnormally long.
    4. It is likely that her progesterone levels rose on day 15.

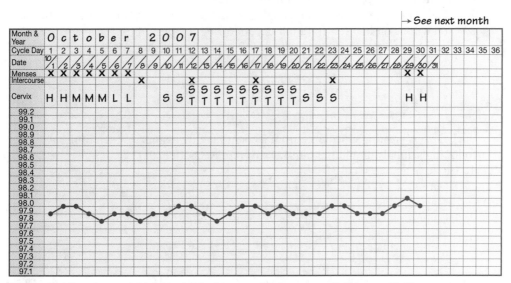

H–heavy period; **M**–moderate period; **L**–light period; **S**–sticky mucus; **SL**–slippery mucus; **T**–thick mucus; **Th**–thin mucus; **C**–clear mucus; **W**–white mucus

40. Which instruction by the nurse should be included in the teaching plan for an infertile woman who has been shown to have a 28-day biphasic menstrual cycle?
    1. Douche with a cider vinegar solution immediately before having intercourse.
    2. Schedule intercourse every day from day 8 to day 14 of the menstrual cycle.
    3. Be placed on follicle-stimulating hormone therapy by the fertility specialist.
    4. Assess the basal body temperature pattern for at least 6 more months.

41. A couple has been told that the male partner, who is healthy, is producing no sperm "because he has cystic fibrosis." Which of the following explanations is accurate in relation to this statement?
    1. Since the man is healthy, he could not possibly have cystic fibrosis.
    2. Men with cystic fibrosis often have no epididymis.
    3. The expressivity of cystic fibrosis is variable.
    4. Cystic fibrosis is a respiratory illness having nothing to do with reproduction.

42. A female client seeks care at an infertility clinic. Which of the following tests may the client undergo to determine what, if any, infertility problem she may have? **Select all that apply.**
    1. Chorionic villus sampling.
    2. Endometrial biopsy.
    3. Hysterosalpingogram.
    4. Serum progesterone assay.
    5. Postcoital test.

43. A client is hospitalized in the acute phase of severe ovarian hyperstimulation syndrome. The following nursing diagnosis has been identified: Fluid volume excess (extravascular) related to third spacing. Which of the following nursing goals is highest priority in relation to this diagnosis?
    1. Client's weight will be within normal limits by date of discharge.
    2. Client's skin will show no evidence of breakdown throughout hospitalization.
    3. Client's electrolyte levels will be within normal limits within one day.
    4. Client's lung fields will remain clear throughout hospitalization.

44. A client is receiving Pergonal (menotropins) intramuscularly for ovarian stimulation. Which of the following is a common side effect of this therapy?
    1. Piercing rectal pain.
    2. Mood swings.
    3. Visual disturbances.
    4. Jerky tremors.

45. A client is to have a hysterosalpingogram. Which of the following information should the nurse provide the client prior to the procedure?
    1. "The test will be performed through a small incision next to your belly button."
    2. "You will be on bed rest for a full day following the procedure."
    3. "An antibiotic fluid will be instilled through a tube in your cervix."
    4. "You will be asked to move from side to side so that x-ray pictures can be taken."

Genetics

46. The nurse is creating a pedigree from a client's family history. Which of the following symbols should the nurse use to represent a female?
    1. Circle.
    2. Square.
    3. Triangle.
    4. Diamond.

47. A woman has been advised that the reason she has had a number of spontaneous abortions is because she has an inheritable mutation. Which of the following situations is consistent with this statement?
    1. A client developed skin cancer after being exposed to the sun.
    2. A client developed colon cancer from an inherited dominant gene.
    3. A reciprocal translocation was reported on a client's genetic analysis.
    4. A client's left arm failed to develop when she was a fetus.

48. Which of the following client responses indicates that the nurse's teaching about care following chorionic villus sampling (CVS) has been successful?
    1. If the baby stops moving, the woman should immediately go to the hospital.
    2. The woman should take oral terbutaline every 2 hours for the next day.
    3. If the woman starts to bleed or to contract, she should call her physician.
    4. The woman should stay on complete bed rest for the next 48 hours.

49. A pregnant woman and her husband are both heterozygous for achondroplastic dwarfism, an autosomal dominant disease. The nurse advises the couple that their unborn child has which of the following probabilities of being of normal stature?
    1. 25% probability.
    2. 50% probability.
    3. 75% probability.
    4. 100% probability.

50. A couple inquires about the inheritance of Huntington's disease (HD) because the prospective father's mother is dying of the illness. There is no history of the disease in his partner's family. The man has never been tested for HD. Which of the following responses by the nurse is appropriate?
    1. "Because HD is an autosomal dominant disease, each and every one of your children will have a 1 in 4 chance of having the disease."
    2. "Because only one of you has a family history of HD, the probability of any of your children having the disease is less than 10%."
    3. "Because HD is such a devastating disease, if there is any chance of passing the gene along, it would be advisable for you to adopt."
    4. "Because neither of you has been tested for HD, the most information I can give you is that each and every one of your children may have the disease."

51. A client, G4 P4004, states that her husband has just been diagnosed with polycystic kidney disease (PKD), an autosomal dominant disease. The husband is heterozygous for PKD, while the client has no PKD genes. The client states, "I have not had our children tested because they have such a slim chance of inheriting the disease. We intend to wait until they are teenagers to do the testing." The nurse should base her reply on which of the following?
    1. Because affected individuals rarely exhibit symptoms before age 60, the children should be allowed to wait until they are adults to be tested.
    2. The woman may be exhibiting signs of denial since each of the couple's children has a 50/50 chance of developing the disease.
    3. Because the majority of the renal cysts that develop in affected individuals are harmless, it is completely unnecessary to have the children tested.
    4. The woman's husband should be seen by a genetic specialist since he is the person who is carrying the affected gene.

52. A woman is a carrier for hemophilia A, an X-linked recessive illness. Her husband has a normal genotype. The nurse can advise the couple that the probability that their daughter will have the disease is:
    1. 0% probability.
    2. 25% probability.
    3. 50% probability.
    4. 75% probability.

53. At her first prenatal visit, a woman relates that her maternal aunt has cystic fibrosis (CF), an autosomal recessive illness. Which of the following comments is appropriate for the nurse to make at this time?
    1. "We can check to see whether or not you are a carrier for cystic fibrosis."
    2. "It is unnecessary for you to worry since your aunt is not a direct relation."
    3. "You should have an amniocentesis to see whether or not your child has the disease."
    4. "Please ask your mother whether she has ever had any symptoms of cystic fibrosis."

54. A woman asks the nurse, "My nuchal fold scan results were abnormal. What does that mean?" Which of the following comments is appropriate for the nurse to make at this time?
    1. "I am sorry to tell you that your baby will be born with a serious deformity."
    2. "The results show that your child will have cri du chat syndrome."
    3. "The test is done to see if you are high risk for preterm labor."
    4. "An abnormal test indicates that your baby may have Down syndrome."

55. A 10-week gravid states that her sister's son has been diagnosed with an X-linked recessive disease, Duchenne muscular dystrophy. She questions the nurse about the disease. Which of the following responses is appropriate for the nurse to make?
    1. "Because Duchenne muscular dystrophy is inherited through the woman, it is advisable for you to see a genetic counselor."
    2. "Duchenne muscular dystrophy usually occurs as a spontaneous mutation. It is very unlikely that your fetus is affected."
    3. "Your child could acquire Duchenne muscular dystrophy only if both you and your husband carried the gene. You need to check your husband's family history."
    4. "If you were to have an amniocentesis and it were to be positive for Duchenne muscular dystrophy, I could recommend you to an excellent abortion counselor."

56. The genetic counselor informs a couple that they have a 25% probability of getting pregnant with a child with a severe genetic disease. The couple asks the nurse exactly what that means. Which of the following responses by the nurse is appropriate?
    1. Their first child will have the genetic disease.
    2. If they have four children, one of the children will have the disease.
    3. Their fourth child will have the genetic disease.
    4. Whenever they get pregnant, the fetus may have the disease.

57. A client has just had an amniocentesis to determine whether her baby has an inheritable genetic disease. Which of the following interventions is highest priority at this time?
    1. Assess the fetal heart rate.
    2. Check the client's temperature.
    3. Acknowledge the client's anxiety about the possible findings.
    4. Answer questions regarding the genetic abnormality.

58. Once oogenesis is complete, the resultant gamete cell contains how many chromosomes?
    1. 23.
    2. 46.
    3. 47.
    4. 92.

59. Based on the karyotype shown below, which of the following conclusions can the nurse make about the female baby?
    1. She has a genetically normal karyotype.
    2. She has trisomy 21.
    3. She has fragile X syndrome.
    4. She has an autosomal monosomy.

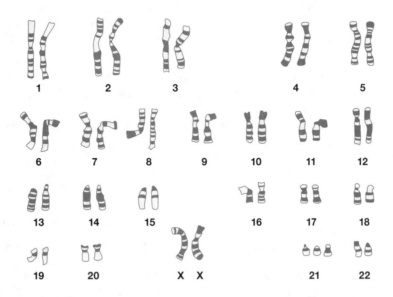

60. A genetic counselor's report states, "The genetic nomenclature for this fetus is 46, XX." How should the nurse who reads this report interpret the cytogenetic results?
    1. The baby is female with a normal number of chromosomes.
    2. The baby is hermaphroditic male with female chromosomes.
    3. The baby is male with an undisclosed genetic anomaly.
    4. There is insufficient information to answer this question.

61. The nurse is analyzing the three-generation pedigree below. In which generation is the proband?
    1. I.
    2. II.
    3. III.
    4. There is not enough information to answer this question.

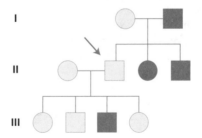

62. A woman is seeking genetic counseling during her pregnancy. She has a strong family history of diabetes mellitus. She wishes to have an amniocentesis to determine whether she is carrying a baby who will "develop diabetes." Which of the following replies would be most appropriate for the nurse to make?
    1. "Doctors don't do amniocenteses to detect diabetes."
    2. "Diabetes cannot be diagnosed by looking at the genes."
    3. "Although diabetes does have a genetic component, diet and exercise also determine whether or not someone is diabetic."
    4. "Even if the baby doesn't carry the genes for diabetes, the baby could still develop the disease."

63. A 25-year-old woman, G0 P0000, enters the infertility clinic stating that she has just learned she is positive for the *BRCA1* and the *BRCA2* genes. She asks the nurse what her options are for getting pregnant and breastfeeding her baby. The nurse should base her reply on which of the following?
    1. Fertility of women who carry the *BRCA1* and *BRCA2* genes is similar to that of unaffected women.
    2. Women with these genes should be advised not to have children because the children could inherit the defective genes.
    3. Women with these genes should have their ovaries removed as soon as possible to prevent ovarian cancer.
    4. Lactation is contraindicated for women who carry the *BRCA1* and *BRCA 2* genes.

64. A woman asks a nurse about presymptomatic genetic testing for Huntington's disease. The nurse should base her response on which of the following?
    1. There is no genetic marker for Huntington's disease.
    2. Presymptomatic testing cannot predict whether or not the gene will be expressed.
    3. If the woman is positive for the gene for Huntington's, she will develop the disease later in life.
    4. If the woman is negative for the gene, her children should be tested to see whether or not they are carriers.

65. A woman, who has undergone amniocentesis, has been notified that her baby is XX with a 14/21 robertsonian chromosomal translocation. The nurse helps the woman to understand which of the following?
    1. The baby will have a number of serious genetic defects.
    2. It is likely that the baby will be unable to have children when she grows up.
    3. Chromosomal translocations are common and rarely problematic.
    4. An abortion will probably be the best decision under the circumstances.

66. A woman who has had multiple miscarriages is advised to go through genetic testing. The client asks the nurse the rationale for this recommendation. The nurse should base his or her response on which of the following?
    1. The woman's pedigree may exhibit a mitochondrial inheritance pattern.
    2. The majority of miscarriages are caused by genetic defects.
    3. A woman's chromosomal pattern determines her fertility.
    4. There is a genetic marker that detects the presence of an incompetent cervix.

67. A nurse has just taken a family history on a 10-week gravid client and created the family pedigree shown below. Each of the darkened symbols represents a person with a serious illness. Which of the following actions should the nurse take at this time?
    1. Advise the woman that she should have an amniocentesis.
    2. Encourage the doctor to send her for genetic counseling.
    3. Ask the woman if she knew any of the relatives who died.
    4. Inform the woman that her pedigree appears normal.

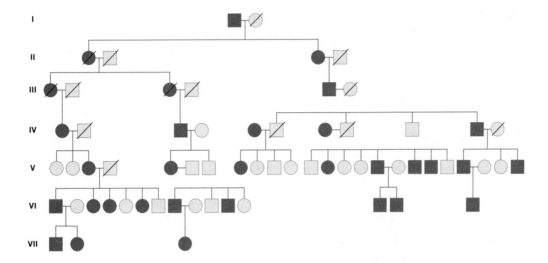

68. A woman is informed that she is a carrier for Tay-Sachs disease, an autosomal recessive illness. What is her phenotype?
    1. She has one recessive gene and one normal gene.
    2. She has two recessive genes.
    3. She exhibits all symptoms of the disease.
    4. She exhibits no symptoms of the disease.

69. During a genetic evaluation, it is discovered that the woman is carrying one autosomal dominant gene for a serious late adult–onset disease, while her partner's history is unremarkable. Based on this information, which of the following family members should be considered high risk and in need of genetic counseling? **Select all that apply.**
    1. The woman's fetus.
    2. The woman's sisters.
    3. The woman's brothers.
    4. The woman's parents.
    5. The woman's partner.

70. Which statement by a gravid client who is a carrier for Duchenne muscular dystrophy, an X-linked recessive disease, indicates that she understands the implications of her status?
    1. "If I have a girl, she will be healthy."
    2. "None of my children will be at risk of the disease."
    3. "If I have a boy, he will be a carrier."
    4. "I am going to abort my fetus because it will be affected."

71. A man has inherited the gene for familial adenomatous polyposis (FAP), an autosomal dominant disease. He and his wife wish to have a baby. Which of the following would provide the couple with the highest probability of conceiving a healthy child?
    1. Amniocentesis.
    2. Chorionic villus sampling.
    3. Pre-implantation genetic diagnosis.
    4. Gamete intrafallopian transfer.

72. A woman asks the obstetrician's nurse about cord blood banking. Which of the following responses by the nurse would be best?
    1. "I think it would be best to ask the doctor to tell you about that."
    2. "The cord blood is frozen in case your baby develops a serious illness in the future."
    3. "The doctors could transfuse anyone who gets into a bad accident with the blood."
    4. "Cord blood banking is very expensive and the blood is rarely ever used."

73. A 3-month-old baby has been diagnosed with cystic fibrosis (CF). The mother says, "How could this happen? I had an amniocentesis during my pregnancy and everything was supposed to be normal!" What must the nurse understand about this situation?
    1. Cystic fibrosis cannot be diagnosed by amniocentesis.
    2. The baby may have an uncommon genetic variant of the disease.
    3. It is possible that the laboratory technician made an error.
    4. Instead of obtaining fetal cells the doctor probably harvested maternal cells.

74. The nurse discusses the results of a 3-generation pedigree with the proband who has breast cancer. Which of the following information must the nurse consider?
    1. The proband should have a complete genetic analysis done.
    2. The proband is the first member of the family to be diagnosed.
    3. The proband's first degree relatives should be included in the discussion.
    4. The proband's sisters will likely develop breast cancer during their lives.

75. The nurse is analyzing the pedigree shown below. How should the nurse interpret the genotype of the individual in location II-4?
    1. Affected male.
    2. Unaffected female.
    3. Stillborn child.
    4. Child of unknown sex.

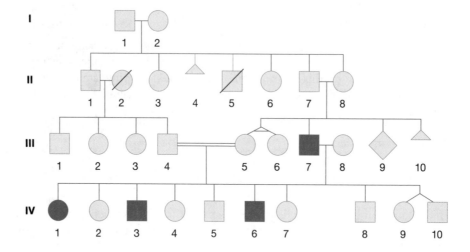

76. The nurse is analyzing the pedigree shown below. How should the nurse interpret the genotype of the individuals in locations IV-9 and IV-10?
    1. Fraternal twins.
    2. Unaffected couple.
    3. Proband and sister.
    4. Known heterozygotes.

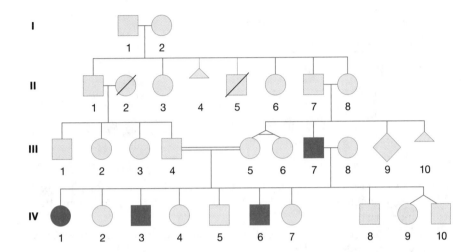

77. A woman who is a carrier for sickle cell anemia is advised that if her baby has two recessive genes, the penetrance of the disease is 100%, but the expressivity is variable. Which of the following explanations will clarify this communication for the mother? All babies with 2 recessive sickle cell genes will:
    1. Develop painful vaso-occlusive crises during their first year of life.
    2. Exhibit at least some signs of the disease while in the neonatal nursery.
    3. Show some symptoms of the disease but the severity of the symptoms will be individual.
    4. Be diagnosed with sickle cell trait but will be healthy and disease-free throughout their lives.

78. Analyze the pedigree below. Which of the following inheritance patterns does the pedigree depict?
    1. Autosomal recessive.
    2. Mitochondrial inheritance.
    3. X-linked recessive.
    4. Y-linked trait.

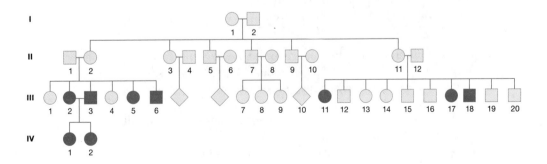

79. Analyze the pedigree below. Which of the following inheritance patterns does the pedigree depict?
    1. Autosomal dominant.
    2. Mitochondrial inheritance.
    3. X-linked recessive.
    4. Y-linked trait.

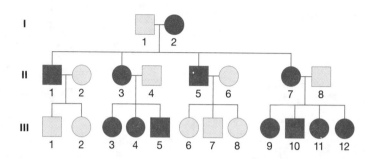

80. The nurse is counseling a pregnant couple who are both carriers for phenylketonuria (PKU), an autosomal recessive disease. Which of the following comments by the nurse is appropriate?
    1. "I wish I could give you good news, but because this is your first pregnancy, your child will definitely have PKU."
    2. "Congratulations, you must feel relieved that the odds of having a sick child are so small."
    3. "There is a 2 out of 4 chance that your child will be a carrier like both of you."
    4. "There is a 2 out of 4 chance that your child will have PKU."

81. A male client has green color blindness, an X-linked recessive genetic disorder. His wife has no affected genes. Which of the following statements by the nurse is true regarding the couple's potential for having a child who is color blind?
    1. All male children will be color blind.
    2. All female children will be color blind.
    3. All male children will be carriers for color blindness.
    4. All female children will be carriers for color blindness.

82. A woman whose blood type is O– (negative) states, "My husband is AB+ (positive)." The mother queries the nurse about what blood type the baby will have. Which of the following blood types should the nurse advise the mother that the baby may have? **Select all that apply.**
    1. "Your baby could be type O+ (positive)."
    2. "Your baby could be type O– (negative)."
    3. "Your baby could be type AB– (negative)."
    4. "Your baby could be type A+ (positive)."
    5. "Your baby could be type B– (negative)."

83. A client's amniocentesis results were reported as 46, XY. Her obstetrician informed her at the time that everything "looks good." Shortly after birth the baby is diagnosed with cerebral palsy. Which of the following responses will explain this result?
    1. It is likely that the client received the wrong amniocentesis results.
    2. Cerebral palsy is not a genetic disease.
    3. The genes that cause cerebral palsy have not yet been discovered.
    4. The genetics lab failed to test for cerebral palsy.

84. Most children born into families look similar but are not exactly the same. The children appear different because homologous chromosomes exchange genetic material at which of the following?
    1. Centromere.
    2. Chiasma.
    3. Chromatid.
    4. Codon.

85. A client is being interviewed prior to becoming pregnant. She states that she has a disease that is transmitted by mitochondrial inheritance. Which of the following statements is consistent with the client's disease?
    1. 100% of her children will be affected.
    2. Only her female children will be affected.
    3. Each fetus will have a 50% probability of being affected.
    4. A fetus will be affected only if it inherits a similar gene from its father.

86. A client wants to undergo amniocentesis because she has a family history of breast cancer. Which of the following choices is the most important information for the nurse to discuss with the client regarding the request?
    1. The breast cancer gene is highly penetrant.
    2. The breast cancer gene has moderate expressivity.
    3. The amniocentesis could result in a miscarriage.
    4. The majority of breast cancers are not inherited.

87. A woman is pregnant. During amniocentesis it is discovered that her child has Down syndrome with a mosaic chromosomal configuration. She asks the nurse what that means. What is the nurse's best response?
    1. "Instead of two number 21 chromosomes, your child has three."
    2. "Your baby's number 21 chromosomes have black and white bands on them."
    3. "Some of your baby's number 21 chromosomes are longer than others."
    4. "Some of your baby's cells have two number 21 chromosomes and some have three."

88. Which of the following is an attainable short-term goal for an 8-week gravid client who has a family history of cystic fibrosis?
    1. Have a sweat chloride test done.
    2. Seek out genetic counseling.
    3. Undergo chorionic villus sampling.
    4. Be seen by a pulmonologist.

89. What is the rationale for testing all neonates for maple syrup urine disease (MSUD) when only 1 in 100,000–300,000 children will be born with the disease?
    1. To encourage the parents to have genetic testing done.
    2. To prevent neurological disease in affected children.
    3. To reduce the amount of money insurance companies must pay for sick MSUD children.
    4. To persuade pharmaceutical companies to develop medications to treat children with MSUD.

The correct answer number and rationale for why it is the correct answer are given in boldface blue type. Rationales for why the other possible answer options are incorrect also are given, but they are not in boldface type.

Sexuality

1. 1. The vas deferens is the internal structure through which the semen passes from the testes to the urethra. Its shape is unaffected by sexual arousal.
   2. The parasympathetic nerves are stimulated during sexual arousal, not the sympathetic nerves.
   3. **When arousal occurs, the penile blood vessels become engorged and an erection is achieved.**
   4. The prepuce, or foreskin, does not increase in length during arousal.

   TEST-TAKING TIP: It is unlikely that the nurse would use some of the terminology included in the responses when speaking with the boys. For example, she might replace the term "prepuce" with the word "foreskin." The test taker should not choose the incorrect response simply because he or she does not understand or disagrees with the terminology in the response. Note that the responses are not direct quotes since they are not surrounded by quotation marks and the stem states, "Which of the following should the nurse base her reply on?"

2. 1. **This statement is true and the discomfort, at the location of the ovary where ovulation occurs, is called mittelschmerz. Ovulation usually occurs 14 days before the first day of the menses.**
   2. The history given by the woman is not indicative of ovarian cancer.
   3. The timing of the pain is more significant than the type of pain.
   4. The timing of the pain is more significant than the type of pain.

   TEST-TAKING TIP: Although the stem includes the fact that the woman is concerned about ovarian cancer, this question is actually testing what the test taker knows about ovulation. The test taker should try not to be confused by extraneous information included in a stem.

3. **2, 1, 3, 4. Gonadotropin-releasing hormone stimulates the production of follicle-stimulating hormone (FSH) and lutenizing hormone (LH). FSH rises first and LH follows. After ovulation, progesterone rises.**

   TEST-TAKING TIP: To remember the hormones of the female menstrual cycle, it is important to know definitions, especially of prefixes and suffixes. Gonadotropin is a hormone that stimulates the gonads—that is, the ovaries or the testes. Follicle-stimulating hormone stimulates the follicle, or ovum sac, to mature, while luteinizing hormone stimulates the release of the ovum from the ovary and heralds the luteal phase of the menstrual cycle (when the corpus luteum is functioning). Finally, progesterone, which is produced by the corpus luteum, rises in the woman's bloodstream.

4. 1. **The fact that the client had intercourse in the last 3 days likely led to the symptoms she is reporting, which are symptoms of a urinary tract infection (UTI).**
   2. Returning from a recent trip abroad is not likely related to the symptoms the client is reporting, which are symptoms of a UTI.
   3. Stopping hormone replacement therapy (HRT) is unlikely related to the symptoms reported by the client.
   4. It is unlikely that starting a weight-lifting program is related to the symptoms of a UTI that the client is reporting.

   TEST-TAKING TIP: The urinary meatus is often manipulated during foreplay and rubbed against during intercourse. To prevent a UTI, women are encouraged to urinate immediately after having intercourse to flush any bacteria from the urethral opening.

5. 1. Estrogen begins to elevate before ovulation. It is not responsible for the temperature elevation.
   2. **Progesterone elevation occurs after ovulation and spikes at about 5–6 days after ovulation. Progesterone is thermogenic—that is, heat producing. Progesterone is the reason women's temperatures are elevated following ovulation.**
   3. LH spikes at the time of ovulation.
   4. FSH promotes the maturation of the ovum.

TEST-TAKING TIP: This question asks the test taker to explain a temperature rise that occurs 2 weeks prior to menstruation. It is essential for the test taker to know that ovulation usually takes place approximately 14 days before the onset of the menses. That eliminates estrogen and FSH since the temperature would have been elevated much earlier in the cycle if those hormones were responsible. LH spikes and then drops at the time of ovulation; that hormone, too, can be eliminated as a possible answer. The only hormone that becomes elevated during the latter part of the menstrual cycle is progesterone.

6. 1. When the ovum is not fertilized, both estrogen and progesterone levels drop. The drop in hormones is followed by menstruation.
   2. When the ovum is not fertilized, both estrogen and progesterone levels drop. The drop in hormones is followed by menstruation.
   3. When the ovum is not fertilized, both estrogen and progesterone levels drop. The drop in hormones is followed by menstruation.
   4. When the ovum is not fertilized, both estrogen and progesterone levels drop. The hormonal drop is followed by menstruation.

TEST-TAKING TIP: Menstruation begins the menstrual cycle. Since pregnancy has not occurred, the test taker can deduce that the hormones of pregnancy did not remain elevated. Option 4, that both estrogen and progesterone are low, is, therefore, the correct response.

7. 1. The temperature does elevate after ovulation, but the elevation is not defined as spinnbarkeit.
   2. The breasts do become sensitive and some women do palpate tender nodules in the breasts at the time of ovulation, but those changes are not spinnbarkeit.
   3. The nipples may tingle and become sensitive, but the sensations are not indicative of spinnbarkeit.
   4. Spinnbarkeit is defined as the "thread" that is created when the vaginal discharge is slippery and elastic at the time of ovulation. The changes are in response to high estrogen levels. The woman inserts her index and middle fingers into her vagina and touches her cervix. After removing her fingers, she separates her fingers and "spins a thread" between her fingers. When

she is not in her fertile period, the mucus is thick and gluey.

TEST-TAKING TIP: It is important for the test taker to be familiar with self-help techniques to assist clients to understand their bodies. *Spinnbarkeit* is a German term that literally means "the ability to create a thread."

8. 1. The ages of a client's children may be important, but it is not the most important information for the nurse to ask about.
   2. Whether or not the client had intercourse the preceding night is important, but it is not the most important information for the nurse to ask about.
   3. This question is the most important for the nurse to ask. The nurse is trying to learn whether or not the client is having intercourse with more than one partner and/or whether the client has intercourse with men, women, or both.
   4. Whether or not the client uses vaginal lubricant is important, but it is not the most important information for the nurse to ask about.

TEST-TAKING TIP: Clients who engage in sex with multiple sex partners are high risk for infection and pregnancy. Women who have intercourse with same-sex partners are high risk for some sexually transmitted infections (STIs), especially bacterial vaginosis. And because there is no risk of pregnancy, women in lesbian relationships may be less likely to protect themselves from infection.

9. 1. FSH is elevated during the follicular phase and the graafian follicle matures.
   2. The fimbriae are located at the ends of the fallopian tubes. They do not multiply in number.
   3. The hormone hCG is not produced during the menstrual cycle. It is produced by the fertilized egg in early pregnancy.
   4. Endometrial proliferation occurs during the secretory phase of the menstrual cycle.

TEST-TAKING TIP: The test taker should always try to find a clue in the stem for the answer to the question. In this question, the test taker is requested to choose "the most important change that happens during the follicular phase." In general, things are named logically, and this case is no different. The follicular phase is the period of the menstrual cycle when the follicle matures.

10. 1. This statement is true. Breast tenderness and mittelschmerz often occur at the time of ovulation.
    2. Breast tenderness and mittelschmerz are symptoms of ovulation, not of abnormal hormonal levels.
    3. Menstruation occurs approximately 14 days after ovulation.
    4. The breast changes are normal and often are felt by women at the time of ovulation.

    TEST-TAKING TIP: There are two hints to the answer in this question. First, the woman has a 31-day cycle and it is day 17. It is, therefore, 14 days before the woman usually menstruates. Women usually ovulate 14 days before their menstrual periods begin. The one-sided lower quadrant pain is also a clue. Women often feel a twinge, called mittelschmerz, near the site of the ovary at the time of ovulation.

11. The test-taker should place an "X" on the testes.

    TEST-TAKING TIP: The test taker should be familiar with the anatomy and physiology of both the male and female reproductive systems. Spermatogenesis occurs in the testes, which is where the "X" should be placed. When the vas deferens is ligated during a vasectomy, the sperm are no longer able to migrate from the testes to the female reproductive tract, and the man becomes sterile.

12. 1. This answer is correct. Meiosis I occurs during puberty.
    2. This response is not true. At the completion of oogenesis only 1 ovum is created. At the completion of spermatogenesis, 4 sperm are created.
    3. This response is not true. Each ovum contains the haploid number of chromosomes.
    4. This response is not true. Sperm have flagella that propel them through the woman's reproductive system. Ova, however, do not have the ability to propel themselves, but rather are propelled externally by the cilia in the fallopian tubes.

    TEST-TAKING TIP: The test taker should be familiar with the fact that meiosis begins during puberty and that the ova age during the following years. This is the likely reason women who attempt to become pregnant after 35 years of age have an increased incidence of infertility as well as an increased probability of becoming pregnant with a Down syndrome fetus.

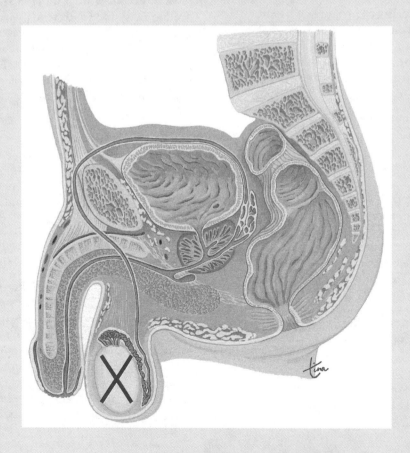

13. 1. If the young woman exercises excessively—for example, as a competitive gymnast or runner—her body fat index will be so low she will become amenorrheic.
    2. Vaccination history has not been shown to be related to secondary amenorrhea.
    3. Pet ownership has not been shown to be related to secondary amenorrhea.
    4. History of asthma has not been shown to be related to secondary amenorrhea.

    TEST-TAKING TIP: If unsure of the definition, the test taker should be able to deduce what is meant by secondary amenorrhea. The prefix "a" means "not" and the remainder of the word refers to the menses. A problem that is labeled "primary" is one that occurs initially. A secondary problem occurs later. A client with primary amenorrhea, therefore, is a young woman who has never had a period. A client with secondary amenorrhea is a young woman who did have periods, but whose periods have stopped. The most common cause of secondary amenorrhea is pregnancy. Many other causes, including a low body fat index, such as can result from excessive or very strenuous exercises, can also lead to amenorrhea.

14. 1. The seminal vesicles, which are not highlighted in the diagram, produce a fluid that nourishes the sperm.
    2. The prostate gland, which is not highlighted in the diagram, secretes a fluid that neutralizes the acidic environment of the vagina.
    3. The highlighted organ is the epididymis, which is the reservoir where sperm mature.
    4. The pubococcygeal muscles are not highlighted in the diagram. These muscles and others contract during ejaculation, forcing the sperm and fluid out of the urethra.

    TEST-TAKING TIP: If the test taker is unfamiliar either with the location of the structures cited in the question or with the name and function of any of the components of the male reproductive system, he or she should review the anatomy and physiology of the male reproductive system.

Infertility

15. 1. This response is incorrect because exposing the testes to the heat of the sauna can alter the normal morphology of the sperm.
    2. Alcohol consumed in excessive amounts can alter spermatogenesis, but one beer per day has not been shown to be a problem.
    3. The high temperature of the sauna could alter the number and morphology of the sperm.
    4. Chemotherapy has been shown to affect the ability of males to create sperm.

    TEST-TAKING TIP: The test taker should try not to be fooled by quantities and numbers when they are included in the stem or answer options. The stem states that the male consumes one beer each evening. That quantity has not been shown to affect fertility.

16. 3, 1, 5, 2, 4. The sperm are produced in the testes (3). They then proceed to the epididymis (1) where they mature. The vas deferens (5) is the conduit through which the sperm first travel during ejaculation. The prostate (2), encircling the neck of the urethra, produces a fluid that protects the sperm, and, finally, the sperm exit the male body via the urethra (4).

    TEST-TAKING TIP: This is an alternate-form question. The test taker is required to place the items in the required sequence. It is essential that the test taker knows and understands normal anatomy and physiology. If the normal functioning of the body is not understood, it will be very difficult for the test taker to learn and remember abnormalities. Although maternity is often viewed as a topic in women's health, it must be remembered that the male's contribution to the embryo is as important to a healthy pregnancy outcome as the woman's. Understanding the male reproductive system is, therefore, a necessary requirement.

17. The student should place an "X" on the outer third of the fallopian tube (see page 34).

    TEST-TAKING TIP: Although the question discusses the fimbriae or fimbriated

ends, the question is actually asking where fertilization takes place—which is in the outer third of the tube. The test taker must be sure to answer the specific question that is being asked.

19. 1. Use of vaginal lubricants is not recommended. Vaginal lubricants may alter the pH of the reproductive system, adversely affecting the couple's potential of becoming pregnant.

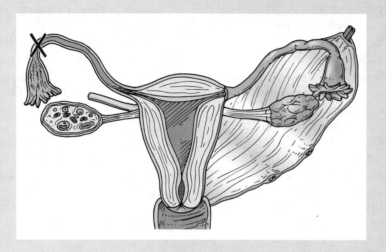

18. 1, 2, 3, 4 are the correct choices.
    1. Condoms should be worn during sexual contacts to prevent infection with a sexually transmitted disease, which can affect the long-term health of the woman's reproductive system.
    2. Women who smoke have a higher incidence of infertility than those who do not smoke. (See http://asrm.org/search/detail.aspx?id=2356&q=smoking)
    3. Women who are either overweight or underweight have increased incidence of infertility.
    4. Body mass index (BMI) is related to the amount of exercise a woman engages in. Those who exercise excessively are more likely to have a very low BMI and those who rarely exercise, to be obese. Since fertility is related to body weight, it is recommended that women exercise in moderation.
    5. There is some evidence that caffeine in large quantities may affect fertility, but decaffeinated carbonated beverages have never been cited as affecting one's fertility.

    TEST-TAKING TIP: There are a number of factors that can affect fertility. Some of the factors are beyond a woman's control. For example, a woman may not marry until she is in her 30s and, consequently, may delay conception. Other factors, such as smoking cigarettes and exercising, are controllable.

    2. Delaying intercourse until the day of ovulation is a poor recommendation. The sperm live for about 3 days. If the couple has daily intercourse beginning 5 or 6 days before ovulation (the "fertile window") and continuing until the day of ovulation, they will maximize their potential of becoming pregnant. In addition, although the practice has not been studied, researchers theorize that abstaining from intercourse for 5 days prior to the fertile window should increase the male's sperm count and therefore increase the potential for fertilization (see Stanford, J.B., White, G.L., & Hatasaka, H. Timing intercourse to achieve pregnancy: Current evidence. [2002]. *Obstetrics & Gynecology*, *100*(6), 1333–1341).
    3. The woman should refrain from douching. Douching can change the normal flora and the pH in the vagina, making the environment hostile to the sperm.
    4. The position of the couple during intercourse will not affect the potential fertility of the woman.

    TEST-TAKING TIP: There is a great deal of false information in the community regarding ways to maximize one's ability to become pregnant. For example, some couples believe that they should have intercourse less frequently when trying to become pregnant because sperm potency drops with frequent ejaculations. This notion has not been shown to be true. Clients need fact-based information regarding ways to maximize their ability to conceive.

20. 1. It is important for the couple to be provided with all relevant information. Adoption is a viable alternative to infertility treatments.
    2. Although there are moral/ethical issues surrounding artificial insemination, there are no legal controversies. Artificial insemination is a legal procedure.
    3. Although it is not without merit, marriage counseling is not mandatory before seeking infertility treatments.
    4. This response is not true. Although up to 10% of couples appear to have no physical cause of their infertility, in the majority of cases a cause is found: 1/3 of cases related to female problems, 1/3 of cases related to male problems, and 1/3 of cases a combination of male and female problems.

TEST-TAKING TIP: Whenever clients seek assistance from health care professionals, it is the obligation of the professional to provide the clients with all options of care. In the case of infertility, clients should be advised regarding infertility counseling, testing, and interventions as well as adoption strategies. The couple should determine for themselves which route(s) they wish to pursue.

21. 1. Kosher diets are complete, providing all nutrients, vitamins, and minerals, needed by the body.
    2. There are no specific positions mandated by Jewish law that inhibit fertilization.
    3. Although Jews do exhibit a large number of genetic diseases, they are not prone to infertility in higher numbers than the general population.
    4. Jewish law does prohibit intercourse during the menses and for 7 days following menses. The woman then goes through a cleansing bath called a *mikvah* before she and her husband may have intercourse. With such a short cycle, she is ovulating during the time frame in which intercourse is restricted.

TEST-TAKING TIP: Remember to consider cultural differences when making nursing assessments and considering nursing interventions. There are three main Jewish traditions: Orthodox, Conservative, and

Reform. Orthodox Jews strictly adhere to the Laws set forth in the Torah, the first 5 books of the Bible. Conservative Jews are observant but less restrictive in their beliefs, while Reform Jews are the most liberal in their traditions. When asked about Jewish traditions, it is important for the test taker to be aware of which group of Jews is being discussed.

22. 1. Endometriosis is characterized by the presence of endometrial tissue outside the uterine cavity. The tissue may be on, for example, the tubes, ovaries, or colon. Adhesions develop from the monthly bleeding at the site of the misplaced endometrial tissue, often resulting in infertility.
    2. Endometriosis is not characterized by hormonal imbalances. Hormonal imbalances can, however, lead to infertility.
    3. A benign tumor of the muscle of the uterus is called a fibroid. It can interfere with pregnancy, but it is not related to endometriosis.
    4. Endometriosis is not caused by an infection.

TEST-TAKING TIP: This question is essentially a knowledge-level question. All of the answer options relate to infertility problems, but only one is specifically related to endometriosis. It is important to have an understanding of gynecological issues since many do affect a woman's fertility.

23. 1, 2, 3, and 4 are the correct choices.
    1. Masturbation and the use of a condom, even for the express purpose of creating life, are considered sins in the Catholic tradition.
    2. Procreation with the man's sperm alone is unlikely. The addition of the donor sperm makes this unacceptable in the eyes of the Catholic Church since a woman should become pregnant only by her husband.
    3. According to the precepts of the Catholic church, fertilization may take place only within the body of the woman.
    4. It is immoral in the Catholic tradition to create more embryos than are needed to conceive.
    5. The medications alone would not be contraindicated per the Catholic Church. The medications are condoned if the ova are being ripened in order for them to become fertilized within her own body.

TEST-TAKING TIP: This is an alternate-form question. It is critical to heed the notation, "Select all that apply." When discussing reproductive rights and practices, religious imperatives are often important issues to consider. (See *Guidelines for Catholics on the Evaluation and Treatment of Infertility*. [n.d.]. Catholic infertility. Retrieved from: http://catholicinfertility.org/guidelines.html)

24. 1. Diabetes has been shown to affect a woman's fertility, but infertility has not been shown to increase a woman's risk of developing diabetes.
    2. Infertility has not been shown to increase a woman's risk of developing nystagmus.
    3. Infertility has not been shown to increase a woman's risk of developing cholecystitis.
    4. Infertility has been shown to increase a woman's risk of developing ovarian cancer.

TEST-TAKING TIP: For a number of years, an association was noted between the long-term use of Clomid (clomiphene) to treat infertility and the incidence of ovarian cancer. It has also been shown that infertility itself is a contributing factor for ovarian cancer. The reason for the association is not yet known. (See http://cancer.org/Cancer/Ovarian-Cancer/DetailedGuide/ovarian-cancer-risk-factors)

25. 1. The luteal phase occurs after ovulation. Pergonal is given to induce ovulation.
    2. Pergonal is administered to infertile women to increase follicular growth and maturation of the follicles and to stimulate ovulation.
    3. Pergonal does not suppress menstruation or promote cervical mucus production.
    4. Pergonal does not suppress menstruation or promote cervical mucus production.

TEST-TAKING TIP: It is possible that the test taker would not know the action of Pergonal. When the generic name is seen, however, an educated guess can be made. A "tropin" is a substance that stimulates an organ to do something. The only answer that states that an organ is being stimulated is choice 2.

26. 1. On the Web, there are sites that promote the intake of ginseng as a therapy for both male and female infertility, although there is no strong evidence to show that either is true. In addition, there is nothing in the question to suggest that the infertility problem is caused by the poor quality of the man's sperm.
    2. There is no evidence that ginseng causes mutations; rather, there is some evidence to show that it is antimutagenic.
    3. There is cause for concern for this woman since she is 35 years old and has been unable to get pregnant for over 6 months.
    4. Because fertility drops as a woman ages, it is advisable to encourage the couple to use conventional therapies in conjunction with the complementary therapy to maximize their potential of becoming pregnant.

TEST-TAKING TIP: Complementary therapies are becoming more and more popular among clients. Although many have not been shown to have direct effects, it can be counterproductive to discourage clients from using complementary therapies. This may alienate the clients from the health care provider. Unless they are known to be dangerous, it is much better to encourage clients to combine standard and complementary methods rather than to dissuade clients from using them.

27. 1. The eggs of an older woman (for reproductive purposes considered 35 years +) do age and fertility is reduced.
    2. Age 13 at the time of menarche is not a significant factor.
    3. Working as a dental hygienist has not been shown to affect fertility.
    4. Excessive exercise can interrupt hormonal function, but jogging 2 miles a day is a moderate exercise pattern.

TEST-TAKING TIP: The woman was 13 years old at menarche, an age that is well within normal limits. Working as a dental hygienist has not been shown to increase one's chances of developing infertility. An excessive exercise schedule is a problem, but jogging 2 miles a day is well within the definition of moderate exercise. When women are over 35 years of age, however, their fertility often drops.

28. 1. Spermatogenesis occurs in the testes. High temperatures harm the development of the sperm.
    2. When the vas deferens is ligated, a man has had a vasectomy and is sterile. The sterility is not, however, due to impaired spermatogenesis, but rather to the inability

of the sperm to migrate to the woman's reproductive tract.

3. The prostate does not affect spermatogenesis. An enlarged or hypertrophied prostate is usually a problem that affects older men.

4. The flagella are the "tails" of the sperm. They are normally divided into a middle and an end segment.

TEST-TAKING TIP: A knowledge of language will help the test taker to answer this question. The suffix "genesis" means "the beginning of, origin of, or the creation of." Therefore, the question is asking which of the factors listed will affect the creation of sperm.

29. 1. Clients who "schedule" intercourse often complain that their sexual relationship is unsatisfying.

2. Years of marriage are not directly related to a couple's sexual relationship. Clients may have a very healthy relationship after many years of marriage.

3. The fact that the couple lives with one set of parents is unlikely related to their sexual relationship.

4. Although it can be very difficult to be around couples who have become pregnant and/or have healthy babies, this factor is not usually related to a couple's sexual relationship.

TEST-TAKING TIP: When answering questions about the nursing process, it is important for the test taker to make sure that each diagnosis is independent. For example, when the nurse identifies sexual dysfunction related to decreased libido as a diagnosis, then the assessments, as well as the goals, interventions, and evaluations, must relate directly to that problem.

30. 1. A diagnosis of herpes simplex 2 is not a contraindication for taking Viagra.

2. It is unsafe to take Viagra while also taking nitroglycerin for angina.

3. Viagra is often prescribed for clients with erectile dysfunction (ED) from diabetes mellitus.

4. Viagra is often prescribed for clients with ED from prostate resection.

TEST-TAKING TIP: Viagra has been shown to increase the hypotensive effects of nitrate-containing medications. It should not be taken in conjunction with any medication that contains nitrates, including nitroglycerin.

31. 1. This response is not true. Physicians usually want a number of eggs to reach maturation.

2. Preimplantation genetic assessment, when done, is performed on the fertilized ova, not on the sperm or unfertilized ova.

3. Artificial insemination will not be performed because the client's tubes are blocked.

4. This response is correct. Since multiple embryos are usually created during the in vitro process, there are often more embryos created than are implanted. The couple may preserve the embryos.

TEST-TAKING TIP: The preserved embryos may be implanted in the future. For example, if the first transfer fails to result in a pregnancy, the remaining embryos may be transferred within a few months. If a pregnancy and a delivery do result, the couple may choose to implant the remaining embryos in the future when they choose to have another child.

32. 1. This statement is true. Although the gametes are placed in the fallopian tubes artificially, fertilization does occur within the woman's body.

2. This statement is true of zygote intrafallopian transfer (ZIFT), not of gamete intrafallopian transfer (GIFT).

3. This statement is not true. Although donor eggs and sperm can be used, usually the couple's own gametes are used. When they are harvested, the gametes are placed directly into the woman's fallopian tubes.

4. This statement describes surrogacy. A surrogate is usually impregnated via artificial insemination.

TEST-TAKING TIP: The best way for the test taker to remember the various forms of infertility therapies is to remember the definitions of the components. For example, when GIFT is being discussed, the term "gamete" (G) refers to the male or female reproductive cell—that is, the sperm or ovum. When ZIFT is being considered, the term "zygote" (Z) refers to the fertilized ovum. The prefix "intra" means "within" and the term "fallopian" refers to the fallopian tube. When GIFT (or ZIFT) is discussed, the method of transfer into the fallopian tube is via laparoscope.

33. 1. It is unlikely that this woman has a urinary tract infection.

2. It is unlikely that the client is already pregnant.

3. This client should be seen by her infertility doctor.
4. Abdominal bloating is a sign of ovarian hyperstimulation.

TEST-TAKING TIP: This client is exhibiting signs of ovarian hyperstimulation. This is a serious complication. The client is likely third spacing her fluids (the fluids in her body are shifting into her interstitial spaces), resulting in abdominal distention, oliguria, and concentrated urine. The client should be evaluated by her physician.

34. 2, 3, and 4 are correct.
    1. A 30-day menstrual cycle is well within normal limits.
    2. Dyspareunia, or pain during intercourse, may be a symptom of a sexually transmitted infection (STI) or of endometriosis. Both STIs and endometriosis can adversely affect a woman's fertility.
    3. A woman who has had pelvic inflammatory disease (PID) is much more likely to have blocked fallopian tubes than a woman who has never had PID.
    4. Women who have facial hair (hirsutism) often have polycystic ovarian syndrome (PCOS). PCOS patients frequently have irregular menses, elevated serum cholesterol, and insulin resistance. Women with PCOS are very often infertile.
    5. A 5-day menstrual period is well within normal limits.

TEST-TAKING TIP: Women with PCOS have many symptoms: hirsutism, insulin resistance, high levels of circulating testosterone, and infertility, to name a few. To improve the chances of a woman with PCOS becoming pregnant, she is frequently prescribed Clomid (clomiphene) for the infertility and Glucophage (metformin) for the insulin resistance. Sexually transmitted infections and endometriosis may also impair a woman's fertility.

35. 1. When a woman's cervical mucus is estrogen rich, it is slippery and elastic (thread-like), and when assessed under a microscope, the practitioner will observe "ferning"—that is, an image that looks like a fern. The woman is then in her fertile period. When she is not in her fertile period, the mucus is thick and gluey.
    2. Basal body temperature assessments are performed to determine if and when ovulation occurs.

3. Culposcopy is a procedure performed to examine the cervix closely. It is not performed to evaluate the receptivity of a woman's cervical mucus to sperm.
4. A hysterotomy is a procedure in which an incision is made into the uterus.

TEST-TAKING TIP: When estrogen levels are high, a woman's cervical mucus is most receptive to a man's sperm. At that time, the pH of the vaginal and cervical environments is most conducive to the sperm's successful migration into the uterus and into the fallopian tubes.

36. 1, 2, 4, and 5 are correct.
    1. Infertility clients often express anger at others who are able to conceive.
    2. Infertility clients often express a feeling of personal failure.
    3. Infertility clients often express an aversion to sex because of the many restrictions/schedules/intrusions that are placed on their sexual relationship.
    4. Sadness is another common feeling expressed by infertility clients.
    5. Guilt is commonly expressed by infertility clients.

TEST-TAKING TIP: Couples who are experiencing infertility express many emotions. One common thread that connects all of the emotions is grief. Infertile couples grieve their inability to conceive. They experience all of the stages of grief including denial, anger, bargaining, and depression. Acceptance, if it is ever reached, often takes many years.

37. 1. The postcoital test is done 1 or 2 days prior to ovulation.
    2. No dye is administered and there are no x-ray pictures taken during a postcoital test.
    3. The test is performed a few hours after a couple has intercourse.
    4. The client will undergo a speculum examination when cervical mucus will be harvested.

TEST-TAKING TIP: The postcoital test is a simple assessment done to see whether the sperm are able to navigate the woman's cervical mucus to ascend into the uterus and fallopian tubes. A few hours postcoitus, immediately before ovulation, the practitioner harvests cervical mucus to assess whether the sperm are still motile and to assess the ferning patterns of the mucus.

38. 1. Only the uterus and the fallopian tubes are evaluated during a hysterosalpingogram.
     2. Tumors and other gross assessments of the uterus can be made out, but the vascularization of the endometrium is beyond the scope of the test.
     3. The competency of the cervix cannot be evaluated during a hysterosalpingogram.
     4. The primary goal of a hysterosalpingogram is to learn whether or not the fallopian tubes are patent.

TEST-TAKING TIP: During a hysterosalpingogram, a dye is inserted through the vagina into the uterine cavity. The dye, visualized on x-ray, then travels up into the fallopian tubes. If the tubes are blocked owing to scarring or endometriosis, the dye does not ascend.

39. 1. When no temperature shifts are noted, it is likely that the client has not ovulated.
     2. If the client is not ovulating, she has no fertile period.
     3. A 7-day menstrual period is not abnormally long.
     4. There is no evidence of a progesterone elevation.

TEST-TAKING TIP: The test taker should be able to make basic interpretations of BBT charts. There is usually a slight dip in the temperature at the LH surge with a rise in temperature for the remainder of the cycle because of the thermogenic effect of progesterone. When no temperature changes are seen, it is likely that the client is not experiencing normal hormonal changes and is not ovulating.

40. 1. Unless medically indicated, douching should never be performed. A vinegar solution is especially inappropriate since sperm are unable to survive in an acidic environment.
     2. This action is recommended. Pregnancy is most likely to occur with daily intercourse from 6 days before ovulation up to the day of ovulation.
     3. If a client is experiencing a biphasic cycle, FSH therapy is probably not indicated.
     4. The basal body temperature (BBT) chart need not be monitored for 6 more months, although it can be used to help time intercourse.

TEST-TAKING TIP: A biphasic cycle on a BBT chart is evidenced by a relatively stable temperature at the beginning of the cycle, a slight dip in temperature at the time of ovulation, and a sustained rise in temperature—of at least 0.4°F for the remainder of the cycle.

41. 1. The man may have both recessive genes for cystic fibrosis even though he is not ill.
     2. This answer is incorrect. Some men with cystic fibrosis, however, have no vas deferens.
     3. This statement is correct. Cystic fibrosis can be expressed in a number of ways. Some affected individuals have very serious illness resulting in early death, while others experience few symptoms.
     4. This statement is incorrect. Some males with cystic fibrosis have no vas deferens and, even if the vas is present, if the man is producing large amounts of thick mucus, the vas may become obstructed. Similarly, in women, the fallopian tubes may become obstructed with thick mucus.

TEST-TAKING TIP: Infertility and genetics are often related. In this situation, the genetic disease cystic fibrosis has resulted in aspermia. In addition, many miscarriages are caused by inborn genetic defects. In general, clients who are infertile should be referred for genetic counseling.

42. 2, 3, 4, and 5 are correct.
     1. Chorionic villus sampling is done to assess for genetic disease in the fetus.
     2. Endometrial biopsy is performed about 1 week following ovulation to detect the endometrium's response to progesterone.
     3. Hysterosalpingogram is performed after menstruation to detect whether or not the fallopian tubes are patent.
     4. Serum progesterone assay is performed about 1 week following ovulation to determine whether or not the woman's corpus luteum produces enough progesterone to sustain a pregnancy.
     5. Postcoital tests are performed about 1–2 days before ovulation to determine whether or not healthy sperm are able to survive in the cervical mucus.

TEST-TAKING TIP: There are a number of tests that are performed to assess fertility in couples. It is important to remember that many of the assessments are invasive, painful, embarrassing, and, depending on the results, may label one of the partners as the cause of the infertility. The knowledge of who is responsible for the infertility can be very difficult for some clients to learn.

43. 1. This is an important goal, but it is not the priority nursing goal.
    2. This is an important goal, but it is not the priority nursing goal.
    3. This is an important goal, but it is not the priority nursing goal.
    4. This is the priority nursing goal related to ovarian hyperstimulation syndrome.

TEST-TAKING TIP: A client who is suffering from ovarian hyperstimulation syndrome experiences intravascular hypovolemia, and a related extravascular hypervolemia. Although the exact cause of the shift in fluids is unknown, the client may experience very serious complications, including pulmonary edema and ascites. The client is hospitalized and palliative therapy is provided until the client's fluid and electrolytes stabilize. It is essential throughout the client's acute phase to make sure that her pulmonary function remains intact.

44. 1. Piercing rectal pain has not been cited as a side effect of Pergonal.
    2. Mood swings and depression are common side effects of the hormonal therapy.
    3. Visual disturbances have not been cited as a side effect of Pergonal.
    4. Jerky tremors have not been cited as a side effect of Pergonal.

TEST-TAKING TIP: The test taker must be aware that not only is infertility itself a psychological stressor but the therapy used to treat it is also a stressor. The client is given daily injections of Pergonal (a mixture of FSH and LH) for 10 days to 2 weeks. The impact of the hormonal injections can be very disruptive to the woman's psyche, leading to mood swings and, in some cases, severe depression.

45. 1. No incision is created when clients have hysterosalpingograms.
    2. The client will be able to ambulate normally after the procedure.
    3. A dye is instilled into the uterine cavity. Some doctors do prescribe oral antibiotics following the procedure to prevent infection.
    4. This statement is correct. A number of pictures will be taken throughout the procedure. The client, who will be awake, is asked to move into positions for the x-rays.

TEST-TAKING TIP: A hysterosalpingogram is one of the many tests performed during a standard infertility work-up. The test taker should be familiar with the rationale for each of the tests as well as the procedures themselves and the information that should be conveyed to each client who is to undergo one of the procedures.

Genetics

46. 1. The circle is the symbol used to represent the female.
    2. The square is the symbol used to represent the male.
    3. The triangle is the symbol used to represent a stillborn.
    4. The diamond is the symbol used to represent a child of unknown sex.

TEST-TAKING TIP: When the same symbols are used in all pedigrees, readers are able to analyze the results easily. Symbols that are light colored or completely uncolored depict healthy individuals. Those that are dark colored depict individuals with disease.

47. 1. The DNA in the client's skin cells did mutate, but the mutation will not affect the client's fertility because the woman's ovaries were not affected.
    2. The inherited gene affects a client's risk of contracting colon cancer. It will not affect fertility.
    3. A reciprocal translocation can result in infertility.
    4. Failure of one arm to develop in utero is related to an environmental insult rather than a genetic insult.

TEST-TAKING TIP: Clients who have reciprocal translocations are usually phenotypically normal. When they produce gametes, however, the eggs (or sperm) have nuclei that are composed of an unbalanced amount of genetic material. Because their offspring are often nonviable, their pregnancies end in miscarriage.

48. 1. CVS is performed well before mothers feel quickening.
    2. Tocolytics, such as terbutaline, are not routinely administered following CVS.
    3. The mother should notify the doctor if she begins to bleed or contract.
    4. It is unnecessary for the mother to stay on complete bed rest following a CVS.

TEST-TAKING TIP: The test taker, if familiar with normal pregnancy changes, can immediately eliminate choice 1 since CVS is performed between 10 and 12 weeks' gestation and quickening rarely occurs before 16 weeks' gestation, even in multiparous pregnancies. Spontaneous abortion is the most common complication of CVS; therefore, the woman should report any bleeding or contractions.

49. 1. The child has a 25% probability of being of normal stature.
    2. The child has a 25% probability of being of normal stature.
    3. The child has a 25% probability of being of normal stature.
    4. The child has a 25% probability of being of normal stature.

After doing a Punnett square,

	Father: A	a
Mother: A	AA	Aa
a	Aa	aa

It can be seen that the probability of the child being of normal stature is 1 in 4, or 25%.

TEST-TAKING TIP: Because both parents are heterozygous ("hetero" meaning "different"), they each have one dominant gene or allele (A) and one recessive gene or allele (a). Therefore, the genotype of each parent is Aa. Because achondroplasia is a dominant disease, the recessive allele in this scenario is the normal gene. Only 1 of the 4 boxes contains 2 recessive (normal) genes; therefore, their child has a 1 in 4, or 25%, chance of being of normal stature.

50. 1. If the prospective father possesses the gene, the probability of their children inheriting the gene is 1 in 2, or 50%. As the man has not been tested, it is impossible to determine the probabilities.
    2. This statement is completely false.
    3. It is improper for the nurse to recommend that the clients not have children. It is the couple's choice whether or not to get pregnant. It is the nurse's responsibility to give information that is as accurate as possible.
    4. This statement is correct. No specific information can be given until or unless the potential father decides to be tested.

TEST-TAKING TIP: It is important for the test taker to know the clinical course of Huntington's disease (HD), a deteriorating

disease of the brain. Affected patients slowly succumb to abnormal movements, behavioral changes, and dementia. There is no cure for this devastating disease. Many clients are reluctant to be tested for the gene since they then end up waiting for the dreaded symptoms to appear. It is not uncommon, therefore, for clients to have no definitive knowledge of their genetic makeup in relation to HD.

51. 1. Symptoms usually appear in affected individuals in their 30s or 40s, but the symptoms can appear as early as childhood.
    2. This response is correct. As can be seen by the Punnett square results, the children have a 50/50 chance of developing PKD. Since the capital A connotes the dominant gene, the child needs only one affected gene to exhibit the disease.

	Father: A	a
Mother: a	Aa	aa
a	Aa	aa

3. This statement is untrue. PKD can be a very serious illness. Some patients with the disease will require dialysis and/or kidney transplants.
    4. This statement is inappropriate. The husband's genotype is already known.

TEST-TAKING TIP: Remember to look to see which inheritance pattern is being discussed in the stem and ALWAYS complete a Punnett square before answering a question. It is very easy to become confused when being asked about Mendelian inheritance patterns.

52. 1. The probability of the couple having a daughter with hemophilia A is 0%.
    2. The probability of the couple having a daughter with hemophilia A is 0%.
    3. The probability of the couple having a daughter with hemophilia A is 0%.
    4. The probability of the couple having a daughter with hemophilia A is 0%.

After doing a Punnett square,

	Father: X	Y
Mother: X	XX	XY
"x"	X"x"	"x"Y

(Affected X is depicted as "x")

It can be seen that the probability of the couple having a daughter with hemophilia A is 0%; in recessive X-linked inheritance, girls would have to have 2 affected "x" genes to exhibit the disease.

TEST-TAKING TIP: It is essential when discussing X-linked recessive inheritance that the probability of boys and girls be assessed separately. Because males carry only one X, they only need one affected "x" to exhibit the X-linked recessive disease. The four offspring depicted in the Punnett square include one unaffected girl (XX), one girl who carries the gene but does not have the disease since the gene is recessive (X"x"), one normal boy (XY), and one boy who has the affected gene and therefore the disease ("x"Y). Girls must carry the affected gene on two "x" chromosomes to exhibit the disease. Thus, the probability of a girl having the disease is 0. It is important to note, however, that the probability of the daughters being carriers is 1 in 2, or 50%.

53. 1. It is possible that this woman is a carrier for cystic fibrosis. A genetic evaluation can be done to determine that possibility.
    2. The affected gene could have been transmitted to both the woman's mother and to the aunt.
    3. Only if both this woman and her partner are carriers is there a possibility of their child having CF. And even if that were the case, the probability of the fetus having the disease would be 1 in 4, or 25%, because CF is an autosomal recessive disease.
    4. This response is inappropriate. The mother could be a carrier of the CF gene (carriers are symptom free) so the client should be tested.

TEST-TAKING TIP: The test taker must remember that just because there is a history of a genetic disease in the family, it does not mean that every member of the family will be affected. It is much less invasive, as well as much less expensive, to do a test on the client's blood to see whether she is carrying the CF gene than to do an amniocentesis to see whether the baby is affected. If both the father and the mother were found to be carriers, then it would be advisable to offer fetal genetic counseling to the couple.

54. 1. This response is inappropriate. The nuchal fold scan is done either late in the first trimester or with the quad second trimester screen. A fetal genetic evaluation

(amniocentesis or percutaneous umbilical blood sampling [PUBS]) must be done before a definitive diagnosis can be made. A genetic analysis is the only absolute diagnostic tool.
    2. Cri du chat syndrome is a mental retardation disease caused by a deletion on chromosome 5. The nuchal fold scan does not screen for chromosomal deletions. It is done to assess for trisomy chromosomal diseases.
    3. The first-trimester assessment screens for Down syndrome. It does not screen for preterm labor risk.
    4. This statement is true, but the definitive diagnosis can be made only via genetic testing.

TEST-TAKING TIP: The first-trimester screen is performed to assess for Down syndrome and other trisomy chromosomal syndromes. It is important for the test taker to remember that screening tests are NOT diagnostic. They are relatively inexpensive tests that are performed on the majority of clients to identify those who are likely to exhibit a disease process. If screening test results are positive, more sophisticated diagnostic tests are performed to make definitive diagnoses.

55. 1. **Because Duchenne muscular dystrophy is X-linked, if her sister is a carrier, she too may be a carrier. She should see a genetic counselor.**
    2. It is unlikely that Duchenne muscular dystrophy developed as a spontaneous mutation.
    3. Duchenne muscular dystrophy is X-linked, so the father's genetics will not affect the outcome.
    4. This response is inappropriate. The decision to abort a child with a disease is up to the parents. Each set of parents must be allowed to make the decision for themselves. Their decision is likely to be based on many things, including their ability to care for a mentally retarded child and the knowledge that their child is affected by a genetic disease. The nurse cannot make the assumption that the parents will decide to abort an affected child.

TEST-TAKING TIP: It is important for the test taker to realize that clients who find out that their child has a genetic disease through amniocentesis do not learn of the results until well into the second trimester. These clients, therefore, may be deciding

whether to abort when they are able to feel fetal movement. Even for clients who are pro-choice, the decision to abort so late in the pregnancy can be a very difficult one.

56. 1. Each pregnancy has its own probability so it is impossible to predict which, if any, child will or will not have the disease.
2. Each pregnancy has its own probability so it is possible for all or none of the children to have the disease.
3. Each pregnancy has its own probability so it is impossible to predict which, if any, child will or will not have the disease.
4. This is true. Every time the woman gets pregnant there is a possibility (25% chance) that she is carrying a child with the disease.

TEST-TAKING TIP: The term "probability" refers to the likelihood of something occurring, rather than to whether something definitely will occur. This concept is often misunderstood by a layperson. It is very important that nurses communicate to parents who carry gene mutations that every time the woman is pregnant, she has the possibility of carrying a baby with the defect.

57. 1. Assessing the fetal heart rate is the highest priority since, although rare, the fetus may have been injured during the procedure.
2. Taking the client's temperature is not the most important action to take at this time.
3. Psychosocial issues are always significant, but they must take a back seat to physiological assessments.
4. It is important to answer all questions posed by clients but, again, these should be answered only after physiological interventions are completed.

TEST-TAKING TIP: This is a prioritizing question. All answers, therefore, are correct. It is the test taker's responsibility to determine which response is of highest priority. The test taker should remember Maslow's Hierarchy of Needs and established procedures for providing first aid and CPR when answering prioritizing questions.

58. 1. The haploid number of chromosomes is 23, the normal number of chromosomes in the gamete—in this case, in the ovum.
2. The diploid number of chromosomes is 46, the normal number of chromosomes in the somatic cells of human beings.

3. Aneuploidy is characterized by a chromosomal number that is not equal to a multiple of the haploid number—that is, the number of chromosomes in the cell is NOT equal to 23, 46, 69, 92, and so on. Trisomy 21 (47 chromosomes) is an example of an aneuploid number, as is a chromosome number of 48 or 49.
4. Polyploidy is characterized by a chromosomal number that is equal to twice, three times, four times, and so on, of the diploid number—that is, the number of chromosomes in the cell is equal to 92 (2 × 46), 138 (3 × 46), and so on.

TEST-TAKING TIP: The test taker should use his or her understanding of language to answer the question. Oogenesis is the development of the female egg, or ovum. (Spermatogenesis is the development of the male sperm.) In order for the fertilized egg (which is created once the ovum and sperm combine) to have the diploid or normal number of chromosomes, the ovum and sperm must each have the haploid number of chromosomes, or 23 in each.

59. 1. This response is incorrect. The baby has Down syndrome.
2. This response is correct. The baby has 3 number 21 chromosomes.
3. This response is incorrect. The fetus has an aneuploid number of chromosomes. There is no evidence of a fragile segment on the long arm of the X chromosome.
4. This response is incorrect. All of the autosomes are paired.

TEST-TAKING TIP: Karyotypes that show translocations, deletions, and other abnormalities can be very difficult to interpret, but it is relatively easy to discern monosomy and trisomy defects. The test taker must simply count the number of chromosomal pairs. If any chromosome is missing its mate or if there are 3 of any of the chromosomes, the fetus will usually exhibit a distinct syndrome. One exception to the rule is the fetus that carries multiple Y chromosomes with 1 X—for example, XYY or XYYY. In that situation, the baby will appear and, in the vast majority of cases, act normally.

60. 1. This response is correct. The normal number of chromosomes is present—46—and the child is a female—XX.
2. This response is incorrect. Hermaphrodites exhibit both male and female organs and characteristics. Hermaphroditism may be

caused by a number of things, including an environmental insult or a genetic mutation.

3. This response is incorrect. An example of a male with a genetic defect is 46,XY,16p13.3. The child is a male—XY—and the defect, as indicated in the nomenclature, is on the p arm of the 16th chromosome at location 13.3.

4. There is sufficient information to answer this question.

TEST-TAKING TIP: When reading genetic nomenclature, the test taker should first look for the number of chromosomes in the cells, then the sex makeup of the cells. If there is a mosaic genotype, the information will be separated by a slash mark. If there is a genetic defect, the information will follow the baseline data.

61. 1. The proband is not in generation I.
2. The proband is in generation II. The proband, or first member of a family to be diagnosed with a specific medical/genetic problem, is identified in a pedigree by an arrow.
3. The proband is not in generation III.
4. There is sufficient information to answer the question. The proband is the member of the family who is identified by an arrow.

TEST-TAKING TIP: There are symbols that have been accepted in the scientific community for labeling pedigrees. The arrow pointing to one member in a pedigree labels the proband, or the first member of the family to be diagnosed with the specific medical/genetic problem.

62. 1. Although this response is accurate, it is an inappropriate response for the nurse to make.
2. Although this response is accurate, it is an inappropriate response for the nurse to make.
3. This response is accurate. Diabetes is one of the many diseases that has both a genetic and an environmental component.
4. Although this response is accurate, it is an inappropriate response for the nurse to make.

TEST-TAKING TIP: Although virtually 100% of some diseases are genetically determined, most diseases have both genetic and environmental components. In other words, they have multifactorial etiologies. Diabetes mellitus, cancer, asthma, and the like are examples of diseases with multifactorial etiologies.

63. 1. This statement is true. Female clients who are *BRCA1* or *BRCA2* positive have similar fertility rates to those who are *BRCA1* or *BRCA2* negative.
2. This statement is incorrect. Nurses provide information. It is inappropriate for nurses to counsel clients whether or not to have children based on the client's genotype.
3. The decision to have an oophorectomy is the client's. The nurse's role is to provide the client with information regarding the genetic profile.
4. Lactation is not contraindicated for these women.

TEST-TAKING TIP: Many women who have been found to carry a *BRCA* gene decide to have mastectomies and/or oophorectomies. Other women choose to have children and then have the procedures and still others choose to have frequent diagnostic tests to monitor for the development of cancer. Whichever path the client takes must be her decision based on accurate information provided by health care professionals.

64. 1. There is a genetic marker for Huntington's disease.
2. In the case of Huntington's disease, if a person has the gene and lives long enough, there is virtually a 100% probability he or she will develop the disease. The gene has a high degree of expressivity, or, in other words, people who carry the gene will develop the disease.
3. This answer is correct, if a person has the gene and lives long enough, virtually 100% of the time the disease will develop and progress.
4. There is no carrier state when a disease is transmitted via a dominant inheritance pattern, as is Huntington's disease.

TEST-TAKING TIP: The test taker must understand the difference between recessive and dominant illnesses. There is a carrier state in recessive illnesses because two affected genes must be present in the genome for the disease to be expressed. Only one affected gene must be present for a dominant disease to be expressed.

65. 1. This response is incorrect. The child will likely be a normal-appearing female.
2. Because there is a translocation in the child's chromosomal pattern, the child's gametes will likely contain an abnormal amount of genetic material and the child will be infertile.

3. Translocations are usually not problematic for the first generation, but they can lead to significant defects and/or infertility in the next generation.
4. The client must decide for herself whether or not to abort the fetus.

TEST-TAKING TIP: When a reciprocal translocation has occurred, part of the chromosomal material from one chromosome improperly attaches to another chromosome and vice versa. In the case of a robertsonian translocation, the affected individual is aneuploid since the centromeres of two chromosomes fuse while the genetic material from the short arms of the chromosomes is lost. Affected individuals usually appear normal and will develop normally even, as in the case of the robertsonian translocation, some genetic material is lost. When the child's gametes develop via meiosis, however, each of the eggs will contain an abnormal quantity of genetic material.

66. 1. The pedigree should be analyzed for any and all abnormal inheritance patterns.
2. This is true. The incidence of miscarriage is very high, about 1 out of every 5 pregnancies, and the majority of miscarriages are related to a genetic defect.
3. A woman's fertility is determined by many factors.
4. This statement is not true. There is no genetic marker for incompetent cervix.

TEST-TAKING TIP: If a client has had more than two miscarriages, she and her partner should be referred to a genetic counselor. Either one of the couple may have a genetic anomaly that is affecting the viability of the fetus. In addition, a DNA sample of the products of each miscarriage should be sent for genetic analysis. Often a diagnosis can be made from the analyses.

67. 1. It is too soon to advise a client to have amniocentesis. Although the pedigree shows an autosomal dominant inheritance pattern, a genetic counselor should analyze the pedigree.
2. This is appropriate. All nurses should have a basic understanding of genetic information, but genetic counselors are the experts in this area.
3. This information may be relevant but should be asked carefully within a counseling session. It is best for a genetic counselor to ask the questions.

4. This response is inappropriate. The pedigree shows an autosomal dominant inheritance pattern.

TEST-TAKING TIP: The nurse should encourage clients' primary care providers to refer clients to special care providers when indicated. The area of genetics is one that is highly specialized and new information is being developed each day. A genetic counselor possesses the specialized knowledge. Another area that often requires specialized knowledge is nutrition. Although most, if not all, nurses take a nutrition course during basic nursing education, nurses are generally not experts in the field.

68. 1. This is the woman's genotype. It is not the woman's phenotype.
2. This is the genotype of a person with Tay-Sachs disease.
3. This is the phenotype of a person with Tay-Sachs disease.
4. This is the woman's phenotype.

TEST-TAKING TIP: A person's genotype refers to a person's genetic code. A person who is a carrier for an autosomal recessive disease will have a heterozygous genotype—Aa. A person's phenotype refers to the person's observable characteristics. A person who is a carrier for an autosomal recessive disease will have a normal phenotype. Only persons who have a genotype of aa would express the disease.

69. 1, 2, 3, and 4 are correct.
1. The woman's fetus has a 1 in 2, or 50%, probability of having the gene.
2. The woman's sisters have a 1 in 2, or 50%, probability of having the gene.
3. The woman's brothers have a 1 in 2, or 50%, probability of having the gene.
4. One of the woman's parents definitely has the gene. Since the age of onset can be as late as age 50, the parents' symptoms may not yet have appeared.
5. It is unlikely that the woman's partner has the gene.

TEST-TAKING TIP: This question requires the test taker to do a reverse genetic analysis. If a woman is carrying one autosomal dominant gene, then her genotype is Aa. She received the affected gene from one of her parents and a normal gene from her other parent. One of her parents, therefore, definitely carries the gene. Because one of her parents carries the gene, each of her siblings has a 50/50

probability of carrying the gene. Because she carries the gene, her fetus has a 50/50 probability of carrying the gene. Since the woman's partner's history is unremarkable, it is unlikely that he carries the gene.

70. 1. This response is correct. As can be seen on the Punnett square, female children of carriers may carry the disease but do not express the disease.
    2. This response is incorrect. Male children are at risk of the disease.
    3. This response is incorrect. Only females are carriers of X-linked diseases.
    4. This response is incorrect. When reviewing X-linked recessive inheritance, the test taker must discuss the male and female probabilities independently. If the fetus is a female, she will be healthy—either with two normal genes or as a carrier. The probability of the males being affected, however, is 50/50—either healthy with two normal genes or with disease because of the normal Y mated with an affected "x." Accordingly, as can be seen in the square below, the probability of a male being affected is 50%.

	Father: X	Y
Mother: X	XX	XY
"x"	X"x"	"x"Y

(Affected X is depicted "x")

TEST-TAKING TIP: It is often especially difficult for women who carry X-linked diseases. While they, as females, are always healthy, it is their bodies that transmit the defective genes to their sons. As a result, the mothers often express a great deal of guilt.

71. 1. Amniocentesis will provide the couple with information regarding the genetics of a fetus in utero.
    2. CVS will provide the couple with information regarding the genetics of a fetus in utero.
    3. Pre-implantation genetic diagnosis will provide the couple with the highest probability of conceiving a healthy child.
    4. GIFT is a type of infertility procedure.

TEST-TAKING TIP: Pre-implantation genetic diagnosis (PGD) is a form of genetic assessment. The assessment is performed prior to the transfer of the embryo into the woman's fallopian tubes. The embryos that are assessed via PGD are conceived via assisted reproductive technology. Since only healthy embryos are implanted,

a couple will not have to decide whether or not to terminate affected pregnancies (see http://pgdis.org/).

72. 1. This response is inappropriate. The client has asked the nurse for information regarding cord blood banking.
    2. This statement is correct. The baby's umbilical cord blood is kept by a cord blood bank to be used if and when the baby should develop a serious illness like leukemia.
    3. The blood is not used in the same way that general blood donations are used. It is used to treat catastrophic illnesses.
    4. This response is true, but it does not provide the client with the information she needs to make an informed decision.

TEST-TAKING TIP: Umbilical cord blood contains stem cells that are used to treat cancers and other catastrophic illnesses, like sickle cell anemia. It is administered in the same way that a bone marrow transplant is administered.

73. 1. This statement is not accurate. Cystic fibrosis can be detected via amniocentesis.
    2. This response is likely. The genetic tests that are performed check only for the most common genetic variants of many diseases, including CF. If the baby were positive for an uncommon variant, it would be missed.
    3. It is unlikely that the lab tech made a mistake.
    4. Although it is possible, it is unlikely that maternal cells were harvested rather than fetal cells.

TEST-TAKING TIP: There are more than 1000 genetic variants of CF. It is impossible to test for all the variants. Unfortunately, clients do not realize that amniocentesis is not 100% reliable in identifying genetic problems. In addition, not all variants are tested on the newborn screen.

74. 1. Until the pedigree is fully analyzed, the need for a complete genetic analysis is uncertain.
    2. This statement is true. The proband is the first individual in any family to be identified with a disorder.
    3. This is not correct. Genetic information is confidential. Only if the proband agrees can others be included in the discussion. Plus, the proband's relatives may or may not be interested in discussing their potential of acquiring a genetic disease.

4. It is virtually impossible to determine if and when someone will develop breast cancer even if a genetic screen has been performed.

TEST-TAKING TIP: Per HIPAA (Health Insurance and Portability Accountability Act of 1996), a nurse who works for a health care organization must not discuss any information about a client's health information unless given express permission to do so by the patient. A patient's right to privacy includes the right to keep information confidential from relatives as well as strangers. In addition, anyone who has a genetic disease is further covered by GINA (Genetic Information Nondiscrimination Act of 2008), which requires that insurance companies and employers not discriminate against those with genetic illnesses (see http://hhs.gov/ocr/privacy/hipaa/understanding/index.html). It is important to remember that the genetic information of one family member may affect others in the family since they, too, may carry defective genes. This knowledge can be very difficult for some family members as well as for the proband. In essence, the nurse must remember that client information must be kept confidential.

75. 1. An affected male would be depicted as a darkened square without a hash mark.
2. An unaffected female would be depicted as a light-colored or uncolored circle without a hash mark.
3. A stillborn child is depicted as a triangle. If the child is known to have had the defect, the triangle would be a darkened triangle.
4. A child of unknown sex is depicted as a diamond. If the child is known to have had the defect, the symbol would be a darkened diamond.

TEST-TAKING TIP: For nurses to interpret pedigrees, they must be familiar with the symbols and terminology used. The Roman numerals at the left of pedigrees depict the generations pictured. Each individual in each generation is then numbered, from left to right. The 4th individual from the left in the second generation, therefore, is at location II-4.

76. 1. The individuals are fraternal twins.
2. An unaffected couple would be depicted as a square and circle connected by a single line. The square and circle would both be light colored or uncolored.

3. The proband is always identified by an arrow.
4. Known heterozygotes are half dark colored and half light colored. For example, a male who is a known heterozygote would be depicted as a square half of which is dark colored and half of which is light colored.

TEST-TAKING TIP: As seen in the pedigree, a y-connector is used to attach the twins to their parents' offspring line. If the twins were monozygotic, they would be of the same sex and there would be an additional line between the legs of the "y."

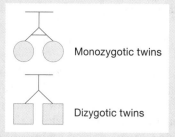

Monozygotic twins

Dizygotic twins

77. 1. This response is incorrect. No one can make such a prediction.
2. Neonates virtually never exhibit signs of sickle cell because fetal hemoglobin does not sickle.
3. This response is correct. Babies with two recessive sickle cell genes will show some symptoms of the disease but the severity of the symptoms will be individual.
4. This response is incorrect. Virtually all children with sickle cell anemia will exhibit some symptoms during their lives.

TEST-TAKING TIP: The test taker must be familiar with common terms used to describe genetic diseases, like penetrance and expressivity. *Penetrance:* When a disease is 100% penetrant, 100% of the individuals who have the gene(s) for the disease will exhibit the disease. Similarly, if a disease is 80% penetrant, only 80% of the individuals who have the gene(s) for the disease will exhibit the disease. *Expressivity:* This term refers to the range of severity—or phenotypes—of a particular genetic disease.

78. 1. The pedigree is an example of autosomal recessive inheritance.

2. The pedigree is not an example of mito-chondrial inheritance.
3. The pedigree is not an example of X-linked recessive inheritance.
4. The pedigree is not an example of Y-linked trait inheritance.

TEST-TAKING TIP: An autosomal recessive inheritance pattern is characterized by 4 things: (1) parents of affected children are usually disease free; (2) about 1 out of every 4 children in large families exhibit the disease; (3) boys and girls are affected equally; and (4) all the children are affected when both parents have the disease.

79. 1. The pedigree is not an example of autoso-mal dominant inheritance.
2. **The pedigree is an example of mito-chondrial inheritance.**
3. The pedigree is not an example of X-linked recessive.
4. The pedigree is not an example of Y-linked trait.

TEST-TAKING TIP: A mitochondrial inheri-tance pattern is characterized by the fact that all of an affected woman's children, whether male or female, exhibit the dis-ease. None of an affected male's children is ever affected. Mitochondrial DNA is transmitted only from mothers.

80. 1. This response is inappropriate. Each and every pregnancy carries the same probability of being affected.
2. This response is inappropriate. It is impos-sible for a nurse to know how a couple will respond to the probability that their fetus will be affected.
3. **This response is accurate.**
4. This response is inaccurate. There is a 1 out of 4 chance that the baby will inherit both recessive genes and have the disease.

	Father: A	a
Mother: A	AA	Aa
a	Aa	aa

TEST-TAKING TIP: As can be seen by the Punnett square, there is a 3 out of 4 probability that their child will be healthy (AA and Aa)—a 1 out of 4 probability that their child with carry no abnormal genes for PKU (AA), a 2 out of 4 probability that their child will be a carrier (Aa)—and a 1 out of 4 probability that their child will have the disease (aa).

81. 1. This response is incorrect. None of their male children will be green color blind.
2. This response is incorrect. None of their female children will be green color blind.
3. This response is incorrect. Males do not carry X-linked recessive traits.
4. **This response is correct. All of the females will be carriers.**

TEST-TAKING TIP: The male client has a genotype of "x"Y, the "x" being the recessive gene responsible for green color blindness. The female has a genotype of XX; both of her genes are normal.

As can be seen by the Punnett square,

	Father: "x"	Y
Mother: X	X"x"	XY
X	X"x"	XY

(Affected X is depicted as "x")

all of the daughters will carry one affected "x" gene from their father, but none of the sons will carry an affected "x" gene.

82. 4 and 5 are correct.
1. This response is incorrect. The baby will be either type A or type B. Type O is the recessive.
2. This response is incorrect. The baby will be either type A or type B. Type O is the recessive.
3. This response is incorrect. The offspring cannot be type AB since the mother is type O.
4. **The baby could be blood type AO (type A) and, if the father is heterozy-gous for the Rh factor, the baby could be either Rh+ (positive) or Rh– (negative).**
5. **The baby could be type BO (type B) and, if the father is heterozygous for the Rh factor, the baby could be either Rh+ (positive) or Rh– (negative).**

TEST-TAKING TIP: To answer this question, the test taker must be familiar with the concept of codominance. In addition, the test taker must create separate Punnett squares. Codominance refers to the fact that both blood type A and type B dominate. If a person possesses the gene for both types, he or she will, therefore, be type AB. Three Punnett squares are needed to determine the answer to this question because the father's Rh genotype could be either homozygous or heterozy-gous and because a person's blood type is independent or a person's Rh factor.

Punnett square to determine blood type:

	Father: A	B
Mother: O	AO (type A)	BO (type B)
O	AO (type A)	BO (type B)

If father is homozygous for Rh⁺ (positive):

	Father: +	+
Mother: −	+−(RH⁺)	+−(RH⁺)
−	+−(RH⁺)	+−(RH⁺)

If father is heterozygous for Rh:

	Father: +	−
Mother: −	+−(RH⁺)	−−(RH⁻)
−	+−(RH⁺)	−−(RH⁻)

83. 1. This information is unsupported by the scenario. Cerebral palsy is not a genetic defect and is not detected through amniocentesis.
    2. Cerebral palsy is not a genetic disease. It is caused by a hypoxic injury that can occur at any time during pregnancy, labor and delivery, or the postdelivery period.
    3. Cerebral palsy is not a genetic disease. It is caused by a hypoxic injury that can occur at any time during pregnancy, labor and delivery, or the postdelivery period.
    4. Cerebral palsy is not a genetic disease. It is caused by a hypoxic injury that can occur at any time during pregnancy, labor and delivery, or the postdelivery period.

TEST-TAKING TIP: Some couples believe that if an amniocentesis result shows that the chromosomes and genes are normal, then the baby will be normal. This is not true. Some problems are caused by teratogens, some are caused by birth injuries, and some genetic diseases are not tested for. Indeed, only a discreet number of defects can be assessed during amniocentesis. It would be financially impossible to test every fetus for every one of the thousands of genetic defects.

84. 1. The centromere is the site where sister chromatids attach during cell division.
    2. A chiasma is the site where crossing over between nonsister chromatids takes place. At this site, genetic material is swapped between the chromatids.
    3. A chromatid is one strand of a duplicated chromosome. Sister chromatids are attached at the chromosome's centromere.

4. A codon is a triad of messenger RNA that encodes for a specific amino acid in a protein.

TEST-TAKING TIP: Crossing over at the chiasmata is an essential process during meiosis. DNA is exchanged between non-sister chromatids—one from the mother and one from the father. This results in the genetic variance of the species.

85. 1. This statement is accurate. All of the woman's children will be affected.
    2. This statement is incorrect. All of the woman's children will be affected.
    3. This statement is incorrect. All of the woman's children will be affected.
    4. This statement is incorrect. All of the woman's children will be affected.

TEST-TAKING TIP: Mitochondrial DNA is inherited through the mother only. Since all of the woman's gametes contain her mitochondrial DNA, all of her offspring will be affected.

86. 1. The breast cancer genes are highly penetrant, but this is not the most important information
    2. The breast cancer genes are moderately expressive, but this is not the most important information.
    3. Amniocentesis does, although rarely, end in miscarriage, but this is not the most important information.
    4. The most important information for the nurse to provide the client is that the vast majority of cases of breast cancer are not inherited.

TEST-TAKING TIP: Every year about 200,000 cases of breast cancer are diagnosed, but only 5%–10% of the cases are inherited. It would be inappropriate to perform an amniocentesis for breast cancer unless the mother has been found to carry one of the genes. In addition, it must be remembered that even inherited breast cancer has a strong environmental component.

87. 1. This is the definition of Down syndrome, but not of Down syndrome with mosaic chromosomal configuration.
    2. All chromosomes are banded.
    3. The number 21 chromosomes are of normal length in Down syndrome
    4. Mosaicism is characterized by the fact that some of the cells of the body have the abnormal number of chromosomes

but some of the cells have the normal number. This may happen with rapid disjunction. In Down syndrome, it means that some of the cells have three number 21 chromosomes and some have the normal number of two number 21 chromosomes. Mosaicism is not specific to Down syndrome but can occur with other chromosomal abnormalities.

TEST-TAKING TIP: The concept of mosaicism can be remembered by thinking about a mosaic piece of art. Mosaic tiles are bits of glass or ceramic that are different colors and shapes, but when put into a design create a piece of art. In genetics, mosaicism refers to the fact that various cells of the body have different numbers of chromosomes.

88. 1. This goal is inappropriate. The client has a family history of cystic fibrosis. She does not have the disease.
    2. This goal is appropriate. Since the client has a family history of the disease, she should seek genetic counseling.
    3. This goal is inappropriate. It is unnecessary to have CVS unless both the mother and the father are found to be carriers of cystic fibrosis.
    4. This goal is inappropriate. The client has a family history of cystic fibrosis. She does not have the disease.

TEST-TAKING TIP: Cystic fibrosis is an autosomal-recessive disease. If the woman has a family history of CF, she may be a carrier for the disease. If her partner also is a carrier, there would be a 1 in 4, or 25%, probability of the fetus having the disease and a 1 in 2, or 50%, chance of the child being a carrier. It is important for the woman to seek genetic counseling.

89. 1. Although the parents should seek genetic counseling before getting pregnant in the future, this is not the rationale for newborn testing.
    2. This is the rationale for newborn testing for maple syrup urine disease. It is done to prevent neurological disease in affected children.
    3. This is a benefit of many of the newborn tests, but it is not the primary rationale. The cost-benefit ratio (in terms of money) does not always support newborn testing. In very rare diseases like MSUD, the cost of testing is often higher than the cost of care for any affected children.
    4. This is not a rationale for newborn testing.

TEST-TAKING TIP: When children with inborn metabolic diseases follow strict diets they have the potential to grow into normal adulthood. It is essential that the tests be performed during the neonatal period because the children's diets must be altered as quickly as possible to prevent the adverse affects. When children with MSUD eat restricted foods, their brains are severely affected, leading to mental retardation, coma, and death.

Women's Health Issues

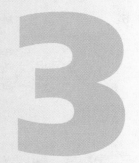

Although this book focuses on issues related to maternity, specifically the antepartum, intrapartum, and postpartum periods, there are a number of other issues that nurses must be familiar with, especially since many of these issues affect women of childbearing age. Among the issues are domestic violence, eating disorders, and sexually transmitted infections. Many of the problems are related to women's relationships, either heterosexual or homosexual. The nurse must be able to assume a number of roles when caring for women: educator, counselor, caregiver, and the like. For example, the nurse must be able to provide teaching on ways to prevent disease and on contraceptive choices, to counsel newly pregnant women, and to administer medications knowledgeably when a woman is diagnosed with a sexually transmitted infection. This chapter focuses on some of the more common issues faced by nurses caring for women of childbearing age.

KEYWORDS

The following words include English vocabulary, nursing/medical terminology, concepts, principles, or information relevant to content specifically addressed in the chapter or associated with topics presented in it. English dictionaries, your nursing textbooks, and medical dictionaries such as *Taber's Cyclopedic Medical Dictionary* are resources that can be used to expand your knowledge and understanding of these words and related information.

anorexia nervosa

bacterial vaginosis

bilateral tubal ligation

birth control pills

bone density

breast cancer

breast self-examination

bulimia

calendar method

cervical cancer

cervical cap

child abuse

chlamydia

confidence interval

contraceptive patch (Ortho Evra)

contraceptive sponge

Depo-Provera (medroxyprogesterone acetate)

domestic violence

endometriosis

endometritis

female condom

fibrocystic breasts

GHB (*gamma*-hydroxybutyric acid)

gonorrhea

hepatitis B

herpes simplex 2

hormone replacement therapy

human immunodeficiency virus (HIV)

human papillomavirus (HPV)

intrauterine device (IUD)

lactation amenorrhea method (LAM)

lesbian

male condom

mammogram

maternal mortality rate

Mifeprex (misepristone/misoprostol [formerly RU-486])

NuvaRing

osteoporosis

ovarian cancer

pelvic inflammatory disease (PID)

perimenopause

plan B (levonorgestrol)

pubic lice

rape (including date rape)

risk ratio

Rohypnol (flunitrazepam)

Seasonale (ethinyl estradiol and levonorgestrel)

sexual assault

sexually transmitted infections

significant difference

syphilis

toxic shock syndrome

trichomoniasis

vasectomy

withdrawal (coitus interruptus)

QUESTIONS

1. The nurse in a pediatric clinic is caring for a 9-year-old girl who has been diagnosed with gonorrhea. Which of the following actions is appropriate for the nurse to take?
   1. Notify the physician so the child can be admitted to the hospital.
   2. Discuss with the girl the need to stop future sexual encounters.
   3. Question the mother about her daughter's menstrual history.
   4. Report the girl's medical findings to child protective services.

2. A 19-year-old client with multiple sex partners is being counseled about the hepatitis B vaccination. During the counseling sessions, which of the following should the nurse advise the client to receive?
   1. Hepatitis B immune globulin before receiving the vaccine.
   2. Vaccine booster every 10 years.
   3. Complete series of three intramuscular injections.
   4. Vaccine as soon as she becomes 21.

3. A postpartum client has decided to use Depo-Provera (medroxyprogesterone acetate) as her contraceptive method. What should the nurse advise the client regarding this medication?
   1. Take the pill at the same time each day.
   2. Refrain from breastfeeding while using the method.
   3. Expect to have no periods as long as she takes the medicine.
   4. Consider switching to another birth control method in a year or so.

4. The nurse is administering Depo-Provera (medroxyprogesterone acetate) to a postpartum client. Which of the following data must the nurse consider before administering the medication?
   1. The capsule must be taken at the same time each day.
   2. The client must be taught to use sunscreen whenever in the sunlight.
   3. The medicine is contraindicated if the woman has lung or esophageal cancer.
   4. The client must use an alternate form of birth control for the first two months.

5. Which statement by the client indicates that she understands the teaching provided about the intrauterine device (IUD)?
   1. "The IUD can remain in place for a year or more."
   2. "I will not menstruate while the IUD is in."
   3. "Pain during intercourse is a common side effect."
   4. "The device will reduce my chances of getting infected."

6. A client has been diagnosed with pubic lice. Which of the following signs/symptoms would the nurse expect to see?
   1. Macular rash on the labia.
   2. Pruritus.
   3. Hyperthermia.
   4. Foul-smelling discharge.

7. The nurse is teaching a client regarding the treatment for pubic lice. Which of the following should be included in the teaching session?
   1. The antibiotics should be taken for a full 10 days.
   2. All clothing should be pretreated with bleach before wearing.
   3. Shampoo should be applied for at least 2 hours before rinsing.
   4. The pubic hair should be combed after shampoo is removed.

TABLE 3-1. Comparison of Self-Reported Sources of Hepatitis B Virus Information by Group

Source	Group Intervention —% Who Received the Vaccine (n = 137)	Control—% Who Did Not Receive the Vaccine (n = 126)	Risk Ratio	95% Confidence Interval (CI)	P
Read/Heard	87.7	70.2	1.25	1.12–1.40	<0.001
School paper	11.7	11.9	0.98	0.51–1.90	0.95
Mass media	24.8	36.5	0.68	0.47–0.99	0.4
Bulletin board	38.7	42.9	0.90	0.67–1.21	0.49
Fliers	50.4	44.4	1.13	0.88–1.46	0.34
Letters	48.9	11.1	4.40	2.61–7.42	<0.001
Parents	33.6	21.4	1.57	1.04–2.36	0.03
University Health Service Providers	2.2	5.6	0.39	0.10–1.49	0.15
Family doctor	25.5	29.4	0.87	0.59–1.29	0.49
Friends	20.4	34.1	0.60	0.40–0.90	0.01
Health History Form	38.7	23.8	1.62	1.11–2.37	0.01

From: Marron, R.L., Lanphear, B.P., Kouides, R., Dudman, L., Manchester, R.A., & Christy, C. (1998). Efficacy of informational letters on hepatitis B immunizations rates in university students. *Journal of American College Health, 47*(3), 123–127.

8. The parent of a newborn angrily asks the nurse, "Why would the doctor want to give my baby the vaccination for hepatitis B? It's a sexually transmitted disease, you know!" Which of the following is the best response by the nurse?
   1. "The hepatitis B vaccine is given to all babies. It is given because many babies get infected from their mothers during pregnancy."
   2. "It is important for your baby to get the vaccine in the hospital because the shot may not be available when your child gets older."
   3. "Hepatitis B can be a life-threatening infection that is contracted by contact with contaminated blood as well as sexually."
   4. "Most parents want to protect their children from as many serious diseases as possible. Hepatitis B is one of those diseases."

9. A nurse is reading the research article "Efficacy of Informational Letters on Hepatitis B Immunization Rates in University Students" (Marron, R.L., Lanphear, B.P., Kouides, R., Dudman, L., Manchester, R.A., & Christy, C. [1998]. *Journal of American College Health, 47*(3), 123–127). In the article, the researchers analyzed the means by which the students learned about the hepatitis B vaccine and compared that information with whether or not the students actually received the vaccine. Table 3-1 describes the data.

Which of the following interpretations of the data from Table 3-1 is correct?
   1. When one considers those who "read/heard" about the vaccine, there is no significant difference between the percentage of students who received the immunization and those who did not receive the immunization.
   2. The likelihood of students who receive the vaccine when they learned about it from the "health history form" was about 1.6 times that of the "health history form" students who did not receive the vaccine.
   3. 44.4% of those who were not vaccinated received their information from "Letters."
   4. The largest percentage of students who received the vaccine learned about it from the "University Health Service (UHS) providers."

10. A nurse is reading a research article on the incidence of sexually transmitted diseases in one population as compared with a second population. The relative risk (RR) is reported as 0.80 and the 95% confidence interval (CI) is reported as 0.62 to 1.4. How should the nurse interpret the results?
    1. Because the CI of the RR includes the value of 1, the difference between the groups is meaningless.
    2. A 95% confidence interval is a statistically significant finding.
    3. A relative risk of 0.80 is moderately powerful.
    4. Because there is no P value reported for the CI, the nurse is unable to make any conclusions about the data.

11. A gravid, married client, 24 weeks' gestation, is found to have bacterial vaginosis. Her health care practitioner has ordered metronidazole (Flagyl) to treat the problem. Which of the following educational information is important for the nurse to provide the woman at this time?
    1. The woman must be careful to observe for signs of preterm labor.
    2. The woman must advise her partner to seek therapy as soon as possible.
    3. A common side effect of the medicine is a copious vaginal discharge.
    4. A repeat culture should be taken two weeks after completing the therapy.

12. A nonpregnant young woman has been diagnosed with bacterial vaginosis (BV). The nurse questions the woman regarding her sexual history, including her frequency of intercourse, how many sexual partners she has, and her use of contraceptives. What is the rationale for the nurse's questions?
    1. Clients with BV can infect their sexual partners.
    2. The nurse is required by law to ask the questions.
    3. Clients with BV can become infected with HIV and other sexually transmitted infections more easily than uninfected women.
    4. The laboratory needs a full client history to know for which organisms and antibiotic sensitivities it should test.

13. A woman is noted to have multiple soft warts on her perineum and rectal areas. The nurse suspects that this client is infected with which of the following sexually transmitted infections?
    1. Human papillomavirus (HPV).
    2. Human immunodeficiency virus (HIV).
    3. Syphilis.
    4. Trichomoniasis.

14. A woman is to receive 2.4 million units of penicillin G benzathine IM to treat syphilis. The medication is available as 1,200,000 units/mL. How many mL should the nurse administer?
    _____ mL

15. Four women who use superabsorbent tampons during their menses are being seen in the medical clinic. The woman with which of the following findings would lead the nurse to suspect that the woman's complaints are related to her use of tampons rather than to an unrelated medical problem?
    1. Diffuse rash with fever.
    2. Angina.
    3. Hypertension.
    4. Thrombocytopenia with pallor.

16. A woman, seen in the emergency department, is diagnosed with pelvic inflammatory disease (PID). Before discharge, the nurse should provide the woman with health teaching regarding which of the following?
    1. Endometriosis.
    2. Menopause.
    3. Ovarian hyperstimulation.
    4. Sexually transmitted infections.

17. A woman has contracted herpes simplex 2 for the first time. Which of the following signs/symptoms is the client likely to complain of?
    1. Flu-like symptoms.
    2. Metrorrhagia.
    3. Amenorrhea.
    4. Abdominal cramping.

18. Which of the following sexually transmitted infections is characterized by a foul-smelling, yellow-green discharge that is often accompanied by vaginal pain and dyspareunia?
    1. Syphilis.
    2. Herpes simplex.
    3. Trichomoniasis.
    4. Condylomata acuminata.

19. The nurse is educating a group of adolescent women regarding sexually transmitted infections (STIs). The nurse knows that learning was achieved when a group member states that the most common sign/symptom of sexually transmitted infections is which of the following?
    1. Menstrual cramping.
    2. Heavy menstrual periods.
    3. Flu-like symptoms.
    4. Lack of signs or symptoms.

20. A woman has been diagnosed with pelvic inflammatory disease (PID). Which of the following organisms are the most likely causative agents? **Select all that apply.**
    1. *Gardnerella vaginalis*.
    2. *Candida albicans*.
    3. *Chlamydia trachomatis*.
    4. *Neisseria gonorrhoeae*.
    5. *Treponema pallidum*.

21. The public health nurse calls a woman and states, "I am afraid that I have some disturbing news. A man who has been treated for gonorrhea by the health department has told them that he had intercourse with you. It is very important that you seek medical attention." The woman replies, "There is no reason for me to go to the doctor! I feel fine!" Which of the following replies by the nurse is appropriate at this time?
    1. "I am sure that you are upset by the disturbing news, but there is no reason to be angry with me."
    2. "I am sorry. We must have received the wrong information."
    3. "That certainly could be the case. Women often report no symptoms."
    4. "All right, but please tell me your contacts because it is possible for you to pass the disease on even if you have no symptoms."

22. A woman has been diagnosed with primary syphilis. Which of the following physical findings would the nurse expect to see?
    1. Cluster of vesicles.
    2. Pain-free lesion.
    3. Macular rash.
    4. Foul-smelling discharge.

23. A woman has been diagnosed with syphilis. Which of the following nursing interventions is appropriate?
    1. Council the woman about how to live with a chronic infection.
    2. Question the woman regarding symptoms of other sexually transmitted infections.
    3. Assist the primary health care practitioner with cryotherapy procedures.
    4. Educate the woman regarding the safe disposal of menstrual pads.

24. After a sex education class, the school nurse overhears an adolescent woman discussing safe sex practices. Which of the following comments by the young woman indicates that teaching about infection control was effective?
    1. "I don't have to worry about getting infected if I have oral sex."
    2. "Teen women are most high risk for sexually transmitted infections (STI)."
    3. "The best thing to do if I have sex a lot is to use spermicide each and every time."
    4. "Boys get human immunodeficiency virus (HIV) easier than girls do."

25. An asymptomatic woman is being treated for HIV infection at the women's health clinic. Which of the following comments by the woman shows that she understands her care?
    1. "If I get pregnant, my baby will be HIV positive."
    2. "I should have my viral load and antibody levels checked every day."
    3. "Since my partner and I are both HIV positive, we use a condom."
    4. "To be safe, my partner and I engage only in oral sex."

26. A female client asks the nurse about treatment for human papilloma viral warts. The nurse's response should be based on which of the following?
    1. An antiviral injection cures approximately fifty percent of cases.
    2. Aggressive treatment is required to cure warts.
    3. Warts often spread when an attempt is made to remove them surgically.
    4. Warts often recur a few months after a client is treated.

27. A triage nurse answers a telephone call from the male partner of a woman who was recently diagnosed with cervical cancer. The man is requesting to be tested for human papillomavirus (HPV). The nurse's response should be based on which of the following?
    1. There is currently no approved test to detect HPV in men.
    2. A viral culture of the penis and rectum is used to detect HPV in men.
    3. A Pap smear of the meatus of the penis is used to detect HPV in men.
    4. There is no need for a test because men do not become infected with HPV.

28. A client who is sexually active is asking the nurse about Gardasil, one of the vaccines that is given to prevent human papillomavirus (HPV). Which of the following should be included in the counseling session?
    1. Gardasil is not recommended for women who are already sexually active.
    2. Gardasil protects recipients from all strains of the virus.
    3. The most common side effect from the vaccine is pain at the injection site.
    4. Anyone who is allergic to eggs is advised against receiving the vaccine.

29. A man has been diagnosed with a chlamydial infection. The nurse would expect the client to complain of pain at which of the following times?
    1. When urinating.
    2. When ejaculating.
    3. When the penis becomes erect.
    4. When the testicles are touched.

30. A couple seeking contraception and infection-prevention counseling state, "We know that the best way for us to prevent both pregnancy and infection is to use condoms plus spermicide every time we have sex." Which of the following is the best response by the nurse?
    1. "That is correct. It is best to use a condom with spermicide during every sexual contact."
    2. "That is true, except if you have intercourse twice in one evening. Then you do not have to apply more spermicide."
    3. "That is not true. It has been shown that condoms alone are very effective and that the spermicide might increase the transmission of some viruses."
    4. "That is not necessarily true. Spermicide has been shown to cause cancer in men and women who use it too frequently."

31. The nurse is teaching an uncircumcised male to use a condom. Which of the following information should be included in the teaching plan?
1. Apply mineral oil to the shaft of the penis after applying the condom.
2. Pull back the foreskin before applying the condom.
3. Create a reservoir at the tip of the condom after putting it on.
4. Wait five minutes after ejaculating before removing the condom.

32. The nurse is teaching a young woman how to use the female condom. Which of the following should be included in the teaching plan?
1. Reuse female condoms no more than five times.
2. Refrain from using lubricant because the condom may slip out of the vagina.
3. Wear both female and male condoms together to maximize effectiveness.
4. Remove the condom by twisting the outer ring and pulling gently.

33. A woman has a history of toxic shock syndrome. Which of the following forms of birth control should she be taught to avoid? **Select all that apply.**
1. Diaphragm.
2. Intrauterine device.
3. Birth control pills (estrogen-progestin combination).
4. Contraceptive sponge.
5. Depo-Provera (medroxyprogesterone acetate).

34. During a counseling session on natural family planning techniques, how should the nurse explain the consistency of cervical mucus at the time of ovulation?
1. It becomes thin and elastic.
2. It becomes opaque and acidic.
3. It contains numerous leukocytes to prevent vaginal infections.
4. It decreases in quantity in response to body temperature changes.

35. A client is being taught about the care and use of the diaphragm. Which of the following comments by the woman shows that she understands the teaching that was provided?
1. "I should regularly put the diaphragm up to the light and look at it carefully."
2. "This is one method that can be used during menstruation."
3. "I can leave the diaphragm in place for a day or two."
4. "The diaphragm should be well powdered before I put it back in the case."

36. A woman, who wishes to use the calendar method for contraception, reports that her last 6 menstrual cycles were 28, 32, 29, 36, 30, and 27 days long, respectively. In the future, if used correctly, she should abstain from intercourse on which of the following days of her cycle?
1. Days 9 to 25.
2. Days 10 to 15.
3. Days 11 to 20.
4. Days 12 to 17.

37. The nurse teaches a couple that the diaphragm is an excellent method of contraception providing that the woman does which of the following?
1. Does not use any cream or jelly with it.
2. Douches promptly after its removal.
3. Leaves it in place for 6 hours following intercourse.
4. Inserts it at least 5 hours prior to having intercourse.

38. The nurse is working with a client who states that she has multiple sex partners. Which of the following contraceptive methods would be best for the nurse to recommend to this client?
1. Intrauterine device.
2. Female condom.
3. Bilateral tubal ligation.
4. Birth control pills.

39. A woman has gotten pregnant with a Copper T intrauterine device (IUD) in place. The physician has ordered an ultrasound to be done to evaluate the pregnancy. The client asks the nurse why this is so important. The nurse should tell the woman that the ultrasound is done primarily for which of the following reasons?
    1. To assess for the presence of an ectopic pregnancy.
    2. To check the baby for serious malformations.
    3. To assess for pelvic inflammatory disease.
    4. To check for the possibility of a twin pregnancy.

40. An adolescent woman confides to the school nurse that she is sexually active. The young woman asks the nurse to recommend a "very reliable" birth control method, but she refuses to be seen by a gynecologist. Which of the following methods would be best for the nurse to recommend?
    1. Contraceptive patch.
    2. Withdrawal method.
    3. Female condom.
    4. Contraceptive sponge.

41. The nurse is developing a teaching plan for a client undergoing a bilateral tubal ligation. Which of the following should be included in the plan?
    1. The surgical procedure is easily reversible.
    2. Menstruation usually ceases after the procedure.
    3. Libido should remain the same after the procedure.
    4. The incision will be made endocervically.

42. The nurse is developing a plan of care for clients seeking contraception information. Which of the following issues about the woman must the nurse consider before suggesting contraceptive choices? **Select all that apply.**
    1. Age.
    2. Ethical and moral beliefs.
    3. Sexual patterns.
    4. Socioeconomic status.
    5. Childbearing plans.

43. A woman is being issued a new prescription for a low-dose combination birth control pill. What advice should the nurse give the woman if she ever forgets to take a pill?
    1. Take it as soon as she remembers, even if that means taking two pills in one day.
    2. Skip that pill and refrain from intercourse for the remainder of the month.
    3. Wear a pad for the next week because she will experience vaginal bleeding.
    4. Take an at-home pregnancy test at the end of the month to check for a pregnancy.

44. A couple is seeking family planning advice. They are newly married and wish to delay childbearing for at least 3 years. The woman, age 26, G0 P0000, has no medical problems and does not smoke. She states, however, that she is very embarrassed when she touches her vagina. Which of the following methods would be most appropriate for the nurse to suggest to this couple?
    1. Diaphragm.
    2. Cervical cap.
    3. Intrauterine device (IUD).
    4. Birth control pills (BCP).

45. What is essential for the nurse to teach a woman who has just had an intrauterine device (IUD) inserted?
    1. Palpate her lower abdomen each month to check the patency of the device.
    2. Remain on bed rest for 24 hours after insertion of the device.
    3. Report any complaints of painful intercourse to the physician.
    4. Insert spermicidal jelly within 4 hours of every sexual encounter.

46. A 16-year-old woman who had unprotected intercourse 24 hours ago has entered the emergency department seeking assistance. Which of the following responses by the nurse is appropriate?
    1. "You can walk into your local pharmacy and buy Plan B (levonorgestrel)."
    2. "I am sorry but because of your age I am unable to assist you."
    3. "The emergency room doctor can prescribe high-dose birth control pills (BCP) for you."
    4. The nurse's response is dependent upon which state he or she is practicing in.

47. A young woman is seen in the emergency department. She states, "I took a pregnancy test today. I'm pregnant. My parents will be furious with me!! I have to do something!" Which of the following responses by the nurse is most appropriate?
    1. "You can take medicine to abort the pregnancy so your parents won't know."
    2. "Let's talk about your options."
    3. "The best thing for you to do is to have the baby and to give it up for adoption."
    4. "I can help you tell your parents."

48. A breastfeeding woman is requesting that she be prescribed Seasonale (ethinyl estradiol and levonorgestrel) as a birth control method. Which of the following information should be included in the patient teaching session?
    1. The woman will menstruate every 8 to 9 weeks.
    2. The pills are taken for 3 out of every 4 weeks.
    3. Breakthrough bleeding is a common side effect.
    4. Breastfeeding is compatible with the medication.

49. Five women wish to use the Ortho Evra (patch) for family planning. Which of the women should be carefully counseled regarding the safety considerations of the method? **Select all that apply.**
    1. The woman who smokes 1 pack of cigarettes each day.
    2. The woman with a history of lung cancer.
    3. The woman with a history of deep vein thrombosis.
    4. The woman who runs at least 50 miles each week.
    5. The woman with a history of cholecystitis.

50. A postpartum woman is using the lactational amenorrhea method of birth control. The nurse should advise the client that the method is effective only if which of the following conditions is present? **Select all that apply.**
    1. Being less than 6 months postpartum.
    2. Being amenorrheic since delivery of the baby.
    3. Supplementing with formula no more than once per day.
    4. Losing less than 10% of weight since delivery.
    5. Sleeping at least 8 hours every night.

51. A woman is being taught how to use the diaphragm as a contraceptive device. Which of the following statements by the woman indicates that the teaching was effective? **Select all that apply.**
    1. Petroleum-based lubricants may be used with the device.
    2. The device must be refitted if the woman gains or loses 10 pounds or more.
    3. The anterior lip must be pushed under the symphysis pubis.
    4. Additional spermicide must be added if the device has been in place over 6 hours.
    5. The diaphragm should be cleaned with a 10% bleach solution after every use.

52. Four women with significant health histories wish to use the diaphragm as a contraceptive method. The nurse should counsel the woman with which of the following histories that the diaphragm may lead to a recurrence of her problem?
    1. Urinary tract infections.
    2. Herpes simplex infections.
    3. Deep vein thromboses.
    4. Human papilloma warts.

53. A woman is using the contraceptive sponge as a birth control method. Which of the following actions is it important for her to perform to maximize the sponge's effectiveness?
    1. Insert the sponge at least one hour before intercourse.
    2. Thoroughly moisten the sponge with water before inserting.
    3. Spermicidal jelly must be inserted at the same time the sponge is inserted.
    4. A new sponge must be inserted every time a couple has intercourse.

54. A man has just had a vasectomy. Which of the following post-procedure teachings should the nurse provide the client? **Select all that apply.**
    1. Complete sterility will occur approximately 1 week post-surgery.
    2. Bed rest should be maintained for a full 24 hours after the vasectomy.
    3. The surgeon should be contacted immediately if marked enlargement of the scrotal sac is noted after the procedure.
    4. An athletic supporter should be worn to protect the surgical site.
    5. Prostate-specific antigen testing (PSA) should be performed every year after a vasectomy.

55. The nurse has given postvasectomy teaching to a client. Which of the following responses by the client indicates that the teaching was effective?
    1. "I will measure my urinary output for two days."
    2. "I will ejaculate the same amount of semen as I did before the surgery."
    3. "I will refrain from having an erection until next week."
    4. "I will irrigate the wound twice today and once more tomorrow."

56. The nurse is providing education to a couple regarding the proper procedure for male condom use. The nurse knows that the teaching was effective when the couple states that which of the following procedures should be taken if the man's penis becomes flaccid immediately after ejaculation?
    1. The woman should douche with white vinegar and water.
    2. The woman should consider taking a postcoital contraceptive.
    3. The man should hold the edges of the condom during its removal.
    4. The man should apply spermicide to the upper edges of the condom.

57. The nurse is developing a standard care plan for the administration of Mifeprex (misepristone/misoprostol; formerly known as RU-486). Which of the following information should the nurse include in the plan?
    1. Women should be evaluated by their health care practitioners 2 weeks after taking the medicine.
    2. This is the preferred method for terminating an ectopic pregnancy when an intrauterine device is in place.
    3. The only symptom clients should experience is bleeding 2 to 3 days after taking the medicine.
    4. Women who experience no bleeding within 3 days should immediately take a home pregnancy test.

58. The nurse has provided a single, perimenopausal woman, G3 P2012, with contraceptive counseling. The woman has four sex partners and smokes 1 pack of cigarettes per day. Which of the following methods is best suited for this client?
    1. Male condom.
    2. Intrauterine device.
    3. NuvaRing.
    4. Oral contraceptives.

59. A client who has been taking birth control pills for 2 months calls the clinic with the following complaint: "I have had a bad headache for the past couple of days and I now have pain in my right leg." Which of the following responses should the nurse make?
    1. "Continue the pill, but take one aspirin tablet with it each day from now on."
    2. "Stop taking the pill, and start using a condom for contraception."
    3. "Come to the clinic this afternoon so that we can see what is going on."
    4. "Those are common side effects that should disappear in a month or so."

60. The nurse has taught a couple about the temperature rhythm method of fertility control. Which of the following behaviors would indicate that the teaching was effective?
    1. The woman takes her basal body temperature before retiring each evening.
    2. The couple charts information from at least six menstrual cycles before using the method.
    3. The couple resumes having intercourse as soon as they see a rise in the basal body temperature.
    4. The woman assesses her vaginal discharge daily for changes in color and odor.

61. A nurse is providing contraceptive counseling to a perimenopausal client, G3 P2012, who is in a monogamous relationship. Which of the following comments by the woman indicates that further teaching is needed?
    1. "The calendar method is the most reliable method for me to use."
    2. "If I use the IUD, I am at minimal risk for pelvic inflammatory disease."
    3. "I should still use birth control even though I had only 2 periods last year."
    4. "The contraceptive patch contains both estrogen and progesterone."

62. The nurse is interviewing a client regarding contraceptive choices. Which of the following client statements would most influence the nurse's teaching?
    1. "I have 2 children."
    2. "My partner and I have sex twice a week."
    3. "I am 25 years old."
    4. "I feel funny touching my private parts."

63. Which of the following clients, who are all seeking a family planning method, is the best candidate for birth control pills?
    1. 19-year-old with multiple sex partners.
    2. 27-year-old who bottle feeds her newborn.
    3. 29-year-old with chronic hypertension.
    4. 37-year-old who smokes one pack per day.

64. The nurse met four clients in the family planning clinic today. It would be most appropriate for the nurse to recommend the intrauterine device (IUD) to which of the clients?
    1. Unmarried, 22-year-old, recent college graduate.
    2. Married, 24-year-old, G0 P0000.
    3. Unmarried, 25-year-old, history of chlamydia.
    4. Married, 26-year-old, G3 P2102.

65. A nurse is educating a group of women in her parish about osteoporosis. The nurse should include in her discussion that which of the following is a risk factor for the disease process?
    1. Multiparity.
    2. Increased body weight.
    3. Late onset of menopause.
    4. Heavy alcohol intake.

66. A woman is taking Fosamax (alendronate) for osteoporosis. The nurse should advise the woman about which of the following when taking the medication?
    1. Remain upright for 30 minutes after taking the medication.
    2. Take only after eating a full meal.
    3. Take medication in divided doses 3 times each day.
    4. Do not break or crush the tablet.

67. A client is put on calcium supplements to maintain bone health. To maximize absorption, the client is also advised to take which of the following supplements?
    1. Vitamin D.
    2. Vitamin E.
    3. Folic acid.
    4. Iron.

68. A client asks a nurse to express an opinion on the value of taking hormone replacement therapy (HRT). The nurse should be aware that it is recognized that HRT is effective in which of the following situations?
    1. No woman should ever take hormone replacement therapy.
    2. Women experiencing severe menopausal symptoms.
    3. Women with severe coronary artery disease.
    4. Women with a history of breast cancer.

69. A woman states that she feels "dirty" during her menses so she often douches to "clean myself." The nurse advises the woman that it is especially important to refrain from douching while menstruating because douching will increase the likelihood of her developing which of the following gynecological complications?
    1. Fibroids.
    2. Endometritis.
    3. Cervical cancer.
    4. Polyps.

70. Women who are on hormone replacement therapy (HRT) for an extended period of time have been shown to be high risk for which of the following complications?
    1. Endometrial cancer.
    2. Gynecomastia.
    3. Renal dysfunction.
    4. Mammary hypertrophy.

71. The nurse is counseling a woman who has been diagnosed with mild osteoporosis. Which of the following lifestyle changes should the nurse recommend? **Select all that apply.**
    1. Eat yellow and orange vegetables.
    2. Go on daily walks.
    3. Stop smoking.
    4. Consume dairy products.
    5. Sleep at least eight hours a night.

72. The nurse should suspect that a client is bulimic when the client exhibits which of the following signs/symptoms?
    1. Significant weight loss and hyperkalemia.
    2. Respiratory acidosis and hypoxemia.
    3. Dental caries and scars on her knuckles.
    4. Hyperglycemia and large urine output.

73. A client has been admitted to the hospital with a diagnosis of bulimia from forced vomiting. Which of the following serum laboratory reports would the nurse expect to see? **Select all that apply.**
    1. Potassium 3.0 mEq/L.
    2. Bicarbonate 30 mmol/L.
    3. Platelet count 450,000 cells/mm^3.
    4. Hemoglobin A$_1$C 9%.
    5. Sodium 150 mEq/L.

74. A client has been admitted to the hospital with a diagnosis of bulimia. Which of the following physical findings would the nurse expect to see?
    1. Mastoiditis.
    2. Hirsutism.
    3. Gynecomastia.
    4. Esophagitis.

75. A school nurse notices that a young woman with scars on the knuckles of her right hand runs to the bathroom each day immediately after eating a high-calorie lunch. Which of the following actions by the nurse is appropriate at this time?
    1. Nothing, because her behavior is normal.
    2. Question the young woman to see if she is being abused.
    3. Recommend that the young woman be seen by her doctor.
    4. Follow the young woman to the bathroom.

76. The clinic nurse is interviewing a client preceding her annual checkup. Which of the following findings would make the nurse suspicious that the client is an anorexic?
    1. Aversion to exercise and food allergies.
    2. Significant weight loss and amenorrhea.
    3. Respiratory distress and thick oral mucus.
    4. Cardiac arrhythmias and anasarca.

77. An 18-year-old client is being evaluated for school soccer by the school nurse. The expected weight for the young woman's height is 120 lb. Her actual weight is 96 lb. The client states that she runs 6 miles every morning and swims 5 miles every afternoon. Which of the following actions should the nurse take at this time?
    1. Ask the client the date of her last menstrual period.
    2. Encourage the client to continue her excellent exercise schedule.
    3. Congratulate the client on her ability to maintain such a good weight.
    4. Advise the client that she will have to stop swimming once soccer starts.

78. A woman is being seen in the gynecology clinic. The nurse notes that the woman has a swollen eye and a bruise on her cheek. Which of the following is an appropriate statement for the nurse to make?
    1. "I am required by law to notify the police department of your injuries."
    2. "Women who are abused often have injuries like yours."
    3. "You must leave your partner before you are injured again."
    4. "It is important that you refrain from doing things that anger your partner."

79. Which of the following questions should be asked of women during all routine medical examinations? **Select all that apply.**
    1. "Has anyone ever forced you to have sex?"
    2. "Are you sexually active?"
    3. "Are you ever afraid to go home?"
    4. "Does anyone you know ever hit you?"
    5. "Have you ever breastfed a child?"

80. The nurse suspects that a client has been physically abused. The woman refuses to report the abuse to the police. Which statement by the client suggests to the nurse that the relationship may be in the "honeymoon phase"?
    1. "My partner said that he will never hurt me again."
    2. "My partner drinks alcohol only on the weekends."
    3. "My partner yells less than he used to."
    4. "My partner has frequent bouts of insomnia."

81. A woman who has been abused for a number of years is finally seeking assistance in leaving her relationship. Identify the actions that the nurse should take at this time. **Select all that apply.**
    1. Comment that the victim could have left long ago.
    2. Assist the victim to develop a safety plan.
    3. Remind the victim that the abuse was not her fault.
    4. Assure the victim that she will receive support for her decision.
    5. Help the victim to contact a domestic violence center.

82. A woman with multiple bruises on her arms and face is seen in the emergency department, accompanied by her partner. When asked about the injuries, the partner states, "She ran into a door." Which of the following actions by the nurse is of highest priority?
    1. Take the woman's vital signs.
    2. Interview the woman in private.
    3. Assess for additional bruising.
    4. Document the location of the bruises.

83. Which of the following behaviors would indicate to a nurse that a gravid woman may be being abused? **Select all that apply.**
    1. Denies that any injuries occurred, even when bruising is visible.
    2. Gives an implausible explanation for any injuries.
    3. Gives the nurse eye contact while answering questions.
    4. Allows her partner to answer the nurse's questions.
    5. Frequently calls to change appointment times.

84. A client is being seen following a sexual assault. A rape examination is being conducted. Which of the following specimens may be collected from the victim during the examination? **Select all that apply.**
    1. Buccal swab for genetic analysis.
    2. Samples of pubic hair.
    3. Toenail scrapings.
    4. Samples of head hair.
    5. Sputum for microbiological analysis.

85. The nurse is conducting a seminar with young adolescent women regarding date rape. Which of the following guidelines are essential to include in the discussion? **Select all that apply.**
    1. The girls should consume drinks from enclosed containers.
    2. The girls should keep extra money in their shoes or bras.
    3. The girls should keep condoms in their pocketbooks.
    4. The girls should meet a new date in a public place.
    5. The girls should go on group dates whenever possible.

86. A young woman in a disheveled state is admitted to the emergency department. She states that she awoke this morning without her underwear on but with no memory of what happened the evening before. She thinks she may have been raped. Which of the following assessments by the nurse is most likely accurate?
    1. The woman is spoiled and is exhibiting attention-seeking behavior.
    2. The woman is experiencing a psychotic break.
    3. The woman regrets having had consensual sex.
    4. The woman unknowingly ingested a date rape drug.

87. A woman has just entered an emergency department after a stranger rape. Which of the following interventions is highest priority at this time?
    1. Create a safe environment.
    2. Offer postcoital contraceptive therapy.
    3. Provide sexually transmitted disease prophylaxis.
    4. Take a thorough health history.

88. The nurse at Victims Assistance Services is speaking with a young woman who states that she was sexually assaulted at a party the evening before. The victim states, "I ran home and took a shower as soon as it happened. I felt so dirty." Which of the following responses should the nurse make first?
    1. "The evidence kit may still reveal important information."
    2. "It was important for you to do that for yourself."
    3. "Have you washed your clothes? If not, we might be able to obtain evidence from them."
    4. "Do you remember what happened? If not, someone may have put a drug in your drink."

89. A young woman was a victim of a sexual assault. After the rape examination was concluded, the client requests to be given emergency contraception (EC). Which of the following information should the nurse teach the client regarding the therapy?
    1. EC is illegal in all 50 states.
    2. The most common side effect of EC is excessive vaginal bleeding.
    3. The same medicine that is used for EC is used to induce abortions.
    4. EC is best when used within 72 hours of contact.

90. A nurse is caring for a client who states that she is a lesbian. Which of the following should the nurse consider when caring for this client?
    1. Lesbian women are usually less sexually active than straight women.
    2. Lesbian women need not be asked about domestic violence issues.
    3. Lesbian women should be tested for cervical cancer every three to seven years.
    4. Lesbian women are at higher risk for bacterial vaginosis than are straight women.

91. The nurse advises the women to whom she is providing health care teaching at a local church that they should see their health care provider to be assessed for ovarian cancer if they experience which of the following signs/symptoms?
    1. Vaginal bleeding and weight loss.
    2. Frequent urination, breast tenderness, and extreme fatigue.
    3. Abdominal pain, bloating, and a constant feeling of fullness.
    4. Hardness on one side of the abdomen.

92. A client states that she has been diagnosed with fibrocystic breast disease. She asks the nurse, "Does that mean that I have breast cancer?" Which of the following statements by the nurse is appropriate at this time?
    1. "I am so sorry. I am sure that the doctor will do everything possible to cure you of the cancer."
    2. "I am not the best person to ask about your diagnosis. I suggest that you ask the doctor."
    3. "If your lumps are round and mobile they are not cancerous, but if they are hard to the touch you probably do have cancer."
    4. "You do not have cancer, but it is especially important for you to have regular mammograms to monitor for any changes."

93. The nurse is educating a group of women on how to perform a breast self-examination (BSE). Which of the following actions should the nurse advise the women to take?
    1. Use the fingertips of their index, middle, and ring fingers.
    2. Use pressure in two intensities, light and deep.
    3. Look for dimpling while bending forward from the waist.
    4. Feel for lumps while encircling the breast from nipple outward.

94. Please draw the pattern that women should use when doing a breast self-examination (BSE).

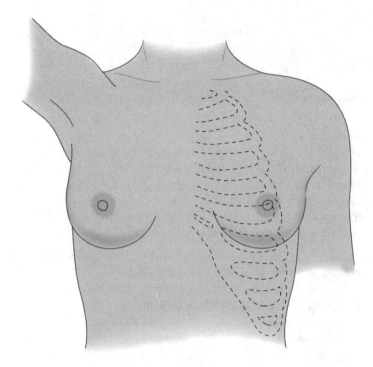

The correct answer number and rationale for why it is the correct answer are given in boldface blue type. Rationales for why the other possible answer options are incorrect also are given, but they are not in boldface type.

1. 1. The child need not be admitted to the hospital.
   2. This assumes that the child has control over the sexual encounter. It is likely that this child is a victim of sexual abuse.
   3. The child's menstrual history is irrelevant. It is possible that she has yet to reach menarche.
   4. **This child must be reported to child protective services.**

   TEST-TAKING TIP: Any time a sexually transmitted disease is discovered in a minor, the nurse has the legal obligation to report the finding to a child protection agency. In addition, if required by law, the health department should also be notified to track and follow up on sexually transmitted infections.

2. 1. The immune globulin is not administered before giving the vaccine.
   2. The vaccine is administered in a series of 3 injections. There are no booster shots being administered at this time.
   3. **To be immunized against hepatitis B, a three-injection vaccine series is administered.**
   4. The vaccine can be administered at any age.

   TEST-TAKING TIP: The current recommendation by the Centers for Disease Control and Prevention (CDC) is that the hepatitis B vaccine series be administered during the neonatal period. For those who have not received the vaccine in infancy, it can be administered at any age. The second and third shots are administered 1 month and 6 months after the first, respectively.

3. 1. Depo-Provera is either administered via intramuscular (150 mg) or subcutaneous (Depo-SubQ Provera, 104 mg) injection every 3 months.
   2. Depo-Provera is a progesterone-based contraceptive. It is safe for use and should not adversely affect the ability to breastfeed.
   3. Both amenorrhea and menorrhagia are side effects of the medication. The client should be advised to notify her health care practitioner regarding any significant menstrual pattern changes.

   4. **Many women who use Depo-Provera for over 2 years have been found to suffer from loss of bone density. Some of the changes in bone density may be irreversible.**

   TEST-TAKING TIP: There is a black box recommendation on the Depo-Provera label. A black box warning is placed on some prescription medications that have been found to have significant side effects. The Food and Drug Administration (FDA) has the power to require pharmaceutical companies to include a black box on a medication that, although approved for use, carries risks when taken. In the case of Depo-Provera, there is an increased risk of osteoporosis.

4. 1. Depo-Provera is either administered via intramuscular (150 mg) or subcutaneous (Depo-SubQ Provera, 104 mg) injection every 3 months.
   2. **The client should use sunscreen while receiving Depo-Provera for birth control.**
   3. The medication is contraindicated for use by women who have breast cancer or who are pregnant. It is not contraindicated for use by those suffering from lung or esophageal cancer.
   4. There is no need to use another contraceptive method. The client should know, however, that Depo-Provera will not protect her from sexually transmitted infections.

   TEST-TAKING TIP: Women can develop dark patches on their skin when using Depo-Provera. The patches often become darker in women who are in the sun without protection. It is strongly recommended that women who use Depo-Provera use sunscreen whenever they are exposed to the sun.

5. 1. IUDs can remain in place for extended periods of time.
   2. The client should expect to menstruate regularly while the IUD is in place.
   3. If dyspareunia occurs, the client should contact her health care practitioner.
   4. **Women who have IUDs in place are at risk of developing pelvic infections.**

   TEST-TAKING TIP: Not only does the IUD not reduce the likelihood of a woman developing a pelvic infection, there are clients who are particularly at high risk for pelvic

inflammatory disease following insertion of an IUD. Women who have multiple sex partners or who have a recent history of a sexually transmitted infection should be considered at high risk for infection. It is recommended that the IUD be placed in these women with caution.

6. 1. A macular rash is not indicative of pubic lice.
   2. Pruritus is, by far, the most common symptom of pubic lice.
   3. Hyperthermia is not commonly seen with an infestation of pubic lice.
   4. Foul-smelling discharge is not commonly seen with an infestation of pubic lice.

TEST-TAKING TIP: Pubic lice, not to be confused with head lice, are commonly called crabs. They are insects, usually sexually transmitted, that invade the pubic hair. Although they are not the same as head lice, the pubic infestation is treated with the same pediculicidal shampoos.

7. 1. Lice are not treated with antibiotics.
   2. Clothing should be washed thoroughly in hot water (at or hotter than 130°F) and dried in a hot dryer for at least 20 minutes.
   3. The over-the-counter shampoo should be applied for 10 minutes and then rinsed off.
   4. To remove the nits, or eggs, the pubic hair should be combed with a fine-tooth nit comb after the shampoo is removed.

TEST-TAKING TIP: Nits are very small, white eggs that are about the size of a period at the end of a sentence. They adhere firmly to the shaft of the pubic hair and take about 1 week to hatch. It is very important, therefore, that the nits be removed with a fine-tooth nit comb to prevent reinfestation.

8. 1. This statement is inappropriate. The hepatitis B vaccine is not administered to prevent all babies from contracting hepatitis B vertically. The majority of babies receive the vaccine to prevent them from contracting the virus in the future. If a pregnant woman is hepatitis B positive, her baby would receive the hepatitis B immune globulin (HBIG), in addition to the vaccine, within 12 hours of delivery. This protocol minimizes the incidence of vertical transmission.
   2. This statement is inappropriate. Vaccines are not administered simply because they are available.

3. This is the best answer. Hepatitis B is a very serious disease that can be transmitted sexually or via contact with blood and blood products. The vaccine is given in infancy to prevent future infections.
4. This response implies that the mother in the scenario is not interested in protecting her child. That is very unlikely.

TEST-TAKING TIP: A number of individuals who contract the hepatitis B virus become long-term carriers of the disease and are able to transmit it to others. They are also at high risk for the development of chronic liver disease and liver cancer (see http://cdc.gov/hepatitis/HBV/index.htm).

9. 1. There was a significant difference between the vaccinated and unvaccinated students in the "read/heard" group—$P < 0.001$.
   2. This is true. The risk ratio for the "Health History form" category is 1.62.
   3. Of those who learned about the vaccine from "Letters," 11.1% were not vaccinated.
   4. The smallest percentage of students in both the vaccinated and unvaccinated groups learned about the vaccine from the UHS providers.

TEST-TAKING TIP: To provide evidence-based nursing, it is very important to be able to read tables and interpret data from scholarly articles. Risk ratios, confidence intervals, and significance data are especially critical and must be understood. It is of interest to note that in the study in question, the health care providers were the poorest source of information about the hepatitis B vaccine.

10. 1. This is true. Relative risk connotes the probability of an experimental event occurring in relation to the control. An $RR = 1$ means that the rate of an experimental event occurring is the same as the rate of the control event occurring. An $RR < 1$ means that the rate of an experimental event occurring is less than the rate of the control event occurring. An $RR > 1$ means that the rate of an experimental event occurring is greater than the rate of the control event occurring.
    2. The values in a 95% confidence interval provide the reader with a range of possible results for the information being given. For example, as in the scenario, although the researchers report the result as one number—0.80—they are 95% confident that the result is between 0.62 and 1.4.

3. An RR of 0.80 means that the rate of an experimental event occurring is only 80% as likely as the likelihood of the control event occurring.
4. This is false. When the RR and CI values are provided for the reader, an interpretation of the data can be made.

TEST-TAKING TIP: Confidence intervals are often reported in relation to relative risk (also called risk ratios) or odds ratios. They also are often reported to interpret raw data. For example, a mean may be reported as 15 with a 95% CI of 10 to 17. The researchers are then stating that the calculated mean is 15 and they are 95% confident that the mean is between 10 and 17. Consulting a statistics text when reading research studies is an excellent practice.

11. 1. Clients with bacterial vaginosis are high risk for preterm labor.
2. Male partners rarely need treatment. Female partners in lesbian relationships may, however, need to be treated.
3. Bacterial vaginosis is characterized by a discharge that is often foul-smelling. The discharge is not related to the therapy.
4. An initial, diagnostic microscopic and culture assessment is done. It is not required that a repeat test be done 2 weeks later.

TEST-TAKING TIP: Bacterial vaginosis is quite common. The problem is characterized by a shift in the bacterial flora of the vagina, resulting in a copious, foul-smelling vaginal discharge. When cultured, the usual findings show a decrease in lactobacilli with an increase in *Gardnerella vaginalis* or other anaerobic bacteria (see http:// cdc.gov/std/BV/STDFact-Bacterial-Vaginosis.htm).

12. 1. Unless the partner is female, the transmission to partners is low.
2. There is no law that requires the nurse to ask these questions.
3. **This statement is true. The change in normal flora increases the woman's susceptibility to other organisms.**
4. There is no need to provide the laboratory with this information.

TEST-TAKING TIP: Once the information regarding the client's history and lifestyle is ascertained, the nurse must provide needed care and teaching. If the client has had multiple partners, other sexually transmitted illnesses (STIs), including HIV, should be considered. The nurse should counsel the client to seek further testing. In addition, the nurse should encourage the client to use contraceptive methods that will protect her from infection as well as pregnancy.

13. 1. Human papillomavirus (HPV) is characterized by flat warts on the vaginal and rectal surfaces.
2. HIV/AIDS is characterized by nonspecific symptoms like weight loss, dry cough, and fatigue.
3. Primary syphilis is characterized by a non-painful lesion, called a chancre.
4. Trichomoniasis is characterized by a yellowish green vaginal discharge that usually has a very strong, offensive odor.

TEST-TAKING TIP: The nurse should be familiar with the primary symptoms of sexually transmitted infections. A woman may confide in the nurse about symptoms that she is experiencing. The nurse must be able to determine when symptoms require medical attention.

14. **2 mL**
The formula for determining the quantity of a medication that must be given is:

$$\frac{\text{Known dosage}}{\text{Known volume}} = \frac{\text{Ordered dosage}}{\text{Needed volume}}$$

$$\frac{1,200,000 \text{ units}}{1 \text{ mL}} = \frac{2,400,000 \text{ units}}{x \text{ mL}}$$

$$12 : 1 = 24 : x$$
$$x = 2$$

TEST-TAKING TIP: The important lesson for the test taker to learn from this example is that math principles do not change simply because numbers are large. Penicillin is ordered in millions of units. That should not frighten the test taker. Simply proceed slowly with each step of the process and the correct result will be found.

15. 1. A diffuse rash with fever should be taken very seriously. These are symptoms of toxic shock syndrome (TSS).
2. Angina is not related to tampon use.
3. Hypertension is not related to tampon use. Hypotension, however, is related.
4. Thrombocytopenia is not related to tampon use.

TEST-TAKING TIP: This client is likely developing TSS. It is associated with the use of superabsorbent tampons. *Staphylococcus aureus*, a bacterium that colonizes the skin, proliferates in the presence of the tampons. Women with the disorder develop a rash, fever, severe vomiting and diarrhea, muscle aches, and chills. The problem must be treated quickly. It is important to note that 5 out of every 100 women who develop TSS will die from the syndrome (see http://cdc.gov/ncidod/dbmd/diseaseinfo/toxicshock_t.htm).

16. 1. PID is not related to endometriosis.
    2. PID is not related to menopause.
    3. PID is not related to ovarian hyperplasia.
    4. PID usually occurs as a result of an ascending sexually transmitted infection.

TEST-TAKING TIP: The most common organisms to cause PID are the organisms that cause gonorrhea and chlamydia. In the early stages of these infections, women often experience only minor symptoms. It is not uncommon, therefore, for the organisms to proliferate and ascend into the uterus and fallopian tubes. The woman must be taught health care practices to decrease her likelihood of a recurrence of the problem (see http://cdc.gov/std/PID/STDFact-PID.htm).

17. 1. The initial infection of herpes simplex 2 is often symptom free but, if symptoms do occur, the client may complain of flu-like symptoms as well as vesicles at the site of the viral invasion.
    2. Metrorrhagia is not associated with herpes simplex 2.
    3. Amenorrhea is not associated with herpes simplex 2.
    4. Abdominal cramping is not associated with herpes simplex 2.

TEST-TAKING TIP: Both herpes simplex 1 and herpes simplex 2 can infect the mucous membranes of the gynecological tract and the oral cavity. The viruses can be transmitted when a vesicle comes in contact with broken skin or mucous membranes. Although outbreaks do resolve, the virus stays dormant in the body and recurrences are often seen during periods of physical and/or emotional stress (see http://cdc.gov/std/Herpes/STDFact-Herpes.htm).

18. 1. Syphilis is caused by the spirochete *Treponema pallidum*. If untreated, syphilis is a three-stage illness. The primary symptom is a pain-free lesion called a chancre.
    2. The primary symptom of herpes simplex is the presence of a cluster of painful vesicles.
    3. Trichomoniasis is characterized by a yellowish green, foul-smelling discharge.
    4. Condylomata are vaginal warts.

TEST-TAKING TIP: Trichomoniasis is a sexually transmitted infection caused by a protozoan. Women who develop the infection during pregnancy may develop preterm labor. Women who are infected with trichomoniasis have an increased risk of contracting HIV if exposed (see http://cdc.gov/std/trichomonas/STDFact-Trichomoniasis.htm).

19. 1. Menstrual cramping is not usually related to sexually transmitted infections.
    2. Heavy menstrual periods are not usually related to sexually transmitted infections.
    3. Flu-like symptoms are not usually related to sexually transmitted infections.
    4. Most commonly, women experience no signs or symptoms when they have contracted a sexually transmitted infection.

TEST-TAKING TIP: Women are usually symptom free when they initially contract gonorrhea or chlamydia. In addition, since the primary infection of syphilis, the chancre, is pain free, women may not realize they have been infected with the spirochete. As a result, it is very important that women, especially those with multiple sex partners, be seen yearly by a gynecologist or nurse practitioner to be tested for STIs.

20. 3 and 4 are correct.
    1. *Gardnerella vaginali* do not cause PID.
    2. *Candida albicans* does not cause PID.
    3. *Chlamydia trachomatis* is a common cause of PID.
    4. *Neisseria gonorrhoeae* is a common cause of PID.
    5. *Treponema pallidum* does not cause PID.

TEST-TAKING TIP: It is important for the test taker to have a working knowledge of pathogens that cause infectious diseases. PID is caused by a bacterium. *Candida* is a yeast, and *Treponema*, the agent that causes syphilis, is a spirochete. The two bacterial organisms listed—*Chlamydia trachomatis* and *Neisseria gonorrhoeae*—are the most common causes of PID. Although *Gardnerella vaginali* is a bacterium, it is not a common cause of PID.

21. 1. This is not appropriate. Instead of reprimanding the client, the nurse should acknowledge how difficult it is to hear the news and continue the discussion.
    2. This is not appropriate. The nurse must pursue the discussion since women often have no symptoms when infected with gonorrhea.
    3. This is true. Women often have no symptoms when infected with gonorrhea.
    4. This is not appropriate. The nurse must pursue the discussion since women often have no symptoms when infected with gonorrhea.

TEST-TAKING TIP: This client is exhibiting signs of denial. The nurse must empathize with the woman regarding the unexpected and unwanted news, but the nurse also must convince the woman to seek care. Giving her the information that many women have no signs of symptoms of disease is essential.

22. 1. A cluster of vesicles is consistent with a diagnosis of herpes, not primary syphilis.
    2. A pain-free lesion, called a chancre, is consistent with a diagnosis of primary syphilis. A reddish brown rash is seen with stage 2 syphilis.
    3. A macular rash is not seen with primary syphilis. A reddish brown rash is seen with stage 2 syphilis.
    4. A foul-smelling discharge is not seen with primary syphilis. It is seen with trichomoniasis.

TEST-TAKING TIP: Syphilis is caused by a spirochete and, like other spirochetal illnesses, has a 3-stage course. The first stage of the disease is the chancre stage. A chancre is a small, round, painless lesion that will disappear, even without treatment, after a month or so. If the client is not treated, the disease will progress to stage 2, during which a reddish brown rash, usually on the palms and soles; sores on the mucous membranes; and flu-like symptoms develop. If the client is still left untreated, the disease will progress to stage 3, the symptoms of

which often appear years later: dementia, paralysis, numbness, and blindness. The damage caused in the tertiary stage of syphilis is not reversible (see http://cdc.gov/std/syphilis/STDFact-Syphilis.htm).

23. 1. Syphilis is treatable. The treatment of choice is penicillin.
    2. Any time someone is infected with one sexually-transmitted infection (STI), it is recommended that he or she be assessed for other STIs.
    3. Cryotherapy is not performed on clients with syphilis.
    4. This is an inappropriate response.

TEST-TAKING TIP: Clients who have become infected with an STI are engaging in risk-taking behavior. Either they or their partners are sexually intimate with at least one other partner. And it is likely that the clients or the partners are not engaging in safe sex. It is important, therefore, that clients who have one disease be further evaluated for the presence of other infections.

24. 1. This is a fallacy. Both men and women can become infected from oral sex.
    2. This is true. The mucous membranes of the female and of the teenager are more permeable to STIs than are the mucous membranes of adults and of men.
    3. The best thing a sexually active man or woman can do is to use a condom—male or female—during intercourse. The only way absolutely to stay disease free is to become celibate.
    4. This is a fallacy. Females are more susceptible to disease than are males.

TEST-TAKING TIP: There are a number of fallacies being communicated among unknowledgeable people. One of the most commonly heard fallacies is that oral sex is safe. It is not. Rather than infecting the reproductive system, the STI will infect the mucous membranes of the mouth. For example, genital warts have been seen in the mouth and throat, and herpes simplex 2 can infect the oral cavity.

25. 1. This is not true. When clients with HIV receive therapy during pregnancy and labor and delivery and their babies receive oral therapy after delivery, the transmission rate of HIV is almost zero.
    2. The viral load and CD4 counts should be monitored regularly but they need not be assessed daily.

3. This is true. She and her partner should use condoms during sexual intercourse.
4. Even though the transmission of HIV via oral sex is likely much lower than it is from genital or rectal intercourse, it is still a dangerous practice.

TEST-TAKING TIP: The human immunodeficiency virus is prone to mutation. It is important that clients use condoms whenever they have intercourse because if the virus mutates and the client becomes infected with two strains of virus, the progression to AIDS is hastened.

26. 1. There are no injections for treating warts. There are gels and creams that can be applied to the warts.
2. This statement is incorrect. Warts usually spontaneously disappear after a period of time.
3. This statement is incorrect. It is a common practice to remove warts surgically.
4. This statement is true. It is not uncommon for warts to return a few months after an initial treatment.

TEST-TAKING TIP: Genital warts are caused by the human papillomavirus. There are more than 100 viral types of HPV. Most of them are harmless, but unfortunately, some high-risk types can cause cancer. Some of the topical treatments for genital warts can be applied at home by the individual or can be administered by a practitioner. Surgery and cryotherapy, also used to treat warts, must be performed by a skilled practitioner (see http://cdc.gov/std/treatment/2010/genital-warts.htm).

27. 1. This is true. The CDC has not approved any tests to detect HPV in men.
2. The CDC has not approved any tests to detect HPV in men.
3. The CDC has not approved any tests to detect HPV in men.
4. The CDC has not approved any tests to detect HPV in men.

TEST-TAKING TIP: Some gay men do have anal Pap smears done to attempt to detect cancer cells in the rectum. This practice is controversial and has not been accepted by the CDC (see http://cdc.gov/std/hpv/STDFact-HPV-and-men.htm).

28. 1. This statement is not true. The vaccine can be administered to women as young as 9 and up to age 26, whether sexually active or not.

2. This statement is not true. The vaccine does not protect against many strains of HPV.
3. This statement is true. There are very few side effects experienced by those who receive the vaccine.
4. This statement is not true.

TEST-TAKING TIP: The CDC Advisory Committee on Immunization Practices recommends that the HPV vaccine—Gardasil—be given to all young men and women between the ages of 11 and 12, or as young as age 9, and up to age 26. There is also a second HPV vaccine on the market, Cervarix. Both Gardasil and Cervarix effectively protect recipients against HPV types 16 and 18—the two types that cause most HPV-related cancers. Only Gardasil®, however, also protects against two additional strains of HPV—types 6 and 11—that cause most cases of genital warts (see http://cdc.gov/vaccines/vpd-vac/hpv/vac-faqs.htm).

29. 1. Men infected with *Chlamydia* often complain of pain on urination.
2. Painful ejaculation is not a common sign of chlamydial infection.
3. Painful erections are not commonly seen when men are infected with *Chlamydia*.
4. It is not common for men infected with *Chlamydia* to experience pain when their testes are touched.

TEST-TAKING TIP: Because chlamydia is usually a silent infection in women, it is often their male partners who are first identified as being infected because they complain of painful urination. Health department practitioners, after being notified of the infection, work to track down the males' contacts so that they can be treated. It is important to note, however, that many men are also symptom free. This is why the disease is so prevalent (see http://cdc.gov/std/chlamydia/STDFact-Chlamydia.htm).

30. 1. This statement is false. Spermicidal creams have been shown actually to increase the transmission of some sexually transmitted infections.
2. This statement is false. Spermicidal creams have been shown actually to increase the transmission of some sexually transmitted infections.
3. This statement is true. Spermicidal creams have been shown actually to increase the transmission of some sexually transmitted infections.

4. This statement is false. Spermicidal creams have not been shown to be cancer-causing agents.

TEST-TAKING TIP: This question is a lesson in changing practice. For many years, it was recommended that men and women always use condoms with spermicide to prevent the spread of STIs, including HIV. It has been shown, however, that latex and polyurethane condoms alone are as effective as condoms with spermicide. In addition, there is evidence to show that spermicides increase the permeability of the mucous membranes to HIV. The test taker must be sure to read the literature to remain current (see Workowski, K.A., & Berman, S.M. [2010]. Sexually transmitted diseases treatment guidelines, 2010. *MMWR, 59*(RR-12), 5–6).

31. 1. Oil- and petroleum-based products can destroy the latex in condoms.
    2. The foreskin should be pulled back before applying the condom.
    3. Before beginning to put the condom on, a reservoir should be created by pinching the end of the condom.
    4. The condom should be removed immediately after ejaculation.

TEST-TAKING TIP: Latex condom use is an excellent means of infection control as well as the prevention of an unwanted pregnancy. This is true, however, only when the condom is applied correctly. In addition to the items noted above, the condom should be applied before any contact between partners has been made, the rim of the condom should be held when removing to keep the semen from spilling, and the male and female condoms should not be used simultaneously because the friction that is caused by the two devices can cause one of them to come off or break (see Workowski & Berman, 2010, pp. 5–6).

32. 1. Female condoms, like male condoms, should be used only once.
    2. Water-based lubricants can be used with female condoms. The same is true of male condoms.
    3. Using both the male and female condom together is not recommended.
    4. The female condom should be removed by twisting the outer ring and pulling gently.

TEST-TAKING TIP: The goal of condom use is to prevent contact of the mucous membranes with sperm and with infectious secretions. The best way to prevent these situations from happening is by enclosing the fluid in the condom as quickly as possible. The male should hold the rim of the male condom while removing the penis from the vagina. Similarly, the female should twist and hold the rim of her condom while removing it from the vagina.

33. 1 and 3 are correct.
    1. Toxic shock syndrome (TSS) is associated with diaphragm use.
    2. TSS is not associated with IUD use.
    3. Toxic shock syndrome (TSS) is associated with contraceptive sponge use.
    4. TSS is not associated with the use of birth control pills.
    5. TSS is not associated with the use of Depo-Provera.

TEST-TAKING TIP: TSS is associated with women who use tampons, especially superabsorbent tampons, and those who use barrier types of contraceptives. It is important, therefore, that anyone who has already experienced an episode of TSS be warned against using those items (see http://cdc.gov/mmwr/preview/mmwrhtml/rr5904a8.htm).

34. 1. The cervical mucus does become thin and elastic at the time of ovulation.
    2. The cervical mucus becomes almost transparent and alkaline at the time of ovulation.
    3. The mucus is leukocyte poor.
    4. The quantity of cervical mucus increases at the time of ovulation.

TEST-TAKING TIP: At the time of ovulation, the cervical mucus is most receptive to the migration of sperm into the uterine cavity. It is thin, slippery, and alkaline, making it most hospitable to the sperm. Women can monitor the consistency of their cervical mucus daily to predict their most fertile periods.

35. 1. The woman should regularly check the diaphragm by looking at it with a good light source.
    2. The diaphragm should not be used during menstruation.
    3. If the diaphragm is left in place for extended periods of time, then the woman is much higher risk for serious complications, especially toxic shock syndrome.

4. The diaphragm should never be powdered because of the possibility of irritation or infection.

TEST-TAKING TIP: The diaphragm is only as good as the barrier that it creates. If there are any holes or breaks in the material, sperm will be able to ascend into the uterine cavity. The woman, therefore, must carefully check for pin-sized holes by regularly examining the diaphragm with a good light source.

36. 1. The woman would abstain from intercourse from day 9 of her menstrual cycle until day 25.
2. The woman would abstain from intercourse from day 9 of her menstrual cycle until day 25.
3. The woman would abstain from intercourse from day 9 of her menstrual cycle until day 25.
4. The woman would abstain from intercourse from day 9 of her menstrual cycle until day 25.

TEST-TAKING TIP: The nurse must be able to advise clients about all types of birth control methods, including natural family planning methods. To calculate the period of abstinence when using the calendar method, the nurse must subtract 18 from the shortest cycle length and 11 from the longest cycle length. The woman must abstain for the entirety of that period to be certain of not becoming pregnant. At least 6 cycle lengths are needed to be able to have some confidence in the method. In the current scenario, therefore, 27 – 18 = 9 and 36 – 11 = 25. The period of abstinence is, therefore, days 9 to 25. As can be seen, women with irregular menstrual periods must abstain for extended periods of time.

37. 1. The diaphragm provides insufficient protection when used without spermicide.
2. It is recommended that women not douche unless medically advised to do so.
3. The diaphragm should be left in place for at least 6 hours after intercourse has ended.
4. The diaphragm should be inserted no earlier than 4 hours before intercourse. If put in place before that time, additional spermicide must be inserted before intercourse begins.

TEST-TAKING TIP: It is important to note that recent evidence has indicated that vaginal spermicides containing nonoxynol-9 (N-9) are not effective in preventing cervical gonorrhea, chlamydial infection, or HIV infection. Although spermicide is not recommended to be used with condoms, diaphragms that are being used for contraception are not effective without the addition of spermicidal gels or creams (see Workowski & Berman, 2010, pp. 5–6).

38. 1. The intrauterine device is an effective contraceptive device, but it will not protect against sexually transmitted infections.
2. The female condom is recommended both for contraception and for infection control.
3. Bilateral tubal ligation is an effective contraceptive method, but it will not protect against sexually transmitted infections.
4. Birth control pills are effective contraceptive methods, but they will not protect against sexually transmitted infections.

TEST-TAKING TIP: The key to answering this question is the fact that the client has multiple sex partners. The client is high risk for becoming pregnant, but as important is also high risk for acquiring a sexually transmitted infection. It is important for the nurse to consider that fact when providing family planning information.

39. 1. When pregnancy occurs with an IUD in place, an ectopic pregnancy should be ruled out.
2. Malformations of the fetus are uncommon.
3. Symptoms of PID are not similar to those of early pregnancy. The most common symptoms of PID are abdominal pain, dyspareunia, foul-smelling vaginal discharge or bleeding, and fever.
4. Twin pregnancies are no more common with a failed IUD than in general.

TEST-TAKING TIP: There are two main reasons pregnancies occurring with an IUD in place are frequently ectopic. First, because the IUD affects the receptivity of the endometrium to the embryo, the fertilized egg often stops its migration and implants in the fallopian tube. Second, sometimes the fallopian tubes become narrowed, preventing the migration of the embryo to the uterine cavity.

40. 1. To obtain the contraceptive patch, the client must obtain a prescription for the device from a health care practitioner.
    2. The withdrawal method (coitus interruptus) is an unreliable method, especially for teenage males.
    3. The female condom is about 95% effective as a contraceptive device and is also effective as an infection-control device.
    4. Although no prescription is needed to use the contraceptive sponge, it is only about 80% effective. In addition, since it uses a spermicide as its means of contraception and infection control, its use may actually be dangerous.

    TEST-TAKING TIP: Adolescents' sex practices are often different from adults'. Teens rarely plan to have intercourse. They "hook up," often having sex on the spur of the moment. It is important, therefore, that they use a method that is immediately effective. In addition, it is not uncommon for adolescents to have more than one sexual partner. Infection control must be a consideration. Female condoms meet both needs.

41. 1. The surgical procedure is not easily reversible.
    2. Menstruation will not cease.
    3. The woman's libido should remain unchanged.
    4. The procedure is usually performed laparoscopically.

    TEST-TAKING TIP: Many men and women have misunderstandings regarding tubal ligations. The surgery merely disrupts the ability of the sperm to travel to the egg to complete fertilization. The fallopian tube is cut, tied, and often cauterized. The ovary and uterus are untouched; therefore, the woman's hormones are unaffected and menstruation does not stop.

42. All choices—1, 2, 3, 4, and 5—are correct.
    1. The woman's age should be considered.
    2. The woman's ethical and moral beliefs should be considered.
    3. The woman's sexual patterns should be considered.
    4. The woman's socioeconomic status should be considered.
    5. The woman's childbearing plans should be considered.

    TEST-TAKING TIP: Each and every one of these factors must be considered when providing family planning counseling. The age of the client will affect, for example, natural family planning, which is not the most appropriate means for young women or for women who are perimenopausal. The woman's beliefs can markedly affect her choices. If the woman has multiple sex partners, an infection-control device should be considered. Some choices are quite expensive and, depending on the client's access to insurance, may not be feasible. If a woman has completed her childbearing, she may wish a permanent form of birth control versus a woman who is young and still interested in having children.

43. 1. This is correct. To maintain the hormonal levels in the bloodstream, the woman should take the pill as soon as she remembers.
    2. This is incorrect. If one pill is missed, it should be taken as soon as possible. If two or more pills are missed, an alternate form of contraception should be used for the remainder of the month.
    3. Breakthrough bleeding can happen at any time, but it rarely happens when one pill is taken a little late.
    4. This is not necessary unless the client is concerned that she may have become pregnant.

    TEST-TAKING TIP: Women who take low-dose birth control pills experience many fewer side effects than women who take high-dose pills. It is important, however, that the pills be taken regularly, ideally at the same time each day. If one pill is missed, it should be taken as soon as possible. If two or more are missed, an alternate form of contraception should be used and the doctor should be questioned regarding whether or not the rest of the pills should be taken (see http://acog.org/~/media/Departments/Adolescent%20Health%20Care/Teen%20Care%20Tool%20Kit/SuggestedResponsesLT2.pdf?dmc=1&ts=20120227T1605503280).

44. 1. Diaphragm is not appropriate. The woman must touch her vagina to insert the device.
    2. Cervical cap is not appropriate. She must touch her vagina to insert the device.
    3. Intrauterine device is effective and the client is in a monogamous relationship, but nulliparous women often complain of cramping and have a relatively high

incidence of spontaneous rejection of the device. Plus, the client will need to palpate for the string after each menses. This requires vaginal manipulation.

4. The birth control pill would be the best choice for this client. She has no medical contraindications to the pill, she wishes to bear children in the future, and it requires no vaginal manipulation.

TEST-TAKING TIP: As in the scenario, the nurse must take multiple factors into consideration before making suggestions about a contraception choice for a client. Because of the number of choices available, the nurse must narrow the choices to those that are best in each situation.

45. 1. The client should palpate for the presence of the string at the external cervical os after each menses.
2. It is not necessary to go on bed rest after an IUD insertion.
3. Reports of dyspareunia should be communicated to the physician.
4. There is no need to insert spermicidal jelly when an IUD is in place.

TEST-TAKING TIP: The sudden onset of dyspareunia can indicate the development of PID. The client should be examined to determine whether or not she has developed an infection.

46. 1. This is true in some states but not in all.
2. There are some states, like New York, that enable adolescents to obtain contraception, including emergency contraception, without a parent's consent. However, that is not true in all states.
3. This is true in some states but not in all.
4. This statement is true. Access to health care by adolescents, including access to birth control methods, is determined by individual states.

TEST-TAKING TIP: It is essential that the nurse knows and understands the rights of clients in his or her state. It is important to note, however, that because the NCLEX-RN® is a national examination, state-specific information will not be asked.

47. 1. This response is inappropriate. The nurse must provide the client with all of her options.
2. This is correct. The nurse should discuss with the young woman all of her possible choices.

3. This response is inappropriate. The nurse must provide the client with all of her options.
4. This is an appropriate follow-up comment. Once the options are provided for the young woman, she may decide to maintain the pregnancy and be in need of assistance to tell her parents. However, it is not appropriate as an initial response.

TEST-TAKING TIP: Unless working in an environment that precludes the nurse from discussing the possibility of an abortion, the nurse is obligated to provide the young woman with all of her choices— maintaining the pregnancy and keeping the baby, maintaining the pregnancy and giving the baby up for adoption, and terminating the pregnancy. If the nurse has a personal bias against abortion, he or she should refer the client to another nurse who will discuss the option.

48. 1. Women who take Seasonale menstruate every 3 months.
2. Seasonale is a daily birth control pill.
3. Women who take Seasonale frequently do experience breakthrough bleeding.
4. Breastfeeding is not compatible with this pill.

TEST-TAKING TIP: Women who wish to breastfeed can take some types of birth control pills (BCPs), but not pills that contain an estrogen medication. Seasonale contains an estrogen. Estrogen inhibits milk production. If they wish to take BCPs, breastfeeding women should take progestin-only pills.

49. 1 and 3 are correct.
1. Women who smoke should be counseled against using the patch.
2. A history of lung cancer is not a contraindication to the patch.
3. Women who have a history of deep venous thrombosis (DVT) should be counseled against using the patch.
4. Being a runner is not a contraindication to the patch.
5. A history of cholecystitis is not a contraindication to the patch.

TEST-TAKING TIP: Women who use the patch are particularly high risk for the development of thrombi. Women with certain medical conditions, such as diabetes or DVT, or with lifestyle issues, like smoking, that place them at high risk for thrombi should be counseled against use of the patch (see http://cdc.gov/mmwr/pdf/rr/rr5904.pdf).

50. 1 and 2 are correct.
    1. The lactational amenorrhea method (LAM) can be effective until 6 months postpartum.
    2. As long as the woman has had no period since delivery, the LAM can be effective.
    3. If the mother gives any supplementation, the LAM is not reliable.
    4. There are no weight loss restrictions when using the LAM.
    5. There are no sleep requirements when using the LAM.

    TEST-TAKING TIP: The LAM is a natural family planning method that is highly effective for postpartum women. However, there are three criteria that must be in place for the method to be effective. (1) The woman must be exclusively breastfeeding her baby. (2) The woman's baby must be less than 6 months old. (3) The woman must not yet have regained her menses after the delivery (see http://waba.org.my/resources/lam/index.htm#LAM).

51. 2, 3, and 4 are correct.
    1. This response indicates that further teaching is needed. Only water-based lubricants should be used with the diaphragm.
    2. This is true. If a woman's weight either increases or decreases by 10 lb or more, the device must be refitted.
    3. This is true. For the diaphragm to fit appropriately, the anterior lip must be pushed snugly under the symphysis.
    4. This is true. Although the device is a type of barrier, it is ineffective without spermicide and the action of spermicide is only effective for 6 hours.
    5. This response indicates that further teaching is needed. The diaphragm should be cleaned with mild soap and water after each use.

    TEST-TAKING TIP: The diaphragm is an excellent device if it is used properly. In addition to the factors cited in the question, the device must be refitted after a client has given birth, it must remain in place for at least 6 hours after intercourse, and, if the couple should decide to engage in intercourse again within the 6-hour period, additional spermicide must be inserted into the vagina before penile penetration.

52. 1. Women who use the diaphragm have increased incidence of urinary tract infections.
    2. Diaphragm may be used with a history of herpes simplex infections, but the device will not protect the woman's partner from contracting the virus.
    3. A woman with a history of DVT can safely use the diaphragm.
    4. Diaphragm may be used with a history of HPV, but the device will not protect the woman's partner from contracting the virus.

    TEST-TAKING TIP: Because the lip of the diaphragm must be inserted under the symphysis, the woman's urethra is sometimes pinched. This makes it difficult to completely empty the bladder when urinating. As a result, the woman is high risk for developing urinary tract infections.

53. 1. The sponge may be inserted any time between 24 hours and a few minutes before intercourse.
    2. The sponge must be moistened with water until it is foamy.
    3. Additional spermicide need not be used.
    4. This is not true. The sponge offers contraceptive protection for up to 24 hours no matter how many times a couple has intercourse.

    TEST-TAKING TIP: Because of its ability to protect a client from becoming pregnant for up to a full day, no matter how many times a couple should have intercourse, the sponge is a very popular method. It must be remembered, however, that the sponge does not protect against sexually transmitted infections and its effectiveness is not as high as the effectiveness of other methods like condoms.

54. 3 and 4 are correct.
    1. This is not true. The man must ejaculate a number of times before his semen will be aspermic. Most urologists assess a man's ejaculate 3 months after the procedure to check for the presence of sperm.
    2. This is not true. Although men are encouraged to rest for at least a day after the procedure, there is no need for them to be on complete bed rest.
    3. This is true. Bleeding into the scrotal sac is a rare complication of vasectomy. Men, therefore, are advised to report any marked swelling to their urologist.

4. This is true. To reduce the pain and swelling, men are encouraged to wear athletic supporters for a few days after the surgery.
5. This is not true. There is no evidence to show that the incidence of prostate cancer is higher in men who have had vasectomies.

TEST-TAKING TIP: A vasectomy procedure is much less invasive than a tubal ligation. A tubal ligation is done in the hospital via laparoscope with the patient under anesthesia, while a vasectomy is done in a physician's office with the patient under local anesthesia. There are few complications associated with the vasectomy: pain at the site and, rarely, infection at the site and/or bleeding into the scrotal sac.

55. 1. This is unnecessary. The client need not measure his urinary output.
    2. This is true. The seminal vesicles and the prostate are untouched.
    3. If he feels comfortable, there is no contraindication to having an erection.
    4. This is not true. There is no need to irrigate the wound.

TEST-TAKING TIP: The vas deferens is ligated during a vasectomy. This will prevent all sperm in the future from migrating from the testes through the vas deferens to the urethra. The blockage is made before the seminal vesicles and prostate, however, so the client will still ejaculate the same amount of fluid.

56. 1. Douching not only is not effective as a contraceptive but also can adversely change the pH in the vagina.
    2. This is not necessary if the man carefully removes the condom.
    3. This is true. The man should carefully remove the condom while holding its edges.
    4. This is not appropriate. While attempting to apply the spermicide, sperm could easily spill from the condom.

TEST-TAKING TIP: The penis becomes flaccid very rapidly after ejaculation. The man should carefully remove the penis from the vagina before the penis becomes flaccid while holding the edges of the condom or, if it does become flaccid, he should be especially careful during its removal.

57. 1. This is true. It is very important that women be evaluated to make sure that the pregnancy is terminated. Even

when bleeding occurs, the pregnancy may still be intact.
2. This is not true. Mifeprex should not be used when an IUD is in place. The IUD should be removed before the medication is administered.
3. This is not true. Women usually complain of cramping, nausea, vomiting, and fatigue. A number of other complaints have also been made.
4. This is unnecessary. If there is no bleeding, she should be seen by the physician for additional treatment.

TEST-TAKING TIP: Mifeprex is available for use for terminating unwanted pregnancies, for completing incomplete spontaneous abortions, and for terminating ectopic pregnancies. If the medicine should be ineffective and the pregnancy survives, there is a strong possibility that the fetus will be damaged. It is very important, therefore, that the client be assessed to make sure that she truly aborted the conceptus (see http://fda.gov/drugs/drugsafety/postmarketdrugsafetyinformationfor patientsandproviders/ucm111323.htm).

58. 1. The male condom is the best device for this client.
    2. Because she has multiple sex partners, the IUD is not the best choice for this client.
    3. The NuvaRing is a hormonal device. Because this client is over 35 years old and is a smoker, the NuvaRing is not the best choice for her.
    4. Oral contraceptives are hormonally based. Because this client is over 35 years old and is a smoker, birth control pills are not the best choice for her.

TEST-TAKING TIP: Even when perimenopausal clients are being counseled, the nurse must ask about drug use, smoking, sexual patterns, and the like. It cannot be assumed that simply because a woman is in her 50s or more that she is asexual or that she is engaging in safe lifestyle choices.

59. 1. This is inappropriate. This client should be seen by her health care practitioner.
    2. This is inappropriate. This client should be seen by her health care practitioner.
    3. This is an appropriate statement. This client should be seen by her health care practitioner.
    4. This is inappropriate. This client should be seen by her health care practitioner.

TEST-TAKING TIP: Clients who use hormonally based contraceptive methods are high risk for clot formation. This client is communicating symptoms that may indicate the presence of a clot. She should be seen by her practitioner to rule out deep vein thrombosis and a possible stroke.

60. 1. This is not appropriate. The basal body temperature (BBT) should be taken upon awakening in the morning.
    2. **The couple should chart temperatures for at least 6 months.**
    3. This is not appropriate. The couple should wait to engage in intercourse until the woman's temperature has been elevated above preovulation baseline for at least 3 days.
    4. An additional action that can be taken as a complement to the temperature rhythm method is cervical mucus assessment, but it is not required. The elasticity of the mucus should be assessed, however, not the color and odor of the mucus.

TEST-TAKING TIP: It is essential that a full 6 months of information be obtained before using the rhythm method as a birth control device. All activities should be recorded on the BBT sheet. For example, the couple should document when the woman has a period, when they have intercourse, when they sleep late, and when the woman feels ill. Each of these situations, and many more, can affect the woman's temperature.

61. 1. This is not true. The menstrual cycle of perimenopausal women is very irregular. It is very difficult to identify safe and unsafe periods for these women.
    2. This is true. This client is a multigravida in a monogamous relationship. She is low risk for infections as well as spontaneous expulsion of the device.
    3. This is true. Even with very irregular menses the client may still be ovulating.
    4. This is true. The patch contains both an estrogen and a progesterone medication.

TEST-TAKING TIP: After providing any kind of teaching, including teaching about contraceptive measures, it is very important to evaluate the client's understanding. A client's misunderstanding could easily result in injury to her or, if she were to become pregnant, to the unborn baby.

62. 1. The fact that the client has two children will not necessarily affect her contraceptive choice. Some couples with two children have completed their childbearing while others wish to have many more children.
    2. The frequency of intercourse is usually not a consideration unless the client has intercourse with a number of partners.
    3. This client's age does not preclude her from using any device. Clients over age 35, especially if they smoke, should not use any of the hormonally based contraceptive methods.
    4. **This statement is very important. If the client refuses to touch her genital area, she is an unlikely candidate for a number of contraceptive devices: female condom, diaphragm, sponge, cervical cap, and IUD.**

TEST-TAKING TIP: It is very important for the nurse to listen very carefully to clients' comments. Many of their statements will influence the nurse's teaching in only minor ways, while other patient comments will dramatically affect the nurse's choices.

63. 1. Although this client has no medical contraindications to using birth control pills, she is having intercourse with a number of partners and, therefore, needs a method that will protect her from infection.
    2. **Of the 4 clients listed, this client is the best candidate for the use of the birth control pill.**
    3. This client has chronic hypertension. She is already high risk for thrombus formation and stroke and birth control pills would increase her risk.
    4. This client is over 35 years old and smokes. She is already high risk for thrombus formation and stroke and the birth control pill would increase her risk.

TEST-TAKING TIP: Birth control pills that contain both estrogen and progesterone are inappropriate for clients who breastfeed because the estrogen inhibits milk production. There is no such contraindication for mothers who bottle feed. It is important to remember, however, that women who breastfeed can use progestin-only pills.

64. 1. The likelihood of this client having multiple sex partners is relatively high. She is not the best candidate for the IUD.

2. This client is in a stable relationship but she has never been pregnant. She is not the best candidate for the IUD.

3. This client is unmarried and has a history of a sexually transmitted infection. She is not the best candidate for the IUD.

4. **This client is in a stable relationship and has had children. She is the best candidate for the IUD.**

TEST-TAKING TIP: This question requires the test taker to use previously learned information. To know facts is not sufficient for the nurse. Nurses must be able to assess the needs of clients in their care and act appropriately.

65. 1. Early-onset menopause is a risk factor for osteoporosis, but not multiparity.
2. Not only does obesity not cause osteoporosis, but some believe that obesity is a protective factor against loss of bone density.
3. Early-onset menopause is a risk factor for osteoporosis.
4. **Alcohol consumption is a contributing factor to osteoporosis.**

TEST-TAKING TIP: Daily consumption of alcohol is a contributing factor to the development of osteoporosis because alcohol interferes with the absorption of vitamin D and calcium in the body. As adequate consumption of the vitamin and mineral is essential for strong bones, alcohol should be consumed in moderation.

66. 1. **This is a true statement. Clients are to take the medication on an empty stomach, immediately after awakening and remain upright for at least 30 minutes.**
2. This statement is incorrect. Clients should take the medication on an empty stomach.
3. Depending on the dosage, the medication is given either once weekly or once daily.
4. This statement is not true. The medication comes in tablet form with no precautions against breaking or crushing.

TEST-TAKING TIP: Fosamax must be consumed with a full glass of water on an empty stomach. It is especially important that the client sit upright for at least 30 minutes after taking the medication because severe upper gastrointestinal irritation can result when reclining. Esophageal irritation, ulceration, and erosions can develop when the medication is taken improperly.

67. 1. **Calcium absorption is enhanced dramatically when vitamin D is also consumed.**
2. Calcium absorption is not directly related to vitamin E consumption.
3. Calcium absorption is not directly related to folic acid consumption.
4. Calcium consumption can inhibit iron absorption.

TEST-TAKING TIP: To maintain proper bone health, it is important for clients, especially women, to consume sufficient quantities of both calcium and vitamin D. The recommended intake of vitamin D per day is from age 1 to 70: 600 IU per day, and after the age of 70: 800 IU per day. The recommended calcium intake per day is for young adult to age 50: 1000 mg per day and after the age of 50: 1200 mg per day (see http://ods.od.nih.gov/factsheets/VitaminD-HealthProfessional/ and http://ods.od.nih.gov/factsheets/Calcium-HealthProfessional/).

68. 1. This is not true. There are situations when hormone replacement therapy (HRT) is recommended.
2. **Women who are experiencing severe menopausal symptoms can benefit from HRT therapy. However, it is recommended that they not be on the medication for an extended period of time.**
3. HRT should not be given to women to prevent or treat coronary artery disease.
4. Women with a history of breast cancer should not take HRT.

TEST-TAKING TIP: Although it was once thought that HRT protected women from coronary artery disease, new evidence shows that is not the case. HRT does help to protect women from osteoporosis, but the incidence of breast cancer in women who take the medication does increase. The recommendation by the FDA is that women who need to take HRT for menopausal symptom relief should do so at the lowest dose possible for the shortest period of time possible. Those who are prone to osteoporosis should use other means—for example, exercise, plus calcium and vitamin D intake—to prevent bone loss (see http://fda.gov/ForConsumers/ByAudience/ForWomen/ucm118624.htm).

69. 1. Fibroids are benign tumors of the myometrium. Douching does not increase the incidence of fibroids.
    2. **Douching can increase a client's potential for endometritis.**
    3. Cervical cancer is almost exclusively caused by the human papillomavirus that is contracted through sexual contact.
    4. Polyps are abnormal tissue growths. They do not develop as a result of douching.

    TEST-TAKING TIP: The act of douching can cause serious gynecological infections up to and including PID. When a woman douches she disrupts the normal flora in her vagina. Pathogens can then invade the area and be pushed upward into the upper gynecological system. Douching should never be performed unless ordered by a health care practitioner.

70. 1. **Women on HRT are high risk for gynecological cancers, especially endometrial and breast cancers.**
    2. Women on HRT are not high risk for gynecomastia.
    3. Women on HRT are not high risk for renal dysfunction.
    4. Women on HRT are not high risk for mammary hypertrophy.

    TEST-TAKING TIP: If the test taker is unaware of the risks associated with HRT, he or she could deduce the correct answer to this question. First, if the test taker is familiar with prefixes and suffixes, he or she would realize that two responses are saying the same thing: "gyne" means "female" and "mastia" means "breast." Gynecomastia usually refers to males who develop breast tissue, but can also refer to women whose breasts are hypertrophied. The test taker, therefore, can easily eliminate choices 2 and 4. Second, since response 1 relates to the gynecological system, it is the logical choice between responses 1 and 3.

71. 2, 3, and 4 are correct.
    1. Yellow and orange vegetables are rich in vitamin A. There is no recommendation to increase one's intake of vitamin A to prevent osteoporosis.
    2. **Daily exercise does help to prevent the development of osteoporosis.**
    3. **Smoking is associated with the development of osteoporosis.**
    4. **Dairy products contain calcium and many have vitamin D added. Both of these nutrients are essential for preventing osteoporosis.**

5. There is no evidence that the lack of sleep is a contributing factor to the development of osteoporosis.

TEST-TAKING TIP: There are a number of factors that clients are unable to control in relation to the development of osteoporosis—for example, sex (women are more at risk than are men), age (older women are more at risk than younger women), and genetics (family history plays a role). Any client who is at risk because of the preceding factors should be especially counseled to eat well, stop smoking, drink in moderation, and get daily exercise.

72. 1. Bulimic clients often experience little fluctuation in weight and are usually hypokalemic.
    2. Bulimia is not related to respiratory acidosis or hypoxemia.
    3. **Dental caries and scars on the knuckles are classic signs of bulimia.**
    4. Hyperglycemia with polyuria is associated with diabetes mellitus.

    TEST-TAKING TIP: Bulimic clients force themselves to vomit. The dentition is adversely affected because of the repeated vomiting. The knuckle scarring, called Russell's sign, develops from tissue injury during the act of jamming the fingers down the throat to force vomiting. Bulimics are also known to take large quantities of cathartics.

73. 1 and 2 are correct.
    1. **The nurse would expect to see a low potassium level.**
    2. **The nurse would expect to see a high bicarbonate level.**
    3. The nurse would not expect to see a high platelet count.
    4. Unless the patient were a diabetic, the nurse would not expect to see a high glycosylated hemoglobin level.
    5. The nurse would not expect to see a high sodium level.

    TEST-TAKING TIP: Because bulimic clients force themselves to vomit, they are losing electrolytes and hydrochloric acid from their stomachs. Because of the low potassium levels, the clients are high risk for cardiac arrhythmias. Their cardiac status should be carefully monitored.

74. 1. Mastoiditis is inflammation of the mastoid bones. This usually results from the progression of a middle ear infection.

2. Hirsutism is characterized by excessive hair growth. Alopecia, or loss of hair, is commonly seen in bulimic clients.
3. Gynecomastia is the hypertrophy of the breast tissue. This is not related to bulimia.
4. Esophagitis is a common finding in people with bulimia.

TEST-TAKING TIP: Because bulimics repeatedly induce themselves to vomit, their esophagi are repeatedly exposed to the acids from the stomach. They, therefore, develop many upper gastrointestinal complications, including esophagitis. Those bulimics who also abuse laxatives may be found to have guaiac-positive stools.

75. 1. The nurse should follow up on her observations.
2. The evidence does not suggest that the young woman is being abused.
3. The nurse should not simply refer the young woman to a doctor.
4. The nurse should follow the young woman into the bathroom to see if she is vomiting.

TEST-TAKING TIP: This young woman is exhibiting classic signs of bulimia: Russell's sign, gorging (eating a calorie-filled meal), and proceeding to the bathroom immediately after eating. It is very likely that the young woman will purge herself of the large meal (by self-induced vomiting). The nurse should then discuss her observations with the young woman and, if appropriate, with her parents.

76. 1. Anorexics commonly engage in excessive exercise regimes.
2. Significant weight loss and amenorrhea are characteristic signs of anorexia.
3. These symptoms are related to severe upper respiratory illnesses, such as cystic fibrosis.
4. Cardiac arrhythmias are more characteristic of bulimia and anasarca is related to congestive heart failure among other illnesses.

TEST-TAKING TIP: The diagnostic criteria for anorexia nervosa are a body weight that is less than 85% of that expected, a pathological fear of gaining weight, a disturbed body image, and the failure to have a menstrual period for 3 or more cycles. Clients, usually women, who are anorexic often are high achievers who also exercise to excess.

77. 1. This is the best response. The school nurse should also note that the client's weight is very low and that her exercise schedule is extreme.
2. This is inappropriate. This young woman is exhibiting clear signs of anorexia nervosa.
3. This is inappropriate. This young woman is exhibiting clear signs of anorexia nervosa.
4. This is inappropriate. This young woman is exhibiting clear signs of anorexia nervosa.

TEST-TAKING TIP: This question requires the test taker to calculate the percentage of the young woman's weight in relation to her expected weight. Once it is noted that she is more than 15% below her expected weight ($120 - 96/120 \times 100 = 20\%$) and that she exercises excessively, the nurse needs to assess whether or not she is exhibiting another sign of anorexia nervosa—namely, amenorrhea.

78. 1. The nurse is not required by law to report the injuries.
2. This is an appropriate statement.
3. The nurse must develop a rapport with the client before accusing the partner of abuse.
4. This statement implies that the partner was justified in abusing the client. This is inappropriate.

TEST-TAKING TIP: Women who are being abused will often deny the abuse. It is not uncommon for abused women to enter the health care system numbers of times before making the decision to terminate the relationship with the abuser. The nurse must discuss his or her observations with the young woman—always in private—and provide the client with possible options at each visit. It is essential that the nurse not ignore the signs, no matter how many times the woman denies that she is being abused.

79. 1, 2, 3, and 4 are correct.
1. This is a question that should be asked at each health care contact.
2. This is a question that should be asked at each health care contact.
3. This is a question that should be asked at each health care contact.
4. This is a question that should be asked at each health care contact.
5. It is not necessary to ask this question every time a female client is seen for a health care visit.

TEST-TAKING TIP: Women (or men) who are being abused rarely discuss their relationships unless asked directly. To identify clients who are being threatened, physically abused, and/or sexually abused, it is essential that nurses query them at each and every visit. The questioning can be done during a face-to-face interview or via a paper and pencil questionnaire. If the client states that he or she is being abused, the nurse should be ready to provide information on safe environments, police contacts, and the like. To be able to provide comprehensive care, the nurse must also know if his or her client is sexually active.

80. 1. This is an example of a comment made during the "honeymoon phase."
    2. Some abusers have set patterns to their behavior, like drinking and abusing only on weekends.
    3. During the "tension-building" phase, abusers often abuse verbally and may even engage in some physical abuse.
    4. Insomnia is not typically part of the "cycle of violence."

TEST-TAKING TIP: The test taker must realize that when an abusive couple first dated, there was love and commitment in the relationship. That love and commitment last well into the time when the relationship becomes violent. In addition, it is important for the test taker to realize that the feelings generated by both parties during the "honeymoon phase"—the period of love and intimacy that immediately follows the abusive phase—revisit that early period of the relationship. It is essential, therefore, for the nurse to develop a rapport with the victim and to remind her that no one deserves to be abused. Options must then be provided to her. Even if she refuses to acknowledge her situation at first, the nurse must revisit the discussion every time the woman revisits the health care system.

81. 2, 3, 4, and 5 are correct.
    1. This is inappropriate. The victim should be praised for making the decision to leave even if it took many years.
    2. It is very important to assist the victim to develop a safety plan. The victim will likely be in danger once the abuser learns that she has decided to leave.
    3. It is very important to remind the victim that the abuse was not her fault.

Many victims believe that they deserve the violence.
    4. It is very important to assure the victim that she will receive support for her decision. It is very scary to decide to break off a relationship, especially if the abuser is the victim's source of financial support.
    5. It is very important to help the victim to contact a domestic violence center. This is a very difficult step for victims to take.

TEST-TAKING TIP: After many years of abuse, victims often have very low self-esteem and are very frightened of their abusers. They need a great deal of emotional support as well as clear, structured guidance in how to leave the relationship. Nurses must be prepared to supply the support (see http://mysistersplacedc.org/).

82. 1. This action is not the highest priority.
    2. This is essential. The client must be interviewed in private.
    3. This action is not the highest priority.
    4. This action is not the highest priority.

TEST-TAKING TIP: This client is exhibiting classic signs of physical abuse. The partner is domineering and the client has injuries that are not supported by the history. To obtain a more accurate history, the nurse must interview the client alone. This can often take place in the women's restroom since, unless this is a lesbian relationship, the partner is unable to follow.

83. 1, 2, 4, and 5 are correct.
    1. Women who skip appointments, delay reporting injuries, or simply do not report injuries should be suspected of being abused.
    2. The history should be assessed very carefully. Often the injuries are not supported by the story.
    3. Victims of abuse frequently refuse to make eye contact with health care practitioners.
    4. Abusers frequently dominate conversations with their victims. When asked questions by the nurse, abusers frequently respond rather than allowing their partners to respond.
    5. Women who frequently skip prenatal or other follow-up appointments must be queried regarding the reason for the absences. There are many possible explanations—for example, they may have no transportation to the site or

they may be forced to remain at home because of visible injuries. A visiting nurse should be sent to the home to determine the reason for the absences.

TEST-TAKING TIP: Nurses must use all their senses when interviewing clients. A physical assessment should be conducted as well as questions asked to check for evidence of abuse. In addition, the client's communications must be critically assessed. Women who always defer to their partners may be exhibiting a sign of abuse. Plus, the history provided by the client and/or her partner must be evaluated for its credibility. If any injuries do not coincide with the story provided, the nurse must investigate the situation further.

84. 1, 2, and 4 are correct.
    1. A buccal swab may be taken. The woman's DNA must be ruled out when compared to any specimens obtained.
    2. Pubic hair samples may be obtained. These are compared with any specimens taken.
    3. Toenail scrapings are not usually obtained, but fingernail scrapings may be.
    4. Head hair samples are obtained. These are compared with any specimens taken.
    5. Sputum is usually not analyzed.

TEST-TAKING TIP: In many ways, a rape examination is another form of invasion for a woman who has been raped. The examiner, only after being given permission by the victim, will take a number of samples, including those mentioned above. Other samples that may be obtained include vaginal smears, any and all clothing worn by the victim, and pictures of any and all injuries. If the perpetrator were to go to trial, it would be far in the future. By that time the victim will no longer have any outward signs of assault. It is important to provide the prosecution with as much evidence as possible if a conviction is to be obtained. It is essential to remember, however, that the victim must be allowed to refuse any examinations (see http://www.rainn.org).

85. 1, 4, and 5 are correct.
    1. It is essential that young women remember to drink liquids only from containers that they have opened themselves and that have never been out of their possession.

2. Although this is a good idea, it will not protect a young woman from a sexual assault.
3. It is an excellent idea for young women to keep condoms in their pocketbook in case they decide, unexpectedly, to engage in consensual sexual intercourse. However, this is not a suggestion that should be given as a protection against sexual assault.
4. Young women should be encouraged to meet new dates in a public place. It is unlikely that an assault will occur in a place where others are present.
5. When a mixed group goes out together, it is unlikely that an assault will take place.

TEST-TAKING TIP: It is very important that young women protect themselves from date rape. Being in a crowd is one excellent way to prevent the potential for being a victim of sexual assault. And because odorless and tasteless date rape drugs—namely, GHB or Rohypnol—can be added to beverages, it is important for young women to consume drinks that have not been out of their sight.

86. 1. It is likely that this woman has been a victim of a sexual assault.
    2. It is likely that this woman has been a victim of a sexual assault.
    3. It is likely that this woman has been a victim of a sexual assault.
    4. It is likely that this woman has been a victim of a sexual assault after ingesting a date rape drug.

TEST-TAKING TIP: Women who have ingested date rape drugs often experience some amnesia afterward. GHB and Rohypnol decrease a woman's ability to resist sexual aggression. The medications can be detected in urine samples up to 72 hours after ingestion (see http://rainn.org/get-information).

87. 1. This woman has just been violated. It is essential that she be in a location where she feels safe.
    2. The young woman should be offered post-coital contraception, but this is not the priority action at this time.
    3. The young woman should be offered sexually transmitted infection prophylaxis, but this is not the priority action at this time.
    4. A health history should be taken, but this is not the priority action at this time.

TEST-TAKING TIP: The initial action the nurse must perform when caring for a client who has just been sexually assaulted is to provide the woman with an environment that enables her to regain a feeling of control. The nurse should ask permission for all care, including history taking. And the care should take place in a secure location. Only after the client has given permission for care should the nurse and other caregivers discuss other issues like history, postcoital contraception, and prophylaxis for infections.

88. 1. This statement should be made only after the nurse has told the client that her actions were appropriate.
2. This statement acknowledges the fact that the client needed to regain some control over her situation.
3. This statement should be made only after the nurse has told the client that her actions were appropriate.
4. This statement should be made only after the nurse has asked the client if it is all right to ask questions about the assault.

TEST-TAKING TIP: A very common response by women to a sexual assault is the need to cleanse their bodies. They frequently state that they feel "dirty." This action does destroy much of the evidence needed if the case were to go to trial, but the nurse must communicate to the client an understanding and acceptance of the young woman's decisions.

89. 1. This statement is not true. EC is available in the United States.
2. This statement is not true. The most common side effects from EC are nausea, vomiting, and headache.
3. This statement is not true. EC medications are essentially high-dose birth control pills.
4. This statement is true. Although EC works up to 5 days after unprotected intercourse, it is most effective when taken within 72 hours of the exposure.

TEST-TAKING TIP: It is essential that the nurse understand the differences between EC and an abortifacient. EC is used to prevent pregnancy after unprotected intercourse. If the woman is unknowingly pregnant at the time she takes EC, she will not abort the fetus. EC is used up to 5 days following exposure while an abortifacient—Mifeprex (misepristone/

misoprostol), formerly known as RU-486—is used to abort a fetus and is used up to 9 weeks' gestation.

90. 1. This statement is incorrect. Lesbian women are neither more nor less sexually active than straight women.
2. This statement is incorrect. Domestic violence can occur in any relationship, straight or gay.
3. This statement is incorrect. Gay women should have Pap tests at the same frequency as straight women.
4. This statement is true, although the precise reason for the high incidence of bacterial vaginosis in gay women is unknown.

TEST-TAKING TIP: Nurses must be prepared to care for clients in every walk of life. The special needs of gay men and women are often ignored by health care workers. When caring for clients, one question that should be asked is the client's sexual preference. Unless the nurse asks the question, important issues may be missed.

91. 1. This statement is incorrect. Although they are not related to ovarian cancer, the symptoms should be assessed by a health care provider.
2. This statement is incorrect. These symptoms are seen in early pregnancy.
3. This statement is correct. Abdominal pain, bloating, and feeling of fullness are early symptoms of ovarian cancer.
4. This statement is incorrect. Although it is not related to ovarian cancer, the symptom should be assessed by a health care provider.

TEST-TAKING TIP: Ovarian cancer is often called the silent killer because it rarely is diagnosed in its early stages. The following signs/symptoms—along with those above—have been identified as early signs of the disease: pelvic pain, abdominal growth, and difficulty eating. Women should be advised to seek care from their health care providers if they experience the symptoms.

92. 1. This response is inappropriate. The woman does not have cancer at this time.
2. This response is inappropriate. The nurse should provide the information requested by the client.
3. This response is inappropriate. Although breast cysts are usually round and mobile,

any nodule felt by a woman should be assessed by a health care practitioner.

4. This response is correct. This client does not have cancer but should be carefully monitored.

TEST-TAKING TIP: Because women who have fibrocystic breast disease have very dense and nodular breasts it is very difficult to detect cancerous lesions by simple palpation. It is very important, therefore, that these women have regular mammograms and ultrasounds and magnetic resonance images (MRIs), if recommended, to monitor for malignant changes.

93. 1. The flat part of the fingers should be used, not the fingertips.
    2. Three pressure depths should be used—light, middle, and deep.
    3. The breasts should be examined visually in four positions, including bent at the waist.
    4. The breast should be examined thoroughly using an up and down pattern.

TEST-TAKING TIP: The test-taker should be familiar with the BSE and be able to teach women how to perform the skill. Clients are then able to take an active role in their own health. In addition, however, it is important for the nurse to advise women that neither the BSE nor a palpation examination performed by a health care practitioner has been shown to increase survival rates in clients with breast cancer. Only mammography has been shown to increase survival rates. Women who are at risk of developing breast cancer should be strongly encouraged, therefore, to have yearly breast mammograms.

94. The figure depicts the pattern that women should use when doing a breast self-examination (BSE) as recommended by the American Cancer Society (see http://cancer.org/docroot/CRI/content/CRI_2_6x_How_to_perform_a_breast_self_exam_5.asp).

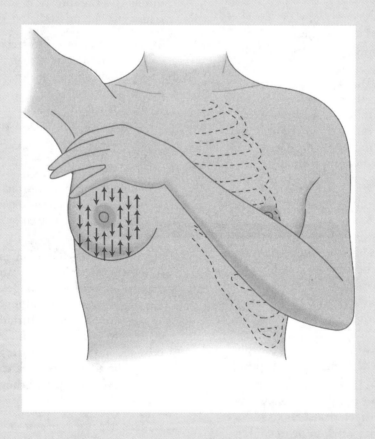

Antepartum

4

Antepartum, or pregnancy, is a 40-week-long period during which the fetus develops inside the uterus of the mother. Because the physiological changes and psychosocial responses that occur during this period tend to be unique during three distinctly different periods of the antepartum, pregnancy has traditionally been divided into three segments, or trimesters. The first trimester, often a period of physical discomfort that includes nausea, vomiting, fatigue, and urinary frequency, is the most important period for fetal development. Indeed, during the first trimester all of the major organ systems of the baby are created. The second trimester is one of physical well-being. The mother feels well, is enthusiastic about eating, and is energetic and happy. The baby, by the middle of the pregnancy, is large enough for the mother to feel movements, and the fetal systems are maturing with each passing day. By the time women enter their third trimester, they are often bothered by discomforts again, including backaches and dyspnea, and, by the time the baby is ready for extrauterine life, mothers are usually more than ready for labor to begin. The nurse must be prepared to counsel, cajole, and inform throughout the antepartum period and even before the pregnancy begins. Indeed, it is especially important for nurses to provide preconception counseling to women so that they enter their pregnancies well, living a healthy lifestyle. Since fetal development begins so early in the pregnancy period, women must plan their pregnancies to make sure they refrain from unhealthy practices when attempting to become pregnant.

KEYWORDS

The following words include vocabulary, nursing/medical terminology, concepts, principles, or information relevant to content specifically addressed in the chapter or associated with topics presented in it. Dictionaries, your nursing textbooks, and medical dictionaries such as *Taber's Cyclopedic Medical Dictionary* are resources that can be used to expand your knowledge and understanding of these words and related information.

ambivalence	embryo
amnion	estrogen
amniotic fluid	fetal development
antepartum	fetus
birth plan	fundal height
blastocyst	fundus
Chadwick's sign	glucose challenge test
chloasma	gravida
chorion	Hegar's sign
chorionic villi	human chorionic gonadotropin
corpus luteum	human placental lactogen
couvade	kyphosis
decidua	lanugo
DHA (docosahexaenoic acid)	lightening
dizygotic twins	linea nigra

Listeria	primigravida
medication pregnancy category	probable signs of pregnancy
melasma	progesterone
monozygotic twins	prostaglandin
Montgomery glands	quickening
morula	spider nevi
mucous plug	striae gravidarum
multigravida	surfactant
nurse midwife	symphysis
organogenesis	teratogen
physiological anemia of pregnancy	trimester
pica	umbilicus
placenta	vegan
positive signs of pregnancy	vernix caseosa
pregnancy	xiphoid process
presumptive signs of pregnancy	

QUESTIONS

1. An antenatal client is informing the nurse of her prenatal signs and symptoms. Which of the following findings would the nurse determine are presumptive signs of pregnancy? **Select all that apply.**
   1. Amenorrhea.
   2. Breast tenderness.
   3. Quickening.
   4. Frequent urination.
   5. Uterine growth.

2. The nurse is assessing the laboratory report of a 40-week gestation client. Which of the following values would the nurse expect to find elevated above prepregnancy levels? **Select all that apply.**
   1. Glucose.
   2. Fibrinogen.
   3. Hematocrit.
   4. Bilirubin.
   5. White blood cells.

3. When analyzing the need for health teaching of a prenatal multigravida, the nurse should ask which of the following questions?
   1. "What are the ages of your children?"
   2. "What is your marital status?"
   3. "Do you ever drink alcohol?"
   4. "Do you have any allergies?"

4. A woman whose prenatal weight was 105 lb weighs 109 lb at her 12-week visit. Which of the following comments by the nurse is appropriate at this time?
   1. "We expect you to gain about 1 lb per week, so your weight is a little low at this time."
   2. "Most women gain no weight during the first trimester, so I would suggest you eat fewer desserts for the next few weeks."
   3. "You entered the pregnancy well underweight, so we should check your diet to make sure you are getting the nutrients you need."
   4. "Your weight gain is exactly what we would expect it to be at this time."

5. Because nausea and vomiting are such common complaints of pregnant women, the nurse provides anticipatory guidance to a 6-week gestation client by telling her to do which of the following?
   1. Avoid eating greasy foods.
   2. Drink orange juice before rising.
   3. Consume 1 teaspoon of nutmeg each morning.
   4. Eat 3 large meals plus a bedtime snack.

6. A client enters the prenatal clinic. She states that she missed her period yesterday and used a home pregnancy test this morning. She states that the results were negative, but "I still think I am pregnant." Which of the following statements would be appropriate for the nurse to make at this time?
   1. "Your period is probably just irregular."
   2. "We could do a blood test to check."
   3. "Home pregnancy test results are very accurate."
   4. "My recommendation would be to repeat the test in one week."

7. A gravida, G1 P0000, is having her first prenatal physical examination. Which of the following assessments should the nurse inform the client that she will have that day? **Select all that apply.**
   1. Pap smear.
   2. Mammogram.
   3. Glucose challenge test.
   4. Biophysical profile.
   5. Complete blood count.

8. The nurse plans to provide anticipatory guidance to a 10-week gravid client who is being seen in the prenatal clinic. Which of the following information should be a priority for the nurse to provide?
   1. Pain management during labor.
   2. Methods to relieve backaches.
   3. Breastfeeding positions.
   4. Characteristics of the newborn.

9. A client asks the nurse what was meant when the physician told her she had a positive Chadwick's sign. Which of the following information about the finding would be appropriate for the nurse to convey at this time?
   1. "It is a purplish stretch mark on your abdomen."
   2. "It means that you are having heart palpitations."
   3. "It is a bluish coloration of your cervix and vagina."
   4. "It means the doctor heard abnormal sounds when you breathed in."

10. A client enters the prenatal clinic. She states that she believes she is pregnant. Which of the following hormone elevations will indicate a high probability that the client is pregnant?
    1. Chorionic gonadotropin.
    2. Oxytocin.
    3. Prolactin.
    4. Luteinizing hormone.

11. A 16-year-old, G1 P0000, is being seen at her 10-week gestation visit. She tells the nurse that she felt the baby move that morning. Which of the following responses by the nurse is appropriate?
    1. "That is very exciting. The baby must be very healthy."
    2. "Would you please describe what you felt for me?"
    3. "That is impossible. The baby is not big enough yet."
    4. "Would you please let me see if I can feel the baby?"

12. A 20-year-old client states that the at-home pregnancy test that she took this morning was positive. Which of the following comments by the nurse is appropriate at this time?
    1. "Congratulations, you and your family must be so happy."
    2. "Have you told the baby's father yet?"
    3. "How do you feel about the results?"
    4. "Please tell me when your last menstrual period was."

13. A client is in the 10th week of her pregnancy. Which of the following symptoms would the nurse expect the client to exhibit? **Select all that apply.**
    1. Backache.
    2. Urinary frequency.
    3. Dyspnea on exertion.
    4. Fatigue.
    5. Diarrhea.

14. The midwife has just palpated the fundal height at the location noted on the picture below. It is likely that the client is how many weeks pregnant?
    1. 12.
    2. 20.
    3. 28.
    4. 36.

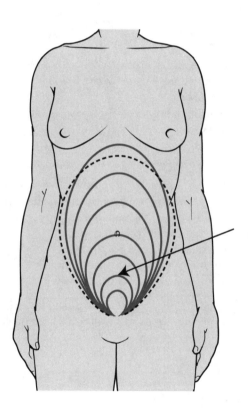

15. When assessing the psychological adjustment of an 8-week gravida, which of the following would the nurse expect to see signs of?
    1. Ambivalence.
    2. Depression.
    3. Anxiety.
    4. Ecstasy.

16. A client makes the following statement after finding out that her pregnancy test is positive, "This is not a good time. I am in college and the baby will be due during final exams!" Which of the following responses by the nurse would be most appropriate at this time?
    1. "I'm absolutely positive that everything will turn out all right."
    2. "I suggest that you e-mail your professors to set up an alternate plan."
    3. "It sounds like you're feeling a little overwhelmed right now."
    4. "You and the baby's father will find a way to get through the pregnancy."

17. The nurse notes each of the following findings in a 10-week gestation client. Which of the findings would enable the nurse to tell the client that she is positively pregnant?
    1. Fetal heart rate via Doppler.
    2. Positive pregnancy test.
    3. Positive Chadwick's sign.
    4. Montgomery gland enlargements.

18. The nurse takes the history of a client, G2 P1001, at her first prenatal visit. Which of the following statements would indicate that the client should be referred to a genetic counselor?
    1. "My first child has cerebral palsy."
    2. "My first child has hypertension."
    3. "My first child has asthma."
    4. "My first child has cystic fibrosis."

19. The nurse has taken a health history on four primigravid clients at their first prenatal visits. It is high priority that which of the clients receives nutrition counseling?
    1. The woman diagnosed with phenylketonuria.
    2. The woman who has Graves' disease.
    3. The woman with Cushing's syndrome.
    4. The woman diagnosed with myasthenia gravis.

20. Which of the following findings in an 8-week gestation client, G2 P1001, should the nurse highlight for the nurse midwife? **Select all that apply.**
    1. Body mass index of 17 kg/ mm^2.
    2. Rubella titer of 1:8.
    3. Blood pressure of 100/60 mm Hg.
    4. Hematocrit of 30%.
    5. Hemoglobin of 13.2 g/dL.

21. A woman, 6 weeks pregnant, is having a vaginal examination. Which of the following would the practitioner expect to find?
    1. Thin cervical muscle.
    2. An enlarged ovary.
    3. Thick cervical mucus.
    4. Pale pink vaginal wall.

22. A pregnant woman must have a glucose challenge test (GCT). Which of the following should be included in the preprocedure teaching?
    1. Fast for 12 hours before the test.
    2. Bring a urine specimen to the laboratory on the day of the test.
    3. Be prepared to have 4 blood specimens taken on the day of the test.
    4. The test should take one hour to complete.

23. The nurse working in an outpatient obstetric office assesses four primigravid clients. Which of the client findings should the nurse highlight for the physician? **Select all that apply.**
    1. 17 weeks' gestation; denies feeling fetal movement.
    2. 24 weeks' gestation; fundal height at the umbilicus.
    3. 27 weeks' gestation; salivates excessively.
    4. 34 weeks' gestation; experiences uterine cramping.
    5. 37 weeks' gestation; complains of hemorrhoidal pain.

24. The following four changes occur during pregnancy. Which of them usually increases the father's interest and involvement in the pregnancy?
    1. Learning the results of the pregnancy test.
    2. Attending childbirth education classes.
    3. Hearing the fetal heartbeat.
    4. Meeting the obstetrician or midwife.

25. The nurse midwife tells a client that the baby is growing and that ballottement was evident during the vaginal examination. How should the nurse explain what the nurse midwife means by ballottement?
    1. The nurse midwife saw that the mucous plug was intact.
    2. The nurse midwife felt the baby rebound after being pushed.
    3. The nurse midwife palpated the fetal parts through the uterine wall.
    4. The nurse midwife assessed that the baby is head down.

26. A multigravid client is 22 weeks pregnant. Which of the following symptoms would the nurse expect the client to exhibit?
    1. Nausea.
    2. Dyspnea.
    3. Urinary frequency.
    4. Leg cramping.

27. The glucose challenge screening test is performed at or after 24 weeks' gestation to assess for the maternal physiological response to which of the following pregnancy hormones?
    1. Estrogen.
    2. Progesterone.
    3. Human placental lactogen.
    4. Human chorionic gonadotropin.

28. A client is 15 weeks pregnant. She calls the obstetric office to request a medication for a headache. The nurse answers the telephone. Which of the following is the nurse's best response?
    1. "Because the organ systems in the baby are developing right now, it is risky to take medicine."
    2. "You can take any of the over-the-counter medications because they are all safe in pregnancy."
    3. "The physician will prescribe a category 'X' medication for you."
    4. "You can take acetaminophen because it is a category 'B' medicine."

29. A 20-week gestation client is being seen in the prenatal clinic. Place an "X" on the place on the abdomen where the nurse would expect the fundal height to be felt.

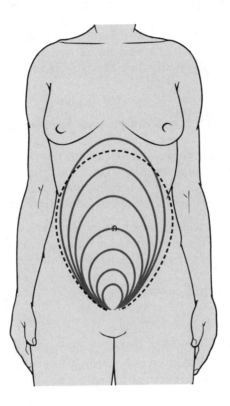

30. A client who was seen in the prenatal clinic at 20 weeks' gestation weighed 128 lb at that time. Approximately how many pounds would the nurse expect the client to weigh at her next visit at 24 weeks' gestation?
    1. 129 to 130 lb.
    2. 131 to 132 lb.
    3. 133 to 134 lb.
    4. 135 to 136 lb.

31. An 18-week gestation client telephones the obstetrician's office stating, "I'm really scared. I think I have breast cancer. My breasts are filled with tumors." The nurse should base the response on which of the following?
    1. Breast cancer is often triggered by pregnancy.
    2. Nodular breast tissue is normal during pregnancy.
    3. The woman is exhibiting signs of a psychotic break.
    4. Anxiety attacks are especially common in the second trimester.

32. A woman states that she frequently awakens with "painful leg cramps" during the night. Which of the following assessments should the nurse make?
    1. Dietary evaluation.
    2. Goodell's sign.
    3. Hegar's sign.
    4. Posture evaluation.

33. Which of the following exercises should be taught to a pregnant woman who complains of backaches?
    1. Kegeling.
    2. Pelvic tilting.
    3. Leg lifting.
    4. Crunching.

34. A woman in her third trimester advises the nurse that she wishes to breastfeed her baby, "but I don't think my nipples are right." Upon examination, the nurse notes that the client has inverted nipples. Which of the following actions should the nurse take at this time?
    1. Advise the client that it is unlikely that she will be able to breastfeed.
    2. Refer the client to a lactation consultant for advice.
    3. Call the labor room and notify them that a client with inverted nipples will be admitted.
    4. Teach the woman exercises to evert her nipples.

35. Which of the following vital sign changes should the nurse highlight for a pregnant woman's obstetrician?
    1. Prepregnancy blood pressure (BP) 100/60 and third trimester BP 140/90.
    2. Prepregnancy respiratory rate (RR) 16 rpm and third trimester RR 22 rpm.
    3. Prepregnancy heart rate (HR) 76 bpm and third trimester HR 88 bpm.
    4. Prepregnancy temperature (T) 98.6°F and third trimester T 99.2°F.

36. A nurse midwife has advised a 39-week gestation gravid to take evening primrose oil 2,500 mg daily as a complementary therapy. This suggestion was made because evening primrose has been shown to perform which of the following actions?
    1. Relieve back strain.
    2. Improve development of colostrum.
    3. Ripen the cervix.
    4. Reduce the incidence of hemorrhoids.

37. A 38-week gestation client, Bishop score 1, is advised by her nurse midwife to take evening primrose daily. The office nurse advises the client to report which of the following side effects that has been attributed to the oil?
    1. Diarrhea.
    2. Pedal edema.
    3. Blurred vision.
    4. Tinnitus.

38. A 37-week gravid client states that she noticed a "white liquid" leaking from her breasts during a recent shower. Which of the following nursing responses is appropriate at this time?
    1. Advise the woman that she may have a galactocele.
    2. Encourage the woman to pump her breasts to stimulate an adequate milk supply.
    3. Assess the liquid because a breast discharge is diagnostic of a mammary infection.
    4. Reassure the mother that this is normal in the third trimester.

39. A 36-week gestation gravid client is complaining of dyspnea when lying flat. Which of the following is the likely clinical reason for this complaint?
    1. Maternal hypertension.
    2. Fundal height.
    3. Hydramnios.
    4. Congestive heart failure.

40. The nurse is providing anticipatory guidance to a woman in her second trimester regarding signs/symptoms that are within normal limits during the latter half of the pregnancy. Which of the following comments by the client indicates that teaching was successful? **Select all that apply.**
    1. "During the third trimester I may experience frequent urination."
    2. "During the third trimester I may experience heartburn."
    3. "During the third trimester I may experience nagging backaches."
    4. "During the third trimester I may experience persistent headache."
    5. "During the third trimester I may experience blurred vision."

41. A client, in her third trimester, is concerned that she will not know the difference between labor contractions and normal aches and pains of pregnancy. How should the nurse respond?
    1. "Don't worry. You'll know the difference when the contractions start."
    2. "The contractions may feel just like a backache, but they will come and go."
    3. "Contractions are a lot worse than your pregnancy aches and pains."
    4. "I understand. You don't want to come to the hospital before you are in labor."

42. Which finding would the nurse view as normal when evaluating the laboratory reports of a 34-week gestation client?
    1. Anemia.
    2. Thrombocytopenia.
    3. Polycythemia.
    4. Hyperbilirubinemia.

43. The nurse asks a 31-week gestation client to lie on the examining table during a prenatal examination. In which of the following positions should the client be placed?
    1. Orthopneic.
    2. Lateral-recumbent.
    3. Sims'.
    4. Semi-Fowler's.

44. A third-trimester client is being seen for routine prenatal care. Which of the following assessments will the nurse perform during the visit? **Select all that apply.**
    1. Blood glucose.
    2. Blood pressure.
    3. Fetal heart rate.
    4. Urine protein.
    5. Pelvic ultrasound.

45. A nurse is working in the prenatal clinic. Which of the following findings seen in third-trimester pregnant women would the nurse consider to be within normal limits? **Select all that apply.**
    1. Leg cramps.
    2. Varicose veins.
    3. Hemorrhoids.
    4. Fainting spells.
    5. Lordosis.

46. A 36-week gestation gravid lies flat on her back. Which of the following maternal signs/symptoms would the nurse expect to observe?
    1. Hypertension.
    2. Dizziness.
    3. Rales.
    4. Chloasma.

47. The nurse is interviewing a 38-week gestation Muslim woman. Which of the following questions would be inappropriate for the nurse to ask?
    1. "Do you plan to breastfeed your baby?"
    2. "What do you plan to name the baby?"
    3. "Which pediatrician do you plan to use?"
    4. "How do you feel about having an episiotomy?"

48. A woman is 36 weeks' gestation. Which of the following tests will be done during her prenatal visit?
    1. Glucose challenge test.
    2. Amniotic fluid volume assessment.
    3. Vaginal and rectal cultures.
    4. Karyotype analysis.

49. A 34-week gestation woman calls the obstetric office stating, "Since last night I have had three nosebleeds." Which of the following responses by the nurse is appropriate?
    1. "You should see the doctor to make sure you are not becoming severely anemic."
    2. "Do you have a temperature?"
    3. "One of the hormones of pregnancy makes the nasal passages prone to bleeds."
    4. "Do you use any inhaled drugs?"

50. The nurse asks a woman about how the woman's husband is dealing with the pregnancy. The nurse concludes that counseling is needed when the woman makes which of the following statements?
    1. "My husband is ready for the pregnancy to end so that we can have sex again."
    2. "My husband has gained quite a bit of weight during this pregnancy."
    3. "My husband seems more worried about our finances now than before the pregnancy."
    4. "My husband plays his favorite music for my belly so the baby will learn to like it."

51. The blood of a pregnant client was initially assessed at 10 weeks' gestation and reassessed at 38 weeks' gestation. Which of the following results would the nurse expect to see?
    1. Rise in hematocrit from 34% to 38%.
    2. Rise in white blood cells from 5,000 cells/mm³ to 15,000 cells/mm³.
    3. Rise in potassium from 3.9 mEq/L to 5.2 mEq/L.
    4. Rise in sodium from 137 mEq/L to 150 mEq/L.

52. A client is 35 weeks' gestation. Which of the following findings would the nurse expect to see?
    1. Nausea and vomiting.
    2. Maternal ambivalence.
    3. Fundal height 10 cm above the umbilicus.
    4. Use of three pillows for sleep comfort.

53. A woman, 26-weeks' gestation, calls the triage nurse stating, "I'm really scared. I tried not to but I had an orgasm when we were making love. I just know that I will go into preterm labor now." Which of the following responses by the nurse is appropriate?
    1. "Lie down and drink a quart of water. If you feel any back pressure at all call me back right away."
    2. "Although oxytocin was responsible for your orgasm, it is very unlikely that it will stimulate preterm labor."
    3. "I will inform the doctor for you. What I want you to do is to come to the hospital right now to be checked."
    4. "The best thing for you to do right now is to take a warm shower, and then do a fetal kick count assessment."

54. A couple is preparing to interview obstetric primary care providers to determine who they will go to for care during their pregnancy and delivery. To make the best choice, which of the following actions should the couple perform first?
    1. Take a tour of hospital delivery areas.
    2. Develop a preliminary birth plan.
    3. Make appointments with three or four obstetric care providers.
    4. Search the Internet for the malpractice histories of the providers.

55. During a preconception counseling session, the nurse encourages a couple to prepare a birth plan. Which of the following is the most important goal for this action?
    1. Promote communication between the couple and health care professionals.
    2. Enable the couple to learn about the types of pain medicine used in labor.
    3. Provide the couple with a list of items that they should take to the hospital for the labor and delivery.
    4. Give the high-risk couple a sense of control over the likelihood of having a surgical delivery.

56. The nurse is assisting a couple to develop decisions for their birth plan. Which of the following decisions should be considered nonnegotiable by the parents?
    1. Whether or not the father will be present during labor.
    2. Whether or not the woman will have an episiotomy.
    3. Whether or not the woman will be able to have an epidural.
    4. Whether or not the father will be able to take pictures of the delivery.

57. During a prenatal visit, a gravid client is complaining of ptyalism. Which of the following nursing interventions is appropriate?
    1. Encourage the woman to brush her teeth carefully.
    2. Advise the woman to have her blood pressure checked regularly.
    3. Encourage the woman to wear supportive hosiery.
    4. Advise the woman to avoid eating rare meat.

58. A gravid woman who recently emigrated from mainland China is being seen at her first prenatal visit. She was never vaccinated in her home country. An injection to prevent which of the following communicable diseases should be administered to the woman during her pregnancy?
    1. Influenza.
    2. Mumps.
    3. Rubella.
    4. Varicella.

59. A gravid woman and her husband inform the nurse that they have just moved into a three-story home that was built in the 1930s. Which of the following is critical for the nurse to advise the woman to protect the unborn child?
    1. Stay out of any rooms that are being renovated.
    2. Drink water only from the hot water tap.
    3. Refrain from entering the basement.
    4. Climb the stairs only once per day.

60. After nutrition counseling, a woman, G3 P1101, proclaims that she certainly can't eat any strawberries during her pregnancy. Which of the following is the likely reason for this statement?
    1. The woman is allergic to strawberries.
    2. Strawberries have been shown to cause birth defects.
    3. The woman believes in old wives' tales.
    4. The premature baby died because the woman ate strawberries.

61. A woman is planning to become pregnant. Which of the following actions should she be counseled to take before stopping birth control? **Select all that apply.**
    1. Take a daily multivitamin.
    2. See a medical doctor.
    3. Drink beer instead of vodka.
    4. Stop all over-the-counter medications.
    5. Stop smoking cigarettes.

62. The nurse discusses sexual intimacy with a pregnant couple. Which of the following should be included in the teaching plan?
    1. Vaginal intercourse should cease by the beginning of the third trimester.
    2. Breast fondling should be discouraged because of the potential for preterm labor.
    3. The couple may find it necessary to experiment with alternate positions.
    4. Vaginal lubricant should be used sparingly throughout the pregnancy.

63. Which of the following skin changes should the nurse highlight for a pregnant woman's health care practitioner?
    1. Linea nigra.
    2. Melasma.
    3. Petechiae.
    4. Spider nevi.

64. A pregnant woman informs the nurse that her last normal menstrual period was on September 20, 2012. Using Nagele's rule, the nurse calculates the client's estimated date of delivery as:
    1. May 30, 2013.
    2. June 20, 2013.
    3. June 27, 2013.
    4. July 3, 2013.

65. A father experiencing couvade syndrome is likely to exhibit which of the following symptoms/behaviors? **Select all that apply.**
    1. Heartburn.
    2. Promiscuity.
    3. Hypertension.
    4. Bloating.
    5. Abdominal pain.

66. A nurse is advising a pregnant woman about the danger signs of pregnancy. The nurse should teach the mother that she should notify the physician immediately if she experiences which of the following signs/symptoms? **Select all that apply.**
    1. Convulsions.
    2. Double vision.
    3. Epigastric pain.
    4. Persistent vomiting.
    5. Polyuria.

67. A woman provides the nurse with the following obstetrical history: Delivered a son, now 7 years old, at 28 weeks' gestation; delivered a daughter, now 5 years old, at 39 weeks' gestation; had a miscarriage 3 years ago, and had a first-trimester abortion 2 years ago. She is currently pregnant. Which of the following portrays an accurate picture of this woman's gravidity and parity?
    1. G4 P2121.
    2. G4 P1212.
    3. G5 P1122.
    4. G5 P2211.

68. The partner of a gravida accompanies her to her prenatal appointment. The nurse notes that the father of the baby has gained weight since she last saw him. Which of the following comments is most appropriate for the nurse to make to the father?
    1. "I see that you are gaining weight right along with your partner."
    2. "You and your partner will be able to go on a diet together after the baby is born."
    3. "I can see that you are a bad influence on your partner's eating habits."
    4. "I am so glad to see that you are taking so much interest in your partner's pregnancy."

69. The nurse is caring for a pregnant client who is a vegan. Which of the following foods should the nurse suggest the client consume as substitutes for restricted foods?
    1. Tofu, legumes, broccoli.
    2. Corn, yams, green beans.
    3. Potatoes, parsnips, turnips.
    4. Cheese, yogurt, fish.

70. When assessing the fruit intake of a pregnant client, the nurse notes that the client usually eats 1 piece of fruit per day and drinks a 12 oz glass of fruit juice per day. Which of the following is the most important communication for the nurse to make?
    1. "You are effectively meeting your daily fruit requirements."
    2. "Fruit juices are excellent sources of folic acid."
    3. "It would be even better if you were to consume more whole fruits and less fruit juice."
    4. "Your fruit intake far exceeds the recommended daily fruit intake."

71. A client states that she is a strong believer in vitamin supplements to maintain her health. The nurse advises the woman that it is recommended to refrain from consuming excess quantities of which of the following vitamins during pregnancy?
    1. Vitamin C.
    2. Vitamin D.
    3. Vitamin B_2 (niacin).
    4. Vitamin B_{12} (cobalamin).

72. A vegan is being counseled regarding vitamin intake. It is essential that this woman supplement which of the following B vitamins?
    1. B_1 (thiamine).
    2. B_2 (niacin).
    3. B_6 (pyridoxine).
    4. B_{12} (cobalamin).

73. A client informs the nurse that she is "very constipated." Which of the following foods would be best for the nurse to recommend to the client?
    1. Pasta.
    2. Rice.
    3. Yogurt.
    4. Celery.

74. A pregnant client is lactose intolerant. Which of the following foods could this woman consume to meet her calcium needs?
    1. Turnip greens.
    2. Green beans.
    3. Cantaloupe.
    4. Nectarines.

75. A nurse, who is providing nutrition counseling to a new gravid client, advises the woman that a serving of meat is approximately equal in size to which of the following items?
    1. Deck of cards.
    2. Paperback book.
    3. Clenched fist.
    4. Large tomato.

76. The nurse is evaluating the 24-hour dairy intake of four gravid clients. Which of the following clients consumed the highest number of dairy servings during 1 day? The client who consumed:
    1. 4 oz whole milk, 2 oz hard cheese, 1 cup of pudding made with milk and 2 oz cream cheese.
    2. 1 cup yogurt, 8 oz chocolate milk, 1 cup cottage cheese, and 1½ oz hard cheese.
    3. 1 cup cottage cheese, 8 oz whole milk, 1 cup buttermilk, and ½ oz hard cheese.
    4. ½ cup frozen yogurt, 8 oz skim milk, 4 oz cream cheese, and 1½ cup cottage cheese.

77. Which of the following choices can the nurse teach a prenatal client is equivalent to one 2 oz protein serving?
    1. 4 tbsp peanut butter.
    2. 2 eggs.
    3. 1 cup cooked lima beans.
    4. 2 ounces mixed nuts.

78. A nurse is discussing the serving sizes in the grain food group with a new prenatal client. Which of the following foods equals 1 ounce serving size from the grain group? **Select all that apply.**
    1. 1 bagel.
    2. 1 slice of bread.
    3. 1 cup cooked pasta.
    4. 1 tortilla.
    5. 1 cup dry cereal.

79. A woman asks the nurse about consuming herbal supplements during pregnancy. Which of the following responses is appropriate?
    1. Herbals are natural substances, so they are safely ingested during pregnancy.
    2. It is safe to take licorice and cat's claw, but no other herbs are safe.
    3. A federal commission has established the safety of herbals during pregnancy.
    4. The woman should discuss everything she eats with a health care practitioner.

80. A Chinese immigrant is being seen in the prenatal clinic. When providing nutrition counseling, which of the following factors should the nurse keep in mind?
    1. Many Chinese eat very little protein.
    2. Many Chinese believe pregnant women should eat cold foods.
    3. Many Chinese are prone to anemia.
    4. Many Chinese believe strawberries can cause birth defects.

81. A nurse has identified the following nursing diagnosis for a prenatal client: Altered nutrition: less than body requirements related to poor folic acid intake. Which of the following foods should the nurse suggest the client consume?
    1. Potatoes and grapes.
    2. Cranberries and squash.
    3. Apples and corn.
    4. Oranges and spinach.

82. A nurse is discussing diet with a pregnant woman. Which of the following foods should the nurse advise the client to avoid consuming during her pregnancy?
    1. Bologna.
    2. Cantaloupe.
    3. Asparagus.
    4. Popcorn.

83. A 12-week gestation client tells the nurse that she and her husband eat sushi at least once per week. She states, "I know that fish is good for me, so I make sure we eat it regularly." Which of the following responses by the nurse is appropriate?
    1. "You are correct. Fish is very healthy for you."
    2. "You can eat fish, but sushi is too salty to eat during pregnancy."
    3. "Sushi is raw. Raw fish is especially high in mercury."
    4. "It is recommended that fish be cooked to destroy harmful bacteria."

84. The nurse is caring for a prenatal client who states she is prone to developing anemia. Which of the following foods should the nurse advise the gravida is the best source of iron?
    1. Raisins.
    2. Hamburger.
    3. Broccoli.
    4. Molasses.

85. It is discovered that a pregnant woman practices pica. Which of the following complications is most often associated with this behavior?
    1. Hypothyroidism.
    2. Iron-deficiency anemia.
    3. Hypercalcemia.
    4. Overexposure to zinc.

86. A woman confides in the nurse that she practices pica. Which of the following alternatives could the nurse suggest to the woman?
    1. Replace laundry starch with salt.
    2. Replace ice with frozen fruit juice.
    3. Replace soap with cream cheese.
    4. Replace soil with uncooked pie crust.

87. A mother is experiencing nausea and vomiting every afternoon. The ingestion of which of the following spices has been shown to be a safe complementary therapy for this complaint?
   1. Ginger.
   2. Sage.
   3. Cloves.
   4. Nutmeg.

88. A woman tells the nurse that she would like suggestions for alternate vitamin C sources because she isn't very fond of citrus fruits. Which of the following suggestions is appropriate?
   1. Barley and brown rice.
   2. Strawberries and potatoes.
   3. Buckwheat and lentils.
   4. Wheat flour and figs.

89. A nurse is providing diet counseling to a new prenatal client. Which of the following dairy products should the client be advised to avoid eating during the pregnancy?
   1. Vanilla yogurt.
   2. Parmesan cheese.
   3. Gorgonzola cheese.
   4. Chocolate milk.

90. A woman asks the nurse about the function of amniotic fluid. Which of the following statements by the woman indicates that the teaching was successful? **Select all that apply.**
   1. The fluid provides fetal nutrition.
   2. The fluid cushions the fetus from injury.
   3. The fluid enables the fetus to grow.
   4. The fluid provides the fetus with a stable thermal environment.
   5. The fluid enables the fetus to practice swallowing.

91. Why is it essential that women of childbearing age be counseled to plan their pregnancies?
   1. Much of the organogenesis occurs before the missed menstrual period.
   2. Insurance companies must preapprove many prenatal care expenditures.
   3. It is recommended that women be pregnant no more than 3 times during their lifetime.
   4. The cardiovascular system is stressed when pregnancies are less than 2 years apart.

92. A woman has just completed her first trimester. Which of the following fetal structures can the nurse tell the woman are well formed at this time? **Select all that apply.**
   1. Genitals.
   2. Heart.
   3. Fingers.
   4. Alveoli.
   5. Kidneys.

93. An ultrasound of a fetus's heart shows that normal fetal circulation is occurring. Which of the following statements should the nurse interpret as correct in relation to the fetal circulation?
   1. The foramen ovale is a hole between the ventricles.
   2. The umbilical vein contains oxygen-poor blood.
   3. The right atrium contains both oxygen-rich and oxygen-poor blood.
   4. The ductus venosus lies between the aorta and pulmonary artery.

94. The nurse is teaching a couple about fetal development. Which statement by the nurse is correct about the morula stage of development?
   1. "The fertilized egg has yet to implant into the uterus."
   2. "The lung fields are finally completely formed."
   3. "The sex of the fetus can be clearly identified."
   4. "The eyelids are unfused and begin to open and close."

95. A woman is carrying dizygotic twins. She asks the nurse about the babies. Which of the following explanations is accurate?
    1. During a period of rapid growth, the fertilized egg divided completely.
    2. When the woman ovulated, she expelled two mature ova.
    3. The babies share one placenta and a common chorion.
    4. The babies will definitely be the same sex and have the same blood type.

96. A mother has just experienced quickening. Which of the following developmental changes would the nurse expect to occur at the same time in the woman's pregnancy?
    1. Fetal heart begins to beat.
    2. Lanugo covers the fetal body.
    3. Kidneys secrete urine.
    4. Fingernails begin to form.

97. A woman who is seen in the prenatal clinic is found to be 8 weeks pregnant. She confides to the nurse that she is afraid her baby may be "permanently damaged because I had at least 5 beers the night I had sex." Which of the following responses by the nurse would be appropriate?
    1. "I would let the doctor know that if I were you."
    2. "It is unlikely that the baby was affected."
    3. "Abortions during the first trimester are very safe."
    4. "An ultrasound will tell you if the baby was affected."

98. A gravida's fundal height is noted to be at the xiphoid process. The nurse is aware that which of the following fetal changes is likely to be occurring at the same time in the pregnancy?
    1. Surfactant is formed in the fetal lungs.
    2. Eyes begin to open and close.
    3. Respiratory movements begin.
    4. Spinal column is completely formed.

99. Below are four important landmarks of fetal development. Please place them in chronological order:
    1. Four-chambered heart is formed.
    2. Vernix caseosa is present.
    3. Blastocyst development is complete.
    4. Testes have descended into the scrotal sac.

100. A client is having an ultrasound assessment done at her prenatal appointment at 8 weeks' gestation. She asks the nurse, "Can you tell what sex my baby is yet?" Which of the following responses would be appropriate for the nurse to make at this time?
    1. "The technician did tell me the sex, but I will have to let the doctor tell you what it is."
    2. "The organs are completely formed and present, but the baby is too small for them to be seen."
    3. "The technician says that the baby has a penis. It looks like you are having a boy."
    4. "I am sorry. It will not be possible to see which sex the baby is for another month or so."

101. Which of the following developmental features would the nurse expect to be absent in a 41-week gestation fetus?
    1. Fingernails.
    2. Eyelashes.
    3. Lanugo.
    4. Milia.

102. A woman delivers a fetal demise that has lanugo covering the entire body, nails that are present on the fingers and toes, but eyes that are still fused. Prior to the death, the mother stated that she had felt quickening. Based on this information, the nurse knows that the baby is about how many weeks' gestation?
    1. 15 weeks.
    2. 22 weeks.
    3. 29 weeks.
    4. 36 weeks.

103. A client asks the nurse, "Could you explain how the baby's blood and my blood separate at delivery?" Which of the following responses is appropriate for the nurse to make?
    1. "When the placenta is born, the circulatory systems separate."
    2. "When the doctor clamps the cord, the blood stops mixing."
    3. "The separation happens after the baby takes the first breath. The baby's oxygen no longer has to come from you."
    4. "The blood actually never mixes. Your blood supply and the baby's blood supply are completely separate."

104. Please place an "X" on the drawing of the cross section of a placenta at the site of gas exchange.

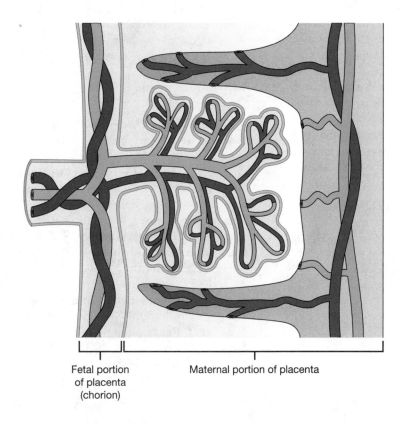

Fetal portion of placenta (chorion)   Maternal portion of placenta

105. The nurse is reading an article that states that the maternal mortality rate in the United States in the year 2000 was 17. Which of the following statements would be an accurate interpretation of the statement?
    1. There were 17 maternal deaths in the United States in 2,000 per 100,000 live births.
    2. There were 17 maternal deaths in the United States in 2,000 per 100,000 women of childbearing age.
    3. There were 17 maternal deaths in the United States in 2,000 per 100,000 pregnancies.
    4. There were 17 maternal deaths in the United States in 2,000 per 100,000 women in the country.

The correct answer number and rationale for why it is the correct answer are given in **boldface blue type.** Rationales for why the other possible answer options are incorrect also are given, but they are not in boldface type.

1. **1, 2, 3, and 4 are correct.**
   1. **Amenorrhea is a presumptive sign of pregnancy.**
   2. **Breast tenderness is a presumptive sign of pregnancy.**
   3. **Quickening is a presumptive sign of pregnancy.**
   4. **Frequent urination is a presumptive sign of pregnancy.**
   5. Uterine growth is a probable sign of pregnancy.

   TEST-TAKING TIP: There are three classifications of signs of pregnancy: presumptive, probable, and positive. Signs that are totally subjective, or *presumptive*, include amenorrhea, breast tenderness, quickening, and frequent urination. Signs that are objective, but not totally absolute, are termed *probable* and include alterations in uterine shape and size and softening of the cervix. Signs that are absolute, or *positive*, include hearing the fetal heartbeat, detecting fetal movement, and seeing ultrasound images of the fetal outline.

2. **2 and 5 are correct.**
   1. Glucose levels should be within normal limits.
   2. **Fibrinogen levels will be elevated slightly in a 40-week-pregnant woman because coagulation factors like fibrinogen increase to help prevent excessive blood loss during delivery.**
   3. Hematocrit levels are usually slightly lower.
   4. Bilirubin levels should be within normal limits.
   5. **A 40-week-pregnant woman's white blood cell count will be elevated above normal as a means of protecting her body from infection.**

   TEST-TAKING TIP: During the latter part of the third trimester, coagulation factors increase in preparation for delivery. It is the body's means of protecting itself against a large loss of blood at delivery. In addition, the white blood cell count rises as a means of protecting the body from infection.

3. 1. This is an important question, but it is not associated with health teaching.
   2. This is an important question, but it is not associated with health teaching.
   3. **This question is important to ask to determine a prenatal client's health teaching needs.**
   4. This is an important question, but it is not associated with health teaching.

   TEST-TAKING TIP: When answering questions, it is essential that the test taker attend to the specific question that is being asked. All of the possible responses are questions that should be asked of a pregnant multigravida, but only one is related to the client's needs for health teaching.

4. 1. Weight gain of 0.8 to 1 lb per week is expected during the second and third trimesters only.
   2. A weight gain of 3 to 5 lb is expected during the entire first trimester.
   3. Since the client's height is not stated, there is no way to know whether or not the client is underweight.
   4. **The weight gain is within normal for the first trimester.**

   TEST-TAKING TIP: One of the assessments that aids health care practitioners in assessing the health and well-being of antenatal clients and their babies is weight gain. For women who enter the pregnancy with a normal weight for height, the expected weight gain is 3 to 5 lb for the entire first trimester and approximately 0.8 to 1 lb per week from weeks 13 to 40. Women with a normal BMI, therefore, should gain between 25 and 35 lb during the entire pregnancy (see http://www.iom.edu/~/media/Files/Report%20Files/2009/Weight-Gain-During-Pregnancy-Reexamining-the-Guidelines/Report%20Brief%20-%20Weight%20Gain%20During%20Pregnancy.pdf).

5. 1. Greasy foods should be avoided.
   2. **Saltine crackers should be eaten before rising. Drinking orange juice has not been recommended.**
   3. Although consuming ginger may help to alleviate the nausea and vomiting of pregnancy, neither cinnamon nor nutmeg has been shown to alleviate the symptoms.
   4. It is recommended that mothers eat small frequent meals throughout the day.

   TEST-TAKING TIP: Although many women experience nausea and vomiting or morning sickness upon rising, many women complain

of nausea and/or vomiting at other times of the day. One theory that has been offered to explain this problem is that the body is ridding itself of teratogens that could potentially harm the fetus.

6. 1. This response is inappropriate. It does not acknowledge the client's concerns.
   2. This response is correct. Serum pregnancy tests are more sensitive than urine tests are.
   3. This statement is correct, but because the woman's period is only 1 day late, the test may not be sensitive enough to detect the pregnancy.
   4. The client could repeat the test, but since the more accurate serum test is available, it would be better for the nurse to recommend that action. At-home tests are reliable only if used correctly.

   TEST-TAKING TIP: Because quantitative pregnancy tests measure the exact quantity of human chorionic gonadotropin in the bloodstream, they are more accurate than urine tests that simply measure whether or not the hormone is present in the urine. Similar to the urine tests on the market, qualitative serum tests detect whether or not the hormone is present, but they are still considered to be more accurate than urine tests are.

7. 1 and 5 are correct.
   1. The client will have a Pap smear done.
   2. A mammogram will not be performed.
   3. A glucose challenge test will likely be performed at the end of the second trimester.
   4. A biophysical profile may be done, but not until the third trimester.
   5. A complete blood count will be performed.

   TEST-TAKING TIP: At the first prenatal visit, pregnant clients will undergo complete obstetrical and medical physical assessments. The assessments are performed to provide the health care practitioner with baseline data regarding the health and well-being of the woman as well as to inform the health care practitioner of any medical problems that the mother has that might affect the pregnancy. A breast exam will be performed by the practitioner to assess for abnormalities, but since mammograms are potentially harm-producing x-rays, they are ordered only in emergent cases.

8. 1. It is too early in the pregnancy to provide anticipatory guidance about pain management during labor.

2. It is appropriate for the nurse to provide anticipatory guidance regarding methods to relieve back pain.
3. It is too early in the pregnancy to provide anticipatory guidance about breastfeeding positions.
4. It is too early in the pregnancy to provide anticipatory guidance about characteristics of the newborn.

   TEST-TAKING TIP: This 10-week gravid client will be entering the second trimester in a couple of weeks. As the uterine body grows, the client is likely to experience backaches. It is appropriate for the nurse to provide information about this possibility and ways to relieve them.

9. 1. Purplish stretch marks are called abdominal striae.
   2. Chadwick's sign is not related to the heart muscle.
   3. A positive Chadwick's sign means that the client's cervix and vagina are a bluish color. It is a probable sign of pregnancy.
   4. Chadwick's sign is not related to the respiratory system.

   TEST-TAKING TIP: Chadwick's sign is a probable sign of pregnancy. The bluish coloration is due to the increase in vascularization of the area in response to the high levels of circulating estrogen in the pregnant woman's system.

10. 1. High levels of the hormone chorionic gonadotropin in the bloodstream and urine of the woman is a probable sign of pregnancy.
    2. Oxytocin is the hormone of labor. It is not measured as a sign of pregnancy.
    3. Prolactin is the hormone that stimulates lactogenesis immediately after delivery. It is not measured as a sign of pregnancy.
    4. Luteinizing hormone is the hormone that stimulates ovulation. It is not measured as a sign of pregnancy.

    TEST-TAKING TIP: Human chorionic gonadotropin is produced by the fertilized egg. Its presence in the bloodstream signals the body to keep the corpus luteum alive. Until the placenta takes over the function of producing progesterone and estrogen, the corpus luteum produces the hormones that are essential to the maintenance of the pregnancy.

11. 1. This is an inappropriate statement to make.
    2. The nurse should query the young woman about what she felt.

3. Even though this statement is correct, it is inappropriate to dismiss the young woman so abruptly.
4. This is an inappropriate statement to make.

TEST-TAKING TIP: Quickening, or subjective fetal movement, occurs between 16 and 20 weeks' gestation. At 10 weeks' gestation it would be impossible for the young woman to feel fetal movement. The nurse, therefore, should elicit more information from the teen to determine what she had felt.

12. 1. It is inappropriate to assume that the client and her family are happy about the pregnancy.
    2. It is inappropriate to assume that the baby's father is still in the young woman's life.
    3. It is important for the nurse to ask the young woman how she feels about being pregnant. She may decide not to continue with the pregnancy.
    4. This information is important, but it is not the best statement to make initially.

TEST-TAKING TIP: Some pregnant women are happy about their pregnancy, some are sad, and still others are frightened. At the initial interview, it is essential that the nurse not assume that the woman will respond in any particular way. The nurse must ask open-ended questions to elicit the woman's feelings about the pregnancy.

13. 2 and 4 are correct.
    1. Backaches usually do not develop until the second trimester of pregnancy.
    2. The woman will likely complain of urinary frequency.
    3. Dyspnea is associated with the third trimester of pregnancy.
    4. Most women complain of fatigue during the first trimester.
    5. Diarrhea is not a complaint normally heard from prenatal clients.

TEST-TAKING TIP: During the first trimester, the body undergoes a number of important changes. The embryo is developing, the hormones of the body are increasing, and the maternal blood supply is increasing. To accomplish each of the tasks, the body uses energy. The mother is fatigued not only because the body is undergoing great change but also because the thyroid gland has not caught up with the increasing energy demands. In addition, because the organs are confined within the bony pelvis, the enlarging uterus prevents the bladder

from expanding with large quantities of urine. As a result, the woman needs to urinate much more frequently than she did prior to becoming pregnant.

14. 1. The client is likely 12 weeks pregnant. At 12 weeks, the fundal height is at the top of the symphysis.
    2. The fundus is at the level of the umbilicus at 20 weeks' gestation.
    3. The fundus is between the umbilicus and the xiphoid process at 28 weeks' gestation.
    4. The fundus is at the level of the xiphoid process at 36 weeks' gestation.

TEST-TAKING TIP: The fundal height is assessed at every prenatal visit. It is an easy, noninvasive means of assessing fetal growth. The nurse should know that the top of the fundus is at the level of the symphysis at the end of the first trimester.

15. 1. It is common for women to be ambivalent about their pregnancy during the first trimester.
    2. The nurse should be concerned if he or she were to see an 8-week-pregnant client who exhibited signs of depression.
    3. The nurse should be concerned if he or she were to see an 8-week-pregnant client who exhibited signs of anxiety.
    4. It is unusual for women at 8 weeks' gestation to exhibit signs of ecstasy.

TEST-TAKING TIP: Even women who stop taking birth control pills to become pregnant are often startled and ambivalent when they actually get pregnant. This is not pathological. The women usually slowly accept the pregnancy and, by 20 weeks' gestation, are happy and enthusiastic about the prospect of becoming a mother.

16. 1. This comment is inappropriate. First of all, everything may not turn out all right. In addition, the comment ignores the client's concerns.
    2. This is a possible plan, but first the nurse should acknowledge the client's feelings.
    3. This is the best comment. It acknowledges the concerns that the client is having.
    4. This comment is inappropriate. First of all, it assumes that the father of the baby is in the picture and second, it ignores the client's concerns.

TEST-TAKING TIP: Nurses have two roles when clients express concerns to them.

First, the nurse must acknowledge the client's concerns so that the client feels accepted and understood. Second, the nurse must help the client to problem solve the situation. It is very important, however, that the acceptance precede the period of problem solving.

17. 1. Hearing a fetal heart rate is a positive sign of pregnancy.
2. A positive pregnancy test is a probable sign of pregnancy.
3. A positive Chadwick's sign is a probable sign of pregnancy.
4. Montgomery gland enlargement is a presumptive sign of pregnancy.

TEST-TAKING TIP: Positive signs of pregnancy are signs that irrefutably show that a fetus is in utero. An ultrasound of a fetus is one positive sign and the fetal heartbeat is another positive sign.

18. 1. Cerebral palsy is not a genetic disease.
2. Hypertensive conditions can be genetically based, but a family history of hypertension does not warrant referral to a genetic counselor.
3. Asthma can be genetically based but a family history of asthma does not warrant referral to a genetic counselor.
4. Cystic fibrosis is an autosomal recessive genetic disease, so the client with a family history of cystic fibrosis should be referred to a genetic counselor.

TEST-TAKING TIP: Virtually all diseases, chronic and acute, have some genetic component, but the ability for the genetic counselor to predict the impact of many diseases is very poor. Those illnesses with clear hereditary patterns, however, do warrant referral to genetic counselors. Cystic fibrosis is inherited via an autosomal recessive inheritance pattern.

19. 1. The client with phenylketonuria (PKU) must receive counseling from a registered dietitian.
2. The client with Graves' disease does not require strict nutrition counseling.
3. The client with Cushing's syndrome does not require strict diet counseling.
4. The client with myasthenia gravis does not require strict diet counseling.

TEST-TAKING TIP: PKU is a genetic disease that is characterized by the absence of the enzyme needed to metabolize phenylalanine, an essential amino acid. When patients with PKU consume phenylalanine,

a metabolite that affects cognitive centers in the brain is created in the body. If a pregnant woman who has PKU were to eat foods high in phenylalanine, her baby would develop severe mental retardation in utero.

20. 1, 2, and 4 are correct.
1. The BMI of 17 is of concern. This client is entering her pregnancy underweight.
2. The rubella titer results should be reported to the nurse midwife.
3. This blood pressure is normal.
4. The hematocrit is below normal.
5. This hemoglobin is normal.

TEST-TAKING TIP: Women who enter their pregnancies underweight are encouraged to gain slightly more—28 to 40 lb—during their pregnancies than are women of normal weight who are encouraged to gain between 25 and 35 lb (see http://iom.edu/~/media/Files/Report%20Files/2009/Weight-Gain-During-Pregnancy-Reexamining-the-Guidelines/Report%20Brief%20-%20Weight%20Gain%20During%20Pregnancy.pdf). A rubella titer of 1:8 or less indicates that the woman is non-immune to rubella. If exposed, she is, therefore, at risk of developing the disease. Because a woman is high risk of becoming anemic during her pregnancy, it is important to identify any woman who enters her pregnancy with a below normal hematocrit.

21. 1. The cervix should be long and thick.
2. The practitioner would expect to palpate an enlarged ovary.
3. The cervical mucus should be thin.
4. The vaginal wall should be bluish in color.

TEST-TAKING TIP: The cervix is long and thick to retain the pregnancy in the uterine cavity. The cervical mucus is thin and the vaginal wall is bluish in color as a result of elevated estrogen levels. The ovary is enlarged because the corpus luteum is still functioning.

22. 1. Although some labs request that patients fast, the GCT is a nonfasting test.
2. It is unnecessary to take a urine sample to the lab on the day of testing.
3. Only one blood specimen is taken on the day of the test.
4. The test does take about 1 hour to complete.

TEST-TAKING TIP: The GCT is done at approximately 24 weeks' gestation to assess the client's ability to metabolize glucose. It is a 1-hour, nonfasting screening test. One hour after a client consumes 50 grams of a concentrated glucose solution, a serum glucose level is done. If the value is 130 mg/dL or higher (some centers are still using 140 mg/dL as the cut off), the client is referred for a 3-hour glucose tolerance test to determine whether or not she has gestational diabetes.

23. 2 and 4 are correct.
    1. It is common for primigravid women not to feel fetal movement until 19 to 20 weeks' gestation.
    2. The fundal height at 24 weeks should be 4 cm above the umbilicus. The fundal height at the level of the umbilicus is expected at 20 weeks' gestation.
    3. Excessive salivation, called ptyalism, is an expected finding in pregnancy.
    4. The woman may be going into preterm labor.
    5. Hemorrhoids are commonly seen in pregnant women.

    TEST-TAKING TIP: It is important for the test taker to know the timing of key pregnancy changes as well as abnormal prenatal findings. The mother should feel fetal movement by 20 weeks' gestation. Primigravidas often feel fetal movement later than multigravidas. Specific fundal height measurements are also expected at key times in the pregnancy. A baby delivered at 34 weeks' gestation is at high risk for many neonatal complications.

24. 1. A positive pregnancy test will not necessarily promote fathers' interests in their partners' pregnancies.
    2. Most fathers are very involved with their partners' pregnancies well before childbirth education classes begin.
    3. Hearing the fetal heartbeat often increases fathers' interests in their partners' pregnancies.
    4. Meeting the health care practitioner is unlikely to promote fathers' interests in their partners' pregnancies.

    TEST-TAKING TIP: Women who are in the first few weeks of pregnancy often experience a number of physical complaints—nausea and vomiting, fatigue, breast tenderness, and urinary frequency. Prospective fathers whose partners experience these complaints are often not very interested in the pregnancies. When the baby becomes "real," with a positive heartbeat or fetal movement, the fathers often become very excited.

25. 1. Ballottement is not related to the mucous plug.
    2. This is the definition of ballottement.
    3. Palpating fetal parts is not related to ballottement.
    4. Fetal position is not related to ballottement.

    TEST-TAKING TIP: Although this question discusses nurse–patient interaction, it is simply a definition question. The test taker is being asked to identify the definition of the word "ballottement."

26. 1. Nausea is commonly seen in the first trimester but should have resolved by the time the second trimester begins.
    2. Dyspnea is commonly seen in the third trimester, not the second trimester.
    3. Urinary frequency is commonly seen in the first trimester and late in the third trimester, but it is not related to the second trimester.
    4. Leg cramping is often a complaint of clients in the second trimester.

    TEST-TAKING TIP: Although clients in the second trimester do experience some physical discomfort, such as leg cramps and backaches, most women feel well. They no longer are fatigued, nauseous, and so on as in the first trimester, but the baby is not so large as to cause significant complaints like dyspnea or the recurrence of urinary frequency.

27. 1. Estrogen levels are not related to glucose metabolism.
    2. Progesterone levels are not related to glucose metabolism.
    3. Human placental lactogen is an insulin antagonist.
    4. Human chorionic gonadotropin levels are not related to glucose metabolism.

    TEST-TAKING TIP: hPL is produced by the placenta. As the placenta grows, the hormone levels rise. At approximately 24 weeks' gestation, the levels are high enough to affect glucose metabolism. If performed earlier, the GCT test may result in a false-negative result.

28. 1. The majority of the organ systems are developed before the end of the first trimester. This client is in her second trimester.

2. There are a number of over-the-counter medications that should be taken with care during pregnancy.
3. Category "X" medications have been shown to be teratogenic.
4. Category "B" medications have been shown to be safe to take throughout pregnancy.

TEST-TAKING TIP: It is important for pregnant women to contact their health care practitioners to find out which medications are safe to take during pregnancy and which medications must be avoided. All medications are assigned a pregnancy category from "A"—research has shown they are safe to be consumed throughout pregnancy—to "X"—a teratogenic agent. Category "B" medications are considered safe because of anecdotal evidence, although controlled research has not been conducted to confirm that evidence. Teratogens are agents that have definitely been shown to cause fetal damage.

29. The "X" should be placed at the level of the umbilicus.

TEST-TAKING TIP: At 20 weeks' gestation, the fundal height should be felt at the umbilicus. About 8 weeks later, it is felt between the umbilicus and xiphoid process and at the xiphoid process at 36 weeks.

30. 1. The woman would be expected to weigh 131 to 132 lb. At this stage of pregnancy, the woman is expected to gain about 0.8 to 1 lb a week.
2. The woman would be expected to weigh 131 to 132 lb. At this stage of pregnancy, the woman is expected to gain about 0.8 to 1 lb a week.
3. The woman would be expected to weigh 131 to 132 lb. At this stage of pregnancy, the woman is expected to gain about 0.8 to 1 lb a week.
4. The woman would be expected to weigh 131 to 132 lb. At this stage of pregnancy, the woman is expected to gain about 0.8 to 1 lb a week.

TEST-TAKING TIP: The incremental weight gain of a client is an important means of assessing the growth and development of the fetus. The nurse would expect that,

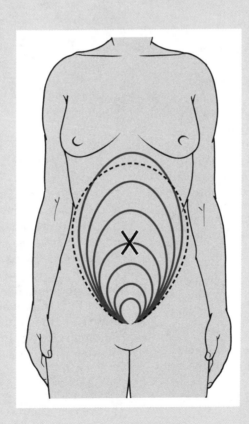

during the second and third trimesters, the woman should gain approximately 0.8 to 1 lb per week.

31. 1. Although breast cancer is hormonally driven, it is rare to see its development during pregnancy.
    2. **Nodular breast tissue is normal in pregnancy.**
    3. The woman is not exhibiting psychotic behavior.
    4. Anxiety attacks are not common during pregnancy.

TEST-TAKING TIP: The high levels of estrogen seen in pregnancy result in a number of changes. The hypertrophy and hyperplasia of the breast tissue, in preparation for neonatal lactation, are two of the changes.

32. 1. **A dietary evaluation is indicated since painful leg cramps can be caused by consuming too little calcium or too much phosphorus.**
    2. Goodell's sign is a physiological finding—a softened cervix.
    3. Hegar's sign is a physiological finding—a softened uterine isthmus.
    4. It is not necessary to evaluate the woman's posture.

TEST-TAKING TIP: Leg cramps can occur as a result of low calcium and/or high phosphorus since they are often related to a poor calcium/phosphorus ratio. A dietary assessment should be done to determine whether or not the client is consuming enough calcium, primarily found in dairy products, or large quantities of phosphorus, found in carbonated beverages and processed sandwich meats.

33. 1. The Kegel exercises are done to promote the muscle tone of the perineal muscles.
    2. **The pelvic tilt is an exercise that can reduce backache pain.**
    3. Leg lifts will not help to reduce backache pain.
    4. Crunches will not help to reduce backache pain.

TEST-TAKING TIP: Pelvic tilt exercises help to reduce backache pain. The client is taught to get into an optimal position—on the hands and knees is often best. She is then taught to force her back out while tucking her head and buttocks under and holding that position for a few seconds, followed by holding the alternate position for a few seconds—arching her back while lifting her head and her buttocks toward

the ceiling. These positions should be alternated repeatedly for about 5 minutes. The exercises are very relaxing while also improving the muscle tone of the lower back.

34. 1. Although some women do have difficulty breastfeeding, many women with inverted nipples are able to breastfeed with little to no problem.
    2. **The client should be referred to a lactation consultant.**
    3. There is no need to telephone the labor unit. However, it would be appropriate to document the finding on the client's prenatal record.
    4. It is not recommended that exercises be done to evert the nipples.

TEST-TAKING TIP: Research on eversion exercises has shown that they are not effective, plus breast manipulation can bring on contractions since oxytocin production is stimulated. Lactation consultants are breastfeeding specialists. A lactation consultant would probably recommend that the client wear breast shields in her bra. The shields are made of hard plastic and have a small hole through which the nipple everts.

35. 1. **The blood pressure should not elevate during pregnancy. This change should be reported to the health care practitioner.**
    2. An increase in the respiratory rate is expected.
    3. An increase in the heart rate is expected.
    4. A slight increase in temperature is expected.

TEST-TAKING TIP: The basal metabolic rate of the woman increases during pregnancy. As a result the nurse would expect to observe a respiratory rate of 20 to 24 rpm. High levels of progesterone in the body result in a decrease in the contractility of the smooth musculature throughout the body. This results in an increase in the pulse rate. In addition, progesterone is thermogenic, resulting in a slight rise in the woman's core body temperature.

36. 1. Evening primrose does not affect back strain.
    2. Evening primrose does not affect lactation.
    3. **Evening primrose converts to a prostaglandin substance in the body. Prostaglandins are responsible for readying the cervix for dilation.**

4. Evening primrose does not affect the development of hemorrhoids.

TEST-TAKING TIP: Nurse midwives often recommend complementary therapies during pregnancy as well as during labor and delivery. Nurse midwives usually believe in promoting natural means for maintaining a healthy pregnancy and for stimulating labor. Evening primrose is one of those interventions.

37. 1. Evening primrose has been shown to cause skin rash in some women.
    2. Evening primrose has not been shown to cause pedal edema.
    3. Evening primrose has not been shown to cause blurred vision.
    4. Evening primrose has not been shown to cause tinnitus.

TEST-TAKING TIP: Even though evening primrose is a "natural" substance, it can cause side effects in some clients. The most common side effect seen from the oil is a skin rash. Headaches and nausea have also been seen.

38. 1. It is unlikely that the client has a galactocele.
    2. The woman should not pump her breasts during pregnancy.
    3. Colostrum is normally seen at this time and naturally can be a number of colors, including whitish, yellowish, reddish, and brownish.
    4. It is normal for colostrum to be expressed late in pregnancy.

TEST-TAKING TIP: Even though colostrum is present in the breasts in the latter part of the third trimester, it is important for women not to pump their breasts. Oxytocin, the hormone that promotes the ejection of milk during lactation, is the hormone of labor. Pumping of the breasts, therefore, could stimulate the uterus to contract.

39. 1. It is unlikely that the woman is hypertensive.
    2. The fundal height is the likely cause of the woman's dyspnea.
    3. It is unlikely that the woman has hydramnios.
    4. It is unlikely that the woman has congestive heart failure.

TEST-TAKING TIP: As the uterus enlarges, the woman's organs are affected. At 36 weeks, the fundus is at the level of the xiphoid process. The diaphragm is elevated and the lungs are displaced.

When a client lies flat she has difficulty breathing. Most women use multiple pillows at night for sleep. Whenever caring for a pregnant woman, the nurse should elevate the head of the bed.

40. 1, 2, and 3 are correct.
    1. Frequency is seen once lightening, or the descent of the fetus into the pelvis, has occurred.
    2. Heartburn is a common complaint of pregnant women.
    3. Backaches are common complaints of pregnant women.
    4. Persistent headache should not be seen in pregnant women.
    5. Pregnant women should not complain of blurred vision.

TEST-TAKING TIP: This question is asking the test taker to differentiate between complaints that are expected during the third trimester and those that are abnormal. Heartburn and backaches are expected complaints. In addition, once lightening has occurred, frequent urination also returns. In each of the 3 cases, the signs do not indicate pathology. Both persistent headache and blurred vision, however, are signs that the woman may have developed a complication of pregnancy. If they should develop, the client should be advised to report them to the health care practitioner.

41. 1. This response ignores and dismisses the client's concerns as unimportant.
    2. This is a true statement.
    3. Although active labor is usually more uncomfortable than the normal aches and pains of pregnancy, that is not necessarily true of prodromal labor or the latent phase of labor.
    4. The nurse is making an assumption here. This may not be the client's concern at all.

TEST-TAKING TIP: Labor contractions often begin in a woman's back, feeling much like a backache. The difference is that labor contractions are intermittent and rhythmic. The client should be advised to attend to any pains that come and go and time them. She may be beginning the labor process.

42. 1. Anemia is an expected finding.
    2. The client should not be thrombocytopenic. Although some women do develop idiopathic thrombocytopenia of pregnancy, this is a complication of pregnancy.

3. The nurse would not expect to see polycythemia.
4. The nurse would not expect to see hyperbilirubinemia

TEST-TAKING TIP: By the end of the second trimester, the blood supply of the woman increases by approximately 50%. This increase is necessary for the client to be able to perfuse the placenta. There is a concurrent increase in red blood cell production, but the vast majority of women are unable to produce the red blood cells in sufficient numbers to keep pace with the increase in blood volume. As a result, clients develop what is commonly called "physiological anemia of pregnancy." A hematocrit of 32% is considered normal for a pregnant woman.

43. 1. Although the orthopneic position is a safe position for the client to be placed in, a prenatal examination cannot be performed in this position.
2. Although the lateral-recumbent position is a safe position for the client to be placed in, a prenatal examination cannot be performed in this position. In addition, the pregnant abdomen may not enable the client fully to attain this position.
3. Although the Sims' position is a safe position for the client to be placed in, a prenatal examination cannot be performed in this position, and the pregnant abdomen may not enable the client fully to attain this position.
4. The client should be placed in a semi-Fowler's position.

TEST-TAKING TIP: Because of the growth of the uterus, it is very difficult for women in the third trimester to breathe in the supine position. During the prenatal visit, the baby's heartbeat will be monitored and the fundal height will be assessed. Both of these procedures can safely be performed in the semi-Fowler's position.

44. 2, 3, and 4 are correct.
1. Urine glucose is performed at each visit, not the blood glucose.
2. The blood pressure is assessed at each prenatal visit.
3. The fetal heart rate is assessed at each prenatal visit. Depending on the equipment available, it will be assessed mechanically via Doppler or manually via fetoscope. The fetal heart is audible via Doppler many weeks before it is audible via fetoscope.

4. Urine protein is performed at each prenatal visit.
5. Ultrasounds are performed only when needed.

TEST-TAKING TIP: The test taker must read the question carefully. Although urine glucose assessments are done at each visit, blood glucoses are assessed only intermittently during the pregnancy. Similarly, although ultrasound assessments may be ordered intermittently during a pregnancy, they are certainly not done at every prenatal visit. As a matter of fact, there is no absolute mandate that a sonogram must be done at all during a pregnancy.

45. 1, 2, 3, and 5 are correct.
1. Leg cramps are normal, although the client's diet should be assessed.
2. Varicose veins are normal, although client teaching may be needed.
3. Hemorrhoids are normal, although client teaching may be needed.
4. Fainting spells are not normal, although the client may feel faint when rising quickly from a lying position.
5. Lordosis, or change in the curvature of the spine, is normal, although patient teaching may be needed.

TEST-TAKING TIP: There are a number of physical complaints that are "normal" during pregnancy. There are interventions, however, that can be taught to help to alleviate some of the discomforts. The test taker should be familiar with patient education information that should be conveyed regarding the physical complaints of pregnancy. For example, clients who complain of hemorrhoids should be encouraged to eat high-fiber foods and drink fluids to produce softer stools. The softer stools should decrease the irritation of the hemorrhoids.

46. 1. The nurse would expect to note hypotension rather than hypertension.
2. Dizziness is an expected finding.
3. The nurse would expect to see dyspnea, not rales.
4. The nurse would not expect to see any skin changes.

TEST-TAKING TIP: Because the weight of the gravid uterus compresses the great vessels, the nurse would expect the client to complain of dizziness when lying supine. The blood supply to the head and other parts of the body is diminished when the great vessels are compressed.

47. 1. This is an appropriate question to ask the client.
    2. It is inappropriate to ask the Muslim client about the name for the baby.
    3. This is an appropriate question to ask the client.
    4. This is an appropriate question to ask the client.

    TEST-TAKING TIP: Traditional Muslim couples will not tell anyone the baby's name until he or she has gone through the official naming ceremony, called *aqiqah.* **Babies are rarely named before a week of age. The parents need time to get to know their baby and decide on an appropriate name for him or her.**

48. 1. The glucose challenge test is performed at approximately 24 weeks' gestation.
    2. Amniotic fluid volume assessment is part of the biophysical profile (BPP). The BPP is performed only when the health care practitioner is concerned about the health and well-being of the fetus.
    3. Vaginal and rectal cultures are done at approximately 36 weeks' gestation.
    4. Karyotype analysis or chromosomal analysis, if performed, is done early in pregnancy.

    TEST-TAKING TIP: Vaginal and rectal cultures are done to assess for the presence of group B streptococcal (GBS) bacteria in the woman's vagina and rectum. If the woman has GBS as part of her normal flora, she will be given IV antibiotics during labor to prevent vertical transmission to her baby at birth. GBS is often called "the baby killer."

49. 1. Unless nosebleeds are excessive, it is rare for them to lead to severe anemia.
    2. Clients with nosebleeds rarely have temperature elevations.
    3. This is an accurate statement. Hormonal changes in pregnancy make the nasal passages prone to bleeds.
    4. Nosebleeds are an expected complication of pregnancy.

    TEST-TAKING TIP: Estrogen, one of the important hormones of pregnancy, promotes vasocongestion of the mucous membranes of the body. Increased vascular perfusion of the mucous membranes of the gynecological system is essential for the developing fetus to survive. The vasocongestion occurs in all of the mucous membranes of the body, however, leading to many complaints including nosebleeds and gingival bleeding.

50. 1. The woman implies that she and her husband are not having sex. There is no need to refrain from sexual intercourse during a normal pregnancy—so the woman and her husband need further counseling.
    2. Some men do gain weight during pregnancy. This is viewed as a sympathetic response to the woman's weight gain.
    3. Men often become much more concerned about the finances of the household during a woman's pregnancy.
    4. The father is exhibiting a strong attachment to the unborn baby.

    TEST-TAKING TIP: *Couvade* **is the term given to a father's physiological responses to his partner's pregnancy. Men have been seen to exhibit a number of physical complaints/changes that simulate their partner's physical complaints/changes—for example, indigestion, weight gain, urinary frequency, and backache.**

51. 1. The nurse would expect the hematocrit to drop.
    2. The nurse would expect to see an elevated white blood cell count.
    3. The nurse would not expect to see an abnormal potassium level.
    4. The nurse would not expect to see an abnormal sodium level.

    TEST-TAKING TIP: At the end of the third trimester and through to the early postpartum period, a normal leukocytosis, or rise in white blood cell count, is seen. This is a natural physiological change that protects the woman's body from the invasion of pathogens during the birth process. The nurse should rely on a temperature elevation to determine whether or not the woman has an infection.

52. 1. 35-week gestation clients should not complain of nausea and vomiting.
    2. 35-week gestation clients should not be ambivalent about their pregnancies.
    3. At 35 weeks, the fundus should be 15 cm above the umbilicus.
    4. The use of three pillows for sleep comfort is often seen in clients who are 35 weeks' gestation.

    TEST-TAKING TIP: It is essential that the test taker differentiate between normal and abnormal findings at various points

during the pregnancy—for example, nausea and vomiting are normal during the first trimester but not during the second or third trimester. The fundal height measurement is also important to remember. From 20 weeks' gestation, when the fundal height is usually at the same height as the umbilicus, to 36 weeks' gestation, when the final height is at the xiphoid process, the height measures are approximately the same number of centimeters above the symphysis as the number of weeks of fetal gestation. For example, at 24 weeks' gestation, the height is usually 24 cm above the symphysis or 4 cm above the umbilicus, and at 35 weeks' gestation, the height is usually 35 cm above the symphysis, or 15 cm above the umbilicus.

53. 1. Unless a woman is high risk for preterm labor, there is no reason to refrain from making love during pregnancy. Therefore, this is an inappropriate statement.
    2. This is an accurate statement.
    3. Unless a woman is high risk for preterm labor, this is an inappropriate statement.
    4. This is an inappropriate statement.

TEST-TAKING TIP: There is no contraindication to intercourse or to orgasm during pregnancy, unless it has been determined that a client is high risk for preterm labor. Until late in pregnancy, there are very few oxytocin receptor sites on the uterine body. The woman will, therefore, not go into labor as a result of an orgasm during sexual relations.

54. 1. Although the tour of the facility is important, this should not be the couple's first step.
    2. It is best that a couple first develop a birth plan.
    3. Although appointments should be made, this should not be the couple's first step.
    4. Although the couple may wish to research the health care practitioner's malpractice history, this should not be the couple's first step.

TEST-TAKING TIP: It is important for a couple's needs and wants to match their obstetrical care practitioner's philosophy of care. If, for example, the couple is interested in the possibility of having a water birth, it is important that the health care provider be willing to perform a water birth. If, however, the woman wants to be "completely pain free," the health care provider must be willing to order pain medications throughout the labor and delivery. A birth plan will list the couples' many wishes.

55. 1. Birth plans help to facilitate communication between couples and their health care providers.
    2. The type of pain medication the woman wishes to have during her labor and birth should be included in the birth plan, but the plan is not the location where the couple will learn about the medications.
    3. The list of items that should be taken to the hospital for labor and delivery is separate from the birth plan, although the plan may include how the items will be used. The items are often placed in what is called a "goody" bag.
    4. The birth plan should give any couple, whether their baby is being delivered vaginally or surgically, a sense of control over the labor and delivery process.

TEST-TAKING TIP: The earlier a birth plan is developed, the better. A pregnant woman and her partner must feel comfortable with the communication methods, physical care, and health care philosophies of their obstetrical health care provider. The birth plan is a means for everyone clearly to understand each step of the birthing process. When the client enters the hospital for delivery, the birth plan should be presented to the nursing staff to facilitate the communication during that transition.

56. 1. The presence of the father at delivery should be nonnegotiable.
    2. Whether or not a client would prefer to have an episiotomy should be discussed, but this may need to be a negotiable issue.
    3. Whether or not a client would prefer to have an epidural should be discussed, but this may need to be a negotiable issue.
    4. Whether or not a father will be allowed to take pictures during the delivery should be discussed, but this may need to be a negotiable issue.

TEST-TAKING TIP: Even though the birth plan should include issues like the use or nonuse of episiotomies, emergent issues during the delivery may lead to a sudden change in plans. For example, if a cesarean is needed for malpresentation, the issue of episiotomy is moot and the client will definitely need anesthesia. However, there are some issues that should be nonnegotiable. If the father wishes to be in the delivery room no matter the type of delivery or whether or not an emergent situation is occurring, that should be stated in the plan and accepted by the health care provider.

57. 1. Clients who experience ptyalism have an excess of saliva. They should be advised to be vigilant in the care of their teeth and gums. Ptyalism is often accompanied by gingivitis and nausea and vomiting.
    2. Ptyalism is not related to a change in blood pressure.
    3. Ptyalism is not related to changes in the lower extremities.
    4. Ptyalism is not related to the meat intake.

TEST-TAKING TIP: Ptyalism is related to the increase in vascular congestion of the mucous membranes from increased estrogen production. Women with increased salivation often also experience gingivitis, which is also related to estrogen production. In addition, ptyalism is seen in women with nausea and vomiting. Because of the caustic effects of gastric juices on the enamel of the teeth, the inflammation seen in the gums, and the increased salivation, it is essential that the pregnant woman take special care of her teeth during pregnancy, including regular visits to the dentist and/or the dental hygienist.

58. 1. The woman should receive the influenza injection. The nasal spray, however, should not be administered to a pregnant woman.
    2. The mumps vaccine should not be administered to the pregnant client.
    3. The rubella vaccine should not be administered to the pregnant client.
    4. The varicella vaccine should not be administered to the pregnant client.

TEST-TAKING TIP: It is very important for pregnant women to be protected from the flu by receiving the inactivated influenza injection. The fetus will not be injured by the shot and the woman will be protected from the many sequelae that can develop from the flu. However, the live nasal flu spray should not be administered to pregnant women. It is contraindicated to vaccinate pregnant women with many other vaccines, including the measles-mumps-rubella (MMR) and the varicella

vaccines (see http://acog.org/Resources_And_Publications/Committee_Opinions/Committee_on_Obstetric_Practice/Influenza_Vaccination_During_Pregnancy).

59. 1. The woman should stay out of rooms that are being renovated.
    2. The water should be tested for the presence of lead. If there is lead in the water, it is recommended that the water from the hot water tap not be consumed.
    3. There is no reason the client should refrain from entering the basement.
    4. As long as she is feeling well, there is no reason the client should refrain from walking up the stairs.

TEST-TAKING TIP: Antique houses often contain lead-based paint and water piping that has been soldered with lead-based solder. Lead, when ingested either through the respiratory tract or the GI tract, can cause permanent damage to the central nervous system of the unborn child. It is very important, therefore, that the woman not breathe in the air in rooms that have recently been sanded. The paint aerosolizes and the lead can be inhaled. In addition, lead leaches into hot water more readily than into cold so water from the cold tap should be consumed—but only after the water has run through the pipes for a minimum of 2 minutes.

60. 1. An allergy to strawberries is not the likely reason.
    2. Strawberries have not been shown to cause birth defects.
    3. The woman believes in old wives' tales.
    4. A previous poor pregnancy outcome is not the likely reason.

TEST-TAKING TIP: There are a number of old wives' tales that pregnant women believe in and live by. One of the common tales relates to the ingestion of strawberries: Women who eat strawberries have babies with strawberry marks on their bodies. Unless belief in old wives' tales has the potential to affect the health of the baby and/or mother, it is ill advised and unnecessary to argue with the mother about her beliefs.

61. 1, 2, and 5 are correct.
    1. It is very important that women before attempting to become pregnant begin taking daily multivitamin tablets.

2. Women who wish to become pregnant should first see a medical doctor for a complete checkup

3. Women who wish to become pregnant should refrain from drinking any alcohol.

4. Women who wish to become pregnant should ask an obstetrician/gynecologist which over-the-counter medications should be avoided. Some—for example, acetaminophen—are safe to take, while others are not.

5. Women who wish to become pregnant should be counseled to stop smoking.

TEST-TAKING TIP: Because the embryo is very sensitive during the first trimester of pregnancy, women should be advised to be vigilant about their health even before becoming pregnant. For example, folic acid, a vitamin in multivitamin tablets, helps to prevent neural tube defects. Women of childbearing age often fail to go for complete physical examinations. It is important to discover the presence of any medical illnesses before the pregnancy begins, however, so women should be counseled to have a complete physical before stopping birth control methods.

62. 1. Unless a woman is high risk for preterm labor, she has been diagnosed with placenta previa, or she has preterm rupture of the membranes, sexual intercourse is not contraindicated.

2. Breast fondling should be discouraged only if the client is high risk for preterm labor.

3. With increasing size of the uterine body, the couple may need counseling regarding alternate options for sexual intimacy.

4. There is no contraindication for vaginal lubricant use in pregnancy. As a matter of fact, with the increased discharge experienced by many mothers, lubricants are often not needed.

TEST-TAKING TIP: Pregnancy lasts 10 lunar months. It is essential that the nurse counsel clients on ways to maintain health and well-being in the many facets of their lives. Sexual intimacy is one of the important aspects of a married couple's life together. The couple can be counseled to use alternate positions, engage in mutual masturbation, or discover other means to satisfy their needs for sexual expression during the pregnancy period.

63. 1. Linea nigra—the darkened area on the skin from the symphysis to the umbilicus—is a normal skin change seen in pregnancy.

2. Melasma—the "mask" of pregnancy—is a normal skin change seen in pregnancy.

3. Petechiae are pinpoint red or purple spots on the skin. They are seen in hemorrhagic conditions.

4. Spider nevi—benign radiating blood vessels—are normal skin changes seen in pregnancy.

TEST-TAKING TIP: There are many skin changes that occur normally during pregnancy. Most of the changes—such as linea nigra, melasma, and hyperpigmentation of the areolae—are related to an increase in the melanin-producing bodies of the skin as a result of stimulation by the female hormones estrogen and progesterone. The presence of petechiae is usually related to a pathological condition, such as thrombocytopenia.

64. 1. The estimated date of delivery is June 27, 2013.
2. The estimated date of delivery is June 27, 2013.
3. The estimated date of delivery is June 27, 2013.
4. The estimated date of delivery is June 27, 2013.

TEST-TAKING TIP: Nagele's rule is a simple method used to calculate a client's estimated date of confinement (EDC) or estimated date of delivery (EDD) from the last normal menstrual period (LMP). The nurse learns the date of the first day of the last menstrual period from the client. He or she then subtracts 3 months from the date, adds 7 days to the date, and adjusts the year, if needed. For the example given:

Last normal menstrual period—September 20, 2012 = 9 - 20 - 2012

$$\frac{-3 + 7}{6\ 27}$$

adjust the year   6 - 27 - 2013
             June 27, 2013

65. 1, 4, and 5 are correct.
1. Heartburn is a common symptom.
2. It is inappropriate for a prospective father to engage in promiscuity.
3. Hypertension in a prospective father should be investigated.
4. Some fathers complain of abdominal bloating.
5. Some fathers complain of abdominal pain.

TEST-TAKING TIP: Heartburn, bloating, and abdominal pain are subjective complaints that fathers often experience during their partners' pregnancies. Fathers who are experiencing couvade symptoms are exhibiting a strong affiliation between themselves and their partners. It is inappropriate for prospective fathers to engage in illicit relationships and/or indifference toward their partners' pregnancies. They should be fully engaged in the process. Hypertension, an objective sign, should be investigated further. The father may have developed a pathological condition.

66. 1, 2, 3, and 4 are correct.
    1. Convulsions are a danger sign of pregnancy.
    2. Double vision is a danger sign of pregnancy.
    3. Epigastric pain is a danger sign of pregnancy.
    4. Persistent vomiting is a danger sign of pregnancy.
    5. Although polyuria may be a sign of diabetes or another illness, it is not highlighted as a danger sign of pregnancy.

TEST-TAKING TIP: The danger signs of pregnancy are signs or symptoms that can occur in an otherwise healthy pregnancy that are likely due to serious pregnancy complications. For example, double vision, epigastric pain, and blurred vision are symptoms of the hypertensive illnesses of pregnancy, and persistent vomiting is a symptom of hyperemesis gravidarum.

67. 1. This does not reflect an accurate picture.
    2. This does not reflect an accurate picture.
    3. This accurately reflects this woman's gravidity and parity—G5 P1122.
    4. This does not reflect an accurate picture.

TEST-TAKING TIP: Gravidity refers to pregnancy and parity refers to delivery. Every time a woman is pregnant, it is counted as one gravida (G). The results of each pregnancy are then documented as a para (P) in the following order. The first number refers to full-term births or births at or greater than 38 weeks' gestation; the second number refers to preterm births or births between 20 and 37 weeks' gestation; the third number refers to abortions, whether spontaneous or therapeutic; and the fourth number refers to the number of living children. The client has been pregnant 5 times (G5); she birthed 1 son,

1 daughter, had 1 miscarriage, had 1 first trimester abortion, and is currently pregnant. Her parity (P1122) accurately reflects her obstetrical history: 1 full-term delivery (daughter at 39 weeks), 1 preterm delivery (son at 28 weeks), 2 abortions (1 miscarriage, 1 first-trimester abortion), and, finally, 2 living children.

68. 1. Although this is an accurate statement, it is inappropriate at this time.
    2. Although this is an accurate statement, it is inappropriate at this time.
    3. It is never appropriate to make this statement.
    4. This is an appropriate comment to make at this time.

TEST-TAKING TIP: This father is exhibiting a sign of couvade, i.e., weight gain. This is a positive response since it shows that he is exhibiting a sympathetic response to his partner's pregnancy. In addition, this father is accompanying his partner to the prenatal visit, another positive sign.

69. 1. Tofu, legumes, and broccoli are excellent substitutes for the restricted foods.
    2. Although corn, yams, and green beans are vegetables, they are not high either in protein or in iron.
    3. Although potatoes, parsnips, and turnips are vegetables, they are not high either in protein or in iron.
    4. These are examples of a vegan's restricted foods.

TEST-TAKING TIP: Vegans are vegetarians who eat absolutely no animal products. Since animal products are most clients' sources of protein and iron, it is necessary for vegans to be very careful to meet their increased needs by eating excellent sources of these nutrients. It is recommended that vegans meet with a registered dietitian early in their pregnancies to discuss diet choices.

70. 1. Although this is an accurate statement, this is not the most important communication for the nurse to make.
    2. Fruit juices are good sources of folic acid, but this is not the most important communication for the nurse to make.
    3. It is recommended that pregnant clients eat whole fruits rather than consume large quantities of fruit juice. This is the most important statement for the nurse to make.

4. Although this is an accurate statement, this is not the most important communication for the nurse to make.

TEST-TAKING TIP: It is recommended that moderately active women of childbearing age consume the equivalent of 2 cups of fruit per day. Approximately 8 oz of fruit juice equals 1 cup of fruit. Fruit juices, however, are rarely made of 100% juice and almost always contain added sugar. In addition, the client is not receiving the benefit of the fiber that is contained in the whole fruit. The nurse should compliment the client on her fruit intake but encourage her to consume whole fruits rather than large quantities of juice (see http://health.gov/dietaryguidelines/dga 2010/DietaryGuidelines2010.pdf).

71. 1. Supplementation of vitamin C has not been shown to be harmful during pregnancy.
    2. **Vitamin D supplementation can be harmful during pregnancy.**
    3. Supplementation of the B vitamins has not been shown to be harmful during pregnancy.
    4. Supplementation of the B vitamins has not been shown to be harmful during pregnancy.

TEST-TAKING TIP: The water-soluble vitamins, if consumed in large quantities, have not been shown to be harmful during pregnancy. The body eliminates the excess quantities through the urine and stool. However, the fat-soluble vitamins— vitamins A, D, E, and K—can build up in the body. Vitamins A and D have been shown to be teratogenic to the fetus in megadoses.

72. 1. Vitamin B_{12} (cobalamin) should be supplemented.
    2. Vitamin B_{12} (cobalamin) should be supplemented.
    3. Vitamin B_{12} (cobalamin) should be supplemented.
    4. Vitamin B_{12} (cobalamin) should be supplemented.

TEST-TAKING TIP: Vitamin B_{12} (cobalamin) is found almost exclusively in animal products—meat, dairy, eggs. Since vegans do not consume animal products, and the vitamin is not in most nonanimal sources, it is strongly recommended that vegans supplement that vitamin. Those who take in too little of the vitamin are susceptible to anemia and nervous system disorders.

In addition, the vitamin is especially important during pregnancy since it is essential for DNA synthesis.

73. 1. Pasta is a low-fiber food.
    2. Rice is a low-fiber food.
    3. Dairy products are low-fiber foods.
    4. **Celery is an excellent food to reverse constipation. It is a high-fiber food.**

TEST-TAKING TIP: Most women complain of constipation during pregnancy. Progesterone, a muscle-relaxant, is responsible for a slowing of the digestive system. It is important, therefore, to recommend foods to pregnant clients that will help to alleviate the problem. Foods high in fiber, like fresh fruits and vegetables, are excellent suggestions.

74. 1. **Turnip greens are calcium rich.**
    2. Green beans are not high in calcium.
    3. Cantaloupes are not high in calcium.
    4. Nectarines are not high in calcium.

TEST-TAKING TIP: There are a number of women who, for one reason or another, do not consume large quantities of dairy products. The nurse must be prepared to suggest alternate sources since dairy products are the best sources for calcium intake. Any of the dark green, leafy vegetables, like kale, spinach, collards, and turnip greens, are excellent sources, as are small fish that are eaten with the bones, like sardines.

75. 1. **This is an accurate statement. A serving of meat—typically a 2 to 3 oz serving—is approximately equal to a deck of cards.**
    2. A paperback book is too large.
    3. A clenched fist is too large.
    4. A large tomato is too large.

TEST-TAKING TIP: The dietary recommendation of the protein group for moderately active women of childbearing age is the equivalent of 5½ oz per day. A 1 oz equivalent is defined as 1 oz of meat, fish, or poultry; 1 egg; 1 tbsp peanut butter; ½ oz nuts or seeds; or ¼ cup cooked beans or peas. The average American diet well exceeds the recommended protein intake since most Americans consider a serving of meat to be much larger than a deck of cards.

76. 1. This client consumed 2⅚ servings: 4 oz whole milk = ½ serving; 2 oz hard cheese = 1⅓ servings; 1 cup pudding made with milk = 1 serving; the 2 oz of

cream cheese = 0 dairy servings since cream cheese is a food in the fat group, not in the dairy group.

2. This client consumed 3½ servings: 1 cup yogurt = 1 serving, 8 oz chocolate milk = 1 serving; 1 cup cottage cheese = ½ serving; and 1½ oz hard cheese = 1 serving.

3. This client consumed 2⅚ servings: 1 cup cottage cheese = ½ serving; 8 oz whole milk = 1 serving; 1 cup buttermilk = 1 serving; and ½ oz hard cheese = ⅓ serving.

4. This client consumed 2¼ servings: ½ cup frozen yogurt = ½ serving, 8 oz skim milk = 1 serving; 4 oz cream cheese = 0 serving; and 1½ cup cottage cheese = ¾ serving.

TEST-TAKING TIP: It is essential that the test taker know which foods are placed in which food groups and the equivalent quantity of food that meets one serving size. For example, 1 cup of any type of milk—whole, skim, butter, or even chocolate—is equal to one dairy serving, while 1½ oz of hard cheese, 1 cup of yogurt, 2 cups of cottage cheese, and 1½ cups of ice cream are all equal to one dairy serving.

77. 1. 4 tbsp of peanut butter = two 2 oz protein servings.
2. 2 eggs = one 2 oz protein serving.
3. 1 cup of cooked lima beans = two 2 oz protein servings.
4. 2 ounces of nuts = two 2 oz protein servings.

TEST-TAKING TIP: The test taker should refer to the U.S. Dietary Association information for up-to-date dietary recommendations. As more research information is forthcoming, dietary recommendations change. The current recommendations can be found at http://health.gov/dietaryguide-lines/dga2010/DietaryGuidelines2010.pdf.

78. 2, 4, and 5 are correct.
1. 1 bagel = two or more 1 oz servings (depending on the size of the bagel).
2. 1 slice bread = one 1 oz serving.
3. 1 cup cooked pasta = two 1 oz servings.
4. 1 tortilla = one 1 oz serving.
5. 1 cup dry cereal = one 1 oz serving.

TEST-TAKING TIP: The test taker should note that moderately active women of childbearing age are recommended to consume six to seven 1 oz servings of grain each day. However, 1 sandwich equals 2 servings since each piece of bread equals 1 serving. Also, it is important to counsel women to eat whole grain foods rather than processed grains. More nutrients as well as more fiber are obtained from whole grain foods.

79. 1. Although herbals are natural substances, there are many herbals that are unsafe for consumption during pregnancy.
2. Both licorice and cat's claw should be avoided during pregnancy. There is evidence that licorice may increase the incidence of preterm labor and cat's claw has been used to prevent and to abort pregnancies.
3. There is not enough evidence to determine whether or not many herbals are safe in pregnancy.
4. Every woman should advise her health care practitioner of what she is consuming, including food, medicines, herbals, and all other substances.

TEST-TAKING TIP: Herbals are not regulated by the Food and Drug Administration (FDA). There is some information on selected herbals at the National Institutes of Health Web site—http://nccam.nih.gov/health—but because research on pregnant women is particularly sensitive there is very little definitive information on the safety of many herbals in pregnancy. No matter what is consumed by the mother, however, the health care practitioner should be consulted.

80. 1. Chinese do consume protein, especially rice and seafood.
2. Many Chinese women do believe in the "hot and cold" theory of life.
3. Chinese women are no more prone to anemia than other groups of women.
4. The belief that strawberries cause birth defects is not particularly associated with the Chinese population.

TEST-TAKING TIP: Whenever a question specifies that a client belongs to a specific cultural or ethnic group, the test taker should attend carefully to that information. It is very likely that the question is asking the test taker to discern cultural/ethnic differences to discern the test taker's cultural competence. Pregnancy is believed by many Chinese, as well as women from other cultures, to be a "hot period." To maintain the equilibrium of the body, therefore, pregnant women consume "cold" foods and drinks.

81. 1. Potatoes and grapes are not high in folic acid.
    2. Cranberries and squash are not high in folic acid.
    3. Apples and corn are not high in folic acid
    4. Oranges and spinach are excellent folic acid sources.

    TEST-TAKING TIP: The intake of folic acid is especially important during the first trimester of pregnancy to help to prevent structural defects, including spina bifida and gastroschisis. The best sources of folic acid are liver and dark green, leafy vegetables. Oranges and orange juice are also good sources.

82. 1. Bologna should not be consumed during pregnancy unless it is thoroughly cooked.
    2. Cantaloupe is an excellent source of vitamins A and C.
    3. Asparagus is an excellent source of vitamin K and folic acid.
    4. Popcorn is an excellent source of fiber, although if loaded with butter and salt is not the most healthy fiber choice.

    TEST-TAKING TIP: Because pregnant women are slightly immunocompromised, they are especially susceptible to certain diseases. Deli meats, unless heated to steaming hot, can cause listeriosis. Pregnant women should avoid these foods. Other foods that contain *Listeria monocytogenes* that should be avoided are unpasteurized milk, soft cheese, and undercooked meats (see http://fda.gov/food/foodsafety/foodborneillness/foodborneillnessfoodbornepathogens naturaltoxins/badbugbook/ucm070064.htm and http://www.health.gov/dietary guidelines/dga2005/document/html/chapter10.htm).

83. 1. Fish is very healthy, but the recommendation is that the fish be well cooked.
    2. Although pregnant women should not overeat salty foods, sushi should be avoided because it is raw, not because of its salt content.
    3. All fish contain methylmercury, but there are some fish with such high levels that they should not be eaten at all: swordfish, tilefish, king mackerel, and shark. The mercury level does not change when a fish is eaten cooked versus raw.
    4. This is correct. It is recommended that during pregnancy the client eat only well-cooked fish.

    TEST-TAKING TIP: Fish is an excellent source of omega-3 oil and protein, but during pregnancy fish should be eaten well cooked to avoid ingestion of pathogens. It is recommended that pregnant women consume 8 to 12 oz of seafood per week. No more than 12 oz per week is recommended, however, to reduce the potential of consuming toxic levels of methylmercury (see www.health.gov/dietaryguidelines/dga2010/DietaryGuidelines2010.pdf).

84. 1. Raisins contain some iron but they are not the best source of iron.
    2. Hamburger contains the most iron.
    3. Broccoli contains some iron but it is not the best source of iron.
    4. Molasses contains some iron but it is not the best source of iron.

    TEST-TAKING TIP: Iron is present in most animal sources—seafood, meats, eggs—although it is not present in milk. There also is iron in vegetable sources, although not in the same concentration as in animal products. If the nurse is caring for a pregnant vegetarian, the nurse must counsel the client regarding good nonanimal sources of all nutrients.

85. 1. Hypothyroidism is not related to pica.
    2. Iron-deficiency anemia is often seen in clients who engage in pica.
    3. Hypercalcemia is not related to pica.
    4. Overexposure to zinc is not related to pica.

    TEST-TAKING TIP: Clients who engage in pica eat large quantities of nonfood items like ice, laundry starch, soap, and dirt. There are a number of problems related to pica, including teratogenesis related to eating foods harmful to the fetus. More commonly, the women fill up on items like ice instead of eating high-quality foods. This practice is often culturally related.

86. 1. This is not an appropriate substitute. High levels of salt can lead to elevated blood pressure and fluid retention.
    2. This is an excellent suggestion. Fruit juice, although high in sugar, does contain vitamins.
    3. This is not an appropriate substitute. Cream cheese has little to no nutritional benefit.
    4. This is not an appropriate substitute. Uncooked pie crust is high in fat and flour. It provides little to no nutritional benefit.

TEST-TAKING TIP: Although the nurse might prefer that a client completely stop a behavior that the nurse deems unsafe or inappropriate, the client may disagree. The nurse, therefore, must attempt to provide a substitute for the client's behavior. Pica is a behavior that should be discouraged because of its potentially detrimental effects. If the client wishes to consume ice, an excellent alternative is ice pops, Italian ices, or iced fruit juice.

87. 1. Ginger has been shown to be a safe antiemetic agent for pregnant women.
    2. Sage has not been shown to reduce nausea and vomiting in pregnant women.
    3. Cloves have not been shown to reduce nausea and vomiting in pregnant women.
    4. Nutmeg has not been shown to reduce nausea and vomiting in pregnant women.

TEST-TAKING TIP: Morning sickness and daytime nausea and vomiting are common complaints of pregnant women during the first trimester. Ginger, consumed as ginger tea, ginger ale, and the like, has been shown to be a safe and an effective anti-nausea agent for many pregnant women.

88. 1. Barley and brown rice are not good vitamin C sources.
    2. **Strawberries and potatoes are excellent sources of vitamin C, as are zucchini, blueberries, kiwi, green beans, green peas, and the like.**
    3. Buckwheat and lentils are not good vitamin C sources.
    4. Wheat flour and figs are not good vitamin C sources.

TEST-TAKING TIP: The test taker must be prepared to answer basic nutrition questions related to the health of the pregnant woman. Even though citrus fruits are commonly thought of as the primary sources of vitamin C, the test taker should realize that virtually all fruits and vegetables contain the vitamin, while grains do not.

89. 1. Yogurt is an excellent dairy source. Its intake should be encouraged.
    2. Parmesan cheese is an excellent dairy source. Its intake should be encouraged.
    3. **The intake of gorgonzola cheese should be discouraged during pregnancy.**
    4. Chocolate milk, although relatively high in calories, is an excellent dairy source. Its intake should be encouraged if the client refuses to drink unflavored milk.

TEST-TAKING TIP: Gorgonzola cheese is a soft cheese. Soft cheeses harbor *Listeria monocytogenes*, the organism that causes listeriosis. Pregnant women are at high risk of developing this infection because they are slightly immunosuppressed. The adult disease can assume many forms, including meningitis, pneumonia, and sepsis. Pregnant women who develop the disease often deliver stillborn babies or babies who are at risk of dying post-delivery from fulminant disease.

90. 2, 3, 4, and 5 are correct.
    1. The umbilical cord, not the amniotic fluid, delivers nutrition to the developing fetus.
    2. **Amniotic fluid does cushion the fetus from injury.**
    3. **Amniotic fluid enables the fetus's limbs and body to move freely so that the baby can grow unencumbered.**
    4. **The amniotic fluid is maintained at the mother's body temperature, providing the fetus with a neutral thermal environment.**
    5. **The fetus does swallow the amniotic fluid while in utero.**

TEST-TAKING TIP: The amniotic fluid is produced primarily by the fetus as fetal urine. In addition to the functions noted above, the baby practices "breathing" the amniotic fluid in and out of the lungs in preparation for breathing air in the extrauterine environment and "drinks" the amniotic fluid in preparation for extrauterine feeding.

91. 1. This statement is true. Organogenesis begins prior to the missed menstrual period.
    2. Insurance companies do not require a woman be preapproved to become pregnant.
    3. This statement is untrue. Only women with specific physical complications may be counseled to limit the numbers of pregnancies that they should carry.
    4. This statement is untrue. The cardiovascular system is stressed during each and every pregnancy.

TEST-TAKING TIP: The test taker may be unfamiliar with the term "organogenesis." To answer the question correctly, however, it is essential that the test taker be able to decipher the definition. It is important that the nurse break the word down into its parts to deduce the meaning. "Organo" means "organ" and "genesis" means "origin." The definition of the term, therefore, is origin, or development, of the organ systems.

92. 1, 2, 3, and 5 are correct.
    1. Although not yet clearly visible on ultrasound, the genitalia are formed by the end of the first trimester.
    2. The heart is formed by the end of the first trimester.
    3. The fingers are formed by the end of the first trimester.
    4. The alveoli will not be formed until well into the second trimester.
    5. The kidneys are formed by the end of the first trimester.

TEST-TAKING TIP: The test taker should be familiar with the basic developmental changes that occur during the three trimesters. In addition, the test taker should be able to develop a basic timeline of developmental milestones that occur during the pregnancy. By the conclusion of the first trimester, all major organs are completely formed. The maturation of the organ systems must, however, still occur.

93. 1. The foramen ovale is a hole between the atria.
    2. The umbilical vein carries oxygen-rich blood.
    3. The right atrium does contain both oxygen-rich and oxygen-poor blood.
    4. The ductus venosus lies between the umbilical vein and the inferior vena cava, not between the aorta and the pulmonary artery.

TEST-TAKING TIP: The test taker should have an understanding of fetal circulation. One principle to remember when studying the circulation of the fetus is that the blood bypasses the lungs since the baby is receiving oxygen-rich blood directly from the placenta via the umbilical vein. The location of the three ducts—ductus venosus, formen ovale, ductus arteriosus—therefore enable the blood to bypass the lungs.

94. 1. This is a true statement. In the morula stage, about 2 to 4 days after fertilization, the fertilized egg has not yet implanted in the uterus.
    2. Lung development occurs much later than the morular stage.

3. The sex of the fetus is identified much later than the morular stage.
4. The fetal eyelids unfuse much later than the morular stage.

TEST-TAKING TIP: The morula is the undifferentiated ball of cells that migrates down the fallopian tube toward the uterine body. The morular stage lasts from about the 2nd to the 4th day after fertilization.

95. 1. This is true of monozygotic twins.
    2. This is a true statement. Dizygotic twins result from two mature ova that are fertilized.
    3. This is true of monozygotic twins.
    4. This is true of monozygotic twins.

TEST-TAKING TIP: The best way for the test taker to differentiate between monozygotic twinning and dizygotic twinning is to remember the meaning of the prefixes to the two words. "Mono" means "1." Monozygotic twins, therefore, originate from one fertilized ovum. The babies have the same DNA; therefore, they are the same sex. They share a placenta and chorion. "Di" means "2." Dizygotic twins arise from 2 separately fertilized eggs. Their genetic relationship is the same as if they were siblings born from different pregnancies.

96. 1. The fetal heart begins to beat during the first trimester, not when quickening is detected at 16 to 20 weeks.
    2. Lanugo does cover the fetal body at approximately 20 weeks' gestation.
    3. The kidneys secrete urine by about week 12, before quickening is detected. Amniotic fluid is composed predominantly of fetal urine.
    4. Fingernails begin to form at about week 10 but do not completely cover the tips of the fingers until mid third trimester.

TEST-TAKING TIP: Although the test taker need not memorize all fetal developmental changes, it is important to have an understanding of major periods of development. For example, organogenesis occurs during the first trimester with all of the major organs functioning at a primitive level by week 12.

97. 1. The woman should be assured that it is unlikely that the fetus was affected.
    2. This statement is true.
    3. It is inappropriate for the nurse to suggest that the client seek an abortion.

4. The woman should be assured that it is unlikely that the fetus was affected.

TEST-TAKING TIP: The 2-week period between ovulation and implantation is often called "the all or nothing period." During that time, the fertilized egg/embryo is floating freely in the woman's fallopian tubes toward the uterine body. The mother is not supplying the embryo with nutrients at this time. Rather, the embryo is self-sufficient. If an insult occurs—for example, a teratogen is ingested or an abdominal x-ray is taken—the embryo is either destroyed or completely spared. And, since the pregnancy of the woman in the scenario was maintained, the nurse can assure her that the embryo was spared insult.

98. 1. Surfactant is usually formed in the fetal lungs by the 36th week.
    2. The eyes open and close at about 28 weeks.
    3. Fetal respiratory movements begin at about 24 weeks.
    4. The spinal column is completely formed well before the end of the first trimester.

TEST-TAKING TIP: The test taker should realize that this question is asking two things. First, the test taker needs to know what stage of pregnancy the woman is in when the fundal height is at the xiphoid process. Once the test taker realizes that this fundal height signifies 36 weeks' gestation, he or she must determine what other change or process is likely to be occurring at 36 weeks. The spinal column is completely formed by the end of the first trimester, fetal respiratory movements begin at about 24 weeks, and the eyes open and close at about 28 weeks. Surfactant, which is essential for mature lung function, forms in the fetal lungs at about 36 weeks. It is important for the nurse to realize that babies who are born preterm are high risk for a number of reasons, including lack of surfactant, lack of iron stores to sustain them during the early months of life, and lack of brown adipose tissue needed for thermoregulation.

99. The correct order is 3, 1, 2, 4.
    3. The blastocyst is developed about 6 days after fertilization and before implantation in the uterus has occurred.
    1. The four-chambered heart is formed during the early part of the first trimester.
    2. Vernix caseosa is present during the latter half of pregnancy.

4. The testes descend in the scrotal sac about mid third trimester.

TEST-TAKING TIP: Before putting these items into chronological order, the test taker should carefully analyze each choice. The blastocyst is developed by about day 6 after fertilization. The egg has yet even to implant into the uterine body at this point. The fetal heart develops during the early part of the first trimester, but after implantation. Vernix is present during the entire latter half of the pregnancy to protect the skin of the fetus. It appears, therefore, at about week 20. And, finally, the testes do not descend into the scrotal sac until mid third trimester. Indeed, male preterm babies are often birthed before the testes descend.

100. 1. This is an inappropriate statement. The nurse should provide clients with accurate information when asked.
     2. The sex is not established yet.
     3. The sex is not established yet.
     4. This statement is true. The sex is not visible yet.

TEST-TAKING TIP: The genitourinary system is the last organ system to fully develop. Before 12 weeks, both female and male genitalia are present. The sex is determined genetically, but it is as yet impossible to determine the sex visually. If the embryo secretes testosterone, the male sex organs mature and the female organs recede. If the embryo does not secrete testosterone, the male sex organs recede and the female organs mature. At 8 weeks, it is not possible to determine the sex of the fetus.

101. 1. Fingernails would likely be quite long.
     2. Eyelashes would be present.
     3. Because this baby is post-term, lanugo would likely not be present.
     4. Milia would be present.

TEST-TAKING TIP: Lanugo is a fine hair that covers the body of the fetus. It begins to disappear at about 38 weeks and very likely has completely vanished by 41 weeks' gestation.

102. 1. 15 weeks is too early for quickening. At 15 weeks, the fetus would not have lanugo.
     2. This fetus is about 22 weeks' gestation. Nails start to develop in the first

trimester, and lanugo starts to develop at about 20 weeks, but eyes remain fused until about 29 weeks. In addition, quickening occurs by week 20.

3. The eyes are unfused by 29 weeks' gestation so the gestation is shorter than that.

4. The eyes are unfused by 29 weeks' gestation so the gestation is shorter than that.

TEST-TAKING TIP: The test taker should not panic when reading a question like the one in the scenario. This is an application question that requires the test taker to take things apart and put them back together again. Each of the signs is unique and relates to a specific period in fetal development. After an analysis, the only response that is plausible is choice 2.

103. 1. This response is incorrect. The circulatory systems are never connected.
2. This response is incorrect. The blood never mixes.

3. This response is incorrect. The systems are never connected.

4. The blood supplies are completely separate.

TEST-TAKING TIP: It is important to understand the relationship between the maternal vascular system and the fetal system. There is a maternal portion to the placenta and a fetal portion of the placenta. By the time the placenta is fully functioning, at about 12 weeks' gestation, fetal blood vessels have burrowed into the decidual lining and maternal vessels have burrowed into the chorionic layer. The vessels, therefore, lie next to each other. Gases and nutrients, then, move across the membranes of the vessels to provide the baby with needed substances and for the mother to dispose of waste products.

104. An "X" will be placed between the neonatal and maternal vessels where gas exchange occurs.

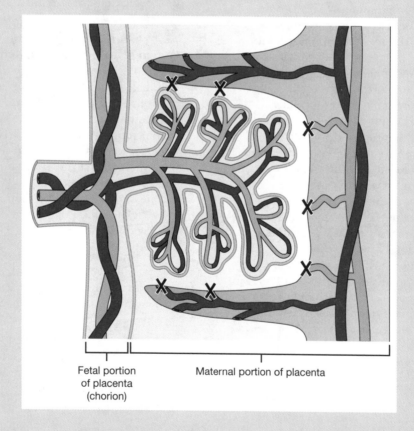

Fetal portion of placenta (chorion)   Maternal portion of placenta

TEST-TAKING TIP: It is important that the test taker have a complete understanding of the anatomy and the physiology of the placenta. Since this is the sole organ that maintains the health and well-being of the fetus, the nurse must be able to differentiate between the maternal portion and the fetal portion as well as the function of the structures.

105. 1. This statement is correct. The maternal mortality rate is the number of deaths of women as a result of the childbearing period per 100,000 live births.
2. This statement is incorrect. The maternal mortality rate is the number of deaths of women as a result of the childbearing period per 100,000 live births, not of women of childbearing age.
3. This statement is incorrect. The maternal mortality rate is the number of deaths of women as a result of the childbearing period per 100,000 live births, not 100,000 pregnancies.
4. This statement is incorrect. The maternal mortality rate is the number of deaths of women as a result of the childbearing period per 100,000 live births.

TEST-TAKING TIP: One important indicator of the quality of health care in a country is its maternal mortality rate. The rate in the United States is very low as compared to many other countries in the world and yet well above other countries. For example, in 2008, the maternal mortality rate in the United States was 24/100,000 live births while in Austria, Belgium, and Denmark the rate was 5/100,000 live births and in both Chad and Somalia the rate was 1200 deaths per 100,000 live births (see http://who.int/en/).

Intrapartum

5

Intrapartum, or labor and delivery, constitutes the birthing process. A pregnant woman enters labor, usually accompanied by her partner and/or other family members. Then, in a matter of hours, she leaves the delivery suite with an additional member of the family. During this period of transition, nurses assist the woman and her significant others to become a newly formed family.

It is a distinct privilege to be part of that process. The nurse must be familiar not only with the many physiological needs of the woman in labor but also of the woman's and her family's psychosocial needs. Birthing is a natural process but, because complications may arise, the nurse must carefully monitor both the mother's and the baby's physiological responses. In addition, the nurse must be prepared to assist the mother with her needs for pain relief and with her cultural, spiritual, and emotional needs.

KEYWORDS

The following words include English vocabulary, nursing/medical terminology, concepts, principles, or information relevant to content specifically addressed in the chapter or associated with topics presented in it. English dictionaries, your nursing textbooks, and medical dictionaries such as *Taber's Cyclopedic Medical Dictionary* are resources that can be used to expand your knowledge and understanding of these words and related information.

acceleration of fetal heart
active phase (phase 2) of the first stage
 of labor
attitude
The Bradley Method®
cardinal moves of labor
   flexion
   descent
   internal rotation
   extension
   external rotation
   expulsion
childbirth education
contraction
delivery
dilation (dilatation)
doula
duration
early deceleration
effacement
effleurage
electronic fetal monitoring
engagement

epidural
fetal heart rate
frequency
intensity
labor
Lamaze®
late deceleration
latent phase (phase 1) of the first stage of
 labor
Leopold's maneuvers
lie
mentum
midwife
pelvic measurements
pelvic rock
placenta
position
presentation
   occipital
   mentum
   sacral
   scapular
regional anesthesia

stage 1 of labor (cervical change to 10 centimeters dilation)

stage 2 of labor (full dilation to birth of the baby)

stage 3 of labor (birth of the baby to birth of the placenta)

station

transition (phase 3) of the first stage of labor

vaginal introitus

variability

variable deceleration

QUESTIONS

1. A client enters the labor and delivery suite stating that she thinks she is in labor. Which of the following information about the woman should the nurse note from the woman's prenatal record before proceeding with the physical assessment? **Select all that apply.**
   1. Weight gain.
   2. Ethnicity and religion.
   3. Age.
   4. Type of insurance.
   5. Gravidity and parity.

2. A woman who states that she "thinks" she is in labor enters the labor suite. Which of the following assessments will provide the nurse with the most valuable information regarding the client's labor status?
   1. Leopold's maneuvers.
   2. Fundal contractility.
   3. Fetal heart assessment.
   4. Vaginal examination.

3. A client in labor, G2 P1001, was admitted 1 hour ago at 2 cm dilated and 50% effaced. She was talkative and excited at that time. During the past 10 minutes she has become serious, closing her eyes and breathing rapidly with each contraction. Which of the following is an accurate nursing assessment of the situation?
   1. The client had poor childbirth education prior to labor.
   2. The client is exhibiting an expected behavior for labor.
   3. The client is becoming hypoxic and hypercapnic.
   4. The client needs her alpha-fetoprotein levels checked.

4. A woman has just arrived at the labor and delivery suite. To report the client's status to her primary health care practitioner, which of the following assessments should the nurse perform? **Select all that apply.**
   1. Fetal heart rate.
   2. Contraction pattern.
   3. Urinalysis.
   4. Vital signs.
   5. Biophysical profile.

5. While performing Leopold's maneuvers on a woman in labor, the nurse palpates a hard round mass in the fundal area, a flat surface on the left side, small objects on the right side, and a soft round mass just above the symphysis. Which of the following is a reasonable conclusion by the nurse?
   1. The fetal position is transverse.
   2. The fetal presentation is vertex.
   3. The fetal lie is vertical.
   4. The fetal attitude is flexed.

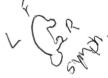

6. When during the latent phase of labor should the nurse assess the fetal heart pattern of a low-risk woman, G1 P0000? **Select all that apply.**
   1. After vaginal exams.
   2. Before administration of analgesics.
   3. Periodically at the end of a contraction.
   4. Every ten minutes.
   5. Before ambulating.

7. The nurse is assessing the fetal station during a vaginal examination. Which of the following structures should the nurse palpate?
   1. Sacral promontory.
   2. Ischial spines.
   3. Cervix.
   4. Symphysis pubis.

8. The labor and delivery nurse performs Leopold's maneuvers. A soft round mass is felt in the fundal region. A flat object is noted on the left and small objects are noted on the right of the uterus. A hard round mass is noted above the symphysis. Which of the following positions is consistent with these findings?
   1. Left occipital anterior (LOA).
   2. Left sacral posterior (LSP).
   3. Right mentum anterior (RMA).
   4. Right sacral posterior (RSP).

9. A nurse is caring for a laboring woman who is in transition. Which of the following signs/symptoms would indicate that the woman is progressing into the second stage of labor? **Select all that apply.**
   1. Bulging perineum.
   2. Increased bloody show.
   3. Spontaneous rupture of the membranes.
   4. Uncontrollable urge to push.
   5. Inability to breathe through contractions.

10. During a vaginal examination, the nurse palpates fetal buttocks that are facing the left posterior and are 1 cm above the ischial spines. Which of the following is consistent with this assessment?
    1. LOA –1 station.
    2. LSP –1 station.
    3. LMP +1 station.
    4. LSA +1 station.

11. The nurse enters a laboring client's room. The client is complaining of intense back pain with each contraction. The nurse concludes that the fetus is likely in which of the following positions?
    1. Mentum anterior.
    2. Sacrum posterior.
    3. Occiput posterior.
    4. Scapula anterior.

12. When performing Leopold's maneuvers, the nurse notes that the fetus is in the left occiput anterior position. Which is the best position for the nurse to place a fetoscope to hear the fetal heartbeat?
    1. Left upper quadrant.
    2. Right upper quadrant.
    3. Left lower quadrant.
    4. Right lower quadrant.

13. On examination, it is noted that a full-term primipara in active labor is right occipitoanterior (ROA), 7 cm dilated, and +3 station. Which of the following should the nurse report to the physician?
    1. Descent is progressing well.
    2. Fetal head is not yet engaged. ✗
    3. Vaginal delivery is imminent.
    4. External rotation is complete.

14. One hour ago, a multipara was examined with the following results: 8 cm, 50% effaced, and +1 station. She is now pushing with contractions and the fetal head is seen at the vaginal introitus. The nurse concludes that the client is now:
    1. 9 cm dilated, 70% effaced, and +2 station.
    2. 9 cm dilated, 80% effaced, and +3 station.
    3. 10 cm dilated, 90% effaced, and +4 station.
    4. 10 cm dilated, 100% effaced, and +5 station.

15. The nurse is caring for a nulliparous client who attended Lamaze childbirth education classes. Which of the following techniques should the nurse include in her plan of care? **Select all that apply.**
    1. Hypnotic suggestion.
    2. Rhythmic chanting.
    3. Muscle relaxation.
    4. Pelvic rocking.
    5. Abdominal massage.

16. Which of the following responses is the primary rationale for the inclusion of the information taught in childbirth education classes?
    1. Mothers who are performing breathing exercises during labor refrain from yelling.
    2. Breathing and relaxation exercises are less exhausting than crying and moaning.
    3. Knowledge learned at childbirth education classes helps to break the fear-tension-pain cycle.
    4. Childbirth education classes help to promote positive maternal–newborn bonding.

17. The childbirth educator is teaching a class of pregnant couples the breathing technique that is most appropriate during the second stage of labor. Which of the following techniques did the nurse teach the women to do?
    1. Alternately pant and blow.
    2. Take rhythmic, shallow breaths.
    3. Push down with an open glottis.
    4. Do slow chest breathing.

18. A nurse is teaching childbirth education classes to a group of pregnant teens. Which of the following strategies would promote learning by the young women?
    1. Avoiding the discussion of uncomfortable procedures like vaginal exams and blood tests.
    2. Focusing the discussion on baby care rather than on labor and delivery.
    3. Utilizing visual aids like movies and posters during the classes.
    4. Having the classes at a location other than high school to reduce their embarrassment.

19. A client who is 7 cm dilated and 100% effaced is breathing at a rate of 50 breaths per minute during contractions. Immediately after a contraction, she complains of tingling in her fingers and some light-headedness. Which of the following actions should the nurse take at this time?
    1. Assess the blood pressure.
    2. Have the woman breathe into a bag.
    3. Turn the woman on her side.
    4. Check the fetal heart rate.

20. A nurse is teaching a class of pregnant couples the most therapeutic breathing technique for the latent phase of labor. Which of the following techniques did the nurse teach?
    1. Alternately panting and blowing.
    2. Rapid, deep breathing.
    3. Grunting and pushing with contractions.
    4. Slow chest breathing.

21. A woman, G2 P0101, 5 cm dilated, and 30% effaced, is doing first-level Lamaze breathing with contractions. The nurse detects that the woman's shoulder and face muscles are beginning to tense during the contractions. Which of the following interventions should the nurse perform first?
    1. Encourage the woman to have an epidural.
    2. Encourage the woman to accept intravenous analgesia.
    3. Encourage the woman to change her position.
    4. Encourage the woman to perform the next level breathing.

22. In addition to breathing with contractions, which of the following actions can help a woman in the first stage of labor to work with her pain?
    1. Lying in the lithotomy position.
    2. Performing effleurage.
    3. Practicing Kegel exercises.
    4. Pushing with each contraction.

23. A client is in the second stage of labor. She falls asleep immediately after a contraction. Which of the following actions should the nurse perform as a result?
    1. Awaken the woman and remind her to push.
    2. Cover the woman's perineum with a sheet.
    3. Assess the woman's blood pressure and pulse.
    4. Administer oxygen to the woman via face mask.

24. A gravid client, G3 P2002, was examined 5 minutes ago. Her cervix was 8 cm dilated and 90% effaced. She now states that she needs to move her bowels. Which of the following actions should the nurse perform first?
    1. Offer the client the bedpan.
    2. Evaluate the progress of labor.
    3. Notify the physician.
    4. Encourage the patient to push.

25. The nurse auscultates a fetal heart rate of 152 on a client in early labor. Which of the following actions by the nurse is appropriate?
    1. Inform the mother that the rate is normal.
    2. Reassess in 5 minutes to verify the results.
    3. Immediately report the rate to the health care practitioner.
    4. Place the client on her left side and apply oxygen by face mask.

110-160

26. The nurse documents in a laboring woman's chart that the fetal heart is being "assessed via intermittent auscultation." To be consistent with this statement, the nurse, using a Doppler electrode, should assess the fetal heart at which of the following times?
    1. After every contraction.
    2. For 10 minutes every half hour.
    3. Periodically during the peak of contractions.
    4. For 1 minute immediately after contractions.

27. While caring for a client in the transition phase of labor, the nurse notes that the fetal monitor tracing shows average short-term and long-term variability with a baseline of 142 beats per minute (bpm). What should the nurse do?
    1. Provide caring labor support.
    2. Administer oxygen via face mask.
    3. Change the client's position.
    4. Speed up the client's intravenous.

28. While evaluating the fetal heart monitor tracing on a client in labor, the nurse notes that there are fetal heart decelerations present. Which of the following assessments must the nurse make at this time?
    1. The relationship between the decelerations and the labor contractions.
    2. The maternal blood pressure.
    3. The gestational age of the fetus.
    4. The placement of the fetal heart electrode in relation to the fetal position.

29. A client is complaining of severe back labor. Which of the following nursing interventions would be most effective?
    1. Assist mother with childbirth breathing.
    2. Encourage mother to have an epidural.
    3. Provide direct sacral pressure.
    4. Move the woman to a hydrotherapy tub.

30. An obstetrician is performing an amniotomy on a gravid woman in transition. Which of the following assessments must the nurse make immediately following the procedure?
    1. Maternal blood pressure.
    2. Maternal pulse.
    3. Fetal heart rate.
    4. Fetal fibronectin level.

31. A nurse has just performed a vaginal examination on a client in labor. The nurse palpates the baby's buttocks as facing the mother's right side. Where should the nurse place the external fetal monitor electrode?
    1. Left upper quadrant (LUQ).
    2. Left lower quadrant (LLQ).
    3. Right upper quadrant (RUQ).
    4. Right lower quadrant (RLQ).

32. Upon examination, a nurse notes that a woman is 10 cm dilated, 100% effaced, and –3 station. Which of the following actions should the nurse perform during the next contraction?
    1. Encourage the woman to push.
    2. Provide firm fundal pressure.
    3. Move the client into a squat.
    4. Monitor for signs of rectal pressure.

33. A woman has decided to hire a doula to work with her during labor and delivery. Which of the following actions would be appropriate for the doula to perform? Select all that apply.
    1. Give the woman a back rub.
    2. Assist the woman with her breathing.
    3. Assess the fetal heart rate.
    4. Check the woman's blood pressure.
    5. Regulate the woman's intravenous.

34. The nurse is assessing a client who states, "I think I'm in labor." Which of the following findings would positively confirm the client's belief?
    1. She is contracting q 5 min × 60 sec.
    2. Her cervix has dilated from 2 to 4 cm.
    3. Her membranes have ruptured.
    4. The fetal head is engaged.

35. The childbirth education nurse is evaluating the learning of four women, 38 to 40 weeks' gestation, regarding when they should go to the hospital. The nurse determines that the teaching was successful when a client makes which of the following statements? **Select all that apply.**
    1. The client who says, "If I feel a pain in my back and lower abdomen every 5 minutes."
    2. The client who says, "When I feel a gush of clear fluid from my vagina."
    3. The client who says, "When I go to the bathroom and see the mucous plug on the toilet tissue."
    4. The client who says, "If I ever notice a greenish discharge from my vagina."
    5. The client who says, "When I have felt cramping in my abdomen for 4 hours or more." – Braxton Hicks

36. A woman, 40 weeks' gestation, calls the labor unit to see whether or not she should go to the hospital to be evaluated. Which of the following statements by the woman indicates that she is probably in labor and should proceed to the hospital?
    1. "The contractions are 5 to 20 minutes apart."
    2. "I saw a pink discharge on the toilet tissue when I went to the bathroom."
    3. "I have had cramping for the past 3 or 4 hours."
    4. "The contractions are about a minute long and I am unable to talk through them."

37. A low-risk 38-week gestation woman calls the labor unit and says, "I have to come to the hospital right now. I just saw pink streaks on the toilet tissue when I went to the bathroom. I'm bleeding." Which of the following responses should the nurse make first?
    1. "Does it burn when you void?"
    2. "You sound frightened."
    3. "That is just the mucous plug."
    4. "How much blood is there?"

38. A gravid client at term called the labor suite at 7:00 p.m. questioning whether she was in labor. The nurse determined that the client was likely in labor after the client stated:
    1. "At 5:00 p.m., the contractions were about 5 minutes apart. Now they're about 7 minutes apart."
    2. "I took a walk at 5:00 p.m., and now I talk through my contractions easier than I could then."
    3. "I took a shower about a half hour ago. The contractions seem to hurt more since I finished."
    4. "I had some tightening in my belly late this afternoon, and I still feel it after waking up from my 2-hour nap."

39. A nurse describes a client's contraction pattern as: frequency every 3 min and duration 60 sec. Which of the following responses corresponds to this description?
    1. Contractions lasting 60 seconds followed by a 1-minute rest period.
    2. Contractions lasting 120 seconds followed by a 2-minute rest period.
    3. Contractions lasting 2 minutes followed by a 60-second rest period.
    4. Contractions lasting 1 minute followed by a 120-second rest period.

40. A nurse determines that a client is carrying a fetus in the vertical lie. The nurse's judgment should be questioned if the fetal presenting part is which of the following?
    1. Sacrum.
    2. Occiput.
    3. Mentum.
    4. Scapula.

41. A nurse is educating a pregnant woman regarding the moves a fetus makes during the birthing process. Please place the following cardinal movements of labor in the order the nurse should inform the client that the fetus will make:
   1. Descent.
   2. Expulsion.
   3. Extension.
   4. External rotation.
   5. Internal rotation.

42. The nurse sees the fetal head through the vaginal introitus when a woman pushes. The nurse, interpreting this finding, tells the client, "You are pushing very well." In addition, the nurse could also state which of the following?
   1. "The baby's head is engaged."
   2. "The baby is floating."
   3. "The baby is at the ischial spines."
   4. "The baby is almost crowning."

43. A midwife advises a mother that her obstetric conjugate is of average size. How should the nurse interpret that information for the mother?
   1. The anterior to posterior diameter of the pelvis will accommodate a fetus with an average-sized head.
   2. The fetal head is flexed so that it is of average diameter.
   3. The mother's cervix is of average dilation for the start of labor.
   4. The distance between the mother's physiological retraction ring and the fetal head is of average dimensions.

44. The frequency of the contractions seen on the monitor tracing below is q _3 min_

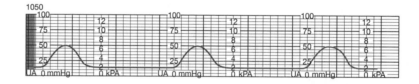

45. The duration of the contractions seen on the monitor tracing below is q _90 sec._

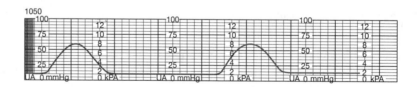

46. Which of the following frequency and duration assessments are consistent with the pattern shown below?

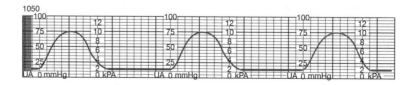

   1. q 2 min × 60 sec.
   2. q 2 min × 90 sec.
   3. q 3 min × 60 sec.
   4. q 3 min × 90 sec.

47. A woman who is in active labor is told by her obstetrician, "Your baby is in the flexed attitude." When she asks the nurse what that means, what should the nurse say?
1. The baby is in the breech position.
2. The baby is in the horizontal lie.
3. The baby's presenting part is engaged.
4. The baby's chin is resting on its chest.

48. An ultrasound report states, "The fetal head has entered the pelvic inlet." What does the nurse interpret this statement to mean?
1. The fetus has become engaged.
2. The fetal head has entered the true pelvis.
3. The fetal lie is horizontal.
4. The fetus is in an extended attitude.

49. Which of the following pictures depicts a fetus in the ROP position?

1.   2.   3.   4.

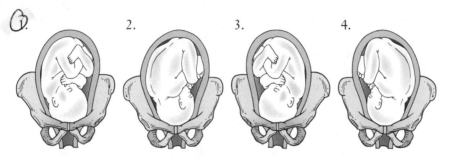

50. Which of the following pictures depicts a fetus in the LSA position?

1.   2.   3.   4.

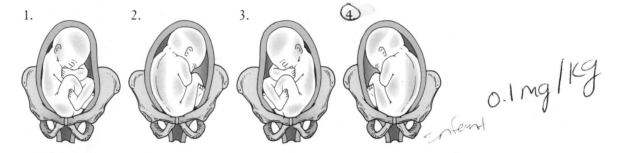

Infant 0.1 mg/kg

51. Which of the following pictures depicts a fetus in the frank breech position?

1.   2.   3.   4.

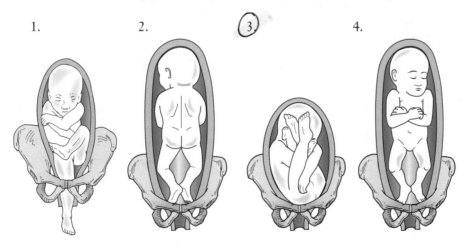

52. During delivery, the nurse notes that the baby's head has just been delivered. The nurse concludes that the baby has just gone through which of the following cardinal moves of labor?
    1. Flexion.
    2. Internal rotation.
    3. Extension.
    4. External rotation.

53. The nurse wishes to assess the variability of the fetal heart rate. Which of the following actions is recommended prior to performing this assessment?
    1. Place the client in the lateral recumbent position.
    2. Insert an internal fetal monitor electrode.
    3. Administer oxygen to the mother via face mask.
    4. Ask the mother to indicate when she feels fetal movement.

54. The nurse is interpreting the fetal monitor tracing below. Which of the following actions should the nurse take at this time?
    1. Provide caring labor support.
    2. Administer oxygen via tight-fitting face mask.
    3. Turn the woman on her side.
    4. Apply the oxygen saturation electrode to the mother.

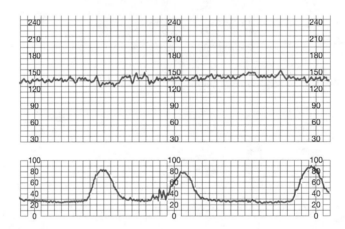

55. After analyzing an internal fetal monitor tracing, the nurse concludes that there is moderate short-term variability. Which of the following interpretations should the nurse make in relation to this finding?
    1. The fetus is becoming hypoxic.
    2. The fetus is becoming alkalotic.
    3. The fetus is in the middle of a sleep cycle.
    4. The fetus has a healthy nervous system.

56. When would the nurse expect to see the monitor tracing shown below?
    1. During latent phase of labor.
    2. During an epidural insertion.
    3. During second stage of labor.
    4. During delivery of the placenta.

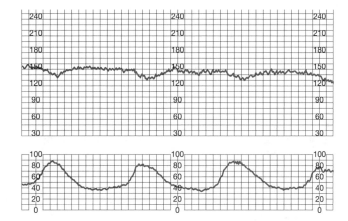

57. When would the nurse expect to see the fetal heart changes noted on the monitor tracing shown below?
    1. During fetal movement.
    2. After the administration of analgesics.
    3. When the fetus is acidotic.
    4. With poor placental perfusion.

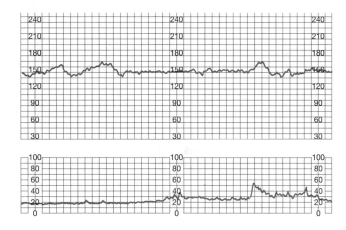

58. A woman is in active labor and is being monitored electronically. She has just received Stadol 2 mg IM for pain. Which of the following fetal heart responses would the nurse expect to see on the internal monitor tracing?
    1. Variable decelerations.
    2. Late decelerations.
    3. Decreased variability.
    4. Transient accelerations.

59. The nurse is assessing an internal fetal heart monitor tracing of an unmedicated, full-term gravida who is in transition. Which of the following heart rate patterns would the nurse interpret as normal?
    1. Baseline of 140 to 150 with V-shaped decelerations to 120 unrelated to contractions.
    2. Baseline of 140 to 150 with decelerations to 100 that mirror each of the contractions.
    3. Baseline of 140 to 142 with decelerations to 120 that return to baseline after the end of the contractions.
    4. Baseline of 140 to 142 with no obvious decelerations or accelerations.

60. A woman is in the second stage of labor with a strong urge to push. Which of the following actions by the nurse is appropriate at this time?
    1. Assess the fetal heart rate between contractions every 60 minutes.
    2. Encourage the woman to grunt during contractions.
    3. Assess the pulse and respirations of the mother every 5 minutes.
    4. Position the woman on her back with her knees on her chest.

61. A nurse is coaching a woman who is in the second stage of labor. Which of the following should the nurse encourage the woman to do?
    1. Hold her breath for twenty seconds during every contraction.
    2. Blow out forcefully during every contraction.
    3. Push between contractions until the fetal head is visible.
    4. Take a slow cleansing breath before bearing down.

62. A primigravida is pushing with contractions. The nurse notes that the woman's perineum is beginning to bulge and that there is an increase in bloody show. Which of the following actions by the nurse is appropriate at this time?
    1. Report the findings to the woman's health care practitioner.
    2. Immediately assess the woman's pulse and blood pressure.
    3. Continue to provide encouragement during each contraction.
    4. Place the client on her side with oxygen via face mask.

63. A multipara, LOA, station +3, who has had no pain medication during her labor, is now in stage 2. She states that her pain is 6 on a 10-point scale and that she wants an epidural. Which of the following responses by the nurse is appropriate?
    1. "Epidurals do not work well when the pain level is above level 5."
    2. "I will contact the doctor to get an order for an epidural right away."
    3. "The baby is going to be born very soon. It is really too late for an epidural."
    4. "I will check the fetal heart rate. You can have an epidural if it is over 120."

64. A pregnant woman is discussing positioning and the use of leg stirrups for delivery with a labor nurse. Which of the following client responses indicates that the client understood the information? **Select all that apply.**
    1. When the client states, "I am glad that deliveries can take place in a variety of places, including a Jacuzzi bathtub."
    2. When the client says, "I heard that for doctors to deliver babies safely, it is essential to have the mother's legs up in stirrups."
    3. When the client states, "I understand that if the fetus needs to turn during labor, I may end up delivering the baby on my hands and knees."
    4. When the client says, "During difficult deliveries it is sometimes necessary to put a woman's legs up in stirrups."
    5. When the client states, "I heard that midwives often deliver their patients either in the side-lying or squatting position."

65. During the third stage, the following physiological changes occur. Please place the changes in chronological order.
    1. Hematoma forms behind the placenta.
    2. Membranes separate from the uterine wall.
    3. The uterus contracts firmly.
    4. The uterine surface area dramatically decreases.

66. A woman had a baby by normal spontaneous delivery 10 minutes ago. The nurse notes that a gush of blood was just expelled from the vagina and the umbilical cord lengthened. What should the nurse conclude?
    1. The woman has an internal laceration.
    2. The woman is about to deliver the placenta.
    3. The woman has an atonic uterus.
    4. The woman is ready to expel the cord bloods.

67. A client is in the third stage of labor. Which of the following assessments should the nurse make/observe for? **Select all that apply.**
    1. Lengthening of the umbilical cord.
    2. Fetal heart assessment after each contraction.
    3. Uterus rising in the abdomen and feeling globular.
    4. Rapid cervical dilation to ten centimeters.
    5. Maternal complaints of intense rectal pressure.

68. A woman is in the transition phase of labor. Which of the following comments should the nurse expect to hear?
    1. "I am so excited to be in labor."
    2. "I can't stand this pain any longer!"
    3. "I need ice chips because I'm so hot."
    4. "I have to push the baby out right now!"

69. A client in labor is talkative and happy. How many centimeters dilated would a maternity nurse suspect that the client is at this time?
    1. 2 cm.
    2. 4 cm.
    3. 8 cm.
    4. 10 cm.

70. A nurse is assessing the vital signs of a client in labor at the peak of a contraction. Which of the following findings would the nurse expect to see?
    1. Decreased pulse rate.
    2. Hypertension.
    3. Hyperthermia
    4. Decreased respiratory rate.

71. A woman, G1 P0000, 40 weeks' gestation, entered the labor suite stating that she is in labor. Upon examination it is noted that the woman is 2 cm dilated, 30% effaced, contracting every 12 min × 30 sec. Fetal heart rate is in the 140s with good variability and spontaneous accelerations. What should the nurse conclude when reporting the findings to the primary health care practitioner?
    1. The woman is high risk and should be placed on tocolytics.
    2. The woman is in early labor and could be sent home.
    3. The woman is high risk and could be induced.
    4. The woman is in active labor and should be admitted to the unit.

72. A nurse concludes that a woman is in the latent phase of labor. Which of the following signs/symptoms would lead a nurse to that conclusion?
    1. The woman talks and laughs during contractions.
    2. The woman complains about severe back labor.
    3. The woman performs effleurage during a contraction.
    4. The woman asks to go to the bathroom to defecate.

73. A G1 P0, 8 cm dilated, is to receive pain medication. The health care practitioner has decided to order an opiate analgesic with an analgesic-potentiating medication. Which of the following medications would the nurse expect to be ordered as the analgesic-potentiating medication?
    1. Seconal (secobarbital).
    2. Vistaril (hydroxyzine).
    3. Benadryl (diphenhydramine).
    4. Tylenol (acetaminophen).

74. On vaginal examination, it is noted that a woman with a well-functioning epidural is in the second stage of labor. The station is –2 and the baseline fetal heart rate is 130 with no decelerations. Which of the following nursing actions is appropriate at this time?
    1. Coach the woman to hold her breath while pushing 3 to 4 times with each contraction.
    2. Administer oxygen via face mask at 8 to 10 liters per minute.
    3. Delay pushing until the baby descends further and the mother has a strong urge to push.
    4. Place the woman on her side and assess her oxygen saturation.

75. A nurse is assisting an anesthesiologist who is inserting an epidural catheter. Which of the following positions should the nurse assist the woman into?
    1. Fetal position.
    2. Lithotomy position.
    3. Trendelenburg position.
    4. Lateral recumbent position.

76. Which of the following actions would the nurse expect to perform immediately before a woman is to have regional anesthesia? **Select all that apply.**
    1. Assess fetal heart rate.
    2. Infuse 1,000 mL of Ringer's lactate.
    3. Place the woman in the Trendelenburg position.
    4. Monitor blood pressure every 5 minutes for 15 minutes.
    5. Have the woman empty her bladder.

77. Immediately following administration of an epidural anesthesia, the nurse must monitor the mother for which of the following?
    1. Paresthesias in her feet and legs.
    2. Drop in blood pressure.
    3. Increase in central venous pressure.
    4. Fetal heart accelerations.

78. A client, G2 P1001, 5 cm dilated and 40% effaced, has just received an epidural. Which of the following actions is important for the nurse to take at this time?
    1. Assess the woman's temperature.
    2. Place a wedge under the woman's side.
    3. Place a blanket roll under the woman's feet.
    4. Assess the woman's pedal pulses.

79. The practitioner is performing a fetal scalp stimulation test. Which of the following fetal responses would the nurse expect to see?
    1. Spontaneous fetal movement.
    2. Fetal heart acceleration.
    3. Increase in fetal heart variability.
    4. Resolution of late decelerations.

80. The nurse is interpreting the results of a fetal blood sampling test. Which of the following reports would the nurse expect to see?
    1. Oxygen saturation of 99%.
    2. Hgb of 11 g/dL.
    3. Serum glucose of 140 mg/dL.
    4. pH of 7.30.

81. Which of the following actions is appropriate for the nurse to perform when caring for a Chinese-speaking woman in active labor?
    1. Apply heat to the woman's back.
    2. Inquire regarding the woman's pain level.
    3. Make sure that the woman's head is covered.
    4. Accept the woman's loud verbalizations.

82. A nurse is caring for women from four different countries. Which of the women is most likely to request that her head be kept covered throughout her hospitalization?
    1. Arabic woman.
    2. Chinese woman.
    3. Russian woman.
    4. Greek woman.

83. The nurse is caring for an Orthodox Jewish woman in labor. It would be appropriate for the nurse to include which of the following in the plan of care?
    1. Encourage the father to hold his partner's hand during labor.
    2. Ask the woman if she would like to speak with her priest.
    3. Provide the woman with a long-sleeved hospital gown.
    4. Place an order for the woman's postpartum vegetarian diet.

84. Which of the following nonpharmacological interventions recommended by nurse midwives may help a client at full term to go into labor? **Select all that apply.**
    1. Engage in sexual intercourse.
    2. Ingest evening primrose oil.
    3. Perform yoga exercises.
    4. Eat raw spinach.
    5. Massage the breast and nipples.

85. The nurse is providing acupressure to provide pain relief to a woman in labor. Where is the best location for the acupressure to be applied? **Select all that apply.**
    1. On the malleolus of the wrist.
    2. Above the patella of the knee.
    3. On the medial aspect of the lower leg.
    4. At the top one third of the sole of the foot.
    5. Below the medial epicondyle of the elbow.

86. To decrease the possibility of a perineal laceration during delivery, the nurse performs which of the following interventions prior to the delivery?
    1. Assists the woman into a squatting position.
    2. Advises the woman to push only when she feels the urge.
    3. Encourages the woman to push slowly and steadily.
    4. Massages the perineum with mineral oil.

87. The physician writes the following order for a newly admitted client in labor: Begin a 1000 mL IV of D5 1/2 NS at 150 mL/hr. The IV tubing states that the drop factor is 10 gtt/mL. Please calculate the drip rate to the nearest whole.
    _____ gtt/min

88. The health care practitioner orders the following medication for a laboring client: Stadol 0.5 mg IV STAT for pain. The drug is on hand in the following concentration: Stadol 2 mg/mL. How many mL of medication will the nurse administer? **Calculate to the nearest hundredth.**
    _____ mL

89. The nurse is performing a vaginal examination on a client in labor. The client is found to be 5 cm dilated, 90% effaced, and station –2. Which of the following has the nurse palpated?
    1. Thin cervix.
    2. Bulging fetal membranes.
    3. Head at the pelvic outlet.
    4. Closed cervix.

90. It is 4 p.m. A client, G1 P0000, 3 cm dilated, asks the nurse when the dinner tray will be served. The nurse replies:
    1. "Laboring clients are never allowed to eat."
    2. "Believe me, you will not want to eat by the time it is the dinner hour. Most women throw up, you know."
    3. "The dinner tray should arrive in an hour or two."
    4. "A heavy meal is discouraged. I can get clear fluids for you whenever you would like them, though."

The correct answer number and rationale for why it is the correct answer are given in **boldface blue type**. Rationales for why the other possible answer options are incorrect also are given, but they are not in boldface type.

1. **1, 2, 3, and 5 are correct.**
   1. **Before proceeding with a physical assessment, the nurse should check the client's weight gain reported in her prenatal record.**
   2. **The client's ethnicity and religion should be noted before physical assessment. This allows the nurse to proceed in a culturally sensitive manner.**
   3. **The client's age should also be noted before the physical assessment is begun.**
   4. The type of insurance the woman has is not relevant to the nurse.
   5. **The client's gravidity and parity—how many times she has been pregnant and how many times she has given birth—should also be noted before a physical assessment is begun.**

   TEST-TAKING TIP: The prenatal record is a summary of the woman's history from the time she entered prenatal care until the record was sent to the labor room (usually at about 36 weeks' gestation). Virtually all of the physical and psychosocial information relating to this woman is pertinent to the care by the nurse. For example, if a woman has gained very little weight during her pregnancy, the baby may be small-for-gestational age. The nurse may also have to change his or her care in relation to the woman's ethnicity and religion, etc.

2. 1. Leopold's maneuvers, although performed on a woman in labor, assess for fetal position, not the progress of labor.
   2. Fundal contractility will assess for uterine contractions, but this is not the most valuable information.
   3. Assessment of the fetal heart is critically important in relation to fetal well-being, but it will not determine the progress of labor.
   4. **A vaginal examination will provide the nurse with the best information about the status of labor.**

   TEST-TAKING TIP: Each of the assessments listed is performed on a woman who enters the labor suite for assessment. However, the only assessment that will determine whether or not a woman is in true labor is a vaginal examination. Only when there is cervical change—dilation and/or effacement—is it determined that a woman is in true labor.

3. 1. There is no indication that this woman has had poor preparation for childbirth.
   2. **The woman is showing expected signs of the active phase of labor.**
   3. There is no indication that this woman is showing signs of hypoxia and/or hypercapnia.
   4. The alpha-fetoprotein assessment is a test to screen for Down syndrome and neural tube defects in the fetus. It is done during pregnancy.

   TEST-TAKING TIP: The test taker must be familiar with the different phases of the first stage of labor: latent, active, and transition. The multiparous woman in the scenario entered the labor suite in the latent phase of labor when being talkative and excited is normal, but after 1 hour she has progressed into the active phase of labor in which being serious and breathing rapidly with contractions are expected behaviors.

4. **1, 2, and 4 are correct.**
   1. **The nurse should assess the fetal heart before reporting the client's status to the health care provider.**
   2. **The nurse should assess the contraction pattern before reporting the client's status.**
   3. A complete urinalysis would likely be ordered by the primary health care practitioner once the client has been officially admitted, but the test would not be performed during the initial assessment process.
   4. **The nurse should assess the woman's vital signs before reporting her status.**
   5. A biophysical profile is performed only if ordered by a health care practitioner.

   TEST-TAKING TIP: The fetal heart, contraction pattern, and maternal vitals all should be assessed to provide the health care practitioner with a picture of the health status of the mother and fetus. In some institutions, the nurse may also do a vaginal examination to assess for cervical change.

5. 1. With the palpation findings of a hard round mass in the fundal area and soft round mass above the symphysis, the nurse can conclude that the fetal position in not transverse.
   2. The findings on palpation also indicate that the presentation is not vertex.
   3. With the findings of a hard round mass in the fundal area and soft round mass above the symphysis, the nurse can conclude that the fetal lie is vertical.
   4. The attitude is difficult to determine when performing Leopold's maneuvers.

TEST-TAKING TIP: Many obstetric assessments have a component that is sensual and a component that is an interpretation or concept. Leopold's maneuvers are good examples. The nurse palpates specific areas of the pregnant abdomen, but then must interpret or translate what he or she is feeling into a concept. For example, in the scenario presented, the nurse palpates a hard, round mass in the fundal area of the uterus and must interpret that feeling as the fetal head. Similarly, the nurse palpates a soft round mass above the symphysis and must interpret that feeling as the fetal buttocks. With these findings and interpretations, the nurse will then realize that the fetal lie is vertical.

6. 1, 2, 3, and 5 are correct.
   1. The nurse should assess the fetal heart after all vaginal exams.
   2. The nurse should assess the fetal heart before giving the mother any analgesics.
   3. The fetal heart should be assessed periodically at the end of a contraction.
   4. The fetal heart pattern should be assessed every 1 hour during the latent phase of a low-risk labor. It is not standard protocol to assess every 10 minutes.
   5. The nurse should assess the fetal heart before the woman ambulates.

TEST-TAKING TIP: Except for invasive procedures, assessment of the fetal heart pattern is the only way to evaluate the well-being of a fetus during labor. The fetal heart pattern should, therefore, be assessed whenever there is a potential for injury to the baby or to the umbilical cord. At each of the times noted in the scenario—vaginal exam, analgesic administration, contraction, and ambulation—either the cord could be compressed or the baby could be compromised.

7. 1. Palpating the sacral promontory assesses the obstetric conjugate, not the fetal station.
   2. Station is assessed by palpating the ischial spines.
   3. Palpating the cervix assesses dilation and effacement, not fetal station.
   4. Palpating the symphysis pubis assesses the obstetric conjugate, not the fetal station.

TEST-TAKING TIP: The test taker must be thoroughly familiar with the anatomy of the female reproductive system and the measurements taken during pregnancy and labor. Station is determined by creating an imaginary line between the ischial spines. The descent of the presenting part of the fetus is then compared with the level of that "line."

8. 1. The nurse's findings upon performing Leopold's maneuvers indicate that the fetus is in the left occiput anterior position (LOA)—that is, the fetal back is felt on the mother's left side, the small parts are felt on her right side, the buttocks are felt in the fundal region, and the head is felt above her symphysis.
   2. The findings after the nurse performs Leopold's maneuvers do not indicate that the fetus is in the left sacral posterior (LSP) position; in that position, the fetus's buttocks (S or sacrum) are facing toward the mother's left posterior (LP), a hard round mass is felt in the fundal region, and a soft round mass is felt above the symphysis.
   3. The findings after the nurse performs Leopold's maneuvers do not indicate that the fetus is in the right mentum anterior (RMA) position; in that position, the fetus's face (M or mentum) is facing toward the mother's right anterior (RA) and small objects are felt on the right of the mother's abdomen with a flat area felt on the mother's left side.
   4. The findings after the nurse performs Leopold's maneuvers do not indicate that the fetus is in the right sacral posterior (RSP) position; in that position, the fetus's sacrum (S) is facing the mother's right posterior (RP) and a hard round mass is felt in the fundal region while a soft round mass is felt above the symphysis.

TEST-TAKING TIP: The test taker must review fetal positioning. This is an especially difficult concept to understand. The best way to learn the three-dimensional concept of fetal position is to look at the pictures in a text and then to get a doll and to imitate the pictures by placing the doll into each of the positions.

9. 1, 2, and 4 are correct. As the fetal head descends through a fully dilated cervix, the perineum begins to bulge, the bloody show increases, and the laboring woman usually feels a strong urge to push.
   1. A bulging perineum indicates progression to the second stage of labor.
   2. The bloody show increases as a woman enters the second stage of labor.
   3. The amniotic sac can rupture at any time.
   4. With a fully dilated cervix and bulging perineum, laboring women usually feel a strong urge to push.
   5. The gravida's ability to work with her labor is more dependent on her level of pain and her preparation for labor than on the phases and/or stages of labor.

   TEST-TAKING TIP: It is important that the test taker clearly understands the difference between the three phases of the first stage of labor and the three stages of labor. The three phases of the first stage of labor—latent, active, and transition—are related to changes in cervical dilation and maternal behaviors. The three stages of labor are defined by specific labor progressions—cervical change to full dilation (stage 1), full dilation to birth of the baby (stage 2), birth of the baby to birth of the placenta (stage 3).

10. 1. The LOA position refers to a fetus whose occiput (O) is facing toward the mother's left anterior (LA) and a presenting part at –1 station is 1 cm above the ischial spines.
    2. The LSP position is the correct answer. The fetal buttocks (S or sacrum) are facing toward the mother's left posterior (LP) and buttocks at –1 station are 1 cm above the ischial spines.
    3. The LMP position refers to a fetus whose face (M or mentum) is facing toward the mother's LP and a presenting part at +1 is 1 cm below the ischial spines.
    4. The LSA position refers to a fetus whose buttocks (S) are facing toward the mother's LA and a presenting part at +1 station is 1 cm below the ischial spines.

    TEST-TAKING TIP: If the test taker understands the definition of station, he or she could easily eliminate two of the four

responses in this question. When the presenting part of the fetus is at zero (0) station, the part is at the same level as an imaginary line between the mother's ischial spines. When the presenting part is above the spines, the station is negative (–). When the presenting part has moved past the spines, the station is defined as positive (+). Because the question states that the nurse palpated the buttocks above the spines, the station is negative. This effectively eliminates the two answer options that include a positive station.

11. 1. A fetus in the mentum anterior position is unlikely to elicit severe back pain in the mother.
    2. A fetus in the sacral posterior position is unlikely to elicit severe back pain in the mother.
    3. When a fetus is in the occiput posterior position, mothers frequently complain of severe back pain.
    4. A fetus in the scapula anterior position is unlikely to elicit severe back pain in the mother.

    TEST-TAKING TIP: If the test taker were to view a picture of a baby in the occiput posterior position, he or she would note that the occiput of the baby lies adjacent to the coccyx of the mother. During each contraction, the occiput, therefore, is forced backward into the coccyx. This action is very painful.

12. 1. The left upper quadrant would be the appropriate place to place a fetoscope to hear the fetal heartbeat if the baby were in the LSA position, not the LOA position.
    2. The right upper quadrant would be appropriate if the baby were in the RSA position.
    3. The fetoscope should be placed in the left lower quadrant for a fetus positioned in the LOA position as described in the question.
    4. The right lower quadrant would be appropriate if the baby were in the ROA position.

    TEST-TAKING TIP: The fetal heart is best heard through the fetal back. Because, as determined by doing Leopold's maneuvers, the baby is LOA, the fetal back (and, hence, the fetal heart) is in the left lower quadrant.

13. 1. Descent is progressing well. The presenting part is 3 centimeters below the ischial spines.
2. The fetal head is well past engagement. Engagement is defined as 0 station.
3. The woman, a primipara, is only 7 centimeters dilated. Delivery is likely to be many hours away.
4. External rotation does not occur until after delivery of the fetal head.

TEST-TAKING TIP: This question includes a number of concepts. Descent and station are discussed in answer options 1 and 2. The dilation of the cervix, which is related to the fact that the woman is a primigravida, is discussed in choice 3. And, one of the cardinal moves of labor—external rotation—is included in choice 4. The test taker must be prepared to answer questions that are complex and that include diverse information. In a 7 cm dilated primipara, with a baby at +3 station, vaginal delivery is not imminent, but the fetal head is well past engagement and descent is progressing well. External rotation has not yet occurred because the baby's head has not yet been birthed.

14. 1. This client is still in stage 1 (the cervix is not fully effaced or fully dilated) and the station is high.
2. This client is still in stage 1 (the cervix is not fully effaced or fully dilated) and the station is high.
3. Although this client is fully dilated, the cervix is not fully effaced and the baby has not descended far enough.
4. The cervix is fully dilated and fully effaced and the baby is low enough to be seen through the vaginal introitus.

TEST-TAKING TIP: To answer this question, the test taker must methodically evaluate each of the given responses. Once the nurse determines that a woman is not yet fully dilated or effaced, it can be determined that the woman is still in stage 1 of labor. Choice 3 does show a woman who is fully dilated but who is yet to efface fully and whose baby is still above the vaginal introitus. Only choice 4 meets all criteria set forth in the question.

15. 3, 4, and 5 are correct.
1. Hypnotic suggestion is usually not included in childbirth education based on the Lamaze method.

2. Rhythmic chanting is usually not included in childbirth education based on the Lamaze method.
3. Muscle relaxation is an integral part of Lamaze childbirth education.
4. Pelvic rocking is taught in Lamaze classes as a way of easing back pain during pregnancy and labor.
5. Abdominal massage, called effleurage, is also an integral part of Lamaze childbirth education.

TEST-TAKING TIP: The test taker may have expected to find breathing techniques included in the question related to Lamaze childbirth education. Although breathing techniques are taught, there are a number of other techniques and principles that couples learn in Lamaze classes. The test taker should be familiar with all aspects of childbirth education.

16. 1. Childbirth educators are not concerned with the possible verbalizations that laboring women might make.
2. Breathing exercises can be quite tiring. Simply being in labor is tiring. The goal of childbirth education, however, is not related to minimizing the energy demands of labor.
3. Some of the techniques learned at childbirth education classes are meant to break the fear-tension-pain cycle.
4. Although childbirth educators discuss maternal–newborn bonding, it is not a priority goal of childbirth education classes.

TEST-TAKING TIP: When a frightened woman enters the labor suite, she is likely to be very tense. It is known that pain is often worse when tensed muscles are stressed. Once the woman feels pain, she may become even more frightened and tense. This process becomes a vicious cycle. The information and skills learned at childbirth education classes are designed to break the cycle.

17. 1. The alternate pant-blow technique is used during stage 1 of labor.
2. Rhythmic, shallow breaths are used during stage 1 of labor.
3. Open glottal pushing is used during stage 2 of labor.
4. Slow chest breathing is used during stage 1.

TEST-TAKING TIP: Because the laboring client is in stage 2, the woman will change from using breathing techniques during contractions to pushing during contractions to birth the baby. Open glottal pushing is recommended because pushing against a closed glottis can decrease the mother's oxygen saturation.

18. 1. It is important to include all relevant information in the childbirth class.
2. Baby care should be included, but it is also important to include information about labor and delivery.
3. **Using visual aids can help to foster learning in teens as well as adults.**
4. Having the classes conveniently located in the school setting often enhances teens' attendance.

TEST-TAKING TIP: Because of their classroom experiences, adolescents are accustomed to learning in groups. The school setting is comfortable for them and, because of its location and its familiarity, is an ideal setting for childbirth education programs. In addition, educators often use visual aids to promote learning and, because teens are frequent theatergoers, showing movies is an especially attractive way to convey information to them.

19. 1. Although this client is light-headed, her problem is unlikely related to her blood pressure.
2. **This client is showing signs of hyperventilation. The symptoms will likely subside if she rebreathes her exhalations.**
3. It is unnecessary for this client to be moved to her side.
4. The baby is not in jeopardy at this time.

TEST-TAKING TIP: It is essential that the test taker attend to the clues in the question and not assume that other issues may be occurring. This client is light-headed as a result of being tachypneic during contractions. This fact is essential. Hyperventilation, which can result from tachypnea, is characterized by tingling and light-headedness. Rebreathing her air should rectify the problem.

20. 1. The pant-blow breathing technique is usually used during the transition phase of labor.
2. Rapid, deep breathing is rarely used in labor.
3. Grunting and pushing is often the method that women instinctively use during the second stage of labor.

4. Most women find slow chest breathing effective during the latent phase.

TEST-TAKING TIP: Because the latent phase is the first phase of the first stage of labor, the contractions are usually mild and they rarely last longer than 30 seconds. A slow chest breathing technique, therefore, is effective and does not tire the woman out for the remainder of her labor.

21. 1. It is inappropriate to encourage her to have an epidural at this time.
2. It is inappropriate to encourage her to have an IV analgesic at this time.
3. A change of position might help but will probably not be completely effective.
4. **This woman is in the active phase of labor. The first phase breathing is probably no longer effective. Encouraging her to shift to the next level of breathing is appropriate at this time.**

TEST-TAKING TIP: If a woman has learned Lamaze breathing, it is important to support her actions. Encouraging her to take pain-relieving medications may undermine her resolve and make her feel like she has failed. The initial response by the nurse should be to support her by encouraging her to use her breathing techniques.

22. 1. The lithotomy position is not physiologically supportive of labor and birth.
2. **Effleurage is a light massage that can soothe the mother during labor.**
3. Practicing Kegel exercises can help to build up the muscles of the perineum but will not help the woman to work with her labor.
4. Pushing is not performed until the second stage of labor.

TEST-TAKING TIP: There are a number of actions that mothers can take that can support their breathing during labor. Walking, swaying, and rocking can all help a woman during the process. Effleurage, the light massaging of the abdomen or thighs, is often soothing for the mothers.

23. 1. The woman should not push until the next contraction. She should be allowed to sleep at this time.
2. **The woman's privacy should be maintained while she is resting.**
3. The woman is in no apparent distress. Vital sign assessment is not indicated.
4. The woman is in no apparent distress. Oxygen is not indicated.

TEST-TAKING TIP: Because the woman is in second stage, she is pushing with contractions. If she is very tired, she is likely to fall asleep immediately following a contraction. It is important for the nurse to maintain the woman's privacy by covering her perineum with a sheet between contractions. It would also be appropriate to awaken the woman at the beginning of the next contraction.

24. 1. This client has probably moved into the second stage of labor. Providing a bedpan is not the first action.
    2. The nurse should first assess the progress of labor to see if the client has moved into the second stage of labor.
    3. It is too early to notify the physician.
    4. It is too early to advise the mother to push.

TEST-TAKING TIP: The average length of transition in multiparas is 10 minutes. This client is likely, therefore, to have moved into the second stage of labor. The nurse's first action, therefore, is to assess the progress of labor. If she is in second stage, the physician will be notified and the client will be encouraged to push. If she is not yet in second stage, she may need the bedpan.

25. 1. This is the correct response. A fetal heart rate of 152 is normal.
    2. This woman is in early labor. The fetal heart does not need to be assessed every 5 minutes.
    3. The rate is normal. There is no need to report the rate to the health care practitioner.
    4. The rate is normal. There is no need to institute emergency measures.

TEST-TAKING TIP: It is essential that the test taker know the normal physiological responses of women and their fetuses in labor. The normal fetal heart rate is 110 to 160 bpm. A rate of 152, therefore, is within normal limits. No further action is needed at this time.

26. 1. The frequency of intermittent auscultation is determined by which stage of labor the woman is in, not by contraction pattern.
    2. The frequency of intermittent auscultation is determined by which stage of labor the woman is in.
    3. Intermittent auscultation is performed between contractions, not during the peak of a contraction.

4. Intermittent auscultation should be performed for 1 full minute after contractions end.

TEST-TAKING TIP: Although most babies are monitored via electronic fetal monitoring in labor, there is a great deal of evidence to show that intermittent auscultation is as effective a method of monitoring the fetal heart. It is essential, however, that the fetal heart be monitored immediately after contractions for 1 full minute to identify the presence of any late or variable decelerations.

27. 1. The tracing is showing a normal fetal heart tracing. No intervention is needed.
    2. There is no need to administer oxygen at this time. The tracing is normal.
    3. If the client is comfortable, there is no need to change her position.
    4. There is no need to speed up the intravenous at this time.

TEST-TAKING TIP: The baseline fetal heart variability is the most important fetal heart assessment that the nurse makes. If the baby's heart rate shows average variability, the nurse can assume that the baby is not hypoxic or acidotic. In addition, the normal heart rate of 142 is reassuring.

28. 1. The relationship between the decelerations and the contractions will determine the type of deceleration pattern.
    2. The maternal blood pressure is not related to the scenario in the question.
    3. Although some fetuses are at higher risk for fetal distress, the nurse must first determine which type of deceleration is present.
    4. If the nurse is able to identify that a deceleration is present, the electrode placement is adequate.

TEST-TAKING TIP: Decelerations are defined by their relationship to the contraction pattern. It is essential that the nurse determine which of the three types of decelerations is present. Early decelerations mirror contractions, late decelerations develop at the peak of contractions and return to baseline well after contractions are over, and variable decelerations can occur at anytime and are unrelated to contractions.

29. 1. Breathing will help with contraction pain, but is not as effective when a client is experiencing back labor.

2. It is inappropriate automatically to encourage mothers to have anesthesia or analgesia in labor. There are other methods of providing pain relief.
3. When direct sacral pressure is applied, the nurse is providing a counteraction to the pressure being exerted by the fetal head.
4. Hydrotherapy is very soothing but will not provide direct relief.

TEST-TAKING TIP: Whenever a laboring woman complains of severe back labor, it is very likely that the baby is lying in the occiput posterior position. Every time the woman has a contraction, the head is pushed into the coccyx. When direct pressure is applied to the sacral area, the nurse is providing counteraction to the pressure being exerted by the fetal head.

30. 1. The maternal blood pressure is not the priority assessment after an amniotomy.
2. The maternal pulse is not the priority assessment after an amniotomy.
3. It is essential to assess the fetal heart rate immediately after an amniotomy.
4. Fetal fibronectin is assessed during pregnancy. It is not assessed once a woman enters labor.

TEST-TAKING TIP: Amniotomy, as the word implies, is the artificial rupture of the amniotic sac. During the procedure, there is a risk that the umbilical cord may become compressed. Because there is no direct way to assess cord compression, the nurse must assess the fetal heart rate for any adverse changes.

31. 1. Because the baby's back is facing the mother's right side, the fetal monitor should not be placed in the LUQ.
2. Because the baby's back is facing the mother's right side, the fetal monitor should not be placed LLQ.
3. Because the baby's back is facing the mother's right side and the sacrum is presenting, the fetal monitor should be placed in her RUQ.
4. The monitor electrode should have been placed in the RLQ if the nurse had assessed a vertex presentation.

TEST-TAKING TIP: Although the question does not tell the test taker whether the sacrum is facing anteriorly or posteriorly, it does provide the information that the sacrum is felt toward the mother's right. Because this baby is in the sacral

presentation and the back is toward the right, the best location for the fetal monitor is in the RUQ, at the level of the fetal back.

32. 1. This client is fully dilated and effaced, but the baby is not yet engaged. Until the baby descends and stimulates rectal pressure, it is inappropriate for the client to begin to push.
2. Fundal pressure is inappropriate.
3. Many women push in the squatting position, but it is too early to push at this time.
4. Monitoring for rectal pressure is appropriate at this time.

TEST-TAKING TIP: Although the test taker may see in practice that women are encouraged to begin to push as soon as they become fully dilated, it is best practice to wait until the woman exhibits signs of rectal pressure. Pushing a baby that is not yet engaged may result in an overly fatigued woman or, more significantly, a prolapsed cord.

33. 1 and 2 are correct.
1. An appropriate action by the doula is giving the woman a back massage.
2. An appropriate action by the doula is to assist the laboring woman with her breathing.
3. The nurse, not the doula, should assess the fetal heart.
4. The nurse, not the doula, should assess the blood pressure.
5. The nurse, not the doula, should regulate the IV.

TEST-TAKING TIP: Even if the test taker were unfamiliar with the role of the doula, he or she could deduce the answers to this question. Three of the responses involve physiological assessments or interventions while two of the responses deal with providing supportive care, the role of the doula.

34. 1. Women may contract without being in true labor.
2. Once the cervix begins to dilate, a client is in true labor.
3. Membranes can rupture before true labor begins.
4. Engagement can occur before true labor begins.

TEST-TAKING TIP: Although laboring women experience contractions, contractions alone are not an indicator of true labor. Only

when the cervix dilates is the client in true labor. False labor contractions are usually irregular and mild, but, in some situations, they can appear to be regular and can be quite uncomfortable.

35. 1, 2, and 4 are correct.
   1. True labor contractions often begin in the back and, when the frequency of the contractions is q 5 minutes or less, it is usually appropriate for the client to proceed to the hospital.
   2. Even if the woman is not having labor contractions, rupture of membranes is a reason to go to the hospital to be assessed.
   3. Expelling the mucous plug is not sufficient reason to go to the hospital to be assessed.
   4. Greenish liquid is likely meconium-stained fluid. The client needs to be assessed.
   5. The latent phase of labor can last up to a full day. In addition, Braxton Hicks' contractions can last for quite a while. Even though a woman may feel cramping for 4 hours or more, she may not be in true labor.

TEST-TAKING TIP: The mucous plug protects the uterine cavity from bacterial invasion. It is expelled before or during the early phase of labor. In fact, it may be hours, days, or even a week after the mucous plug is expelled before true labor begins.

36. 1. This client may be in the latent phase of labor or may be experiencing false labor contractions. Either way, unless she is having other symptoms, there is no need to be seen by a health care practitioner.
   2. This client is having some bloody show with the expulsion of the mucous plug, but pink streaks are normal and can be seen hours to a few days before true labor begins.
   3. This client may be in the latent phase of labor, but there is no need to go to the hospital with "cramping."
   4. This client is exhibiting clear signs of true labor. Not only are the contractions lasting a full minute but she is stating that they are so uncomfortable that she is unable to speak through them. She should be seen.

TEST-TAKING TIP: The test taker must remember that nurses interpret the comments made by gravid women who are close to term. Clients, especially

primiparas, are often anxious about the labor process and have difficulty interpreting what they are feeling. Only when the woman is experiencing contractions that are increasing in intensity and duration and decreasing in frequency, or when the woman has ruptured membranes, should she be encouraged to go to the hospital for an evaluation.

37. 1. The client may have a urinary tract infection with blood in the urine. First, however, the nurse should acknowledge the client's concerns.
   2. The nurse is using reflection to acknowledge the client's concerns.
   3. Although the woman's statement is consistent with the expulsion of the mucous plug, this response ignores the fact that the client is frightened by what she has seen.
   4. The nurse will want to clarify that the woman isn't actually bleeding, but the question should follow an acknowledgment of the woman's concerns.

TEST-TAKING TIP: Pregnant women are very protective of themselves and of the babies they are carrying. Any time a change that might portend a problem occurs, a pregnant woman is likely to become concerned and frightened. Certainly, seeing any kind of blood loss from the vagina can be scary. The nurse must acknowledge that fear before asking other questions or making other comments.

38. 1. The frequency of labor contractions decreases. It does not increase.
   2. Labor contractions increase in intensity. They do not become milder.
   3. This response indicates that the labor contractions are increasing in intensity.
   4. This client has slept through the "tightening" and there is no increase in intensity. It is unlikely that she is in true labor.

TEST-TAKING TIP: The test taker should review the labor contraction definitions of frequency, duration, and intensity. As labor progresses, the frequency of contractions decreases but the duration and the intensity, or strength, of the contractions increase. The nurse notes the change in intensity when he or she palpates the fundus of the uterus, and the client subjectively complains of increasing pain.

39. 1. The frequency and duration of this contraction pattern is every 2 minutes lasting 60 seconds.

2. The frequency and duration of this contraction pattern is every 4 minutes lasting 120 seconds.
3. The frequency and duration of this contraction pattern is every 3 minutes lasting 120 seconds.
4. The frequency and duration of this contraction pattern is every 3 minutes lasting 60 seconds.

TEST-TAKING TIP: The test taker must recall that frequency is defined as the time from the beginning of one contraction to the beginning of the next, while duration is defined as the beginning of the increment of a contraction to the end of the decrement. The only choices that include a frequency of 3 minutes are choices 3 and 4, whereas the only choice with a duration of 60 seconds is choice 4.

40. 1. A fetus in a sacral presentation is in a vertical lie.
2. A fetus in an occipital presentation is in a vertical lie.
3. A fetus in a mentum presentation is in a vertical lie.
4. A fetus in a scapular presentation is in a horizontal lie.

TEST-TAKING TIP: Lie is concerned with the relationship between the fetal spine and the maternal spine. When the spines are parallel, the lie is vertical (or longitudinal). When the spines are perpendicular, the lie is horizontal (or transverse). It is physiologically impossible for a baby in the horizontal lie to be delivered vaginally.

41. 1, 5, 3, 4, 2. The correct order of the movements listed is:
1. Descent.
5. Internal rotation.
3. Extension.
4. External rotation.
2. Expulsion.

TEST-TAKING TIP: The test taker must review the cardinal moves of labor. There are a couple of tricks to help the test taker to remember the sequence of the moves of labor. First, descent and flexion must occur. If the baby does not descend into the birth canal and the baby does not flex the head so that his or her chin is on the chest, the baby simply will not be able to traverse through the bony pelvis. Second, internal rotation (rotation of the fetal body when the fetal head is still *inside* the mother's pelvis) must occur

before external rotation (rotation of the fetal body after the fetal head is *outside* the mother). In between the rotational moves is extension, the delivery of the head. And, finally, expulsion must be last because the delivery of the baby's body is simply the last movement.

42. 1. Engagement is equal to 0 station. This fetus is well past 0 station.
2. A baby that is floating is in negative station.
3. When the presenting part is at the ischial spines, the baby is engaged or at 0 station.
4. The baby's head is almost crowning.

TEST-TAKING TIP: The test taker should remember that a baby is crowning when the mother's perineal tissues are stretched around the fetal head at the same location where a crown would sit. The station at this time is past +5 station (or 5 cm past the ischial spines).

43. 1. The obstetric conjugate is the shortest anterior to posterior diameter of the pelvis. When it is of average size, it will accommodate an average-sized fetal head.
2. When the fetal head is flexed, the diameter of the head is minimized. This is not, however, the obstetric conjugate.
3. There is no average dilation for the beginning of labor.
4. The physiological retraction ring is the area of the uterus that forms as a result of cervical effacement. It is not related to the obstetric conjugate.

TEST-TAKING TIP: The obstetric conjugate is measured by the health care practitioner to estimate the potential for the fetal head to fit through the anterior-posterior diameter of the maternal pelvis. It is the internal distance between the sacral promontory and the symphysis pubis.

44. q 3 minutes

TEST-TAKING TIP: The test taker must remember three things when assessing frequency: (1) Frequency is defined as the time from the beginning of one contraction to the beginning of the next contraction, not the time from the end of one contraction to the beginning of the next contraction; (2) time is characterized by a space on the graph, not by a point; and (3) frequency is always expressed in minutes, not seconds.

45. 90 seconds

    TEST-TAKING TIP: The test taker must remember 3 things when assessing duration: (1) Duration of a contraction is measured from the beginning of the increment—where the contraction begins to curve upward from baseline—to the end of the decrement—when the contraction returns to baseline; (2) time is characterized by a space on the graph, not by a point; and (3) duration is always written in seconds, not minutes.

46. 1. The contraction pattern is q 3 min × 90 sec
    2. The contraction pattern is q 3 min × 90 sec
    3. The contraction pattern is q 3 min × 90 sec
    4. The contraction pattern is q 3 min × 90 sec

    TEST-TAKING TIP: First, the test taker should place his or her pencil at the beginning of the increment of the first contraction and the beginning of the increment of the next contraction and then count the number of 10-second spaces. This is the frequency once the time has been converted into minutes. Next, the test taker should place his or her pencil at the beginning of the increment of the first contraction and at the end of the decrement of the same contraction and count the number of 10-second spaces. This is the duration and it should be left in seconds.

47. 1. A baby in the breech presentation may or may not be in the flexed attitude.
    2. A baby in the horizontal lie may or may not be in the flexed attitude.
    3. Engagement is unrelated to attitude.
    4. When the baby's chin is on his or her chest, the baby is in the flexed attitude.

    TEST-TAKING TIP: The diameter of the fetal head is dependent upon whether or not the head is flexed with the chin on the chest or extended with the chin elevated. When the baby is in the flexed attitude, with the chin on the chest, the diameter of the fetal head entering the pelvis averages 9.5 cm (the suboccipitobregmatic diameter), whereas if the baby is in the extended attitude, with the chin elevated, the diameter of the fetal head entering the pelvis can be as large as 13.5 cm (the occipitomental diameter). For the fetal

head to pass through the mother's pelvis, therefore, it is best for the head to be in the flexed attitude.

48. 1. Engagement is achieved when the baby's presenting part reaches an imaginary line between the ischial spines. The station of the fetal head, as described in the question, is past the inlet.
    2. The inlet's boundaries are: the sacral promontory and the upper margins of the ilia, ischia, and the symphysis pubis. This is the entry into the true pelvis.
    3. The baby is physiologically unable to enter the true pelvis when in a horizontal lie.
    4. The attitude of the baby is not discussed in the ultrasound statement.

    TEST-TAKING TIP: It is very important that the test taker be familiar with the many definitions that are used in obstetrics. If any of the definitions is unfamiliar, the test taker may be confused by some of the question stems or by the many answer options.

49. 1. This is a picture of a fetus in the ROP (right occiput posterior) position.
    2. This is a picture of a fetus in the ROA (right occiput anterior) position.
    3. This is a picture of a fetus in the LOP (left occiput posterior) position.
    4. This is a picture of a fetus in the LOA (left occiput anterior) position.

    TEST-TAKING TIP: It is very important, when determining the position of a fetus, to remember that the test taker must consider the posture of the fetal body in relation to the left and/or right side of the maternal body and not in relation to the left and/or right side of the test taker's body.

50. 1. This is a picture of a fetus in the RSP (right sacral posterior) position.
    2. This is a picture of a fetus in the RSA (right sacral anterior) position.
    3. This is a picture of a fetus in the LSP (left sacral posterior) position.
    4. This is a picture of a fetus in the LSA (left sacral anterior) position.

    TEST-TAKING TIP: It is very important when determining the position of a fetus to remember that the maternal aspects of the position—that is, left/right/etc. and anterior/posterior/etc.—must be determined by locating the fetal presenting part. In other words, the test taker must determine toward which part of the mother the presenting part of the fetus is pointing. In this question, for example, the sacrum of the fetus is pointing toward the left anterior of the mother.

51. 1. This is a picture of a fetus in the single footling breech position.
    2. This is a picture of a fetus in the double footling breech position
    3. **This is a picture of a fetus in the frank breech position.**
    4. This is a picture of a fetus in the double footling breech position.

TEST-TAKING TIP: There are three main breech positions: frank, where the buttocks present and both feet are located adjacent to the fetal head; single footling, when one leg is extended through the cervix and vagina while the remaining leg is bent; and double footling, when both legs are extended through the cervix and vagina. It is likely that a woman carrying a breech in any position will have a cesarean section.

52. 1. Flexion is one of the first of the cardinal moves of labor.
    2. Internal rotation occurs while the baby is still in utero.
    3. **During extension, the baby's head is birthed.**
    4. The baby rotates externally after the birth of the head.

TEST-TAKING TIP: The baby must move through the cardinal moves because the fetal head is widest anterior-posterior but the fetal shoulders are widest laterally. On the other hand, the maternal pelvis is widest laterally in the inlet but anterior-posterior at the outlet.

53. 1. When assessing the variability of the fetal heart, the mother can be in any position.
    2. **Before the variability can be accurately assessed, an internal fetal heart electrode should be applied.**
    3. Only after assessing a poor fetal monitor tracing would the nurse administer oxygen.
    4. Variability is unrelated to fetal movement.

TEST-TAKING TIP: There are many important principles related to electronic fetal heart monitoring. Variability is the most important of the baseline data. Variability is a measure of the competition between the sympathetic nervous system, which speeds up the heart rate, and the parasympathetic nervous system, which

slows down the heart rate. When the fetal heart variability is adequate, the nurse can conclude, therefore, that the baby's autonomic nervous system is healthy.

54. 1. **Because the variability is moderate (6 to 25 bpm wide), the nurse can conclude that the baby is well and that caring labor support is indicated.**
    2. Because the variability is moderate (6 to 25 bpm wide), there is no need for the mother to receive oxygen.
    3. Because the variability is moderate (6 to 25 bpm wide), there is no need to move the mother to another position.
    4. Because the variability is moderate (6 to 25 bpm wide), there is no need to measure the mother's oxygen saturation.

TEST-TAKING TIP: A tracing showing moderate variability—that is, 6 to 25 bpm wide—indicates adequate variability and this, in turn, indicates normal pH and oxygenation of the fetus. A flat tracing indicates absent variability, whereas a tracing showing minimal variability exhibits a pattern that is less than or equal to 5 bpm wide. When there is no other explanation for either a flat or minimal tracing, the drop in variability is a sign of fetal hypoxia and acidosis and is an obstetric emergency.

55. 1. Moderate variability is indicative of fetal health, not of hypoxia.
    2. A change in variability indicates acidosis, not alkalosis. In this situation, there is no indication of acidosis.
    3. During sleep cycles, fetal heart rate variability decreases.
    4. **Moderate variability is indicative of fetal health.**

TEST-TAKING TIP: It is important for the test taker to be familiar with situations that can change the fetal heart variability. Normal situations that can decrease the variability include fetal sleep, administration of central nervous system depressant medications, and prematurity. A normal situation that can increase the variability is fetal activity.

56. 1. Early decelerations are rarely seen during the latent phase of labor.
    2. Epidural insertion is not associated with early decelerations.
    3. **Early decelerations are frequently seen during the second stage of labor.**

4. By the time the placenta is being delivered, the baby is already born.

TEST-TAKING TIP: Early deceleration, one of the three types of decelerations, is a drop in fetal heart rate that mirrors the contraction. It is caused by fetal head compression. Early decelerations are noted during the second stage of labor because the fetal head is compressed against the maternal soft tissues during pushing.

57. 1. The fetal heart rate normally accelerates during fetal movement.
    2. When analgesics are administered, the fetal heart rate variability drops and accelerations are rarely seen.
    3. When a fetus is acidotic, the fetal heart rate variability drops and accelerations are rarely seen.
    4. With poor placental perfusion, the fetal heart rate variability drops and accelerations are rarely seen.

TEST-TAKING TIP: Fetal heart accelerations are usually a sign of fetal well-being. When the baby is healthy, they are almost always noted during periods of fetal movement. Similar to what occurs in a runner, with increased movement, the fetal heart rate speeds up to accommodate increasing energy needs.

58. 1. The baby's heart rate should not exhibit variable decelerations after the mother is given pain-relieving medication.
    2. The baby's heart rate should not exhibit late decelerations after the mother is given an analgesic.
    3. **Analgesics are central nervous system (CNS) depressants. The variability of the fetal heart rate, therefore, will be decreased.**
    4. The baby's heart rate is unlikely to exhibit transient accelerations after the mother receives analgesics.

TEST-TAKING TIP: It is important for the test taker to remember the side effects of commonly used medications. The analgesics used in labor are opiates. The CNS-depressant effect of the opiates is therapeutic for the mother who is in pain, but the baby is also affected by the medication, often exhibiting decreased variability.

59. 1. A baseline fetal heart rate (FH) of 140 to 150 is a baseline with moderate variability, but V-shaped decelerations are variable decelerations. These are related to cord compression and are not normal.

2. A baseline FH of 140 to 150 is a baseline showing moderate, or normal, variability. Decelerations that mirror contractions are defined as early decelerations. These are related to head compression and are expected during transition and second stage labor.
3. A baseline with beat to beat changes of only 2 bpm is defined as minimal variability. Also, there are late decelerations. Late decelerations are related to uteroplacental insufficiency. This situation is an obstetric emergency.
4. A baseline with beat to beat changes of only 2 bpm is defined as minimal variability. Even when no decelerations are noted, the nurse should be concerned when the FH is showing minimal variability.

TEST-TAKING TIP: The test taker must be prepared to differentiate between normal situations and obstetric emergencies. Even though there are decelerations in choice 2, the decelerations are expected because the woman is currently in the transition phase of the first stage of labor.

60. 1. The fetal heart should be assessed every 5 minutes during the second stage of labor.
    2. **The woman should be encouraged to grunt during contractions.**
    3. The pulse should be assessed, but it is unnecessary to do so every 5 minutes.
    4. This position is not physiological.

TEST-TAKING TIP: During second stage labor, the woman should push on an open glottis to prevent the vasovagal response. Research has shown that when women push without being coached, they do not hold their breath to bear down, but instead grunt during the second stage.

61. 1. Holding the breath for 20 seconds during each contraction can stimulate the Valsalva maneuver, which can lead to a sudden drop in blood pressure and fainting.
    2. One cannot push and blow out at the same time. This will not facilitate the delivery of the baby.
    3. Pushing should be done only during contractions, not between contractions.
    4. **By taking a slow, cleansing breath before pushing, the woman is waiting until the contraction builds to its peak. Her pushes will be more effective at this point in the contraction.**

TEST-TAKING TIP: It is essential that the test taker read each question and the possible answer options carefully. If the test taker were to read response 3 quickly, he or she might mistakenly choose it as the correct response. Because the woman is being encouraged to push between contractions, however, the answer is incorrect.

62. 1. This is a normal finding. There is no need to notify the health care practitioner at this time.
    2. This is a normal finding. The woman is not in need of immediate cardiovascular assessment.
    3. Because this is a normal finding, the nurse should continue to provide labor support and encouragement.
    4. This finding is normal. There is no need to administer oxygen or to change the woman's position.

TEST-TAKING TIP: The bulging perineum is an indication that the baby is descending in the birth canal and the bloody show results from injury to the capillaries in the mother's cervix. Because this woman is a primigravida, she will likely need to push for many more minutes so it is not necessary to notify the health care provider until additional signs are noted.

63. 1. Epidurals are a form of regional anesthesia. They are used to obliterate pain.
    2. It is inappropriate to encourage the woman to receive an epidural at this time.
    3. Because this woman is a multipara, the position is LOA, and the station is +3, this is an accurate statement.
    4. It is inappropriate to encourage the woman to receive an epidural at this time.

TEST-TAKING TIP: The average length of the second stage of labor for multiparas is about 15 minutes, whereas the average time for an epidural to be inserted and to take effect is approximately 20 minutes. In addition, the fetus in the scenario has already descended to +3 station and is in the optimal position for delivery—LOA. It is very likely that this baby will be born in a few contractions. The nurse should encourage the client to continue pushing with her contractions.

64. 1, 3, 4, and 5 are correct.
    1. This statement is true. A birth may take place in the shower, when the mother is in a soaking tub, in a bed, or even while standing.
    2. The nurse should provide additional information to this client. Many deliveries are performed safely without stirrups.
    3. If the fetus is in the posterior or transverse position, the woman may be encouraged to push while on her hands and knees. This may enable the baby to turn into the anterior position and the delivery may soon follow.
    4. Many mothers deliver in their labor beds without stirrups. Some beds transform into delivery beds and some are regular hospital beds. Still others are double or queen-sized beds so that the father and/or the delivering practitioner can also relax in the bed. When forceps or other interventions are needed for a delivery, however, stirrups may be required.
    5. Midwives deliver their clients in a variety of positions, including the side-lying, squatting, and lithotomy positions, as well as when the clients are on their hands and knees.

TEST-TAKING TIP: Deliveries can be performed in a variety of positions, including lithotomy, squatting, and side-lying; in a variety of locations, including labor bed, delivery bed, toilet, shower, and in a dry environment or in water. It is recommended that mothers consult with their health care practitioners early in the pregnancy regarding the practitioner's delivery practices, including birth positions. The mother's birth preference may influence her choice of caregiver.

65. The order of change during the third stage of labor is: 3, 4, 1, 2.
    3. The contraction of the uterus after delivery of the baby is the first step in the third stage of labor.
    4. As the uterus contracts, its surface area decreases more and more.
    1. A hematoma forms behind the placenta as the placenta separates from the uterine wall after the uterus has contracted and its surface area has decreased.
    2. The membranes separate from the uterine wall after the placenta separates and begins to be born.

TEST-TAKING TIP: The test taker should become familiar with the process of placental separation. Once the baby is born, the uterus contracts. When it does so, the surface area of the internal uterine wall decreases, forcing the placenta to begin to separate. As the placenta separates, a hematoma forms behind it, further promoting placental separation. Once the placenta separates and begins to be born, the membranes peel off the uterine wall and are delivered last.

66. 1. Considering the signs, this is an unlikely reason.
    2. These are signs of placental delivery.
    3. Considering the signs, this is an unlikely reason.
    4. Cord bloods are obtained by the practitioner once the cord is cut. The clamp on the cord that is still attached to the placenta is released and blood is obtained from the cut cord.

TEST-TAKING TIP: Although they sound abnormal, the following are the normal signs of placental separation: The uterus rises in the abdomen and becomes globular, there is a gush of blood expelled from the vagina, and the umbilical cord lengthens. The placenta should be delivered between 5 and 30 minutes after the delivery of the baby.

67. 1 and 3 are correct.
    1. This is a sign of placental separation.
    2. Once second stage is complete, the baby is no longer in utero.
    3. This is a sign of placental separation.
    4. Dilation and effacement are complete before second stage begins.
    5. Rectal pressure is usually a sign of fetal descent. Once the second stage is complete, the baby is no longer in utero.

TEST-TAKING TIP: It is essential that the test taker clearly differentiate between stage 1, stage 2, and stage 3 of labor. Stage 1, what is usually referred to as "labor," ends with full cervical dilation. At the end of stage 2, the baby is born. And at the conclusion of stage 3, the placenta is born.

68. 1. This comment would be consistent with a client in the latent phase of labor.
    2. This comment is consistent with a woman in the transition phase of stage 1.
    3. This comment could be made at a variety of times during the labor.
    4. This comment is consistent with a woman in stage 2 labor.

TEST-TAKING TIP: The test taker must be familiar not only with the physiological

changes that occur during each phase of labor but also with the maternal behaviors that are expected at each phase.

69. 1. The nurse would expect the woman to be 2 cm dilated.
    2. At 4 cm, the woman is entering the active phase of labor.
    3. At 8 cm, the woman is in the transition phase of labor.
    4. At 10 cm, the woman is in the second stage of labor.

TEST-TAKING TIP: In the latent phase of labor, clients are often very excited because the labor has finally begun. They frequently are very talkative and easily distracted from the discomfort of the contractions. The test taker should be familiar with the cervical changes that correlate with the various phases and stages of labor.

70. 1. With pain and increased energy needs, the pulse rate often increases.
    2. The blood pressure rises dramatically.
    3. Although the woman is working very hard, her temperature should remain normal.
    4. With pain and increased energy needs, the respiratory rate often increases.

TEST-TAKING TIP: During contractions, the blood from the placenta is forced into the peripheral vascular system and there is an increase in cardiac output. As a result, the woman's blood pressure rises: an average of 35 mm Hg systolic and 25 mm Hg diastolic. The blood pressure should never be assessed during a contraction because the reading will be a marked distortion of the woman's true blood pressure.

71. 1. The woman is exhibiting no high-risk issues.
    2. The woman is in early labor. There is no need for her to be hospitalized at this time.
    3. The woman is exhibiting no high-risk issues.
    4. The woman is in early labor, not active phase.

TEST-TAKING TIP: The key facts that the test taker should attend to in this question about a primigravida are the cervical dilation, the contraction pattern, and the fetal heart pattern. The woman is clearly in the latent phase because she is only 2 cm dilated, 30% effaced, and is contracting infrequently at q 12 minutes

72. 1. Talking and laughing are characteristic behaviors of the latent phase.
2. Back labor can be experienced during any phase of labor.
3. Women in the latent phase often do perform effleurage, but it can also be performed during other phases of labor.
4. A woman in the latent phase might go to the bathroom but defecating is not indicative of the first phase of labor.

TEST-TAKING TIP: Although effleurage is a massage that women are taught to use during the latent phase of labor, it is important for the test taker to remember that women are individuals and are encouraged to use breathing techniques and other therapies that help them with their labors. Some women enjoy performing massage well into the active and transition phases and others never find it comforting.

73. 1. Seconal is a barbiturate sedative. It is not used as an analgesic potentiator.
2. Vistaril can be used as an analgesic potentiator.
3. Benadryl is an antihistamine that is not used as an analgesic potentiator.
4. Tylenol is a nonsteroidal anti-inflammatory drug that is ineffective as an analgesic in labor.

TEST-TAKING TIP: Vistaril is a valuable analgesic potentiator, not only because it helps to increase the effectiveness of the analgesic but also because it acts as an antiemetic. Women often vomit during transition. Vistaril, as well as other medications like Reglan (metoclopramide), helps to diminish the nausea associated with the analgesic as well as the vomiting associated with transition. Vistaril is also used as an anxiety reducer.

74. 1. It is recommended that women delay pushing until they feel the urge to push.
2. There is no indication for oxygen in this scenario.
3. Once the woman has a strong urge to push, then she should be encouraged to push against an open glottis to birth the baby.
4. There is no indication of maternal compromise in this scenario.

TEST-TAKING TIP: Although the use of an epidural is not high risk, there can be injuries to the maternal birth canal and/or the fetus when pushing is performed by a mother with no feeling. It is recommended that women who have lost all feeling because of an epidural "labor down," or rest and wait, until the urge to push returns. Once that happens, the woman should perform open glottal pushing.

75. 1. The woman should be helped into the fetal position.
2. The lithotomy position is inappropriate.
3. The Trendelenburg position is inappropriate.
4. The lateral recumbent position is inappropriate.

TEST-TAKING TIP: For the anesthesiologist to be able to insert the epidural catheter into the epidural space, the woman must be placed in either the fetal position or sitting with her chin on her chest and her back convex. In both of those positions, the woman's vertebrae separate, providing the anesthesiologist access to the required space.

76. 1, 2, and 5 are correct.
1. Before a woman is given regional anesthesia, the nurse should assess the fetal heart rate.
2. The nurse should receive an order to infuse Ringer's lactate before the woman is given regional anesthesia.
3. It is not necessary to place the woman in the Trendelenburg position.
4. The blood pressure will need to be monitored every 5 minutes for 15 minutes after administration of the anesthesia, but not before.
5. The nurse should ask the woman to empty her bladder.

TEST-TAKING TIP: Before any medication, whether analgesia or anesthesia, is administered during labor, the fetal heart should be assessed to make sure that the baby is not already compromised. Before regional anesthesia administration, a liter of fluid should be infused to increase the woman's vascular fluid volume. This will help to maintain her blood pressure after the epidural insertion. And the woman's bladder should be emptied because she will not have the sensation of a full bladder once the epidural is in place.

77. 1. It is unlikely that the woman will experience adverse feelings in her lower extremities.

2. **Hypotension is a very common side effect of regional anesthesia.**
3. The epidural does not enter the spinal canal. There will be no change, higher or lower, in the central venous pressure.
4. Fetal heart accelerations are positive signs. These are not adverse findings.

TEST-TAKING TIP: The test taker must be familiar with the side effects of all medications. If no other therapeutic interventions are performed, virtually all women will show signs of hypotension after epidural administration. The change is related to two phenomena: dilation of the vessels in the pelvis and increased compression of the vena cava.

78. 1. The temperature does not need to be assessed immediately after the epidural insertion.
2. **A wedge should be placed under one side of the woman.**
3. There is no indication that a blanket roll needs to be placed under the woman's feet at this time.
4. It is not necessary for the nurse to assess the pedal pulses at this time.

TEST-TAKING TIP: The test taker must remember that hypotension is the most common complication of epidural anesthesia in labor. One of the most important reasons for this is the compression of the vena cava by the pregnant uterus. When a wedge is placed under the woman's side—usually the right side—the uterus is tilted, relieving the pressure on the great vessels.

79. 1. Fetal movement is noted during labor, but it is not directly related to the fetal scalp stimulation test.
2. **The fetal heart should accelerate in response to scalp stimulation.**
3. The variability does not change in direct response to the fetal scalp stimulation test.
4. Late decelerations are related to uteroplacental insufficiency. The fetal scalp stimulation test will not affect a late deceleration pattern.

TEST-TAKING TIP: The fetal scalp stimulation test is performed by the health care practitioner when the fetal heart pattern is equivocal. For example, if the variability is questionable, the practitioner may perform the stimulation test. If the fetal heart rate accelerates in response to the test, the nurse interprets the response as a positive sign.

80. 1. Oxygen saturations are noninvasive assessments whereas fetal scalp sampling assessments are performed on blood obtained from the fetal scalp. Fetal oxygen saturation levels are well below those seen in extrauterine life—approximately 50% to 75%.
2. Normal fetal hemoglobin levels are well above those seen in extrauterine life—14 to 20 g/dL.
3. This fetal glucose level is indicative of maternal hyperglycemia.
4. **This fetal pH value is within normal limits.**

TEST-TAKING TIP: It is essential that the test taker be aware that many fetal lab values are much different from those seen in extrauterine life. The nurse would expect to see fetal oxygen saturation of 50% to 75%, not 99%, and fetal hemoglobin levels of 14 to 20 g/dL, not 11 g/dL. The nurse would expect to see a fetal serum glucose level of 140 mg/dL only if the mother had diabetes. The only expected value listed is a pH of 7.30 because this is consistent with a normal, slightly acidic fetal pH. The differences in fetal and extrauterine values reflect the fact that the fetus is not oxygenating efficiently through the lungs, as happens in the extrauterine environment, but rather is "breathing" indirectly via the placenta.

81. 1. Many Chinese believe that labor is a "hot" period. Applying heat at this time would be culturally insensitive.
2. **It is important to inquire about the pain level of all women in labor, but especially those from the Asian culture.**
3. Head covering is important for observant Jewish women and Muslim women, but is not usually important for Chinese women.
4. It is very uncommon for Chinese women to be verbal during labor.

TEST-TAKING TIP: Childbearing and child rearing are fraught with cultural implications. It is essential that the nurse understand the many cultural beliefs of clients for whom they will care. Chinese women are often expected to be quiet during labor. Even when in severe pain, they often remain stoic and uncomplaining. It is essential, therefore, that the nurse repeatedly question them regarding their level of pain using an objective pain scale.

82.
1. Muslim women, who are often from Arabic countries, are expected to keep their heads covered at all times.
2. Chinese women do not usually request that their heads be covered.
3. Russian women do not usually request that their heads be covered unless they are observant Jews.
4. Greek women do not usually request that their heads be covered.

TEST-TAKING TIP: There are two groups of women who are likely to request that their heads be covered at all times—observant Jews and Muslims. Many Arabic women are Muslim; therefore, the nurse should ask whether or not they would like head coverings. Observant or Orthodox Jewish women also will usually request that their heads be covered. It is very important that religious requests be met with acceptance by the health care staff.

83.
1. An Orthodox Jewish man is forbidden by Jewish law from touching his mate whenever she is experiencing vaginal discharge.
2. The religious leader of the Jewish people is the rabbi. A priest is the religious leader of Catholics and some other Christian sects.
3. **Observant Jewish women are expected to have their elbows covered at all times. A long-sleeved gown, therefore, should be provided for them.**
4. Observant Jewish women will follow a kosher diet that may or may not be vegetarian.

TEST-TAKING TIP: There are a number of religious mandates that guide the lives of Jewish couples. The mandates surround everyday life—what to eat, what to wear, when work is allowed, and when it is prohibited—as well as life events—sexuality and birthing. The nurse should have some familiarity with the many precepts of the Jewish religion to care for that population with cultural competence.

84. 1, 2, and 5 are correct.
1. **Nurse midwives sometimes recommend that women at full term engage in sexual intercourse to stimulate labor.**
2. **Ingesting primrose oil is also sometimes recommended. Primrose oil is believed to help ripen the cervix.**
3. Exercise should be encouraged throughout pregnancy, but it is not used for induction.
4. Raw spinach is an excellent source of iron as well as a source of calcium and fiber. It is, however, not used for induction.

5. **Nipple and breast massage is sometimes recommended to help induce labor.**

TEST-TAKING TIP: If the test taker were unfamiliar with nonpharmacological induction methods, he or she could make some educated guesses by remembering that pharmacological medications for labor induction are prostaglandins and oxytocin. When a woman has an orgasm during intercourse, she releases oxytocin. Nipple and breast massage also stimulate oxytocin production. And evening primrose oil contains a fatty acid that converts into a prostaglandin compound.

85. 3 and 4 are correct.
1. The malleolus of the wrist has not been shown to reduce the pain of labor contractions.
2. The area above the patella of the knee has not been shown to reduce the pain of labor contractions.
3. **Pressure applied on the medial surface of the lower leg has been shown to lessen the pain of labor.**
4. **Pressure applied to the depression at the top one third of the sole of the foot has been shown to lessen the pain of labor.**
5. The area below the elbow has not been shown to reduce the pain of labor contractions.

TEST-TAKING TIP: Complementary therapies have been shown to be of value in a number of clinical situations, including labor. The specific acupressure point on the leg is located about 3 cm above the inner malleolus in the calf region. Strong pressure placed at these points has been shown to reduce the pain of labor contractions.

86.
1. Squatting is an alternate position for delivery, but it is not used to decrease perineal tearing.
2. Pushing the fetal head against the perineum is the cause of perineal tearing.
3. Pushing the fetal head against the perineum is the cause of perineal tearing.
4. **Massaging of the perineum with mineral oil does help to reduce perineal tearing.**

TEST-TAKING TIP: During labor, nurses and nurse midwives often massage a woman's perineum to increase the elasticity of the tissue. Because the tissue is more elastic, it is less inclined to tear during the delivery.

In addition, mothers are often encouraged to begin massaging the tissue during their last trimester.

87. 25 gtt/min

Formula for drip rate calculations:

$$\frac{\text{volume in mL} \times \text{drop factor}}{\text{time in minutes}}$$

$$\frac{150 \text{ mL} \times 10 \text{ gtt/mL}}{60 \text{ min}} = \frac{150}{6}$$

$$\frac{150}{6} = 25 \text{ gtt/min}$$

TEST-TAKING TIP: Please note that when the units for each of the numbers is included, the test taker will never make a mistake with drip rate calculations because, as can be seen above, the mL's are cancelled out and what remains is the required units, gtt/min. Drip rates are always calculated to the nearest whole number because it is impossible to administer a fraction of a drop.

88. 0.25 mL

Formula for calculating the volume of medication to be administered:

Known dosage : known value = desired dosage : desired volume

$$2 \text{ mg} : 1 \text{ mL} = 0.5 \text{ mg} : x \text{ mL}$$
$$2 \text{ mg } x = 0.5 \text{ mg}$$
$$x = 0.25 \text{ mL}$$

TEST-TAKING TIP: This is a simple ratio and proportion problem. The known is placed on one side of the equation (2 mg/mL) and the desired is placed on the other side of the equation (0.5 mg/x mL). To solve the problem, the nurse simply must cross multiply.

89. 1. The cervix is thin.
2. There is nothing in the scenario that suggests that the membranes are bulging.
3. At –2 station, the head is well above the ischial spines.
4. The cervix is dilated 5 cm (or approximately 2 inches). The nurse would, therefore, not feel a closed cervix.

TEST-TAKING TIP: During pregnancy and early labor, the cervix is closed, long, and thick. During the labor process, however, the cervix changes shape, becoming paper thin and dilating to 10 cm. This is a universal finding. No matter how tall or short, old or young a woman is, her cervix will dilate to 10 cm and efface 100% if she has a vaginal delivery.

90. 1. Laboring clients are allowed to eat by some practitioners. Midwives are more likely to allow eating than are physicians.
2. This is a very negative statement that does not answer the client's question.
3. It is unlikely that the woman will eat at established meal times. Plus, a regular diet is rarely given to laboring clients, even by midwives.
4. This is the best response.

TEST-TAKING TIP: Peristalsis slows dramatically during labor. Because of this, women rarely become hungry during labor, but they do need fluids and some nourishment. Clear fluids, including ice chips, water, tea, and bouillon, are often allowed. Ultimately, though, it is the health care practitioner's decision what and how much the client may consume.

Normal Newborn

6

Newborn babies emerge from the womb where they have been protected and nourished throughout the pregnancy. Although their bodies may function well in utero, they must transition after birth to an extrauterine existence. Neonates must respire through their lungs, consume food, and excrete their bodily wastes. The nurse is responsible for assessing the newborn baby's changes and reporting any deviations from normal. Newborns' physical characteristics are unique. The nurse, therefore, must also be fully knowledgeable of those many differences and report any deviations from normal. And, as important as the physical care is, so too is the education that nurses must impart to the parents of new babies. Once the babies are discharged, the parents will need to provide full care. Unless nurses provide the parents with the knowledge that allows them to do so, there is the potential for child neglect and abuse.

KEYWORDS

The following words include English vocabulary, nursing/medical terminology, concepts, principles, or information relevant to content specifically addressed in the chapter or associated with topics presented in it. English dictionaries, your nursing textbooks, and medical dictionaries such as *Taber's Cyclopedic Medical Dictionary* are resources that can be used to expand your knowledge and understanding of these words and related information.

anticipatory guidance

Apgar score

Babinski reflex

bilirubin

brown adipose tissue

café au lait spot

caput succedaneum

cephalhematoma

circumcision

colic

colostrum

cryptorchidism

dysplasia

en face

Epstein's pearls

erythema toxicum

frenulum

harlequin sign

hepatitis B vaccine

hypoglycemia

hypothermia

intracostal retractions

jaundice

kernicterus

meconium

milia

mongolian spots

Moro reflex

neonatal abduction

neonatal feeding: breastfeeding and
 bottle-feeding

Neonatal Infant Pain Scale (NIPS)

neonatal mortality rate

neonatal ophthalmic prophylaxis

neonatal screening tests

neonate

ophthalmia neonatorum

Ortolani sign

petechiae

plagiocephaly

pseudomenses

subconjunctival hemorrhages

sudden infant death syndrome (SIDS)

supernumerary nipples

telangiectatic nevi
tonic neck reflex
vernix caseosa

vitamin K (Aquamephyton)
witch's milk

QUESTIONS

1. The nurse is discussing the neonatal blood screening test with a new mother. The nurse knows that the teaching was successful when the mother states that the test screens for the presence in the newborn of which of the following diseases? **Select all that apply.**
   1. Hypothyroidism.
   2. Sickle cell disease.
   3. Galactosemia.
   4. Cerebral palsy.
   5. Cystic fibrosis.

2. The nursery nurse is careful to wear gloves when admitting neonates into the nursery. Which of the following is the scientific rationale for this action?
   1. Meconium is filled with enteric bacteria.
   2. Amniotic fluid may contain harmful viruses.
   3. The high alkalinity of fetal urine is caustic to the skin.
   4. The baby is high risk for infection and must be protected.

3. A full-term newborn was just born. Which nursing intervention is important for the nurse to perform first?
   1. Remove wet blankets.
   2. Assess Apgar score.
   3. Insert eye prophylaxis.
   4. Elicit the Moro reflex.

4. To reduce the risk of hypoglycemia in a full-term newborn weighing 2,900 grams, what should the nurse do?
   1. Maintain the infant's temperature above 97.7°F.
   2. Feed the infant glucose water every 3 hours until breastfeeding well.
   3. Assess blood glucose levels every 3 hours for the first twelve hours.
   4. Encourage the mother to breastfeed every 4 hours.

5. A mother asks the nurse to tell her about the responsiveness of neonates at birth. Which of the following answers is appropriate? **Select all that apply.**
   1. "Babies have a poorly developed sense of smell until they are 2 months old."
   2. "Babies respond to all forms of taste well, but they prefer to eat sweet things like breast milk."
   3. "Babies are especially sensitive to being touched and cuddled."
   4. "Babies are nearsighted with blurry vision until they are about 3 months of age."
   5. "Babies respond to many sounds, especially to the high-pitched tone of the female voice."

6. A mother, 1 day postpartum from a 3-hour labor and a spontaneous vaginal delivery, questions the nurse because her baby's face is "purple." Upon examination, the nurse notes petechiae over the scalp, forehead, and cheeks of the baby. The nurse's response should be based on which of the following?
   1. Petechiae are indicative of severe bacterial infections.
   2. Rapid deliveries can injure the neonatal presenting part.
   3. Petechiae are characteristic of the normal newborn rash.
   4. The injuries are a sign that the child has been abused.

7. A 2-day-old breastfeeding baby born via normal spontaneous vaginal delivery has just been weighed in the newborn nursery. The nurse determines that the baby has lost 3.5% of the birth weight. Which of the following nursing actions is appropriate?
   1. Do nothing because this is a normal weight loss.
   2. Notify the neonatologist of the significant weight loss.
   3. Advise the mother to bottle feed the baby at the next feed.
   4. Assess the baby for hypoglycemia with a glucose monitor.

8. Four newborns are in the neonatal nursery, none of whom is crying or in distress. Which of the babies should the nurse report to the neonatologist?
   1. 16-hour-old baby who has yet to pass meconium.
   2. 16-hour-old baby whose blood glucose is 50 mg/dL.
   3. 2-day-old baby who is breathing irregularly at 70 breaths per minute.
   4. 2-day-old baby who is excreting a milky discharge from both nipples.

9. The pediatrician has ordered vitamin K 0.5 mg IM for a newborn. The medication is available as 2 mg/mL. How many milliliters (mL) should the nurse administer to the baby? **Calculate to the nearest hundredth.**
   _____ mL

10. A nurse is doing a newborn assessment on a new admission to the nursery. Which of the following actions should the nurse make when evaluating the baby for developmental dysplasia of the hip (DDH)? **Select all that apply.**
    1. Grasp the baby's legs with the thumbs on the inner thighs and forefingers on the outer thighs.
    2. Gently adduct and abduct the baby's thighs.
    3. Palpate the trochanter during hip rotation.
    4. Place the baby in a fetal position.
    5. Compare the lengths of the baby's legs.

11. A nurse notes that a 6-hour-old neonate has cyanotic hands and feet. Which of the following actions by the nurse is appropriate?
    1. Place child in an isolette.
    2. Administer oxygen.
    3. Swaddle baby in a blanket.
    4. Apply pulse oximeter.

12. A couple is asking the nurse whether or not their son should be circumcised. On which fact should the nurse's response be based?
    1. Boys should be circumcised for them to establish a positive self-image.
    2. Boys should not be circumcised because there is no medical rationale for the procedure.
    3. Experts from the Centers for Disease Control and Prevention argue that circumcision is desirable.
    4. A statement from the American Academy of Pediatrics asserts that circumcision is optional.

13. A baby boy is to be circumcised by the mother's obstetrician. Which of the following actions shows that the nurse is being a patient advocate?
    1. Before the procedure, the nurse prepares the sterile field for the physician.
    2. The nurse refuses to unclothe the baby until the doctor orders something for pain.
    3. The nurse holds the feeding immediately before the circumcision.
    4. After the procedure, the nurse monitors the site for signs of bleeding.

14. Using the Neonatal Infant Pain Scale (NIPS), a nurse is assessing the pain response of a newborn who has just had a circumcision. The nurse is assessing a change in which of the following signs/symptoms? **Select all that apply.**
    1. Heart rate.
    2. Blood pressure.
    3. Temperature.
    4. Facial expression.
    5. Breathing pattern.

15. A nurse is teaching a mother how to care for her 3-day-old son's circumcised penis. Which of the following actions demonstrates that the mother has learned the information?
    1. The mother cleanses the glans with a cotton swab dipped in hydrogen peroxide.
    2. The mother covers the glans with antifungal ointment after rinsing off any discharge.
    3. The mother squeezes soapy water from the wash cloth over the glans.
    4. The mother replaces the dry sterile dressing before putting on the diaper.

16. Please put an "X" on the site where the nurse should administer vitamin K 0.5 mg IM to the neonate.

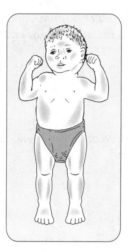 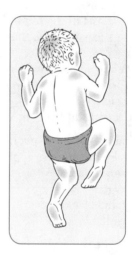

17. The nurse is teaching a mother regarding the baby's sutures and fontanelles. Please put an "X" on the fontanelle that will close at 6 to 8 weeks of age.

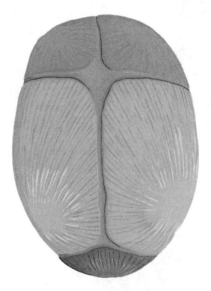

18. A neonate is being admitted to the well-baby nursery. Which of the following findings should be reported to the neonatologist?
    1. Umbilical cord with three vessels.
    2. Diamond-shaped anterior fontanelle.
    3. Cryptorchidism.
    4. Café au lait spot.

19. A female African American baby has been admitted into the nursery. Which of the following physiological findings would the nurse assess as normal? **Select all that apply.**
    1. Purple-colored patches on the buttocks and torso.
    2. Bilateral whitish discharge from the breasts.
    3. Bloody discharge from the vagina.
    4. Sharply demarcated dark red area on the face.
    5. Deep hair-covered dimple at the base of the spine.

20. The nurse is assessing a newborn on admission to the newborn nursery. Which of the following findings should the nurse report to the neonatologist?
    1. Intracostal retractions.
    2. Caput succedaneum.
    3. Epstein's pearls.
    4. Harlequin sign.

21. Four babies have just been admitted into the neonatal nursery. Which of the babies should the nurse assess first?
    1. Baby with respirations 42, oxygen saturation 96%.
    2. Baby with Apgar 9/9, weight 4,660 grams.
    3. Baby with temperature 98.0°F, length 21 inches.
    4. Baby with glucose 55 mg/dL, heart rate 121.

22. A neonate is in the active alert behavioral state. Which of the following would the nurse expect to see?
    1. Baby is showing signs of hunger and frustration.
    2. Baby is starting to whimper and cry.
    3. Baby is wide awake and attending to a picture.
    4. Baby is asleep and breathing rhythmically.

23. A mother asks whether or not she should be concerned that her baby never opens his mouth to breathe when his nose is so small. Which of the following is the nurse's best response?
    1. "The baby does rarely open his mouth but you can see that he isn't in any distress."
    2. "Babies usually breathe in and out through their noses so they can feed without choking."
    3. "Everything about babies is small. It truly is amazing how everything works so well."
    4. "You are right. I will report the baby's small nasal openings to the pediatrician right away."

24. The nursery charge nurse is assessing a 1-day-old female on morning rounds. Which of the following findings should be reported to the neonatologist as soon as possible? **Select all that apply.**
    1. Blood in the diaper.
    2. Grunting during expiration.
    3. Deep red coloring on one side of the body with pale pink on the other side.
    4. Lacy and mottled appearance over the entire chest and abdomen.
    5. Flaring of the nares during inspiration.

25. A mother calls the nurse to her room because "My baby's eyes are bleeding." The nurse notes bright red hemorrhages in the sclerae of both of the baby's eyes. Which of the following actions by the nurse is appropriate at this time?
    1. Notify the pediatrician immediately and report the finding.
    2. Notify the social worker about the probable maternal abuse.
    3. Reassure the mother that the trauma resulted from pressure changes at birth and the hemorrhages will slowly disappear.
    4. Obtain an ophthalmoscope from the nursery to evaluate the red reflex and condition of the retina in each eye.

26. Which of the following full-term babies requires immediate intervention?
    1. Baby with seesaw breathing.
    2. Baby with irregular breathing with 10-second apnea spells.
    3. Baby with coordinated thoracic and abdominal breathing.
    4. Baby with respiratory rate of 52.

27. Which of the following drawings is consistent with a baby who was in the frank breech position in utero?

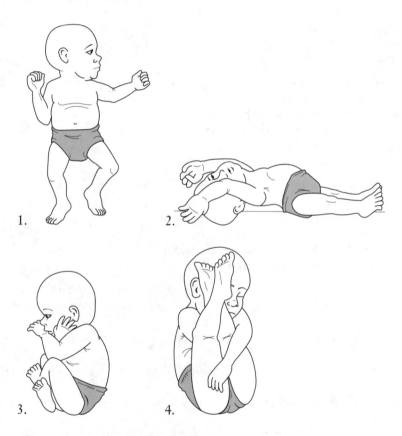

1.   2.

3.   4.

28. The following four babies are in the neonatal nursery. Which of the babies should be seen by the neonatologist?
    1. 1-day-old, HR 100 beats per minute, in deep sleep.
    2. 2-day-old, T 97.7°F, slightly jaundiced.
    3. 3-day-old, breastfeeding every 4 hours, jittery.
    4. 4-day-old, crying, papular rash on an erythematous base.

29. In which of the following situations would it be appropriate for the father to place the baby in the en face position to promote neonatal bonding?
    1. The baby is asleep with little to no eye movement, regular breathing.
    2. The baby is asleep with rapid eye movement, irregular breathing.
    3. The baby is awake, looking intently at an object, irregular breathing.
    4. The baby is awake, placing hands in the mouth, irregular breathing.

30. Four newborns were admitted into the neonatal nursery 1 hour ago. They are all sleeping in overhead warmers. Which of the babies should the nurse ask the neonatologist to evaluate?
    1. The neonate with a temperature of 98.9°F and weight of 3,000 grams.
    2. The neonate with white spots on the bridge of the nose.
    3. The neonate with raised white specks on the gums.
    4. The neonate with respirations of 72 and heart rate of 166.

31. A neonate is admitted to the nursery. The nurse makes the following assessments: weight 3,845 grams, head circumference 35 cm, chest circumference 33 cm, positive Ortolani sign, and presence of supernumerary nipples. Which of the assessments should be reported to the health care practitioner?
    1. Birth weight.
    2. Head and chest circumferences.
    3. Ortolani sign.
    4. Supernumerary nipples.

32. The nurse is about to elicit the Moro reflex. Which of the following responses should the nurse expect to see?
    1. When the cheek of the baby is touched, the newborn turns toward the side that is touched.
    2. When the lateral aspect of the sole of the baby's foot is stroked, the toes extend and fan outward.
    3. When the baby is suddenly lowered or startled, the neonate's arms straighten outward and the knees flex.
    4. When the newborn is supine and the head is turned to one side, the arm on that same side extends.

33. To check for the presence of Epstein's pearls, the nurse should assess which part of the neonate's body?
    1. Feet.
    2. Hands.
    3. Back.
    4. Mouth.

34. The nurse is assessing a neonate in the newborn nursery. Which of the following findings in a newborn should be reported to the neonatologist?
    1. The eyes cross and uncross when they are open.
    2. The ears are positioned in alignment with the inner and outer canthus of the eyes.
    3. Axillae and femoral folds of the baby are covered with a white cheesy substance.
    4. The nostrils flare whenever the baby inhales.

35. A 40-week-gestation neonate is in the first period of reactivity. Which of the following actions should the nurse take at this time?
    1. Encourage the parents to bond with their baby.
    2. Notify the neonatologist of the finding.
    3. Perform the gestational age assessment.
    4. Place the baby under the overhead warmer.

36. The nurse notes that a newborn, who is 5 minutes old, exhibits the following characteristics: heart rate 108 bpm, respiratory rate 29 rpm with lusty cry, pink body with bluish hands and feet, some flexion. What does the nurse determine the baby's Apgar score is?
    1. 6.
    2. 7.
    3. 8.
    4. 9.

37. A neonate, who is being admitted into the well-baby nursery, is exhibiting each of the following assessment findings. Which of the findings should the nurse report to the primary health care provider? **Select all that apply.**
    1. Harlequin sign.
    2. Extension of the toes when the lateral aspect of the sole is stroked.
    3. Elbow moves past the midline when the scarf sign is assessed.
    4. Slightly curved pinnae of the ears that are slow to recoil.
    5. Telangiectatic nevi.

38. The mother notes that her baby has a "bulge" on the back of one side of the head. She calls the nurse into the room to ask what the bulge is. The nurse notes that the bulge covers the right parietal bone but does not cross the suture lines. The nurse explains to the mother that the bulge results from which of the following?
    1. Molding of the baby's skull so that the baby could fit through her pelvis.
    2. Swelling of the tissues of the baby's head from the pressure of her pushing.
    3. The position that the baby took in her pelvis during the last trimester of her pregnancy.
    4. Small blood vessels that broke under the baby's scalp during birth.

39. A nurse is providing discharge teaching to the parents of a newborn. Which of the following should be included when teaching the parents how to care for the baby's umbilical cord?
    1. Cleanse it with hydrogen peroxide if it starts to smell.
    2. Remove it with sterile tweezers at one week of age.
    3. Call the doctor if greenish drainage appears.
    4. Cover it with sterile dressings until it falls off.

40. A mother asks the nurse which powder she should purchase to use on the baby's skin. What should the nurse's response be?
    1. "Any powder made especially for babies should be fine."
    2. "It is recommended that powder not be put on babies."
    3. "There is no real difference except that many babies are allergic to cornstarch so it should not be used."
    4. "As long as you put it only on the buttocks area, you can use any brand of baby powder that you like."

41. The nurse is teaching the parents of a 1-day-old baby how to give a sponge bath. Which of the following actions should be included?
    1. Clean the eyes from outer canthus to inner canthus.
    2. Cleanse the ear canals with a cotton swab.
    3. Assemble all supplies before beginning the bath.
    4. Check the temperature of the bath water with the fingertips.

42. The nurse is teaching the parents of a female baby how to change the baby's diapers. Which of the following should be included in the teaching?
    1. Always wipe the perineum from front to back.
    2. Remove any vernix caseosa from the labial folds.
    3. Put powder on the buttocks every time the baby stools.
    4. Weigh every diaper to assess hydration status.

43. The nurse has provided anticipatory guidance to a couple that has just delivered a baby. Which of the following is an appropriate short-term goal for the care of their new baby?
    1. The baby will have a bath with soap every morning.
    2. During a supervised play period, the baby will be placed on the tummy every day.
    3. The baby will be given a pacifier after each feeding.
    4. For the first month of life, the baby will sleep on its side in a crib next to the parents.

44. A nurse is advising a mother of a neonate being discharged from the hospital regarding car seat safety. Which of the following should be included in the teaching plan? **Select all that apply.**
    1. Place the baby's car seat in the front passenger seat of the car.
    2. Position the car seat rear facing until the baby reaches two years of age.
    3. Attach the car seat to the car at 2 latch points at the base of the car seat.
    4. Check that the installed car seat moves no more than 1 inch side to side or front to back.
    5. Make sure that there is at least a 3-inch space between the straps of the seat and the baby's body.

45. A nurse is providing anticipatory guidance to a couple regarding the baby's immunization schedule. Which of the following statements by the parents shows that the teaching by the nurse was successful? **Select all that apply.**
    1. The first hepatitis B injection is given by 1 month of age.
    2. The first polio injection will be given at 2 months of age.
    3. The MMR (measles, mumps, and rubella) immunization should be administered before the first birthday.
    4. Three DTaP (diphtheria, tetanus, and acellular pertussis) shots will be given during the first year of life.
    5. The Varivax (varicella) immunization will be administered after the baby turns one year of age.

46. A nurse is advising the parents of a newborn regarding when they should call their pediatrician. Which of the following responses show that the teaching was effective? **Select all that apply.**
    1. If the baby repeatedly refuses to feed.
    2. If the baby's breathing is irregular.
    3. If the baby has no tears when he cries.
    4. If the baby is repeatedly difficult to awaken.
    5. If the baby's temperature is above 100.4°F.

47. A nurse is providing anticipatory guidance to a couple before they take home their newborn. Which of the following should be included?
    1. If their baby is sleeping soundly, they should not awaken the baby for a feeding.
    2. If they take their baby outside, they should put sunscreen on the baby.
    3. They should purchase liquid acetaminophen to be used when ordered by the pediatrician.
    4. They should notify their pediatrician when the umbilical cord falls off.

48. A mucousy baby is being left with the parents for the first time after delivery. Which of the following should the nurse teach the parents regarding use of the bulb syringe?
    1. Suction the nostrils before suctioning the mouth.
    2. Make sure to suction the back of the throat.
    3. Insert the syringe before compressing the bulb.
    4. Dispose of the drainage in a tissue or a cloth.

49. Please put an "X" on the site where the nurse should perform a heel stick on the neonate.

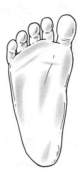

50. A nurse must give vitamin K 0.5 mg IM to a newly born baby. Which of the following needles could the nurse safely choose for the injection?
    1. ⅝ inch, 18 gauge.
    2. ⅝ inch, 25 gauge.
    3. 1 inch, 18 gauge.
    4. 1 inch, 25 gauge.

51. A nurse is practicing the procedures for conducting cardiopulmonary resuscitation (CPR) in the neonate. Which site should the nurse use to assess the pulse of a baby?
    1. Carotid.
    2. Radial.
    3. Brachial.
    4. Pedal.

52. A baby has just been admitted into the neonatal nursery. Before taking the newborn's vital signs, the nurse should warm his or her hands and the stethoscope to prevent heat loss resulting from which of the following?
    1. Evaporation.
    2. Conduction.
    3. Radiation.
    4. Convection.

53. The nurse is developing a teaching plan for parents who are taking home their 2-day-old breastfed baby. Which of the following should the nurse include in the plan?
    1. Wash hands well before picking up the baby.
    2. Refrain from having visitors for the first month.
    3. Wear a mask to prevent transmission of a cold.
    4. Sterilize the breast pump supplies after every use.

54. It is time for a baby who is in the drowsy behavioral state to breastfeed. Which of the following techniques could the mother use to arouse the baby? **Select all that apply.**
    1. Swaddle or tightly bundle the baby.
    2. Hand express milk onto the baby's lips.
    3. Talk with the baby while making eye contact.
    4. Remove the baby's shirt and change the diaper.
    5. Play pat-a-cake with the baby.

55. A bottle-feeding mother is providing a return demonstration of how to burp the baby. Which of the following would indicate that the teaching was successful? **Select all that apply.**
    1. The woman gently strokes and pats her baby's back.
    2. The woman positions the baby in a sitting position on her lap.
    3. The woman waits to burp the baby until the baby's feeding is complete.
    4. The woman states that a small amount of regurgitated formula is acceptable.
    5. The woman remarks that the baby does not need to burp after trying for one full minute.

56. A breastfeeding baby is born with a tight frenulum. Which of the following is an important assessment for the nurse to make?
    1. Integrity of the baby's uvula.
    2. Presence of maternal nipple damage.
    3. Presence of neonatal tongue injury.
    4. The baby's breathing pattern.

57. A mother is told that she should bottle feed her child for medical reasons. Which of the following maternal disease states are consistent with the recommendation? **Select all that apply.**
    1. Untreated, active tuberculosis.
    2. Hepatitis B surface antigen positive.
    3. Human immunodeficiency virus positive.
    4. Chorioamnionitis.
    5. Mastitis.

58. A nurse has brought a 2-hour-old baby to a mother from the nursery. The nurse is going to assist the mother with the first breastfeeding experience. Which of the following actions should the nurse perform first?
    1. Compare mother's and baby's identification bracelets.
    2. Help the mother into a comfortable position.
    3. Teach the mother about a proper breast latch.
    4. Tickle the baby's lips with the mother's nipple.

59. Which short-term goal is appropriate for a full-term, breastfeeding neonate?
    1. The baby will regain birth weight by 4 weeks of age.
    2. The baby will sleep through the night by 4 weeks of age.
    3. The baby will stool every 2 to 3 hours by 1 week of age.
    4. The baby will urinate 6 to 10 times per day by 1 week of age.

60. A mother is attempting to latch her newborn baby to the breast. Which of the following actions are important for the mother to perform to achieve effective breastfeeding? **Select all that apply.**
    1. Place the baby on his or her back in the mother's lap.
    2. Wait until the baby opens his or her mouth wide.
    3. Hold the baby at the level of the mother's breasts.
    4. Point the baby's nose to the mother's nipple.
    5. Wait until the baby's tongue is pointed toward the roof of his or her mouth.

61. The nurse is evaluating the effectiveness of an intervention when assisting a woman whose baby has been latched to the nipple only rather than to the nipple and the areola. Which response would indicate that further intervention is needed?
    1. The client states that the pain has decreased.
    2. The nurse hears the baby swallow after each suck.
    3. The baby's jaws move up and down once every second.
    4. The baby's cheeks move in and out with each suck.

62. The parents and their full-term, breastfed neonate were discharged from the hospital. Which behavior 2 days later indicates a positive response by the parents to the nurse's discharge teaching? **Select all that apply.**
    1. The parents count their baby's diapers.
    2. The parents measure the baby's intake.
    3. The parents give one bottle of formula every day.
    4. The parents take the baby to see the pediatrician.
    5. The parents time the baby's feedings.

63. The nurse does not hear the baby swallow when suckling even though the baby appears to be latched properly to the breast. Which of the following situations may be the reason for this observation?
    1. The mother reports a pain level of 4 on a 5-point scale.
    2. The baby has been suckling for over 10 minutes.
    3. The mother uses the cross-cradle hold while feeding.
    4. The baby lies with the chin touching the under part of the breast.

64. The nurse is concerned that a bottle-fed baby may become obese because of which activity by the mother?
    1. She encourages the baby to finish the bottle at each feed.
    2. She feeds the baby every 3 to 4 hours.
    3. She feeds the baby a soy-based formula.
    4. She burps the baby every ½ to 1 ounce.

65. A 2-day-old, exclusively breastfed baby is to be discharged home. Under what conditions should the nurse teach the parents to call the pediatrician?
    1. If the baby feeds 8 to 12 times each day.
    2. If the baby urinates 6 to 10 times each day.
    3. If the baby has stools that are watery and bright yellow.
    4. If the baby has eyes and skin that are tinged yellow.

66. A nurse who is caring for a mother/newborn dyad on the maternity unit has identified the following nursing diagnosis: Effective breastfeeding. Which of the following would warrant this diagnosis?
    1. Baby's lips are flanged when latched.
    2. Baby feeds every 4 hours.
    3. Baby lost 12% of weight since birth.
    4. Baby's tongue stays behind the gum line.

67. A newborn was born weighing 3,278 grams. On day 2 of life, the baby weighed 3,042 grams. What percentage of weight loss did the baby experience? **Calculate to the nearest hundredth.**
    _____ %

68. A mother is preparing to breastfeed her baby. Which of the following actions would encourage the baby to open the mouth wide for feeding?
    1. Holding the baby in the en face position.
    2. Pushing down on the baby's lower jaw.
    3. Tickling the baby's lips with the nipple.
    4. Giving the baby a trial bottle of formula.

69. A breastfeeding mother mentions to the nurse that she has heard that babies sleep better at night if they are given a small amount of rice cereal in the evening. Which of the following comments by the nurse is appropriate?
    1. "That is correct. The rice cereal takes longer for them to digest so they sleep better and longer."
    2. "It is recommended that babies receive only breast milk for the first 4 to 6 months of their lives."
    3. "It is too early for rice cereal, but I would recommend giving the baby a bottle of formula at night."
    4. "A better recommendation is to give apple sauce at 3 months of age and apple juice 1 month later."

70. On admission to the maternity unit, it is learned that a mother has smoked 2 packs of cigarettes per day and expects to continue to smoke after discharge. The mother also states that she expects to breastfeed her baby. The nurse's response should be based on which of the following?
    1. Breastfeeding is contraindicated if the mother smokes cigarettes.
    2. Breastfeeding is protective for the baby and should be encouraged.
    3. A 2-pack-a-day smoker should be reported to child protective services for child abuse.
    4. A mother who admits to smoking cigarettes may also be abusing illicit substances.

71. A breastfeeding mother who is 2 weeks postpartum is informed by her pediatrician that her 4-year-old has chickenpox (varicella). The mother calls the nursery nurse because she is concerned about having the baby in contact with the sick sibling. The mother had chickenpox as a child. Which of the following responses by the nurse is appropriate?
    1. "The baby received passive immunity through the placenta, plus the breast milk will also be protective."
    2. "The baby should stay with relatives until the ill sibling recovers from the episode of chickenpox."
    3. "Chickenpox is transmitted by contact route so careful hand washing should prevent transmission."
    4. "Because chickenpox is a spirochetal illness, both the child and baby should receive the appropriate medications."

72. A client is preparing to breastfeed her newborn son in the cross-cradle position. Which of the following actions should the woman make?
    1. Place a pillow in her lap.
    2. Position the head of the baby in her elbow.
    3. Put the baby on his back.
    4. Move the breast toward the mouth of the baby.

73. A mother, who gave birth 5 minutes ago, states that she would like to breastfeed. The baby's Apgar score is 9/9. Which of the following actions should the nurse perform first?
    1. Assist the woman to breastfeed.
    2. Dress the baby in a shirt and diaper.
    3. Administer the ophthalmic prophylaxis.
    4. Take the baby's rectal temperature.

74. A 4-day-old breastfeeding neonate whose birth weight was 2,678 grams has lost 100 grams since the cesarean birth. Which of the following actions should the nurse take?
    1. Nothing because this is an acceptable weight loss.
    2. Advise the mother to supplement feedings with formula.
    3. Notify the neonatologist of the excessive weight loss.
    4. Give the baby dextrose water between breast feedings.

75. A 2-day-postpartum breastfeeding client is complaining of pain during feedings. Which of the following may be causing the pain?
    1. The neonate's frenulum is attached to the tip of the tongue.
    2. The baby's tongue forms a trough around the breast during the feedings.
    3. The newborn's feeds last for 30 minutes every 2 hours.
    4. The baby is latched to the nipple and to about 1 inch of the mother's areola.

76. A newly delivered mother states, "I have not had any alcohol since I decided to become pregnant. I have decided not to breastfeed because I would really like to go out and have a good time for a change." Which of the following is the best response by the nurse?
    1. "I understand that being good for so many months can become very frustrating."
    2. "Even if you bottle feed the baby, you will have to refrain from drinking alcohol for at least the next six weeks to protect your own health."
    3. "Alcohol can be consumed at any time while you are breastfeeding."
    4. "You may drink alcohol while breastfeeding, although it is best to wait until the alcohol has been metabolized before you feed again."

77. A physician writes in a breastfeeding mother's chart, "Ampicillin 500 mg q 6 h po. Baby should be bottle fed until medication is discontinued." What should be the nurse's next action?
    1. Follow the order as written.
    2. Call the doctor and question the order.
    3. Follow the antibiotic order but ignore the order to bottle feed the baby.
    4. Refer to a text to see whether the antibiotic is safe while breastfeeding.

78. Four pregnant women advise the nurse that they wish to breastfeed their babies. Which of the mothers should be advised to bottle feed her child?
    1. The woman with a neoplasm requiring chemotherapy.
    2. The woman with cholecystitis requiring surgery.
    3. The woman with a concussion.
    4. The woman with thrombosis.

79. A woman states that she is going to bottle feed her baby because, "I hate milk and I know that to make good breast milk I will have to drink milk." The nurse's response about producing high-quality breast milk should be based on which of the following?
    1. The mother must drink at least 3 glasses of milk per day to absorb sufficient quantities of calcium.
    2. The mother should consume at least 1 glass of milk per day but should also consume other dairy products like cheese.
    3. The mother can consume a variety of good calcium sources like broccoli and fish with bones as well as dairy products.
    4. The mother must monitor her protein intake more than her calcium intake because the baby needs the protein for growth.

80. A client asks whether or not there are any foods that she must avoid eating while breastfeeding. Which of the following responses by the nurse is appropriate?
    1. "No, there are no foods that are strictly contraindicated while breastfeeding."
    2. "Yes, the same foods that were dangerous to eat during pregnancy should be avoided."
    3. "Yes, foods like onions, cauliflower, broccoli, and cabbage make babies very colicky."
    4. "Yes, spices from hot and spicy foods get into the milk and can bother your baby."

81. A woman who has just delivered has decided to bottle feed her full-term baby. Which of the following should be included in the patient teaching?
    1. The baby's stools will appear bright yellow and will usually be loose.
    2. The bottle nipples should be enlarged to ease the baby's suckling.
    3. It is best to heat the baby's bottle in the microwave before feeding.
    4. It is important to hold the bottle to keep the nipple filled with formula.

82. Please choose the picture of the breastfeeding baby that shows correct position and latch on.

1.

2.

3.

4.

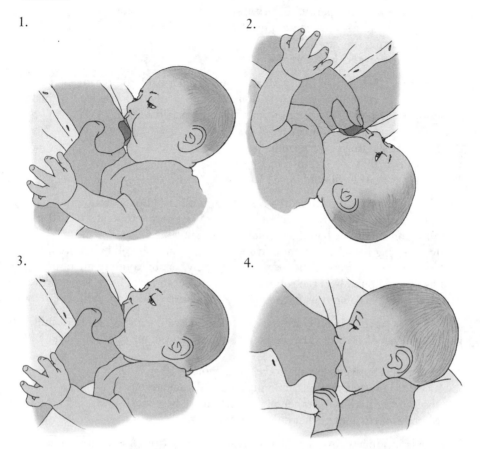

83. A full-term neonate, Apgar 9/9, has just been admitted to the nursery after a cesarean delivery, fetal position LMA, under epidural anesthesia. Which of the following physiological findings would the nurse expect to see?
    1. Soft pulmonary rales.
    2. Absent bowel sounds.
    3. Depressed Moro reflex.
    4. Positive Ortolani sign.

84. A full-term neonate has brown adipose fat tissue (BAT) stores that were deposited during the latter part of the third trimester. What does the nurse understand is the function of BAT stores?
    1. To promote melanin production in the neonatal period.
    2. To provide heat production when the baby is hypothermic.
    3. To protect the bony structures of the body from injury.
    4. To provide calories for neonatal growth between feedings.

85. A neonate has an elevated bilirubin and is slightly jaundiced on day 3 of life. What is the probable reason for these changes?
    1. Hemolysis of neonatal red blood cells by the maternal antibodies.
    2. Physiological destruction of fetal red blood cells during the extrauterine period.
    3. Pathological liver function resulting from hypoxemia during the birthing process.
    4. Delayed meconium excretion resulting in the production of direct bilirubin.

86. The pediatrician writes the following order for a term newborn: Vitamin K 1 mg IM. Which of the following responses provides a rationale for this order?
    1. During the neonatal period, babies absorb fat-soluble vitamins poorly.
    2. Breast milk and formula contain insufficient quantities of vitamin K.
    3. The neonatal gut is sterile.
    4. Vitamin K prevents hemolytic jaundice.

87. A nurse takes a Spanish-speaking Mexican woman her baby to breastfeed. The woman refuses to feed and makes motions that she wants to bottle feed. Which of the following is a likely explanation for the woman's behavior?
    1. She has decided not to breastfeed.
    2. She thinks she must give formula before the breast.
    3. She believes that colostrum is bad for the baby.
    4. She thinks that she should bottle feed.

88. The nurse enters a Latin woman's postpartum room and notes that her neonate is wearing a hat and is covered in three blankets. The room temperature is 70°F. The nurse's action should be based on which of the following?
    1. Overdressing babies is common in some cultures and should be ignored.
    2. The mother has dressed the baby appropriately for the room temperature.
    3. The nurse should drop the room temperature because the baby is overdressed.
    4. Overheating is dangerous for neonates and the extra clothing should be removed.

89. The nurse observes a healthy woman of African descent expressing breast milk into her baby's eyes. Which of the following responses by the nurse is appropriate at this time?
    1. Report the abusive behavior to the social worker.
    2. Advise the mother that her action is potentially dangerous.
    3. Observe the mother for other signs of irrational behavior.
    4. Ask the woman about other cultural traditions.

90. The nurse informs the parents of a breastfed baby that the American Academy of Pediatrics advises that babies be supplemented with which of the following vitamins?
    1. Vitamin A.
    2. Vitamin B_{12}.
    3. Vitamin C.
    4. Vitamin D.

91. A 2-day-old neonate received a vitamin K injection at birth. Which of the following signs/symptoms in the baby would indicate that the treatment was effective?
    1. Skin color is pink.
    2. Vital signs are normal.
    3. Glucose levels are stable.
    4. Blood clots after heel sticks.

92. A nurse is about to administer the ophthalmic preparation to a newly born neonate. Which of the following is the correct statement regarding the medication?
    1. It is administered to prevent the development of neonatal cataracts.
    2. The medicine should be placed in the lower conjunctiva from the inner to outer canthus.
    3. The medicine must be administered immediately upon delivery of the baby.
    4. It is administered to neonates whose mothers test positive for gonorrhea during pregnancy.

93. A mother questions why the ophthalmic medication is given to the baby. Which of the following responses by the nurse would be appropriate to make at this time?
    1. "I am required by law to give the medicine."
    2. "The medicine helps to prevent eye infections."
    3. "The medicine promotes neonatal health."
    4. "All babies receive the medicine at delivery."

94. A neonate is to receive the hepatitis B vaccine in the neonatal nursery. Which of the following must the nurse have available before administering the injection?
    1. Hepatitis B immune globulin in a second syringe.
    2. Sterile water to dilute the vaccine before injecting.
    3. Epinephrine in case of severe allergic reactions.
    4. Oral syringe because the vaccine is given by mouth.

95. A certified nursing assistant (CNA) is working with a registered nurse (RN) in the neonatal nursery. Which of the following actions should the RN perform rather than delegating it to the CNA?
    1. Bathe and weigh a 1-hour-old baby.
    2. Take the apical heart rate and respirations of a 4-hour-old baby.
    3. Obtain a stool sample from a 1-day-old baby.
    4. Provide discharge teaching to the mother of a 4-day-old baby.

96. Four babies with the following conditions are in the well-baby nursery. The baby with which of the conditions is high risk for physiological jaundice?
    1. Cephalhematoma.
    2. Caput succedaneum.
    3. Harlequin coloring.
    4. Mongolian spotting.

97. A full-term baby's bilirubin level is 12 mg/dL on day 3. Which of the following neonatal behaviors would the nurse expect to see?
    1. Excessive crying.
    2. Increased appetite.
    3. Lethargy.
    4. Hyperreflexia.

98. The nursing management of a neonate with physiological jaundice should be directed toward which of the following client care goals?
    1. The baby will exhibit no signs of kernicterus.
    2. The baby will not develop erythroblastosis fetalis.
    3. The baby will have a bilirubin of 16 mg/dL or higher at discharge.
    4. The baby will spend at least 20 hours per day under phototherapy.

99. A 2-day-old baby's blood values are:
    Blood type, O– (negative).
    Direct Coombs, negative.
    Hematocrit, 50%.
    Bilirubin, 1.5 mg/dL.
    The mother's blood type is A+. What should the nurse do at this time?
    1. Do nothing because the results are within normal limits.
    2. Assess the baby for opisthotonic posturing.
    3. Administer RhoGAM to the mother per doctor's order.
    4. Call the doctor for an order to place the baby under bili-lights.

100. A 4-day-old baby born via cesarean section is slightly jaundiced. The laboratory reports a bilirubin assessment of 6.0 mg/dL. Which of the following would the nurse expect the neonatologist to order for the baby at this time?
    1. To be placed under phototherapy.
    2. To be discharged home with the parents.
    3. To be prepared for a replacement transfusion.
    4. To be fed glucose water between routine feeds.

101. A nurse is assessing the bonding of the father with his newborn baby. Which of the following actions by the father would be of concern to the nurse?
    1. He holds the baby in the en face position.
    2. He calls the baby by a full name rather than a nickname.
    3. He tells the mother to pick up the crying baby.
    4. He falls asleep in the chair with the baby on his chest.

102. The nurse is conducting a state-mandated evaluation of a neonate's hearing. Infants are assessed for deficits because hearing-impaired babies are high risk for which of the following?
    1. Delayed speech development.
    2. Otitis externa.
    3. Poor parental bonding.
    4. Choanal atresia.

103. A baby has just been circumcised. If bleeding occurs, which of the following actions should be taken first?
    1. Put the baby's diapers on as tightly as possible.
    2. Apply light pressure to the area with sterile gauze.
    3. Call the physician who performed the surgery.
    4. Assess the baby's heart rate and oxygen saturation.

104. A nurse reads that the neonatal mortality rate in the United States for a given year was 5. The nurse interprets that information as:
    1. 5 babies less than 28 days old per 1,000 live births died.
    2. 5 babies less than 1 year old per 1,000 live births died.
    3. 5 babies less than 28 days old per 100,000 births died.
    4. 5 babies less than 1 year old per 100,000 births died.

105. A mother tells the nurse that because of family history she is afraid her baby son will develop colic. Which of the following colic management strategies should the parents be taught? **Select all that apply.**
    1. Small, frequent feedings.
    2. Prone sleep positioning.
    3. Tightly swaddling the baby.
    4. Rocking the baby while holding him face down on the forearm.
    5. Maintaining a home environment that is cigarette smoke–free.

106. A nurse, when providing discharge teaching to parents, emphasizes actions to prevent plagiocephaly and to promote gross motor development in their full-term newborn. Which of the following actions should the nurse advise the parents to take?
    1. Breastfeed the baby frequently.
    2. Make sure the baby receives vaccinations at recommended intervals.
    3. Change the diapers regularly.
    4. Minimize supine positioning during supervised play periods.

107. A mother and her 2-day-old baby are preparing for discharge. Which of the following situations would require the baby's discharge to be cancelled?
    1. The parents own a car seat that only faces the rear of the car.
    2. The baby's bilirubin is 19 mg/dL.
    3. The baby's blood glucose is 59 mg/dL.
    4. There is a large bluish spot on the left buttock of the baby.

108. A mother confides to a nurse that she has no crib at home for her baby. The mother asks the nurse which of the following places would be best for the baby to sleep. Of the following choices, which location should the nurse suggest?
    1. In bed with his 5-year-old brother.
    2. In a waterbed with his mother and father.
    3. In a large empty dresser drawer.
    4. In the living room on a pull-out sofa.

109. A baby is just delivered. Which of the following physiological changes is of highest priority?
    1. Thermoregulation.
    2. Spontaneous respirations.
    3. Extrauterine circulatory shift.
    4. Successful feeding.

110. A breastfeeding mother refuses to place her unclothed baby face down on her chest because "babies are always supposed to be put on their backs. Babies who are on their stomachs die from SIDS." The nurse's action should be based on which of the following?
    1. Skin-to-skin contact facilitates breastfeeding and helps to maintain neonatal temperature.
    2. The risk of SIDS increases whenever unsupervised babies are placed in the supine position.
    3. SIDS rarely occurs before the completion of the neonatal period.
    4. Back-to-sleep guidelines have been modified for breastfeeding babies.

111. The nursing diagnosis—Risk for suffocation—is included in a standard care plan in the neonatal nursery. Which of the following outcome goals should be included in relation to this diagnosis?
    1. Baby will be placed supine for sleep.
    2. Baby will be breastfed in the side-lying position.
    3. Baby will be swaddled when in the open crib.
    4. Baby will be strapped when seated in a car seat.

112. It has just been discovered that a newborn is missing from the maternity unit. The nursing staff should be watchful for which of the following individuals?
    1. A middle-aged male.
    2. An underweight female.
    3. Pro-life advocate.
    4. Visitor of the same race.

113. Which of the following behaviors should nurses know are characteristic of infant abductors? **Select all that apply.**
    1. Act on the spur of the moment.
    2. Create a diversion on the unit.
    3. Ask questions about the routine of the unit.
    4. Choose rooms near stairwells.
    5. Wear over-sized clothing.

The correct answer number and rationale for why it is the correct answer are given in **boldface blue type**. Rationales for why the other possible answer options are incorrect also are given, but they are not in boldface type.

1. **1, 2, 3, and 5 are correct.**
   1. **Congenital hypothyroidism is a malfunction of or complete absence of the thyroid gland that is present from birth. It is screened for in all 50 states.**
   2. **Sickle cell disease is an autosomal recessive disease resulting in abnormally shaped red blood cells. It is screened for in all 50 states.**
   3. **Galactosemia is an incurable autosomal recessive disease characterized by the absence of the enzyme required to metabolize galactose. It is screened for in all 50 states.**
   4. Cerebral palsy (CP) is a disorder characterized by motor dysfunction resulting from a nonprogressive injury to brain tissue. The injury usually occurs during labor, delivery, or shortly after delivery. Physical examination is required to diagnose CP. Blood screening is not an appropriate means of diagnosis.
   5. **Cystic fibrosis is an autosomal recessive illness characterized by the presence of thick mucus in many organs systems, most notably the respiratory track. It is screened for in all 50 states.**

   TEST-TAKING TIP: It is important to realize that neonatal screening is state-specific. Each state determines which diseases will be screened for. The March of Dimes and other groups have recommended that at least 29 inborn diseases be screened for in all states. (To find which states screen for which diseases, please see the following Web site: http://genes-r-us.uthscsa.edu/nbsdisorders.pdf.)

2. 1. Meconium is a sterile stool. The newborn will not produce gastrointestinal bacteria until a few days after delivery.
   2. **Amniotic fluid is a reservoir for viral diseases like HIV and hepatitis B. If the woman is infected with those viruses, the amniotic fluid will be infectious.**
   3. Fetal urine is not highly alkaline.
   4. Although babies are at high risk for infection, there is no need for nurses to wear gloves routinely when caring for the babies.

   Immediately after delivery the nurse is protecting himself or herself from the baby, not the other way around.

   TEST-TAKING TIP: By wearing gloves the nurse is practicing standard precautions per the Centers for Disease Control and Prevention (CDC) to protect himself or herself from viruses that may be present in the amniotic fluid and on the neonate's body. This question illustrates how important it is for the test taker to read each possible answer very carefully. For example, the test taker may be tempted to choose choice 1 but the fact that the option states that meconium contains "enteric bacteria" makes that answer incorrect.

3. 1. **When newborns are wet they can become hypothermic from heat loss resulting from evaporation. They may then develop cold stress syndrome.**
   2. The first Apgar score is not done until 60 seconds after delivery. The wet blankets should have been removed from the baby well before that time.
   3. Eye prophylaxis can be delayed until after the parents have begun bonding with their baby.
   4. Although the baby's central nervous system must be carefully assessed, reflex assessment should be postponed until after the baby is dried and is breathing on his or her own.

   TEST-TAKING TIP: This is a prioritizing question. Every one of the actions will be performed after the birth of the baby. The nurse must know which action is performed first. Because hypothermia can compromise a neonate's transition to extrauterine life, it is essential to dry the baby immediately to minimize heat loss through evaporation. It is important for the test taker to review cold stress syndrome.

4. 1. **Hypothermia in the neonate is defined as a temperature below 97.7°F. Cold stress syndrome may develop if the baby's temperature is below that level.**
   2. A healthy neonate does not need supplemental feedings. And if supplements are needed, they should be either formula or breast milk.
   3. There is no indication in the stem that glucose assessments are needed for this baby.

4. Babies should be breastfed every 2 to 3 hours. Feedings every 4 hours are not frequent enough.

TEST-TAKING TIP: It is important for the student to know that a baby weighing 2900 grams is an average-sized baby (range 2500 to 4000 grams). In addition, because no other information is included in the stem, the test taker must assume that the baby is healthy. The answers, therefore, should be evaluated in terms of the healthy newborn. Hypoglycemia can result when a baby develops cold stress syndrome because babies must metabolize food to create heat. When they use up their food stores, they become hypoglycemic.

5. 2, 3, and 5 and correct.
   1. All of the babies' senses are well developed at birth.
   2. Babies respond to all forms of taste. They prefer sweet things.
   3. Babies' sense of touch is considered to be the most well-developed sense.
   4. Babies see quite well at 8 to 12 inches. They prefer to look at the human face.
   5. Babies hear quite well once the amniotic fluid is absorbed from the ear canal. Because early intervention benefits babies who are hearing impaired, in most hospitals their hearing is tested prior to discharge from the newborn nursery.

TEST-TAKING TIP: Many parents and students believe that babies are incapable of receptive communication. On the contrary, they are amazingly able. The test taker must review the abilities of neonates to respond appropriately to questions and to teach parents about the abilities of their newborns.

6. 1. Petechiae can be present as a result of an infectious disease, e.g., meningococcemia. In this situation, however, there is no indication that an infection is present.
   2. When neonates speed through the birth canal during rapid deliveries, the presenting parts become bruised. The bruising often takes the form of petechial hemorrhages.
   3. Erythema toxicum, the newborn rash, is characterized by papules or pustules on an erythematous base.
   4. There is nothing in the scenario to suggest that child abuse has occurred.

TEST-TAKING TIP: Although this question is about the neonate, the key to answering the question is knowledge of the normal length of a vaginal labor and delivery. Multiparous labors average about 8 to 10 hours, and primiparous labors can last more than 20 hours. The 3-hour labor noted in the stem of the question is significantly shorter than the average labor. The neonate, therefore, has progressed rapidly through the birth canal and, as a result, is bruised.

7. 1. The baby has lost less than 4% of its birth weight. Babies often lose between 5% and 10% of their birth weight. A loss greater than 10% is considered pathological.
   2. The weight loss is within normal limits.
   3. Supplementation is not needed at this time.
   4. There is no indication in the stem that the baby is high risk for hypoglycemia.

TEST-TAKING TIP: To answer this question correctly, the test taker must be aware that most neonates lose weight after birth and that the weight loss is not considered pathological unless it exceeds 10%. Only then will the test taker know that there is no need to report the baby's weight loss or to begin supplementation.

8. 1. Meconium should pass within 24 hours of delivery.
   2. This baby's glucose level is within normal limits.
   3. Normal neonatal breathing is irregular at 30 to 60 breaths per minute. This baby is tachypneic.
   4. A milky discharge—witch's milk—is normal. It results from the drop in maternal hormones in the neonatal system following delivery.

TEST-TAKING TIP: Unless the test taker understands the characteristics of a normal newborn, it is impossible to answer questions that require him or her to make subtle discriminations on exams or in the clinical area. Careful studying of normal physical neonatal findings is essential.

9. 0.25 mL
   A simple ratio and proportion equation is needed to calculate the volume of vitamin K that should be given to the baby.

   Known volume : known dosage = desired volume : desired dosage
   $$2 : 1 \text{ mL} = 0.5 : x$$
   The means are multiplied together and extremes are multiplied together.
   $$2x = 0.5$$
   $$x = 0.25 \text{ mL}$$

TEST-TAKING TIP: This is an alternate-form question. Test takers will be required to do mathematical calculations and input their answers. Test takers must be familiar with med math calculations and with simple clinical calculations. Note that the units—in this case, mL—are included in the question and that the question indicates how many decimal places to calculate the answer to. There should be no question in the test taker's mind in what units the answer should be or to what decimal place the answer should be calculated.

10. 1, 2, 3, and 5 are correct.
   1. With the baby placed flat on its back, the practitioner grasps the baby's thighs using his or her thumbs and index fingers.
   2. When assessing for Ortolani sign, the baby's thighs are abducted. When performing the Barlow test, the baby's thighs are adducted.
   3. With the baby's hips and knees at 90° angles, the hips are abducted. With DDH, the trochanter dislocates from the acetabulum.
   4. When performing both the Ortolani and Barlow tests, the baby is placed flat on its back. When assessing for symmetry of leg lengths and tissue folds, the baby is placed in both the supine and prone positions.
   5. Legs are extended to assess for equal leg lengths and for equal thigh and gluteal folds.

TEST-TAKING TIP: The test taker should review assessment skills. To assess for developmental dysplasia of the hip, the Ortolani and the Barlow tests are performed. The order of the steps of the Ortolani procedure is (a) the nurse places the baby on its back; (b) the nurse grasps the baby's thighs with a thumb on the inner aspect and forefingers over the trochanter; (c) with the knees flexed at 90° angles, the hips are abducted; and (d) the nurse palpates the trochanter to assess for hip laxity. The Barlow test is performed by: (a) adducting the baby's legs; (b) gently pushing the legs posteriorly; and (c) feeling to note any slippage of the trochanter out of the acetabulum. Galeazzi sign can also be performed.

11. 1. There is no evidence in the stem that would warrant placing the child in an isolette.
   2. Cyanotic hands and feet are not signs of hypoxia in the neonate.
   3. The baby's extremities are cyanotic as a result of the baby's immature circulatory system. Swaddling helps to warm the baby's hands and feet.
   4. There is no evidence in the stem that would warrant monitoring with the pulse oximeter.

TEST-TAKING TIP: The test taker must be familiar with the differences between normal findings of the newborn and those of an older child or adult. Acrocyanosis, bluish/cyanotic hands and feet, is normal in the very young neonate resulting from its immature circulation to the extremities.

12. 1. There is no evidence that circumcision status affects a boy's self-image.
   2. No official statements have been published regarding the rationality of performing circumcisions.
   3. The CDC has made no policy statement on circumcision.
   4. The AAP, although acknowledging that there are some advantages to circumcision, states that there is not enough evidence to suggest that all baby boys be circumcised.

TEST-TAKING TIP: In this question, authorities were cited—namely, the Centers for Disease Control and Prevention (CDC) and the American Academy of Pediatrics (AAP). The student should be familiar with authorities in the field, including the CDC, AAP, and the Association of Women's Health, Obstetric, and Neonatal Nursing (AWHONN). It is helpful to cite authorities when responding to parents' questions about emotionally charged issues like circumcision.

13. 1. Circumcision is a surgical procedure that requires a sterile field and sterile technique. The nurse is performing safe practice in this situation.
   2. The nurse is being a patient advocate because the baby is unable to ask for pain medication. The AAP has made a policy statement that pain medications be used during all circumcision procedures.
   3. If a baby feeds immediately before the circumcision, he may aspirate his feeds. This is safe practice.
   4. Making sure the baby is not hemorrhaging at the incision site is also an example of safe nursing practice.

TEST-TAKING TIP: Nurses perform a variety of roles. Being a safe practitioner is an essential role of the nurse. Just as important, and quite different, however, is the role of patient advocate—that is, providing support for the rights of a client who is unable to speak for or support himself or herself.

14. 4 and 5 are correct.
    1. Although assessed in other pain scales, the heart rate is not part of the NIPS.
    2. Blood pressure is not assessed in any infant pain scale.
    3. Temperature is not assessed in any infant pain scale.
    4. Facial expression is one variable that is evaluated as part of the NIPS.
    5. Breathing pattern is one variable that is evaluated as part of the NIPS.

TEST-TAKING TIP: The student should be familiar with the pain-rating scales and use them clinically because neonates cannot communicate their pain to the nurse. The scoring variables that are evaluated when assessing neonatal pain using the NIPS are facial expression, crying, breathing patterns, movement of arms and legs, and state of arousal. Other pain assessment tools are the Pain Assessment Tool (PAT), the Neonatal Post-op Pain Scale (CRIES), and the Premature Infant Pain Profile (PIPP).

15. 1. Hydrogen peroxide is not used when cleansing the circumcised penis.
    2. Antifungals are not indicated in this situation.
    3. Squeezing soapy water over the penis cleanses the area without irritating the site and causing the site to bleed.
    4. Dry dressings are not applied to the circumcised penis. It is, however, usually recommended to liberally apply petroleum jelly to the site before diapering. The petroleum jelly may be applied directly to the penis via a sterile dressing or via a petroleum jelly–impregnated gauze.

TEST-TAKING TIP: The circumcised penis has undergone a surgical procedure, but to apply a dry dressing is potentially injurious. If the dressing adheres to the newly circumcised penis, the incision could bleed. The test taker should be aware that with routine cleaning, as cited above, circumcisions usually heal quickly and rarely become infected.

16. The "X" should be placed on the baby in the supine position on the vastus lateralis on either the left or right thigh—that is, the anterior-lateral portion of the middle third of the thigh from the trochanter to the patella. This is the only safe site for intramuscular injections in infants.

TEST-TAKING TIP: This is another alternate-form question. The test taker must place the "X" on the appropriate picture—the baby in the supine position—and be careful to place the "X" at the precise location where the injection can safely be given. If the "X" extends past the area of safety, the question will be marked as incorrect.

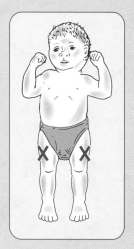 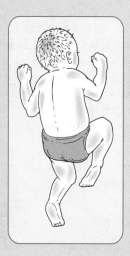

17. The "X" should be placed on the posterior fontanelle or the triangle-shaped area on the occiput of the baby's head.

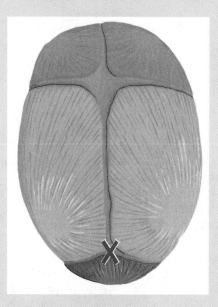

TEST-TAKING TIP: It is important not only to know the shape and size of the fontanelles but also to know the ages when the fontanelles usually close. The nurse will need to know this to provide anticipatory guidance to the parents as well as to be able to assess the child for normal growth and development.

18. 1. A 3-vessel cord is a normal finding.
    2. The anterior fontanelle is diamond-shaped.
    3. Undescended testes—cryptorchidism—is an unexpected finding. It is one sign of prematurity.
    4. Although multiple café au lait spots are seen in some neurological anomalies, the presence of one area of pigmentation is a normal finding.

TEST-TAKING TIP: It is important for the test taker to be able to discriminate between normal and abnormal findings. In addition, it is important for the nurse to be able to discern when the amount or degree of a finding is abnormal, as in the presence of multiple café au lait spots.

19. 1, 2, and 3 are correct.
    1. The patches are called mongolian spots and they are commonly seen in babies of color. They will fade and disappear with time.
    2. The whitish discharge is called witch's milk and is excreted as a result of the drop in maternal hormones in the baby's system. The discharge is temporary.
    3. The bloody discharge is called pseudomenses and occurs as a result of the drop in maternal hormones in the baby's system. The discharge is temporary.
    4. The demarcated area is a port wine stain, or capillary angioma. It is a permanent birthmark.
    5. The dimple may be a pilonidal cyst or a small defect into the spinal cord (spina bifida). An ultrasound should be done to determine whether or not a pathological condition is present.

TEST-TAKING TIP: A multiple-response type of question is often a more difficult type of question to answer than is a standard multiple-choice item because there is not simply one correct response to the question. The test taker must look at each answer option to see whether or not it accurately answers the stem of the question. In this question, purple-colored

patches, a whitish discharge from the breasts, and a bloody discharge in a female African American neonate are all considered normal.

20. 1. Intracostal retractions are a sign of respiratory distress.
    2. Caput succedaneum is a normal finding in a neonate.
    3. Epstein's pearls are often seen in the mouths of neonates.
    4. Harlequin sign, although odd-appearing, is a normal finding in a neonate.

TEST-TAKING TIP: Each of the normal findings is seen in newborns, although not seen later in life. The test taker must be familiar with these age-specific normal findings. It is also important to remember that, based on the hierarchy of needs, respiratory problems always take precedence.

21. 1. Respiratory rate between 30 and 60 and oxygen saturation above 95% are normal findings.
    2. Although the Apgar score—9—is excellent, the baby's weight—4,660 grams—is well above the average of 2,500 to 4,000 grams. Babies who are large for gestational age are at high risk for hypoglycemia.
    3. Temperature 97.7° to 99°F and length 18 to 22 inches are normal findings.
    4. Blood glucose 40 to 60 mg/dL and heart rate 120 to 160 bpm are normal findings.

TEST-TAKING TIP: This is a prioritizing question requiring very subtle discriminatory ability. The test taker must know normal values and conditions as well as the consequences that may occur if findings outside of normal are noted.

22. 1. Showing signs of hunger and frustration describes the active alert or active awake state.
    2. Starting to whimper and cry describes the crying behavioral state.
    3. This describes the quiet alert state; sometimes called wide-awake state.
    4. Sleeping and breathing regularly describe deep or quiet sleep.

TEST-TAKING TIP: Although knowledge-level questions like this are infrequently included in the NCLEX®, it is essential that the test taker be able to discern the differences between the various behaviors of the neonate to teach clients about the inherent behavioral expressions of their babies. Babies are in a transition period during the active alert period. Caregivers often can meet the needs of the baby in the active alert state to preclude the need for the baby to resort to crying.

23. 1. This is actually a true statement. Babies do rarely open their mouths to breathe when they are respiring. However, it is not the best response that the nurse could provide.
    2. **This statement provides the mother with the knowledge that babies are obligate nose breathers so that they are able to suck, swallow, and breathe without choking.**
    3. Again, this statement is inherently true, but it is a meaningless platitude that will not satisfy the mother's need for information.
    4. This response is inappropriate. Healthy newborns have small nares but aerate effectively as obligate nose breathers.

    TEST-TAKING TIP: Some test takers might be tempted to respond to this question by choosing answer 4. It is important, however, to respond to the question as it is posed. There is nothing in the stem that hints that this child is having any respiratory distress. The responder must choose an answer based on the assumption that this is a normal, healthy neonate.

24. 2 and 5 are correct.
    1. Pseudomenses is a normal finding in a 1-day-old female.
    2. Expiratory grunting is an indication of respiratory distress.
    3. This is a description of the harlequin sign, a normal neonatal finding.
    4. Neonates are often mottled when chilled. Unless other signs or symptoms are present, it is a normal finding.
    5. Nasal flaring is an indication of respiratory distress.

    TEST-TAKING TIP: Pseudomenses is seen in many 1-day-old female neonates. Although mottling and the harlequin sign can be present in emergent situations, they are usually normal findings. Expiratory grunting and nasal flaring, however, are not normal. Respiratory difficulties always need to be assessed fully.

25. 1. This is not an emergent problem needing physician intervention.
    2. There is nothing in the stem that implies that the child has been abused.

3. Subconjunctival hemorrhages are a normal finding and are not pathological. They will disappear over time. Explaining this to the mother is the appropriate action.
4. There is nothing in the stem that implies that there has been any intraocular damage.

TEST-TAKING TIP: The key to answering this question is knowing what is normal and what is abnormal in a neonate. Hemorrhages in the sclerae are considered normal, resulting from pressure changes at birth. Although the mother is frantic, the nurse's assessment shows that this is a normal finding. The nurse, therefore, provides the mother with the accurate information.

26. 1. Seesaw breathing is an indication of respiratory distress.
    2. This is the normal breathing pattern of a neonate.
    3. When babies breathe, their abdomens and thoraces rise and fall in synchrony.
    4. The normal respiratory rate is 30 to 60 rpm.

    TEST-TAKING TIP: The test taker must be knowledgeable of the normal variations of neonatal respirations. Apnea spells of 10 seconds or less are normal, but apnea spells longer than 20 seconds should be reported to the neonatologist. Normally, when a baby breathes, his or her abdomen and chest rise and fall in synchrony. When they rise and fall arrhythmically, as in seesaw breathing, it is an indication that the baby is in respiratory difficulty.

27. 1. This is an image of a baby in the tonic neck position.
    2. This is an image of a baby in the opisthotonic posture.
    3. This is an image of a baby in the classic fetal position.
    4. This is an image of a baby in the breech posture.

    TEST-TAKING TIP: Babies often assume a posture after delivery that reflects the posture they were in, in utero. Babies in the frank breech position in utero are bent at the waist with both legs adjacent to the head. That same posture is seen in the baby after delivery.

28. 1. Slight drop in heart rate is normal when babies are in deep sleep.

2. Slight jaundice is within normal limits on day 2. Pathological jaundice appears within the first 24 hours of life, whereas physiological jaundice appears after 24 hours of life. Temperature is within normal limits (97.5° to 99.0°F).

3. Babies who breastfeed fewer than 8 times a day are not receiving adequate nutrition. Jitters are indicative of hypoglycemia.

4. The rash is a normal newborn rash—erythema toxicum. Crying, without other signs and symptoms, is a normal response by babies.

TEST-TAKING TIP: Just because a baby is older does not mean that it is necessarily healthier than a younger baby. A 3-day-old baby breastfeeding every 4 hours, rather than every 2 to 3 hours, is not consuming enough. As a result the baby is jittery, which is a sign of below-normal serum glucose.

29. 1. This baby is asleep. Placing the baby en face will not promote neonatal bonding.
    2. This baby is asleep. Placing the baby en face will not promote neonatal bonding.
    3. This baby is in the quiet alert behavioral state. Placing the baby en face will foster bonding between the father and baby.
    4. This baby is showing hunger cues. The baby likely needs to be fed at this time.

TEST-TAKING TIP: The test taker could make an educated guess regarding this question even if the term "en face" were unfamiliar. The expression means "face to face," which is clearly implied by the term. Because bonding between parent and child is so important, whenever a baby exhibits the quiet alert behavior, the nurse should encourage the interaction. Although the father may bond with a sleeping baby who is in the en face position, the baby is unable to interact or bond with his or her parent.

30. 1. The normal temperature of a neonate is 97.5° to 99.5°F and the weight of a term neonate is between 2,500 and 4,000 grams.
    2. Milia—white spots on the bridge of the nose—are exposed sebaceous glands. They are normal.
    3. Epstein's pearls—raised white specks on the gums or on the hard palate—are normal findings in the neonate.

4. The normal resting respiratory rate of a neonate is 30 to 60 and the normal resting heart rate of a neonate is 110 to 160.

TEST-TAKING TIP: The test taker should not be overwhelmed by descriptions of findings. Although the descriptions of milia and Epstein's pearls appear to be abnormal, the item writer has merely rephrased information in a different way. It is important, therefore, to stay calm and read and decipher the information in each of the possible options.

31. 1. The weight is normal. The normal weight of a term neonate is between 2,500 and 4,000 grams.
    2. The circumferences are within normal limits. The head circumference should be 32 to 37 cm and the chest circumference 1 to 2 cm smaller than the head.
    3. A positive Ortolani sign indicates a likely developmental dysplasia of the hip. In the Ortolani sign, the thighs are gently abducted. If the trochanter displaces from the acetabulum, the result is positive and indicative of developmental dysplasia of the hip.
    4. Supernumerary nipples are normal. They appear on the mammary line. Usually only the primary nipples mature.

TEST-TAKING TIP: In this scenario, the nurse must determine which of a group of findings discovered on a neonatal assessment is unexpected. It is important to realize that a patient may exhibit normalcy in the majority of ways, but still may have a problem that needs further assessment or intervention. It is essential for nurses not to have tunnel vision when caring for clients.

32. 1. This is a description of the rooting reflex.
    2. This is a description of the Babinski reflex.
    3. This is a description of the Moro reflex. When the baby is suddenly lowered or startled, the neonate's arms straighten outward and the knees flex.
    4. This is a description of the tonic neck reflex.

TEST-TAKING TIP: The test taker must be familiar not only with the reason for eliciting reflexes but also with the correct technique for eliciting the actions.

33. 1. Epstein's pearls are not found on the feet.
    2. Epstein's pearls are not found on the hands.

3. Epstein's pearls are not found on the back.
4. Epstein's pearls—small white specks (keratin-containing cysts)—are located on the palate and gums.

TEST-TAKING TIP: The question is not a trick question. Some test takers, when asked a fairly direct question, believe that the questioner is trying to trick them and choose an alternate response to try to outfox the examiner. The test taker should always take each question at face value and not try to read into the question or to out-psych the questioner.

34. 1. Pseudostrabismus—eyes cross and uncross when they are open—is normal in the neonate because of poor tone of the muscles of the eye.
2. Ears positioned in alignment with the inner and outer canthus of the eyes is the normal position. In Down syndrome, ears are low set.
3. Vernix caseosa covers and protects the skin of the fetus. Depending on the gestational age of the baby, there is often some left on the skin at birth.
4. Nasal flaring is a symptom of respiratory distress.

TEST-TAKING TIP: At first glance, the test taker may panic because each of the responses looks abnormal. Again, it is essential that the test taker know and apply neonatal normals.

35. 1. Babies are awake and alert for approximately 30 minutes to 1 hour immediately after birth. This is the perfect time for the parents to begin to bond with their babies.

2. There is no reason to notify the neonatologist.
3. This is a full-term baby. There is no need to perform a gestational age assessment.
4. Warmth can be maintained, preferably by placing the baby skin to skin with the mother or, if required, by swaddling the baby in one or more blankets.

TEST-TAKING TIP: After the first period of reactivity, babies enter a phase of inactivity when they sleep. They may be in the sleep phase for a number of hours. It is important, therefore, for parental bonding to be initiated during the reactivity phase and, if the mother plans to breastfeed, to have the baby go to breast at this time as well.

36. 1. The baby's Apgar is 8.
2. The baby's Apgar is 8.
3. The baby's Apgar is 8.
4. The baby's Apgar is 8.

TEST-TAKING TIP: Apgar scoring is usually a nursing responsibility. To determine the correct response the test taker must know the Apgar scoring scale given below and add the points together: 2 for heart rate, 2 for respiratory rate, 1 for color, 2 for reflex irritability, 1 for flexion. The total is 8.

The test taker must remember that Apgar "normals" are NOT the same as clinical normals. For example, the normal heart rate of a neonate is defined as 110 to 160 bpm. The baby will receive the maximum 2 points for heart rate, however, with a heart rate of greater than or equal to 100 bpm.

The Apgar Score

Assessment	0 points	1 point	2 points
Color	Central cyanosis	Acrocyanosis	All pink
Heart rate	No heart rate	1–99 bpm	≥100 bpm
Respiratory rate	No respirations	Slow and irregular	Good lusty cry
Reflex irritability	No response	Grimace	Good lusty cry
Tone	Flaccid	Some flexion	Marked flexion or active movement

37. 3 and 4 are correct.
    1. Harlequin sign—deep red coloring over one side of the baby's body and pale coloration over the other side—is transient and, in most situations, normal.
    2. Extension of the toes when the lateral aspect of the sole is stroked is the expected Babinski reflex until approximately 2 years of age.
    3. When the scarf sign is assessed, a premature baby would be able to move the elbow past the midline. A full-term baby would not be able to do this.
    4. Ear pinnae that are slightly curved and slow to recoil are seen in preterm babies.
    5. Telangiectatic nevi, or stork bites, are pale pink spots often found on the eyelids and at the nape of the neck. They usually fade by age 2.

    TEST-TAKING TIP: The test taker should not be confused by the mixing of technical terms and descriptions of findings. Even though technical terms were included, the correct responses are actually descriptions—in this case, a description of the scarf sign and the immature pinnae of the ears as seen in preterm babies.

38. 1. Molding is characterized by the overlapping of the cranial bones. It is rarely one sided and would feel like a ridge rather than a bulge.
    2. Swelling of the tissues of the baby's head occurs over the entire cranium and is called caput succedaneum.
    3. Positioning usually results in molding.
    4. Cephalhematomas are subcutaneous swellings of accumulated blood from the trauma of delivery. The bulges may be one-sided or bilateral and the swellings do not cross suture lines.

    TEST-TAKING TIP: The key to the correct response is the fact that the bulge has not crossed the suture lines. Although each of the answer options is a common finding in neonates, only one is consistent with the assessments made by the nurse.

39. 1. There is controversy in the literature regarding what should be used to clean the umbilical cord, but hydrogen peroxide is not one of the recommended agents. Some research actually indicates that nothing should be applied to the umbilical cord and that it should be allowed to air dry.
    2. The cord should fall off on its own. This usually happens 7 to 10 days after birth.
    3. The green drainage may be a sign of infection. The cord should become dried and shriveled.
    4. There is no need to cover the umbilicus.

    TEST-TAKING TIP: The test taker, who has forgotten the substances used to clean cords, like triple dye and alcohol, might be tempted to respond to the question by choosing hydrogen peroxide cleansing. After careful study of the responses, however, it is clear that a sign of infection is definitely the only correct answer.

40. 1. It is recommended that powders, even if advertised for the purpose, not be used on babies.
    2. It is recommended that powders, even if advertised for the purpose, not be used on babies.
    3. There is no evidence that most babies are allergic to cornstarch.
    4. It is irrelevant where the powder is being used; it is recommended that powders, even if advertised for the purpose, not be used on babies.

    TEST-TAKING TIP: Sometimes answer options include qualifiers. For example, in this question, choice 4 includes the qualifier "As long as you put it only on the buttocks area." Test takers should be wary of qualifiers. They are often used to draw one to an incorrect response.

41. 1. To prevent infection, the eye should be cleaned from inner canthus to outer canthus.
    2. To prevent injury, parents should be advised never to put anything smaller than their fingertips into the baby's nose or ears.
    3. If items must be obtained while the bath is being given, the baby may become hypothermic from evaporation resulting from exposure to the air when wet.
    4. The safest way to check the temperature of the water is with a thermometer or, if none is available, with the elbow or forearm.

    TEST-TAKING TIP: Safety issues are especially important when providing parent education. The test taker must be familiar with actions that promote safety as well as those that put the neonate at risk.

42. 1. The perineum of female babies should always be cleansed from front to back to prevent bacteria from the rectum from causing infection.
    2. Vernix may be in the labial folds at delivery. It is a natural lanolin that will be absorbed

over time. Actively removing the vernix can actually irritate the baby's tissues.

3. Powder is not recommended for use on babies, especially in the diaper area. When mixed with urine, powders can produce an irritating paste.

4. The number of a baby's diapers should be counted to assess for hydration, but weighing the diapers of full-term babies is rarely needed.

TEST-TAKING TIP: It is important for nurses to provide needed education to parents for the care of their new baby. Diapering, although often seen as a skill that everyone should know, must be taught. And it is especially important to advise parents that introducing bacteria from the rectum can cause urinary tract infections in their babies, especially female babies.

43. 1. Babies do not need to have a full bath each day. Plus, daily soap baths can dry the newborn's skin.

2. Tummy time, while awake and while supervised, helps to prevent plagiocephaly and to promote growth and development.

3. There is no recommendation that babies be given a pacifier after every feeding. In fact, pacifier use may interfere with the success of breastfeeding.

4. It is strongly recommended that babies always be placed on their backs for sleep.

TEST-TAKING TIP: The test taker must not be confused by recommendations that are made by professional organizations. The recommendations usually are time specific. For example, babies should be placed for sleep on their backs, but should receive tummy time while awake and supervised.

44. 2, 3, and 4 are correct.
1. Because air bag deployment can seriously injure young children, it is recommended that no child under 13 years of age be seated in the front seat of a car.

2. The baby should be facing the rear in the back seat of the car.

3. Since 2002, infant car seats have been designed with 2 attachment points at the base of the car seat. The car seat should be attached to the seat of the car using both attachment points.

4. After being installed, if a car seat moves more than 1 inch back and forth or side to side, it is not installed properly.

5. The straps of a car seat should fit snugly, allowing only 2 fingers to be inserted between them and the baby.

TEST-TAKING TIP: Test takers should be aware that recommendations and guidelines often change over time. In March 2011, the American Academy of Pediatrics came out with updated recommendations on infant and child seat restraint systems (see http://pediatrics.aappublications.org/content/127/4/e1050.full.pdf+html?sid=f7d6a841-052e-4617-bb22-ec2bb4f9e).

45. 1, 2, 4, and 5 are correct.
1. The first of 3 injections of the hepatitis B vaccine is often given in the newborn nursery, but, if not, it is recommended that it be given by 1 month of age.

2. It is recommended that the first of 3 injections of the Salk polio vaccine be given at the 2-month health maintenance checkup.

3. Because the baby has received passive immunity from the mother, the MMR is not given until the second year of life.

4. Three DTaP injections are given during the first year of life and boosters are given as the child grows.

5. Because the baby has received passive immunity from the mother, Varivax is not given until the second year of life.

TEST-TAKING TIP: Many recommendations are time specific. The CDC changes immunization recommendations when new research emerges. The test taker should periodically review reliable sites like www.CDC.gov (Centers for Disease Control and Prevention) and www.aap.org (American Academy of Pediatrics) to check recommendations.

46. 1, 4, and 5 are correct.
1. Babies do not starve themselves. If a baby refuses to eat, it may mean that the baby is seriously ill. For example, babies with cardiac defects often refuse to eat.

2. Newborns normally breathe irregularly. Apnea spells of 10 seconds or less are normal.

3. Newborns do not tear when they cry. If a baby does tear, he or she may have a blocked lacrimal duct.

4. Although babies who are in the deep sleep state are difficult to arouse, the deep sleep state lasts no more than

an hour. If the baby continues to be nonarousable, the pediatrician should be notified.

5. A temperature above 100.4°F is a febrile state for a newborn and the pediatrician should be notified.

TEST-TAKING TIP: The test taker must judge each answer option independently of the others when completing a multiple-response item. These items require more comprehensive knowledge because there is not simply one best response, but rather many correct answers.

47. 1. Some babies do not respond to their own hunger cues. It is especially important to note that breastfed babies must feed at least 8 times in a 24-hour period to grow and for the mother to produce a sufficient milk supply. Parents should awaken a baby if he or she sleeps through a feeding.

2. It is recommended that sunscreen not be applied to babies until they are 6 months old. Babies should always be shielded from direct sunlight.

3. Liquid acetaminophen should be available in the home, but it should not be administered until the parent speaks to the pediatrician.

4. There is no need to notify the doctor when the cord falls off.

TEST-TAKING TIP: A nurse who gives parents anticipatory guidance is providing the couple with knowledge that they will need for the future. Anticipatory guidance can prevent crises from occurring. Here, the nurse is providing accurate information so that the parents will be prepared to ensure that their child feeds often enough and is given medication only when it is needed.

48. 1. The mouth should be suctioned before the nose.

2. If the back of the throat is suctioned, it will stimulate the gag reflex.

3. The bulb should be compressed before it is inserted into the baby's mouth.

4. The drainage should be evaluated by the nurse. The drainage, therefore, should be disposed of in a tissue or cloth.

TEST-TAKING TIP: To remember whether the nose or the mouth should be suctioned first, the test taker should remember "m" comes before "n"—the mouth should be suctioned before the nose.

49. The "X" should be placed on one of the lateral aspects of the heel, the safe sites

for heel sticks. If other sites are used, the baby's nerves, arteries, or fat pad may be damaged.

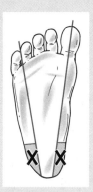

TEST-TAKING TIP: When responding to "X marks the spot" questions, it is essential that the "X" be placed accurately. Trying to fudge the answer by placing the "X" between sites will result in an incorrect response.

50. 1. An 18-gauge needle is too thick to be used.

2. A ⅝-inch, 25-gauge needle is an appropriate needle for a neonatal IM injection.

3. A 1-inch needle is too long and the gauge is too thick.

4. Although the gauge is appropriate, a 1-inch needle is too long.

TEST-TAKING TIP: One way to determine an appropriate length for an intramuscular needle is to grasp the muscle where the injection is to be given, measure the width of the muscle, and then divide by 2. The muscle of a neonate is about 1 to 1½ inches wide. A ½- to ⅝-inch-long needle should be used. Another principle that the test taker should remember regarding needles is the larger the gauge of a needle, the narrower the needle width and vice versa. The 25-gauge needle, therefore, is narrow, whereas the 18-gauge needle is thick.

51. 1. The recommended site for assessing the pulse of a neonate is the brachial pulse. The carotid pulse is used to assess the pulse of an adult as well as that of a child over 1 year of age.

2. The radial pulse is never recommended for use during CPR.

3. The recommended site for assessing the pulse of a neonate undergoing CPR is the brachial pulse.

4. The pedal pulse is never recommended for use during CPR.

TEST-TAKING TIP: The test taker should remember that neonates and infants have very short necks. It is very difficult to access the carotid pulse in them. The brachial pulse is easily accessible and is a relatively strong pulse.

52. 1. Heat loss resulting from evaporation occurs when the baby is wet and exposed to the air.
    2. Heat loss resulting from conduction occurs when the baby comes in contact with cold objects (hands or stethoscope).
    3. Heat loss resulting from radiation occurs when the baby is exposed to cool objects that the baby is not in direct contact with.
    4. Heat loss resulting from convection occurs when the baby is exposed to the movement of cooled air—for example, air-conditioning currents.

TEST-TAKING TIP: The test taker must remember that heat loss can lead to cold stress syndrome in the neonate. All four causes of heat loss must be understood and actions must be taken to prevent the baby from situations that would foster heat loss from any of the causes.

53. 1. Although this baby is being breastfed, he or she is still susceptible to illness. The best way to prevent transmission of pathogens is to wash hands carefully before touching the baby.
    2. Visitors, too, should wash hands before touching the baby, but it is unnecessary to isolate the baby from them.
    3. The best way to prevent the transmission of a cold is to wash hands. Also, this baby is receiving protective antibodies through the breast milk. Masks are not necessary.
    4. Sterilization is not necessary. All washable pieces of the equipment should be washed thoroughly in dish detergent and water and rinsed well. The dishwasher-safe pieces could be cleansed in the dishwasher.

TEST-TAKING TIP: The test taker should choose responses that dictate behavior very carefully. For example, the test taker should realize that "Refrain from having visitors for the first month" is not the best response because there are very few instances when social interaction is prohibited. It is important for the test taker to remember, however, that the most important action that can be taken to prevent communicable disease transmission is washing of the hands.

54. 2, 3, 4, and 5 are correct.
    1. Babies who are in the drowsy behavioral state and who are tightly swaddled often fall asleep rather than become aroused.
    2. The smell and/or the taste of the milk often will arouse a drowsy baby.
    3. Drowsy babies will open their eyes when placed in the en face position and are interacted with.
    4. Performing manipulations like diapering or playing pat-a-cake often will arouse a drowsy baby.
    5. Performing manipulations like diapering or playing pat-a-cake often will arouse a drowsy baby.

TEST-TAKING TIP: It is important to distinguish a drowsy baby from a baby in the quiet alert or active alert state. For example, a baby who is in the active alert state may actually benefit from being swaddled because he or she is upset and needs to be calmed. Conversely, a baby in a drowsy state may need to be stimulated by manipulating or playing with the baby or by expressing milk onto the baby's lips.

55. 1, 2, and 4 are correct.
    1. Stroking and patting the baby's back are very effective ways of burping.
    2. Babies can be burped in many different positions, including over the shoulder, lying flat across the lap, and in a sitting position. When placing the baby in the sitting position, the mother should carefully support the baby's chin. Positioning the baby face down on the lap can be very effective and some mothers feel more secure using this position because the baby is unlikely to be dropped from this position.
    3. In the first few weeks of life, it is important to burp babies frequently throughout feedings. Bottle-fed babies often take in a great deal of air. Babies who burp only at the end of the feed often burp up large quantities of formula. Further teaching is needed.
    4. A small amount of "spit up" is within normal limits. Breastfed babies also often spit up bits of their feeds.
    5. It may take quite a few minutes of patting before the baby burps effectively. If the baby does not burp well, he or she may regurgitate large quantities of the feeding.

TEST-TAKING TIP: It is important to distinguish between babies who are bottle-fed and those who are breastfed. Breastfed babies usually ingest much less air than do bottle-fed babies. Breastfed babies should

be burped at least once in the middle of their feeds, whereas bottle-fed babies should be burped every ½ to 1 ounce.

56. 1. The uvula and frenulum are distinctly different structures in the mouth.
    2. Babies who are tongue-tied—that is, have a tight frenulum—have difficulty extending their tongues while breast-feeding. The mothers' nipples often become damaged as a result.
    3. A tight frenulum does not result in injury to the baby's tongue.
    4. There is no relationship between breathing ability and being tongue-tied.

    TEST-TAKING TIP: The test taker should understand the many actions that the baby's tongue must make to be able to breastfeed successfully. One of the first actions the tongue must make is to extend past the gum line. A tight frenulum precludes the baby from being able to fully extend his or her tongue.

57. 1 and 3 are correct.
    1. A mother with active, untreated TB should be separated from her baby until the mother has been on antibiotic therapy for about 2 weeks. She can, however, pump her breast milk and have it fed to the baby through an alternate feeding method.
    2. Being hepatitis B surface antigen positive (HBsAg+) is not a contraindication to breastfeeding.
    3. Mothers who are HIV positive are advised not to breastfeed because there is an increased risk of transmission of the virus to the infant.
    4. Acute bacterial infections, such as chorioamnionitis, are not contraindications to breastfeeding unless the medication given to the mother is contraindicated. There are, however, very few antibiotics that are incompatible with breastfeeding.
    5. It is recommended that a mother with mastitis continue to breastfeed. She must keep draining her breasts of milk to prevent the development of a breast abscess. Again, only antibiotics compatible with breast-feeding should be administered.

    TEST-TAKING TIP: The test taker should remember that there are very few instances when breastfeeding is contraindicated. Mothers who are hepatitis B positive may breastfeed because it has not been shown that transmission rates increase with breastfeeding.

58. 1. The first action the nurse should always perform is to make sure that the correct baby is being given to the correct mother.
    2. This is an important action but it is not the first action.
    3. This is an important action but it is not the first action.
    4. This is an important action but it is not the first action.

    TEST-TAKING TIP: When establishing priorities, it is essential that the most important action be taken first. Even though the question discusses breastfeeding, the feeding method is irrelevant to the scenario. The most important action is to check the identity of the mother and baby to make sure that the correct baby has been taken to the correct mother.

59. 1. Breastfed babies usually regain their birth weights by about day 10.
    2. Rarely do babies sleep through the night by 4 weeks of age.
    3. By 1 week of age, breastfed babies should have 3 to 4 bright yellow stools in every 24-hour period, although some babies do stool more frequently.
    4. By 1 week of age, breastfed babies should be urinating at least 6 times in every 24-hour period.

    TEST-TAKING TIP: Although the test taker may hear anecdotally that babies should sleep through the night by 4 weeks of age, this should not be an expectation. Even bottle-fed babies usually awaken for feeds during the night.

60. 2, 3, and 4 are correct.
    1. The baby should be placed "tummy to tummy" with the mother. Babies cannot swallow when their heads are turned. They must face the breast for effective feeding.
    2. To achieve an effective latch of both the nipple and the areolar tissue, the baby must have a wide-open mouth.
    3. Because the neonate's mouth muscles are relatively weak, it is important for the baby to be placed at the level of the breast. If the baby is placed lower, he or she is likely to "slip to the tip" of the nipple and cause nipple abrasions.
    4. Babies latch best when they are positioned at the breast, in preparation to opening their mouths, with their noses pointed toward their mothers' nipples.

5. The baby's tongue must be below the nipple to achieve effective suckling.

TEST-TAKING TIP: The test taker must remember that positioning of a baby at the breast is much different from positioning a bottle-fed baby. For example, even though bottle-fed babies feed effectively while lying on their backs, breastfeeding will be unsuccessful in the same position.

61. 1. Unless the nipples have been damaged extensively, once babies are latched correctly pain usually subsides.
    2. Audible swallowing is an excellent indicator of breastfeeding success.
    3. Slow, rhythmic jaw movement is an indicator of breastfeeding success.
    4. Babies whose cheeks move in and out during feeds are attempting to use negative pressure to extract the milk from the breasts. This action is not an indicator of breastfeeding success.

TEST-TAKING TIP: This question tests the last phase of the nursing process—evaluation. When answering this question, the test taker should apply the principles of successful breastfeeding—audible swallowing, rhythmic jaw extrusion, and pain-free feeding. The last choice, although in the abstract may sound plausible, is not an indicator of breastfeeding success.

62. 1 and 4 are correct.
    1. To determine that the baby is consuming sufficient quantities of breast milk, the parents should count the number of wet and soiled diapers the baby has throughout every day.
    2. There is no physical way to measure breastfeeding intake unless the baby is weighed immediately before and immediately after feeds. This action is not routinely recommended.
    3. To promote milk production, it is recommended that babies breastfeed at each feed until at least 1 month of age.
    4. The baby should be seen by the pediatrician.
    5. Breastfeedings should not be timed. Some babies are rapid eaters whereas others eat more slowly. The baby should decide when he or she has finished a feeding.

TEST TAKING TIP: In 2004, the AAP published a statement recommending that babies be seen by the pediatrician at 3 to 5 days of age to assess for the presence of jaundice, dehydration, or other complications. **Because most babies are discharged on day 2 of life, they need to be taken to the pediatrician within 3 days of discharge (see http://pediatrics.aappublications.org/content/114/1/297.full.pdf+html?sid=0ef396fc-b599-4dc7-b68c-ee3344093061).**

63. 1. When the mother is anxious, overly fatigued, and/or in pain, the secretion of oxytocin is inhibited, and this, in turn, inhibits the milk ejection reflex and insufficient milk may be consumed.
    2. If a baby is suckling effectively at the breast, the baby will swallow breast milk even after 10 minutes.
    3. The cross-cradle hold is one of the recommended breastfeeding positions.
    4. Ideally, the baby's chin should touch the underside of the mother's breast.

TEST-TAKING TIP: It is important for the test taker to realize that the breast is never empty of milk. Even if the baby has suckled for a long period of time, the baby will still be able to extract milk from the breast. Also, the role of oxytocin in breastfeeding should be fully understood.

64. 1. It has been shown that bottle-fed babies are at higher risk for obesity than breastfed babies. One of the reasons is the insistence by some mothers that the baby finish the formula in a bottle even if the baby initially rejects it. The increased calorie intake leads to increased weight gain.
    2. Bottle-fed babies usually feed every 3 to 4 hours.
    3. All formulas for full-term babies supply the same number of calories per ounce.
    4. It is recommended that bottle-fed babies burp every ½ to 1 ounce when they are very young.

TEST-TAKING TIP: It is important for the test taker to be familiar with the normal feeding patterns of bottle-fed and breast-fed babies. Bottle-feeding mothers should be strongly encouraged to allow their babies to determine how much formula they wish to consume at each feeding.

65. 1. It is expected that the baby feed 8 to 12 times a day.
    2. It is expected that the baby void a minimum of 6 to 10 times a day.
    3. Breastfed babies' stools are watery and yellow in color.

4. If the baby has yellow sclerae, the baby is exhibiting signs of jaundice and the pediatrician should be contacted.

TEST-TAKING TIP: When nurses discharge patients with their neonates, the nurses must provide anticipatory guidance regarding hyperbilirubinemia. Jaundice is the characteristic skin color of a baby with elevated bilirubin. The parents must be taught to notify their pediatrician if the baby is jaundiced because bilirubin is neurotoxic.

66. 1. Both the upper and lower lips should be flanged.
   2. Breastfed babies usually feed every 2 to 3 hours.
   3. A 12% weight loss is significant in any neonate whether breastfeeding or bottle feeding.
   4. When the tongue stays behind the gum line the baby is unable to strip the breast of milk.

TEST-TAKING TIP: There are very few nursing diagnoses that describe positive events. Effective breastfeeding is one of them. It is essential, therefore, for the test taker to choose the response that indicates a successful breastfeeding experience.

67. To determine how many grams the baby has lost, the test taker must subtract the new weight from the birth weight:

$$\begin{array}{r} 3278 \\ -3042 \\ \hline \end{array}$$
       236 grams of weight loss

Then, to determine the percentage of weight loss, the test taker must divide the difference by the original weight and multiply by 100%:

$$\frac{236}{3278} = 0.0719$$
$$0.0719 \times 100 = 7.19\%$$

TEST-TAKING TIP: To calculate percentage of weight loss, which is needed in a variety of clinical settings as well as in the neonatal nursery, the test taker must subtract the new weight from the old weight, divide the difference by the old weight, and then multiply the result by 100%.

68. 1. The en face position is an ideal position for interacting with a baby who is in the quiet alert behavioral state, but not to encourage a baby to open wide for feeding.
   2. Although sometimes needed, it is not routinely recommended that mothers

push down on their baby's lower jaw to encourage the baby to open his or her mouth for feeding.
   3. Tickling the baby's lips with the nipple is the recommended method of encouraging a baby to open his or her mouth for feeding.
   4. Bottles should not be used to entice babies to breastfeed. Expressing breast milk onto the baby's lips may encourage the baby to open wide.

TEST-TAKING TIP: It is interesting to note that babies have been shown to imitate behavior. For example, in the en face position, if a mother opens her mouth and sticks out her tongue, her baby will often imitate the behavior. The en face position, however, is not conducive to effective breastfeeding.

69. 1. Babies before the age of 4 to 6 months digest cereal poorly and may develop allergies from exposure to the proteins in the cereal.
   2. This is the correct response.
   3. It is recommended that babies receive breast milk at all feedings. When formula feeds are substituted, breastfeeding success is often compromised.
   4. Apple juice is added to the diet when recommended by the pediatrician, usually well after cereals have been introduced.

TEST-TAKING TIP: It is important for the test taker to separate common beliefs from scientific fact. Although many grandmothers strongly encourage the addition of solids early in a baby's diet, it is important for the nurse to provide the parents with up-to-date information followed by a rationale. It is recommended that solid foods not be introduced into a baby's diet until the baby is 4 to 6 months old.

70. 1. Although it is recommended that the mother stop smoking, breastfeeding is not contraindicated when the mother smokes.
   2. This is true. Breastfeeding is protective of the baby and should be encouraged.
   3. Maternal smoking does not warrant a report to Child Protective Services.
   4. This statement is not true. There is no evidence to show that women who smoke at the time they deliver have a high incidence of illicit drug use.

TEST-TAKING TIP: It is important that the test taker not make assumptions about

client behavior. Even though smoking is discouraged because of the serious health risks associated with the addiction, it is a legal act. It is best for the nurse to promote behaviors that will mitigate the negative impact of smoking. Breastfeeding the baby is one of those behaviors. Encouraging the mother to refrain from smoking inside the house is another.

71. 1. This statement is accurate.
2. The baby has already been exposed to the chickenpox, including during the prodromal period. The baby received passive antibodies through the placenta and is now receiving antibodies via the breast milk; therefore, there is no need to remove the baby from the home.
3. Chickenpox is highly contagious via droplet and contact routes.
4. Chickenpox is transmitted via the herpes zoster virus.

TEST-TAKING TIP: One of the important clues to the answer to this question is the age of the baby. Antibodies passed by passive immunity are usually evident in the neonatal system for at least 3 months. Because this baby is only 2 weeks old, the antibodies should protect the baby. Plus, because the baby is breastfeeding, the baby is receiving added protection.

72. 1. This is true. The baby must be at the level of the breast to feed effectively.
2. In the cross-cradle position, the baby's head is in the mother's hand.
3. The baby should be positioned facing the mother—"tummy to-tummy."
4. The baby should be brought to the mother. The mother should not move her body to the baby.

TEST-TAKING TIP: Even if the nurse is unfamiliar with the cross-cradle position, making sure that the baby is at the level of the breast is one of the important principles for successfully breastfeeding a neonate. In addition, "tummy-to-tummy" positioning and having the baby brought to the mother rather than vice versa are also important. Plus, if the nurse had confused the cradle position with the cross-cradle position, it is recommended that when feeding in the cradle position the baby's head be placed on the mother's forearm, not in the antecubital fossa.

73. 1. Breastfeeding should be instituted as soon as possible to promote milk

production, stability of the baby's glucose levels, and meconium excretion, as well as to stabilize the baby's temperature through skin-to-skin contact.
2. Although the baby will eventually need to be dressed in a shirt and diaper, skin-to-skin contact—baby's naked body against mother's naked body—facilitates successful breastfeeding.
3. Ophthalmic prophylaxis should be delayed until after the first feeding. The drops/ointment can impact bonding by impairing the baby's vision.
4. Skin-to-skin contact with the mother during breastfeeding effectively stabilizes neonatal temperatures.

TEST-TAKING TIP: Unless the health of the baby is compromised, one of the first actions that should be made after delivery is placing the baby skin to skin, at the breast, with a warm blanket covering both mother and baby. The baby's temperature will normalize and the baby will receive needed nourishment from the colostrum.

74. 1. This baby has lost only 3.7% of his or her birth weight—100/2,678 × 100% = 3.7%. This is below the accepted weight loss of 5% to 10%.
2. There is no need to supplement this baby's feeds.
3. The weight loss is not excessive.
4. Dextrose water is not recommended for babies.

TEST-TAKING TIP: To answer this question, the test taker can either estimate the maximum accepted weight loss for this baby or calculate the exact weight loss for this baby. The best way to estimate the accepted weight loss is to multiply the birth weight by 0.1 to calculate a 10% weight loss (2678 × 0.1 = 267.8 g) and then to divide 267.8 by 2 (267.8 ÷ 2 = 133.9 g) to calculate the 5% weight loss. A 100-gram loss is below both figures.

75. 1. Babies with short frenulums—tongue-tied babies—are unable to extend their tongues enough to achieve a sufficient grasp. Painful and damaged nipples often result.
2. The baby's tongue should be troughed to feed effectively.
3. This is, on average, the feeding pattern of breastfed babies.
4. Babies should latch to both the nipple and areola.

TEST-TAKING TIP: It is important for test takers not to panic when confronted with unfamiliar terms. If the test taker understands normal breastfeeding behaviors, this question should be easily answered even if the term "frenulum" is not familiar.

76. 1. This response acknowledges the client's feelings but it does not provide her with the information she needs regarding alcohol consumption and breastfeeding.
    2. Alcohol is not restricted during the postpartum period.
    3. Alcohol is found in the breast milk in exactly the same concentration as in the mother's blood. Alcohol consumption is not, however, incompatible with breastfeeding. The woman should breastfeed immediately before consuming a drink and then wait 1 to 2 hours to metabolize the drink before feeding again. If she decides to have more than one drink, she can pump and dump her milk for a feeding or two.
    4. Alcohol is found in the breast milk in exactly the same concentration as in the mother's blood. Alcohol consumption is not, however, incompatible with breastfeeding. The woman should breastfeed immediately before consuming a drink and then wait 1 to 2 hours to metabolize the drink before feeding again. If she decides to have more than one drink, she can pump and dump her milk for a feeding or two.

TEST-TAKING TIP: In relation to alcohol consumption, breastfeeding is different from placental feeding in a very important way: The neonate is on the breast intermittently, not continually, so that the alcohol can be consumed and metabolized in time for the next breastfeeding. The mother can be educated to consume alcohol in moderation and with some minor restrictions.

77. 1. Most medications are safely consumed by the breastfeeding mother. To blindly follow this order is poor practice.
    2. Ultimately, this probably will be the nurse's action but he or she must have a rationale for questioning the order.
    3. It is unacceptable to completely ignore an order even though the nurse may disagree with the order.
    4. Once the reference has been consulted, the nurse will have factual information to relay to the physician—specifically

that ampicillin is compatible with breastfeeding. A call to the doctor would then be appropriate.

TEST-TAKING TIP: Nurses not only are responsible for instituting the orders made by physicians and other primary health care practitioners but also have independent practice for which they are accountable. In this scenario, the nurse is accountable to the client. Because the medication is compatible with breastfeeding, but the physician was apparently unaware of that fact, it is the nurse's responsibility to convey that information to the doctor and to advocate for the client. The NIH has created a Web site—LactMed—where the potential danger of medications during lactation can be checked (see http://toxnet.nlm.nih.gov/cgi-bin/sis/htmlgen?LACT).

78. 1. Breastfeeding is contraindicated when a woman is receiving chemotherapy.
    2. Neither the medical problem—in this case, cholecystitis—nor the planned surgery precludes breastfeeding. The mother may have to pump and dump a few feedings depending on the short-term medications that she will receive, but she will still ultimately be able to breastfeed.
    3. Breastfeeding is not contraindicated with a diagnosis of a concussion. Again, the mother may have to pump and dump a few feedings if she must take any incompatible short-term medications, but she will still ultimately be able to breastfeed.
    4. Breastfeeding is not contraindicated with a diagnosis of thrombosis. Again, the mother may have to pump and dump a few feedings if she must take any incompatible short-term medications, but she will still ultimately be able to breastfeed.

TEST-TAKING TIP: By and large, mothers who wish to breastfeed should be enthusiastically encouraged to do so. It is the responsibility of the nurse to make sure that any medications that the woman is taking are compatible with breastfeeding. A reliable source should be consulted. In addition, it is the nurse's responsibility to advocate for breastfeeding mothers who must undergo surgery or who are diagnosed with acute illnesses that are compatible with breastfeeding.

79. 1. The woman does not have to consume 3 glasses of milk per day.

2. It is unnecessary for the mother to consume any dairy products.
3. Dairy foods provide protein and other nutrients, including the important mineral calcium. The calcium can, however, be obtained from a number of other foods, such as broccoli and fish with bones.
4. Protein can be obtained from many other foods, including meat, poultry, rice, legumes, and eggs.

TEST-TAKING TIP: Breast milk is synthesized in the glandular tissue of the mother from the raw materials in the mother's bloodstream. There is, therefore, no need for the mother to consume milk as long as she receives the needed nutrients in another manner.

80. 1. There are no foods that are absolutely contraindicated during lactation. Some babies may react to certain foods, but this must be determined on a case-by-case basis.
    2. Food restrictions are lifted once the baby is born.
    3. Some babies may be bothered by gas-producing foods, but this is not universal.
    4. Some babies may be bothered by hot and spicy foods, but this is not universal.

TEST-TAKING TIP: There is a popular belief that mothers who breastfeed must restrict their eating habits. This is not true. In fact, it is important for the test taker to realize that breastfed babies often are less fussy eaters because the flavor of breast milk changes depending on the mother's diet. Mothers should be encouraged to have a varied diet, and only if their baby appears to react to a certain food should it be eliminated from the diet. As for everyone, it is important to remind mothers to consume a maximum of two servings of fish per week.

81. 1. Stools in breastfed babies are bright yellow and loose. In bottle-fed babies, they are brownish and pasty.
    2. To prevent aspiration, bottle nipples should not be enlarged.
    3. Microwaving can overheat the formula, causing burns.
    4. **To minimize the ingestion of large quantities of air, the bottle should be held so that the nipple is always filled with formula.**

TEST-TAKING TIP: It is important for the nurse to teach parents never to place formula in the microwave for warming. This is a safety issue. The microwave does not change the composition of the formula, but it can overheat the formula, resulting in severe burns in the baby's mouth.

82. 4. The baby that is latched well should be chosen.

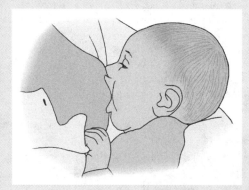

TEST-TAKING TIP: It is important for the test taker not only to be able to choose a correct answer from a word description but also to be able to assess a mother–infant dyad and determine whether or not the breastfeeding positioning is ideal.

83. 1. Soft rales are expected because babies born via cesarean section do not have the advantage of having the amniotic fluid squeezed from the pulmonary system as occurs during a vaginal birth.
    2. The bowel sounds should be normal.
    3. The Moro reflex should be normal.
    4. Babies in the LMA position are not at high risk for developmental dysplasia of the hip. Breech babies are high risk for DDH.

TEST-TAKING TIP: Cesarean section (C/S) babies often respond differently in the immediate postdelivery period than babies born vaginally. Remembering that one of the triggers for neonatal respirations is the mechanical compression of the thorax, which results in the forced expulsion of amniotic fluid from the baby's lungs, is important here. Because C/S babies do not traverse the birth canal, they do not have the benefit of that compression.

84. 1. Melanin production is not related to the presence of BAT.
    2. Babies do not shiver. Rather, to produce heat they utilize chemical thermogenesis, also called nonshivering thermogenesis.

BAT is metabolized during hypothermic episodes to maintain body temperature. Unfortunately, this can lead to metabolic acidosis.

3. BAT is unrelated to injury prevention.
4. Sufficient calories for growth are provided from breast milk or formula.

TEST-TAKING TIP: Neonates have immature thermoregulatory systems. To compensate for their inability to shiver to produce heat, full-term babies have BAT stores that were laid down during the latter part of the third trimester. Preterm babies, however, do not have sufficient BAT stores.

85. 1. This is a description of pathological jaundice resulting from maternal–fetal blood incompatibilities.
2. With lung oxygenation, the neonate no longer needs large numbers of red blood cells. As a result, excess red blood cells are destroyed. Jaundice often results on days 2 to 4.
3. There is nothing in the scenario to suggest that this was a traumatic delivery.
4. There is nothing in the scenario to suggest that meconium excretion was delayed.

TEST-TAKING TIP: One of the important clues to the answer of this question is the age of the baby. The timing of jaundice is very important. Physiological jaundice, seen in a large number of neonates, is observed after the first 24 hours. Pathological jaundice, a much more serious problem, is seen during the first 24 hours.

86. 1. Healthy babies are able to absorb fat-soluble vitamins.
2. Vitamin K is synthesized in the gut in the presence of normal flora.
3. It takes about 1 week for the baby to be able to synthesize his or her own vitamin K. The gut, at birth, is sterile.
4. Vitamin K has no function in relation to the development of pathological jaundice.

TEST-TAKING TIP: It is important for the test taker to review how vitamin K is synthesized by the intestinal flora. Because the neonate is deficient in intestinal flora until 1 week of age, he or she is unable to manufacture vitamin K until that time. Vitamin K is important, especially for babies who will be circumcised, because it is needed to activate coagulation factors synthesized in the liver.

87. 1. It is unlikely that the woman has changed her mind.

2. It is likely that she will bottle feed her baby until her milk comes in.
3. It is a common belief among women of many cultures, including Mexican, some Asian, and some Native Americans, that colostrum is bad for babies.
4. Although some women bottle feed after immigrating to the United States because they see American women bottle feeding their babies, this is an unlikely explanation for the scenario in the question.

TEST-TAKING TIP: Although the scientific community understands that colostrum is the ideal food for the newborn baby, cultural beliefs are very strong and entrenched. To develop strategies for patient education, the nurse must understand why clients may not "comply" with recommended protocols.

88. 1. Overdressing is a cultural characteristic, but it is potentially dangerous. The incidence of SIDS increases when babies are too warm. 70°F is an appropriate room temperature for the baby.
2. 70°F is an appropriate room temperature for the baby. The usual recommendation is to have babies clothed in, at the most, one layer more than is needed by adults.
3. The nurse must educate the mother regarding the need to clothe the baby appropriately.
4. The clothing should be removed and the mother should be educated about SIDS and about the correlation between overheating and SIDS.

TEST-TAKING TIP: Although behavior can sometimes be explained by cultural beliefs, it is important for the nurse to provide necessary education in an attempt to change a behavior that may be dangerous. It is also important for the nurse to provide rationales for change rather than simply to dictate change.

89. 1. This is not an example of abusive behavior.
2. Because the mother is healthy, this is not a potentially dangerous action.
3. This behavior is not irrational for a woman of African descent.
4. In Africa, breast milk is often expressed into babies' eyes to prevent neonatal eye infections. Asking the woman about other cultural traditions is appropriate.

TEST-TAKING TIP: Breast milk contains active anti-infective properties—for example, white blood cells and lactoferrin. In

countries where eye prophylaxis is not available, breast milk is often expressed into the eyes of neonates to prevent ophthalmia neonatorum. It is standard cultural practice.

90. 1. Breast milk contains sufficient quantities of vitamin A.
2. Breast milk contains sufficient quantities of vitamin B$_{12}$.
3. Breast milk contains sufficient quantities of vitamin C.
4. Many babies are vitamin D deficient because of the recommendation that they be kept out of direct sunlight to protect their skin from sunburn. For this reason, supplementation with vitamin D is recommended.

TEST-TAKING TIP: Breast milk is sufficient in vitamins and minerals for the healthy full-term baby. However, an increased incidence of rickets is being seen because many babies are rightfully kept out of direct sunlight. This is especially a problem in babies of color because their skin filters sunlight. The AAP, therefore, recommends that breastfed babies be supplemented with 400 IU of vitamin D per day (see http://pediatrics.aappublications.org/content/129/3/e827.full?sid=ff2bfb9f-9a4b-45cf-89ae-bdc7abaa2f43).

91. 1. The therapeutic action of vitamin K is not related to skin color.
2. The therapeutic action of vitamin K is not related to vital signs.
3. The therapeutic action of vitamin K is not related to glucose levels.
4. Vitamin K is needed for adequate blood clotting.

TEST-TAKING TIP: It is essential that the test taker be familiar with the actions, normal dosages, recommended routes, and so on of all standard medications administered to the neonate.

92. 1. The ophthalmic preparation is administered to prevent ophthalmia neonatorum, which is caused by gonorrhea and/or chlamydial infections. It is not given to prevent cataracts.
2. This is the correct method of instillation of the ophthalmic prophylaxis.
3. The medication can be delayed until the baby has had his or her first feeding and has begun the bonding process.
4. Ophthalmic prophylaxis is given to all neonates at birth whether or not their mothers are positive for gonorrhea.

TEST-TAKING TIP: The eye prophylaxis clouds the vision of the neonate. Even though it is state law in all 50 states that the medication be given, it is best to delay the instillation of the medication for an hour or so after birth so that eye contact and parent–infant bonding can occur during the immediate postuterine period.

93. 1. Although this is a true statement, it does not provide a rationale for the medication administration.
2. This response gives the mother a brief scientific rationale for the medication administration.
3. This response is too vague.
4. Although this is a true statement, it does not provide a rationale for the medication administration.

TEST-TAKING TIP: When asked a direct question by a client, it is important for the nurse to give as complete a response as possible. Trite responses like "All babies receive the medication at birth" do not provide information to the client. It is the right of all clients to receive accurate and complete information about their own treatments and, because the neonate is a dependent, the parents have the right to receive accurate and complete information about their baby's treatments.

94. 1. Hepatitis B immune globulin is given only to babies whose mothers are hepatitis B positive, not to all babies. If the immune globulin is administered, it should be administered via a second syringe in the opposite leg from where the vaccine is administered.
2. The hepatitis B vaccine is not diluted with sterile water.
3. Epinephrine should be available whenever vaccinations are administered in case the recipient should develop anaphylactic symptoms.
4. The vaccine is administered intramuscularly in the vastus lateralis.

TEST-TAKING TIP: Although vaccinations are administered relatively routinely, they are not without their potential side effects. One very serious side effect is anaphylaxis. Therefore, the nurse should always have epinephrine available in case of a severe reaction.

95. 1. With training, unlicensed personnel are able to provide basic patient care,

including taking vital signs, obtaining specimens, and performing activities of daily living (ADLs).

2. With training, unlicensed personnel are able to provide basic patient care, including taking vital signs, obtaining specimens, and performing ADLs.

3. With training, unlicensed personnel are able to provide basic patient care, including taking vital signs, obtaining specimens, and performing ADLs.

4. It is the registered nurse's responsibility to provide discharge teaching to clients. Only the RN knows the scientific rationales as well as the knowledge of teaching-learning principles necessary to provide accurate information and answer questions appropriately.

TEST-TAKING TIP: There are important differences between actions that necessitate professional knowledge and skill and actions that may be performed either by unlicensed personnel or by licensed practical nurses. Patient teaching is a task that the registered nurse cannot delegate.

96. 1. Red blood cells in the cephalhematoma will have to be broken down and excreted. The by-product of the destruction—bilirubin—increases the baby's risk for physiological jaundice.

2. A caput is merely a collection of edematous fluid. There is no relation between the presence of a caput and jaundice.

3. Harlequin coloration is related to the dilation of blood vessels on one side of the baby's body. There is no relation between the presence of harlequin coloring and jaundice.

4. Mongolian spots are hyperpigmented areas primarily seen on the buttocks. There is no relation between the presence of mongolian spots and jaundice.

TEST-TAKING TIP: During the early newborn period, whenever a situation exists that results in the breakdown of red blood cells, the baby is at high risk for hyperbilirubinemia and resulting jaundice. In this case, the baby is at high risk from a cephalhematoma, a collection of blood between the skull and the periosteal membrane. In addition, the neonate is at high risk for hyperbilirubinemia because of the immaturity of the newborn liver.

97. 1. Excessive crying is not a symptom of hyperbilirubinemia.

2. Babies often feed poorly when their bilirubin levels are elevated.

3. Lethargy is one of the most common early symptoms of hyperbilirubinemia.

4. Hyperreflexia is seen with prolonged periods of markedly elevated serum bilirubin.

TEST-TAKING TIP: The test taker should be familiar with the normal bilirubin values of the healthy full-term baby (less than 2 mg/dL in cord blood to approximately 12 to 14 mg/dL on days 3 to 5), as well as those values that may result in kernicterus, an infiltration of bilirubin into neural tissue. Brain damage rarely develops when serum bilirubin levels are below 20 mg/dL.

98. 1. When bilirubin levels elevate to toxic levels, babies can develop kernicterus.

2. Erythroblastosis fetalis is a syndrome resulting from the antigen–antibody reaction related to maternal–fetal blood incompatibility.

3. This bilirubin level is above the level most neonatologists consider acceptable for discharge.

4. Phototherapy is ordered when hyperbilirubinemia is present or when the development of hemolytic jaundice is very likely.

TEST-TAKING TIP: This question asks the test taker to identify a client care goal for a newborn with physiological jaundice. The client care goal reflects the nurse's desired patient care outcome. The development of kernicterus is a potential pathological outcome resulting from hyperbilirubinemia. The client care goal, therefore, is that the neonate not develop kernicterus.

99. 1. These findings are all within normal limits.

2. There is no indication that this child has developed any signs of kernicterus, which is associated with opisthotonic posturing.

3. The mother is Rh-positive. Only mothers who are Rh-negative and who deliver babies who are Rh-positive receive RhoGAM.

4. The bilirubin level is very low. There is no indication that phototherapy is needed.

TEST-TAKING TIP: Blood incompatibilities are seen when the mother is Rh-negative and the baby is Rh-positive or when the mother is type O and the baby is either type A or type B. When the baby is either Rh-negative or type O, there is actually a reduced risk that pathological jaundice will result.

100. 1. A bilirubin level of 6 mg/dL is well within the normal range for a baby who is 4 days old.
2. Because peak bilirubin levels are seen between days 3 and 5, and because the level is well within normal range, the nurse should expect that the baby will be discharged home with the parents.
3. This scenario includes no evidence that a transfusion is needed.
4. Glucose water is not recommended for neonatal feedings. If a neonate needs fluids, he or she should be given either formula or breast milk.

TEST-TAKING TIP: Hemolytic jaundice is seen within the first 24 hours of life. A neonatologist would be concerned about the health of the baby with a bilirubin of 6 mg/dL during that time frame. Physiological jaundice, on the other hand, is seen in about 50% of healthy full-term babies, with bilirubin levels rising after the first 24 hours and peaking at 3 to 5 days. A level of 6 mg/dL at 4 days, therefore, is well within normal limits.

101. 1. With the baby in the en face position, the father is holding the baby "face to face" so that he is looking directly into the baby's eyes.
2. Parents who call their babies by name, whether full or nickname, are exhibiting one sign of positive bonding.
3. A father who expects his partner to quiet a crying baby may not be accepting the parenting role.
4. Although this may not be the safest position for a baby to be sleeping in, the father is showing a sign of positive bonding.

TEST-TAKING TIP: This question should be read carefully. The question is not asking about safe sleep practices—although the nurse should discuss safe sleep practices with this father. Rather, the question is asking about evidence of poor bonding.

102. 1. Babies learn to speak by imitating the speech of others in their environment. If they are hearing impaired, there is a likelihood of delayed speech development.
2. Otitis externa is an inflammation of the ear canal outside of the eardrum. It is often called "swimmer's ear."
3. Parents bond well with babies who are deaf. As a matter of fact, parents are often unaware that their babies have hearing deficits.
4. Choanal atresia is a congenital condition when the nasal passages are blocked. Babies who have choanal atresia often choke during feedings because they are not able to breathe through their noses

TEST-TAKING TIP: It is important that the test taker not be lured to an answer simply because the question includes an unfamiliar technical term, such as otitis externa or choanal atresia. The nurse should remember that speech development is directly related to hearing ability and, therefore, should be chosen as the correct response.

103. 1. Putting the baby's diapers on tightly will put pressure on the area and help to stop the bleeding, but it is not the first or best response.
2. Putting direct pressure on the site is the best way to stop the bleeding.
3. The nurse must first apply pressure and then notify the physician.
4. Only after performing first aid should the nurse assess the vital signs.

TEST-TAKING TIP: This is a prioritizing question. The nurse's first action must be to provide immediate first aid to best stop the bleeding. Then the nurse must obtain assistance and assess the baby's vital signs to see if they have deviated.

104. 1. The neonatal period is defined as the first 28 days of life. The neonatal mortality rate is defined as neonatal deaths per 1,000 live births. Therefore, 5 babies less than 28 days old per 1,000 live births died.
2. The neonatal period is defined as the first 28 days of life, whereas the infancy period is defined as the period between birth and 1 year of life.
3. The neonatal mortality rate is defined as neonatal deaths per 1,000 live births, not per 100,000 live births.
4. The neonatal period is defined as the first 28 days of life, the infancy period is defined as the period between birth and 1 year of life, and the neonatal mortality rate is defined as neonatal deaths per 1,000 live births, not per 100,000 live births.

TEST-TAKING TIP: The term "neonatal" refers to the first 28 days of life. Therefore, answer options 2 and 4 can be eliminated. A neonatal death rate of 5 means that 5 babies less than 28 days old per 1,000 live births died. It is important to be able to interpret statistical data to compare and contrast health care outcomes from state to state and country to country.

105. 1, 3, 4, and 5 are correct.
1. Small, frequent feedings reduce the symptoms of colic in some babies.
2. The prone sleep position is not recommended for babies under 1 year of age.
3. Some babies' symptoms have decreased when they were tightly swaddled.
4. This is called the colic hold. The position does help to soothe some colicky neonates.
5. Babies who live in an environment where adults smoke have a higher incidence of colic than babies who live in a smoke-free environment.

TEST-TAKING TIP: It is essential to read each possible answer option carefully. Even though it has been shown that colicky babies sometimes find relief when they are placed prone on a hot water bottle, it is not recommended that the babies be left in that position for sleep. It is recommended that healthy babies, whether colicky or not, be placed in the prone position only while awake and while supervised.

106. 1. Breastfeeding does not prevent the development of plagiocephaly nor does it promote gross motor development.
2. Vaccinations do not prevent the development of plagiocephaly nor do they promote gross motor development.
3. Changing the baby's diapers will not prevent the development of plagiocephaly nor will it promote gross motor development.
4. Prolonged supine posturing by babies can result in flattening of the backs of babies' heads (plagiocephaly). Being placed in the prone position while awake allows babies to practice gross motor skills like rolling over.

TEST-TAKING TIP: Even if the exact definition of plagiocephaly is unknown, the test taker can surmise that the word is related to the skull because the term "cephalic" pertains to the head. Neither breastfeeding, vaccinations, nor diaper changing is related to head development.

107. 1. The neonate should be placed in a rear-facing car seat.
2. A bilirubin of 19 mg/dL is above the expected level. Therapeutic intervention is needed.
3. A blood glucose level of 59 mg/dL is within normal levels for a neonate.
4. Mongolian spots are normal variations seen on the neonatal skin.

TEST-TAKING TIP: The bilirubin level of 19 mg/dL is well above normal, and because bilirubin levels peak on day 3 to 5, it is likely that the level will rise even higher. It is likely that a therapeutic intervention, like phototherapy, will be ordered for this baby.

108. 1. Sleeping with a sibling has been shown to put babies at high risk for SIDS.
2. Sleeping in an adult bed has been shown to put babies at high risk for SIDS.
3. A large empty drawer has a firm bottom so that the baby is unlikely to rebreathe his or her own carbon dioxide and the sides of the drawer will prevent the baby from falling out of "bed."
4. Pull-out sofas have been shown to put babies at high risk for SIDS.

TEST-TAKING TIP: Creative strategies are sometimes required to meet the needs of clients with limited assets. As compared with the other three responses, the empty drawer provides the baby with the safest possible environment. The nurse should also refer this mother and baby to a social worker for assistance.

109. 1. Thermoregulation is important, but it is not the highest priority.
2. If a baby does not breathe, the remaining physiological transitions cannot successfully take place.
3. Converting from an intrauterine circulatory pattern to an extrauterine circulatory pattern is important, but it is not the highest priority.
4. Successful feeding is important but is not the highest priority.

TEST-TAKING TIP: When answering a prioritizing question that has multiple physiological answers, one good way to approach it is to think of CPR. The priority order when performing CPR is C-A-B, i.e., circulation, airway, breathing. In reviewing the responses, a test taker might be inclined to choose response 3, "Extrauterine circulatory shift." But, because there is mixed oxygenated and deoxygenated blood in fetal circulation, babies can survive even when the circulation fails immediately to shift to the extrauterine pattern. The "A" for airway and "B" for breathing, therefore, are the first priorities for the newborn because oxygenating the blood is essential to survival.

110. 1. Skin-to-skin contact (kangaroo care) has been shown to have many benefits for neonates, including promoting breast latch and stabilizing neonatal temperatures.
    2. Prone positioning, not supine, is contraindicated when babies are not being supervised. A baby being held skin to skin on the mother's chest, however, is being supervised.
    3. Neonates have been diagnosed with SIDS, although the peak incidence of SIDS is between 2 and 4 months of age.
    4. Back-to-sleep guidelines are the same for all babies.

    TEST-TAKING TIP: It is often the responsibility of the nurse to clarify recommended guidelines for parents. Even though unsupervised babies should never be placed in the prone position, those who are supervised should be placed on their stomachs. Skin-to-skin contact facilitates breastfeeding and thermoregulation. In addition, babies who are placed on their stomachs have decreased incidence of plagiocephaly.

111. 1. It has been shown that many neonatal SIDS deaths result from a form of suffocation. Babies breathe in their own exhaled carbon dioxide when they are placed prone for sleep. Babies should be placed supine.
    2. Side-lying position for sleep has not been shown to affect the rate of neonatal suffocation. The side-lying position does facilitate breastfeeding, however.
    3. Swaddling babies does not reduce the risk of their being suffocated. Placing them supine in the crib reduces their risk. Swaddling is performed to maintain a neonate's temperature.

    4. Car seat safety is unrelated to suffocation. Rather, the baby is being protected from injury when strapped into a car seat during a car accident.

    TEST-TAKING TIP: It is very important for the test taker to read the question carefully. Although each of the possible answer options is correct—that is, babies should be fed in the side-lying position, babies are often swaddled when placed supine in their crib, and babies should always be strapped into a car seat when riding in the car—only placing babies supine for sleep will reduce the babies' risk of being suffocated.

112. 1. Males are rarely newborn abductors.
    2. Women who abduct neonates are often overweight. They rarely appear underweight.
    3. Pro-life advocates have not been shown to be high risk for neonatal abduction.
    4. **Abductors usually choose newborns of their same race.**

    TEST-TAKING TIP: An abductor of a newborn is usually a female who is unable to have a child of her own. Because she wishes to have her own child, she targets babies who are similar in appearance to her.

113. 2, 3, 4, and 5 are correct.
    1. Abductors usually plan their strategies carefully before taking the baby.
    2. **A common diversion is pulling the fire alarm to distract the staff.**
    3. **Those who are inquisitive about where babies are at different times of the day may be planning an abduction.**
    4. **Rooms near stairwells provide the abductor with a quick and easy get-away.**
    5. **The abductor is able to hide a baby in oversized clothing or in large bags.**

    TEST-TAKING TIP: The test taker should familiarize himself or herself with the many characteristics of the neonatal abductor including, in addition to those cited above, individuals who are emotionally immature, suffer from low self-esteem, and have a history of manipulative behavior.

Normal Postpartum

7

The postpartum period begins immediately after the delivery of the placenta and lasts until the uterus has fully involuted, about 6 weeks later. The first hour after delivery is often referred to as the fourth stage of labor, but because the assessments and concerns of that hour relate more directly to the postpartum period, those questions have been included in this chapter. The postpartum nurse must be vigilant in monitoring the mother's physiological adjustment to the nonpregnant state, whether the client delivered vaginally or via cesarean section. As important, the nurse must evaluate the mother's and father's emotional adjustment to parenthood. Educational goals include self-care needs and baby care (see Chapter 6, Newborn).

KEYWORDS

The following words include English vocabulary, nursing/medical terminology, concepts, principles, or information relevant to content specifically addressed in the chapter or associated with topics presented in it. English dictionaries, your nursing textbooks, and medical dictionaries such as *Taber's Cyclopedic Medical Dictionary* are resources that can be used to expand your knowledge and understanding of these words and related information.

cesarean section	Methergine (ergonovine)
Colace (docusate sodium)	nonimmune
complementary therapy	patient-controlled analgesia (PCA)
diaphoresis	postpartum
discharge teaching	postpartum blues
engorgement	postpartum depression
epidural anesthesia	postpartum exercises
episiotomy	postpartum psychosis
forceps delivery	puerperium
fourth stage of labor	REEDA scale
fundal assessment	sitz bath
Homan's sign	spinal anesthesia
Kegel exercises	spontaneous vaginal delivery
laceration (1°, 2°, 3°, and 4°)	"taking in" phase
"letting go" phase	"taking hold" phase
lochia (rubra, serosa, alba)	vacuum extraction

QUESTIONS

1. A 3-day-breastfeeding client who is not immune to rubella is to receive the rubella vaccine at discharge. Which of the following must the nurse include in her discharge teaching regarding the vaccine?
   1. The woman should not become pregnant for at least 4 weeks.
   2. The woman should pump and dump her breast milk for 1 week.
   3. Surgical masks must be worn by the mother when she holds the baby.
   4. Antibodies transported through the breast milk will protect the baby.

2. A 3-day-postpartum client questions why she is to receive the rubella vaccine before leaving the hospital. Which of the following rationales should guide the nurse's response?
   1. The client's obstetric status is optimal for receiving the vaccine.
   2. The client's immune system is highly responsive during the postpartum period.
   3. The client's baby will be high risk for acquiring rubella if the woman does not receive the vaccine.
   4. The client's insurance company will pay for the shot if it is given during the immediate postpartum period.

3. A patient, G2 P1102, who delivered her baby 8 hours ago, now has a temperature of 100.2°F. Which of the following is the appropriate nursing intervention at this time?
   1. Notify the doctor to get an order for acetaminophen.
   2. Request an infectious disease consult from the doctor.
   3. Provide the woman with cool compresses.
   4. Encourage intake of water and other fluids.

4. To prevent infection, the nurse teaches the postpartum client to perform which of the following tasks?
   1. Apply antibiotic ointment to the perineum daily.
   2. Change the peripad at each voiding.
   3. Void at least every two hours.
   4. Spray the perineum with povidone-iodine after toileting.

5. A 3-day-postpartum breastfeeding woman is being assessed. Her breasts are firm and warm to the touch. When asked when she last fed the baby her reply is, "I fed the baby last evening. I let the nurses feed him in the nursery last night. I needed to rest." Which of the following actions should the nurse take at this time?
   1. Encourage the woman exclusively to breastfeed her baby.
   2. Have the woman massage her breasts hourly.
   3. Obtain an order to culture her expressed breast milk.
   4. Take the temperature and pulse rate of the woman.

6. A breastfeeding woman has been counseled on how to prevent engorgement. Which of the following actions by the mother shows that the teaching was effective?
   1. She pumps her breasts after each feeding.
   2. She feeds her baby every 2 to 3 hours.
   3. She feeds her baby 10 minutes on each side.
   4. She supplements each feeding with formula.

7. A 2-day-postpartum breastfeeding woman states, "I am sick of being fat. When can I go on a diet?" Which of the following responses is appropriate?
   1. "It is fine for you to start dieting right now as long as you drink plenty of milk."
   2. "Your breast milk will be low in vitamins if you start to diet while breastfeeding."
   3. "You must eat at least 3,000 calories per day in order to produce enough milk for your baby."
   4. "Many mothers lose weight when they breastfeed because the baby consumes about 600 calories a day."

8. A G2 P2002, who is postpartum 6 hours from a spontaneous vaginal delivery, is assessed. The nurse notes that the fundus is firm at the umbilicus, there is heavy lochia rubra, and perineal sutures are intact. Which of the following actions should the nurse take at this time?
   1. Do nothing. This is a normal finding.
   2. Massage the woman's fundus.
   3. Take the woman to the bathroom to void.
   4. Notify the woman's primary health care provider.

9. A client informs the nurse that she intends to bottle feed her baby. Which of the following actions should the nurse encourage the client to perform? **Select all that apply.**
   1. Increase her fluid intake for a few days.
   2. Massage her breasts every 4 hours.
   3. Apply heat packs to her axillae.
   4. Wear a supportive bra 24 hours a day.
   5. Stand with her back toward the shower water.

10. The nurse in the obstetric clinic received a telephone call from a bottle-feeding mother of a 3-day-old. The client states that her breasts are firm, red, and warm to the touch. Which of the following is the best action for the nurse to advise the client to perform?
   1. Intermittently apply ice packs to her axillae and breasts.
   2. Apply lanolin to her breasts and nipples every 3 hours.
   3. Express milk from the breasts every 3 hours.
   4. Ask the primary health care provider to order a milk suppressant.

11. A multigravid, postpartum woman reports severe abdominal cramping whenever she nurses her baby. Which of the following responses by the nurse is appropriate?
   1. Suggest that the woman bottle feed for a few days.
   2. Instruct the patient on how to massage her fundus.
   3. Instruct the patient to feed using an alternate position.
   4. Discuss the action of breastfeeding hormones.

12. The nurse is caring for a breastfeeding mother who asks advice on foods that will provide both vitamin A and iron. Which of the following should the nurse recommend?
   1. ½ cup raw celery dipped in 1 ounce cream cheese.
   2. 8 ounce yogurt mixed with 1 medium banana.
   3. 12 ounce strawberry milk shake.
   4. 1½ cup raw broccoli.

13. A breastfeeding mother states that she has sore nipples. In response to the complaint, the nurse assists with "latch on" and recommends that the mother do which of the following?
   1. Use a nipple shield at each breastfeeding.
   2. Cleanse the nipples with soap 3 times a day.
   3. Rotate the baby's positions at each feed.
   4. Bottle feed for 2 days then resume breastfeeding.

14. Which of the following statements is true about breastfeeding mothers as compared to bottle-feeding mothers?
   1. Breastfeeding mothers usually involute completely by 3 weeks postpartum.
   2. Breastfeeding mothers have decreased incidence of diabetes mellitus later in life.
   3. Breastfeeding mothers show higher levels of bone density after menopause.
   4. Breastfeeding mothers are prone to fewer bouts of infection immediately postpartum.

15. A breastfeeding woman, 1½ months postdelivery, calls the nurse in the obstetrician's office and states, "I am very embarrassed but I need help. Last night I had an orgasm when my husband and I were making love. You should have seen the milk. We were both soaking wet. What is wrong with me?" The nurse should base the response to the client on which of the following?
    1. The woman is exhibiting signs of pathological galactorrhea.
    2. The same hormone stimulates orgasms and the milk ejection reflex.
    3. The woman should have a serum galactosemia assessment done.
    4. The baby is stimulating the woman to produce too much milk.

16. A client who is 3 days postpartum asks the nurse, "When may my husband and I begin having sexual relations again?" The nurse should encourage the couple to wait until after which of the following has occurred?
    1. The client has had her six-week postpartum checkup.
    2. The episiotomy has healed and the lochia has stopped.
    3. The lochia has turned to pink and the vagina is no longer tender.
    4. The client has had her first postpartum menstrual period.

17. A breastfeeding client, 7 weeks postpartum, complains to an obstetrician's triage nurse that when she and her husband had intercourse for the first time after the delivery, "I couldn't stand it. It was so painful. The doctor must have done something terrible to my vagina." Which of the following responses by the nurse is appropriate?
    1. "After a delivery the vagina is always very tender. It should feel better the next time you have intercourse."
    2. "Does your baby have thrush? If so, you should be assessed for a yeast infection in your vagina."
    3. "Women who breastfeed often have vaginal dryness. A vaginal lubricant may remedy your discomfort."
    4. "Sometimes the stitches of episiotomies heal too tight. Why don't you come in to be checked?"

18. The nurse monitors his or her postpartum clients carefully because which of the following physiological changes occurs during the early postpartum period?
    1. Decreased urinary output.
    2. Increased blood pressure.
    3. Decreased blood volume.
    4. Increased estrogen level.

19. A woman, 24 hours postpartum, is complaining of profuse diaphoresis. She has no other complaints. Which of the following actions by the nurse is appropriate?
    1. Take the woman's temperature.
    2. Advise the woman to decrease her fluid intake.
    3. Reassure the woman that this is normal.
    4. Notify the neonate's pediatrician.

20. Which of the following laboratory values would the nurse expect to see in a normal postpartum woman?
    1. Hematocrit, 39%.
    2. White blood cell count, 16,000 cells/mm³.
    3. Red blood cell count, 5 million cells/mm³.
    4. Hemoglobin, 15 grams/dL.

21. A nurse reports that a client has moderate lochia flow. Which of the following pads would be consistent with her evaluation? (Please mark the appropriate pad with an "X.")

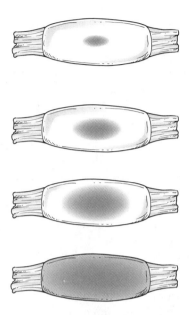

22. The nurse is discussing the importance of doing Kegel exercises during the postpartum period. Which of the following should be included in the teaching plan?
    1. She should repeatedly contract and relax her rectal and thigh muscles.
    2. She should practice by stopping the urine flow midstream every time she voids.
    3. She should get on her hands and knees whenever performing the exercises.
    4. She should be taught that toned pubococcygeal muscles decrease blood loss.

23. The nurse is evaluating the involution of a woman who is 3 days postpartum. Which of the following findings would the nurse evaluate as normal?
    1. Fundus 1 cm above the umbilicus, lochia rosa.
    2. Fundus 2 cm above the umbilicus, lochia alba.
    3. Fundus 2 cm below the umbilicus, lochia rubra.
    4. Fundus 3 cm below the umbilicus, lochia serosa.

24. During a home visit, the nurse assesses a client 2 weeks after delivery. Which of the following signs/symptoms should the nurse expect to see?
    1. Diaphoresis.
    2. Lochia alba.
    3. Cracked nipples.
    4. Hypertension.

25. The day after delivery, a woman, whose fundus is firm at 1 cm below the umbilicus and who has moderate lochia, tells the nurse that something must be wrong: "All I do is go to the bathroom." Which of the following is an appropriate nursing response?
    1. Catheterize the client per doctor's orders.
    2. Measure the client's next voiding.
    3. Inform the client that polyuria is normal.
    4. Check the specific gravity of the next voiding.

26. A breastfeeding client, G10 P6408, delivered 10 minutes ago. Which of the following assessments is most important for the nurse to perform at this time?
    1. Pulse.
    2. Fundus.
    3. Bladder.
    4. Breast.

27. The nurse is caring for a client who had a cesarean section under spinal anesthesia less than 2 hours ago. Which of the following nursing actions is appropriate at this time?
    1. Elevate the head of the bed 60 degrees.
    2. Report absence of bowel sounds to the physician.
    3. Have her turn and deep breathe every 2 hours.
    4. Assess for patellar hyperreflexia bilaterally.

28. The nurse is caring for a postpartum client who experienced a second-degree perineal laceration at delivery 2 hours ago. Which of the following interventions should the nurse perform at this time?
    1. Apply an ice pack to the perineum.
    2. Advise the woman to use a sitz bath after every voiding.
    3. Advise the woman to sit on a pillow.
    4. Teach the woman to insert nothing into her rectum.

29. A woman had a cesarean section yesterday. She states that she needs to cough but that she is afraid to. Which of the following is the nurse's best response?
    1. "I know that it hurts but it is very important for you to cough."
    2. "Let me check your lung fields to see if coughing is really necessary."
    3. "If you take a few deep breaths in, that should be as good as coughing."
    4. "If you support your incision with a pillow, coughing should hurt less."

30. A woman is receiving patient-controlled analgesia (PCA) post–cesarean section. Which of the following must be included in the patient teaching?
    1. The client should monitor how often she presses the button.
    2. The client should report any feelings of nausea or itching to the nurse.
    3. The family should press the button whenever they feel the woman is in pain.
    4. The family should inform the nurse if the client becomes sleepy.

31. The nurse is caring for a client who had an emergency cesarean section, with her husband in attendance, the day before. The baby's Apgar was 9/9. The woman and her partner had attended childbirth education classes and had anticipated having a water birth with family present. Which of the following comments by the nurse is appropriate?
    1. "Sometimes babies just don't deliver the way we expect them to."
    2. "With all of your preparations, it must have been disappointing for you to have had a cesarean."
    3. "I know you had to have surgery, but you are very lucky that your baby was born healthy."
    4. "At least your husband was able to be with you when the baby was born."

32. A postoperative cesarean section woman is to receive morphine 4 mg q 3–4 h subcutaneously for pain. The morphine is available on the unit in premeasured syringes 10 mg/1 mL. Each time the nurse administers the medication, how many milliliters (mL) of morphine will be wasted? Calculate to the nearest tenth.
    _____ mL

33. The obstetrician has ordered that a post-op cesarean section client's patient-controlled analgesia (PCA) be discontinued. Which of the following actions by the nurse is appropriate?
    1. Discard the remaining medication in the presence of another nurse.
    2. Recommend waiting until her pain level is zero to discontinue the medicine.
    3. Discontinue the medication only after the analgesia is completely absorbed.
    4. Return the unused portion of medication to the narcotics cabinet.

34. A client is receiving an epidural infusion of a narcotic for pain relief after a cesarean section. The nurse would report to the anesthesiologist if which of the following were assessed?
    1. Respiratory rate 8 rpm.
    2. Complaint of thirst.
    3. Urinary output of 250 mL/hr.
    4. Numbness of feet and ankles.

35. A client, 2 days postoperative from a cesarean section, complains to the nurse that she has yet to have a bowel movement since the surgery. Which of the following responses by the nurse would be appropriate at this time?
    1. "That is very concerning. I will request that your physician order an enema for you."
    2. "Two days is not that bad. Some patients go four days or longer without a movement."
    3. "You have been taking antibiotics through your intravenous. That is probably why you are constipated."
    4. "Fluids and exercise often help to combat constipation. Take a stroll around the unit and drink lots of fluid."

36. A post–cesarean section, breastfeeding client, whose subjective pain level is 2/5, requests her as needed (prn) narcotic analgesics every 3 hours. She states, "I have decided to make sure that I feel as little pain from this experience as possible." Which of the following should the nurse conclude in relation to this woman's behavior?
    1. The woman needs a stronger narcotic order.
    2. The woman is high risk for severe constipation.
    3. The woman's breast milk volume may drop while taking the medicine.
    4. The woman's newborn may become addicted to the medication.

37. A nurse is assessing a 1-day-postpartum woman who had her baby by cesarean section. Which of the following should the nurse report to the surgeon?
    1. Fundus at the umbilicus.
    2. Nodular breasts.
    3. Pulse rate 60 bpm.
    4. Pad saturation every 30 minutes.

38. The nurse is assessing the midline episiotomy on a postpartum client. Which of the following findings should the nurse expect to see?
    1. Moderate serosanguinous drainage.
    2. Well-approximated edges.
    3. Ecchymotic area distal to the episiotomy.
    4. An area of redness adjacent to the incision.

39. A client, G1 P1, who had an epidural, has just delivered a daughter, Apgar 9/9, over a mediolateral episiotomy. The physician used low forceps. While recovering, the client states, "I'm a failure. I couldn't stand the pain and couldn't even push my baby out by myself!" Which of the following is the best response for the nurse to make?
    1. "You'll feel better later after you have had a chance to rest and to eat."
    2. "Don't say that. There are many women who would be ecstatic to have that baby."
    3. "I am sure that you will have another baby. I bet that it will be a natural delivery."
    4. "To have things work out differently than you had planned is disappointing."

40. The nurse is developing a standard care plan for postpartum clients who have had midline episiotomies. Which of the following interventions should be included in the plan?
    1. Assist with stitch removal on third postpartum day.
    2. Administer analgesics every four hours per doctor's orders.
    3. Teach client to contract her buttocks before sitting.
    4. Irrigate incision twice daily with antibiotic solution.

41. A client, G1 P1001, 1 hour postpartum from a spontaneous vaginal delivery with local anesthesia, states that she needs to urinate. Which of the following actions by the nurse is appropriate at this time?
    1. Provide the woman with a bedpan.
    2. Advise the woman that the feeling is likely related to the trauma of delivery.
    3. Remind the woman that she still has a catheter in place from the delivery.
    4. Assist the woman to the bathroom.

42. A nurse is assessing the fundus of a client during the immediate postpartum period. Which of the following actions indicates that the nurse is performing the skill correctly?
    1. The nurse measures the fundal height using a paper centimeter tape.
    2. The nurse stabilizes the base of the uterus with his or her dependent hand.
    3. The nurse palpates the fundus with the tips of his or her fingers.
    4. The nurse precedes the assessment with a sterile vaginal exam.

43. A 1-day postpartum woman states, "I think I have a urinary tract infection. I have to go to the bathroom all the time." Which of the following actions should the nurse take?
    1. Assure the woman that frequent urination is normal after delivery.
    2. Obtain an order for a urine culture.
    3. Assess the urine for cloudiness.
    4. Ask the woman if she is prone to urinary tract infections.

44. The nurse is assessing the laboratory report on a 2-day postpartum G1 P1001. The woman had a normal postpartum assessment this morning. Which of the following results should the nurse report to the primary health care provider?
    1. White blood cells, 12,500 cells/mm^3.
    2. Red blood cells, 4,500,000 cells/mm^3.
    3. Hematocrit, 26%.
    4. Hemoglobin, 11 g/dL

45. A bottle-feeding woman, 1½ weeks postpartum from a vaginal delivery, calls the obstetric office to state that she has saturated 2 pads in the past 1 hour. Which of the following responses by the nurse is appropriate?
    1. "You must be doing too much. Lie down for a few hours and call back if the bleeding has not subsided."
    2. "You are probably getting your period back. You will bleed like that for a day or two and then it will lighten up."
    3. "It is not unusual to bleed heavily every once in a while after a baby is born. It should subside shortly."
    4. "It is important for you to be examined by the doctor today. Let me check to see when you can come in."

46. A client, 2 days postpartum from a spontaneous vaginal delivery, asks the nurse about postpartum exercises. Which of the following responses by the nurse is appropriate?
    1. "You must wait to begin to perform exercises until after your six-week postpartum checkup."
    2. "You may begin Kegel exercises today, but do not do any other exercises until the doctor tells you that it is safe."
    3. "By next week you will be able to return to the exercise schedule you had during your prepregnancy."
    4. "You can do some Kegel exercises today and then slowly increase your toning exercises over the next few weeks."

47. The nurse is examining a 2-day-postpartum client whose fundus is 2 cm below the umbilicus and whose bright red lochia saturates about 4 inches of a pad in 1 hour. What should the nurse document in the nursing record?
    1. Abnormal involution, lochia rubra heavy.
    2. Abnormal involution, lochia serosa scant.
    3. Normal involution, lochia rubra moderate.
    4. Normal involution, lochia serosa heavy.

48. The nurse palpates a distended bladder on a woman who delivered vaginally 2 hours earlier. The woman refuses to go to the bathroom, "I really don't need to go." Which of the following responses by the nurse is appropriate?
    1. "Okay. I must be palpating your uterus."
    2. "I understand but I still would like you to try to urinate."
    3. "You still must be numb from the local anesthesia."
    4. "That is a problem. I will have to catheterize you."

49. A client, G1 P0101, postpartum 1 day, is assessed. The nurse notes that the client's lochia rubra is moderate and her fundus is boggy 2 cm above the umbilicus and deviated to the right. Which of the following actions should the nurse take first?
    1. Notify the woman's primary health care provider.
    2. Massage the woman's fundus.
    3. Escort the woman to the bathroom to urinate.
    4. Check the quantity of lochia on the peripad.

50. The nurse has taught a new admission to the postpartum unit about pericare. Which of the following indicates that the client understands the procedure? **Select all that apply.**
    1. The woman performs the procedure twice a day.
    2. The woman washes her hands before and after the procedure.
    3. The woman sits in warm tap water for ten minutes three times a day.
    4. The woman sprays her perineum from front to back.
    5. The woman mixes warm tap water with hydrogen peroxide.

51. The nurse informs a postpartum woman that which of the following is the reason ibuprofen (Advil) is especially effective for afterbirth pains?
    1. Ibuprofen is taken every two hours.
    2. Ibuprofen has an antiprostaglandin effect.
    3. Ibuprofen is given via the parenteral route.
    4. Ibuprofen can be administered in high doses.

52. A woman had a 3,000-gram baby via normal spontaneous vaginal delivery 12 hours ago. Place an "X" on the location where the nurse would expect to palpate her fundus.

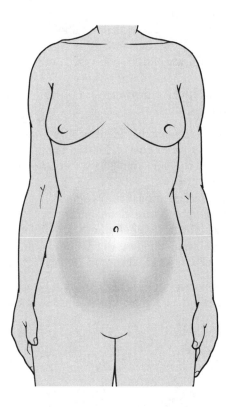

53. A physician has ordered an iron supplement for a postpartum woman. The nurse strongly suggests that the woman take the medicine with which of the following drinks?
    1. Skim milk.
    2. Ginger ale.
    3. Orange juice.
    4. Chamomile tea.

54. On admission to the labor and delivery unit, a client's hemoglobin (Hgb) was assessed at 11.0 g/dL, and her hematocrit (Hct) at 33%. Which of the following values would the nurse expect to see 2 days after a normal spontaneous vaginal delivery?
    1. Hgb 12.5 g/dL; Hct 37%.
    2. Hgb 11.0 g/dL; Hct 33%.
    3. Hgb 10.5 g/dL; Hct 31%.
    4. Hgb 9.0 g/dL; Hct 27%.

55. During a postpartum assessment, it is noted that a G1 P1001 woman, who delivered vaginally over an intact perineum, has a cluster of hemorrhoids. Which of the following would be appropriate for the nurse to include in the woman's health teaching? **Select all that apply.**
    1. The client should use a sitz bath daily as a relief measure.
    2. The client should digitally replace external hemorrhoids into her rectum.
    3. The client should breastfeed frequently to stimulate oxytocin to reduce the size of the hemorrhoids.
    4. The client should be advised that the hemorrhoids will increase in size and quantity with subsequent pregnancies.
    5. The client should apply topical anesthetic as a relief measure.

56. Which of the following is the priority nursing action during the immediate postpartum period?
    1. Palpate fundus.
    2. Check pain level.
    3. Perform pericare.
    4. Assess breasts.

57. Immediately after delivery, a woman is shaking uncontrollably. Which of the following nursing actions is most appropriate?
    1. Provide the woman with warm blankets.
    2. Put the woman in the Trendelenburg position.
    3. Notify the primary health care provider.
    4. Increase the intravenous infusion.

58. One nursing diagnosis that a nurse has identified for a postpartum client is: Risk for intrauterine infection r/t vaginal delivery. During the postpartum period, which of the following goals should the nurse include in the care plan in relation to this diagnosis? **Select all that apply.**
    1. The client will drink sufficient quantities of fluid.
    2. The client will have a stable white blood cell count.
    3. The client will have a normal temperature.
    4. The client will have normal-smelling vaginal discharge.
    5. The client will take two or three sitz baths each day.

59. Which of the following nursing interventions would be appropriate for the nurse to perform to achieve the client care goal: The client will not develop postpartum thrombophlebitis?
    1. Encourage early ambulation.
    2. Promote oral fluid intake.
    3. Massage the legs of the client twice daily.
    4. Provide the client with high-fiber foods.

60. The nurse is developing a plan of care for the postpartum client during the "taking in" phase. Which of the following should the nurse include in the plan?
   1. Teach baby-care skills like diapering.
   2. Discuss the labor and birth with the mother.
   3. Discuss contraceptive choices with the mother.
   4. Teach breastfeeding skills like pumping.

61. The nurse is developing a plan of care for the postpartum client during the "taking hold" phase. Which of the following should the nurse include in the plan?
   1. Provide the client with a nutritious meal.
   2. Encourage the client to take a nap.
   3. Assist the client with activities of daily living.
   4. Assure the client that she is an excellent mother.

62. The nurse takes a newborn to a primipara for a feeding. The mother holds the baby en face, strokes his cheek, and states that this is the first newborn she has ever held. Which of the following nursing assessments is most appropriate?
   1. Positive bonding and client needs little teaching.
   2. Positive bonding but teaching related to newborn care is needed.
   3. Poor bonding and referral to a child abuse agency is essential.
   4. Poor bonding but there is potential for positive mothering.

63. A primipara, 2 hours postpartum, requests that the nurse diaper her baby after a feeding because "I am so tired right now. I just want to have something to eat and take a nap." Based on this information, the nurse concludes that the woman is exhibiting signs of which of the following?
   1. Social deprivation.
   2. Child neglect.
   3. Normal postpartum behavior.
   4. Postpartum depression.

64. A nurse is counseling a woman about postpartum blues. Which of the following should be included in the discussion?
   1. The father may become sad and weepy.
   2. Postpartum blues last about a week or two.
   3. Medications are available to relieve the symptoms.
   4. Very few women experience postpartum blues.

65. A 2-day postpartum mother, G2 P2002, states that her 2-year-old daughter at home is very excited about taking "my baby sister" home. Which of the following is an appropriate response by the nurse?
   1. "It's always nice when siblings are excited to have the babies go home."
   2. "Your daughter is very advanced for her age. She must speak very well."
   3. "Your daughter is likely to become very jealous of the new baby."
   4. "Older sisters can be very helpful. They love to play mother."

66. The home health nurse visits a client who is 6 days postdelivery. The client appears sad, weeps frequently, and states, "I don't know what is wrong with me. I feel terrible. I should be happy, but I'm not." Which of the following nursing diagnoses is appropriate for this client?
   1. Suicidal thoughts related to psychotic ideations.
   2. Post-trauma response related to traumatic delivery.
   3. Ineffective individual coping related to hormonal shifts.
   4. Spiritual distress related to immature belief systems.

67. A Muslim woman requests something to eat after the delivery of her baby. Which of the following meals would be most appropriate for the nurse to give her?
   1. Ham sandwich.
   2. Bacon and eggs.
   3. Spaghetti with sausage.
   4. Chicken and dumplings.

68. The nurse is caring for a Seventh Day Adventist woman who delivered a baby boy by cesarean section. Which of the following questions should be asked regarding this woman's care?
    1. "Would you like me to order a vegetarian clear liquid diet for you?"
    2. "Is there anything special you will need for your Sabbath on Sunday?"
    3. "Would you like to telephone your clergy to set up a date for the baptism?"
    4. "Will a rabbi be performing the circumcision on your baby?"

69. An Asian client's temperature 10 hours after delivery is 100.2°F, but when encouraged she refuses to drink her ice water. Which of the following nursing actions is most appropriate?
    1. Replace the ice water with hot water.
    2. Notify the client's health care provider.
    3. Reassess the temperature in one half hour.
    4. Remind the client that drinking is very important.

70. A medication order reads: Methergine (ergonovine) 0.2 mg po q 6 h × 4 doses. Which of the following assessments should be made before administering each dose of this medication?
    1. Apical pulse.
    2. Lochia flow.
    3. Blood pressure.
    4. Episiotomy.

71. Which of the following complementary therapies can a nurse suggest to a multiparous woman who is complaining of severe afterbirth pains?
    1. Lie prone with a small pillow cushioning her abdomen.
    2. Contract her abdominal muscles for a count of ten.
    3. Slowly ambulate in the hallways.
    4. Drink ice tea with lemon or lime.

72. The nurse should warn a client who is about to receive Methergine (ergonovine) of which of the following side effects?
    1. Headache.
    2. Nausea.
    3. Cramping.
    4. Fatigue.

73. The third stage of labor has just ended for a client who has decided to bottle feed her baby. Which of the following maternal hormones will increase sharply at this time?
    1. Estrogen.
    2. Prolactin.
    3. Human placental lactogen.
    4. Human chorionic gonadotropin.

74. The nurse has provided teaching to a post-op cesarean client who is being discharged on Colace (docusate sodium) 100 mg po tid. Which of the following would indicate that the teaching was successful?
    1. The woman swallows the tablets whole.
    2. The woman takes the pills between meals.
    3. The woman calls the doctor if she develops a headache.
    4. The woman understands that her urine may turn orange.

75. The nurse hears the following information on a newly delivered client during shift report: 21 years old, married, G1 P1001, 8 hours post-spontaneous vaginal delivery over an intact perineum; vitals 110/70, 98.6°F, 82, 18; fundus firm at umbilicus; moderate lochia rubra; ambulated to bathroom to void 4 times; breastfeeding every 2 hours. Which of the following nursing diagnoses should the nurse include in this client's nursing care plan?
    1. Fluid volume deficit r/t excess blood loss.
    2. Impaired skin integrity r/t vaginal delivery.
    3. Impaired urinary elimination r/t excess output.
    4. Knowledge deficit r/t lack of parenting experience.

76. A client who delivered a 3,900-gram baby vaginally over a right mediolateral episiotomy states, "How am I supposed to have a bowel movement? The stitches are right there!" Which of the following is the best response by the nurse?
    1. "I will call the doctor to order a stool softener for you."
    2. "Your stitches are actually far away from your rectal area."
    3. "If you eat high-fiber foods and drink fluids you should have no problems."
    4. "If you use your topical anesthetic on your stitches you will feel much less pain."

77. After a client's placenta is birthed, the obstetrician states, "Please add 20 units of oxytocin to the intravenous and increase the drip rate to 250 mL/hr." The client has 750 mL in her IV and the IV tubing delivers fluid at the rate of 10 gtt/mL. To what drip rate should the nurse set the intravenous?
    _____ gtt/min

78. A client has just been transferred to the postpartum unit from labor and delivery. Which of the following nursing care goals is of highest priority?
    1. The client will breastfeed her baby every 2 hours.
    2. The client will consume a normal diet.
    3. The client will have a moderate lochial flow.
    4. The client will ambulate to the bathroom every 2 hours.

79. A client has just been transferred to the postpartum unit from labor and delivery. Which of the following tasks should the registered nurse delegate to the nursing care assistant?
    1. Assess client's fundal height.
    2. Teach client how to massage her fundus.
    3. Take the client's vital signs.
    4. Document quantity of lochia in the chart.

80. A client, G2 P1102, is 30 minutes postpartum from a low forceps vaginal delivery over a right mediolateral episiotomy. Her physician has just finished repairing the incision. The client's legs are in the stirrups and she is breastfeeding her baby. Which of the following actions should the nurse perform?
    1. Assess her feet and ankles for pitting edema.
    2. Advise the client to stop feeding her baby while her blood pressure is assessed.
    3. Lower both of her legs at the same time.
    4. Measure the length of the episiotomy and document the findings in the chart.

81. A maternity nurse knows that obstetric clients are most at high risk for cardiovascular compromise during the one hour immediately following a delivery because of which of the following?
    1. Weight of the uterine body is significantly reduced.
    2. Excess blood volume from pregnancy is circulating in the woman's periphery.
    3. Cervix is fully dilated and the lochia flows freely.
    4. Maternal blood pressure drops precipitously once the baby's head emerges.

82. The nurse must initiate discharge teaching with the couple regarding the need for an infant car seat for the day of discharge. Which of the following responses indicates that the nurse acted appropriately? The nurse discussed the need with the couple:
    1. On admission to the labor room.
    2. In the client room after the delivery.
    3. When the client put the baby to the breast for the first time.
    4. The day before the client and baby are to leave the hospital.

83. The nurse is preparing to place a peripad on the perineum of a client who delivered her baby 10 minutes earlier. The client states, "I don't use those. I always use tampons." Which of the following actions by the nurse is appropriate at this time?
    1. Remove the peripad and insert a tampon into the woman's vagina.
    2. Advise the client that for the first two days she will be bleeding too heavily for a tampon.
    3. Remind the client that a tampon would hurt until the soreness from the delivery resolves.
    4. State that it is unsafe to place anything into the vagina until involution is complete.

84. A client has been transferred to the post–anesthesia care unit from a cesarean delivery. The client had spinal anesthesia for the surgery. Which of the following interventions should the nurse perform at this time?
    1. Assess the level of the anesthesia.
    2. Encourage the client to urinate in a bedpan.
    3. Provide the client with the diet of her choice.
    4. Check the incision for signs of infection.

85. The surgeon has removed the surgical cesarean section dressing from a post-op day 1 client. Which of the following actions by the nurse is appropriate?
    1. Irrigate the incision twice daily.
    2. Monitor the incision for drainage.
    3. Apply steristrips to the incision line.
    4. Palpate the incision and assess for pain.

86. A nurse is performing a postpartum assessment on a newly delivered client. Which of the following actions will the nurse perform? **Select all that apply.**
    1. Palpate the breasts.
    2. Auscultate the carotid.
    3. Check vaginal discharge.
    4. Assess the extremities.
    5. Inspect the perineum.

87. During a postpartum assessment, the nurse assesses the calves of a client's legs. The nurse is checking for which of the following signs/symptoms? **Select all that apply.**
    1. Pain.
    2. Warmth.
    3. Discharge.
    4. Ecchymosis.
    5. Redness.

The correct answer number and rationale for why it is the correct answer are given in **boldface blue type**. Rationales for why the other possible answer options are incorrect also are given, but they are not in boldface type.

1. 1. **This statement is correct. The rubella vaccine is a live attenuated vaccine. Severe birth defects can develop if the woman becomes pregnant within 4 weeks of receiving the injection.**
   2. This is unnecessary. There is no risk to the baby whether the mother is bottle feeding or breastfeeding.
   3. This statement is incorrect. There is no risk to the baby.
   4. This statement is incorrect.

   TEST-TAKING TIP: If rubella is contracted during pregnancy, the fetus is at very high risk for injury. Whenever gravid clients are found to be nonimmune to rubella—defined as a titer of 1:8 or lower—they are advised to receive the vaccine during the early postpartum period and are counseled regarding the teratogenic properties of the vaccine.

2. 1. **This statement is correct. Because the vaccine is teratogenic, the best time to administer it is when the client is not pregnant.**
   2. This statement is incorrect. The immune systems of women during their pregnancies and immediately postpartum are slightly depressed.
   3. This statement is incorrect. The baby will be susceptible to rubella whether or not the woman receives the vaccine.
   4. In general, insurance companies will pay for vaccinations whenever they are needed.

   TEST-TAKING TIP: The correct answer did not explicitly state that the vaccine is administered during the immediate postpartum period because the woman is not pregnant and is unlikely to become pregnant within the next 4 weeks. But the test taker must know that a woman's obstetric status immediately after delivery is optimal for receiving the medication precisely because she is not pregnant and very unlikely to become pregnant.

3. 1. A temperature of 100.2°F is not a febrile temperature. It is unlikely that this client needs acetaminophen.
   2. A temperature of 100.2°F is not a febrile temperature. It is unlikely that this client is infected.
   3. A temperature of 100.2°F is not a febrile temperature. It is unlikely that this client needs cool compresses.
   4. **It is likely that this client is dehydrated. She should be advised to drink fluids.**

   TEST-TAKING TIP: In the early postpartum period, up to 24 hours after delivery, the most common reason for clients to have slight temperature elevations is dehydration. During labor, clients work very hard, often utilizing breathing techniques as a form of pain control. As a result, the clients lose fluids through insensible loss via the respiratory system.

4. 1. It is unnecessary to apply antibiotic ointment to the perineum after delivery.
   2. **Clients should be advised to change their pads at each voiding.**
   3. The clients should void about every 2 hours, but this action is not an infection control measure.
   4. It is unnecessary to spray the perineum with a povidone-iodine solution. Plain water, however, should be sprayed on the perineum.

   TEST-TAKING TIP: Postpartum women should be advised to perform three actions to prevent infections: (1) change their peripads at each toileting because blood is an excellent medium for bacterial growth; (2) spray the perineum from front to back with clear water to cleanse the area; and (3) wipe the perineum after toileting from front to back to prevent the rectal flora from contaminating sterile sites.

5. 1. **Clients should be strongly encouraged exclusively to breastfeed their babies to prevent engorgement.**
   2. Massaging of the breast will stimulate more milk production. That is not the best action to take.
   3. It is unnecessary to culture the breast. This client is engorged; she does not have an infection.

4. It is unnecessary to assess this client's temperature and pulse rate. This client is engorged; she is not infected.

TEST-TAKING TIP: The lactating breast produces milk in response to being stimulated. When a feeding is skipped, milk is still produced for the baby. When the baby is not fed, breast congestion or engorgement results. Not only is engorgement uncomfortable, it also gives the body the message to stop producing milk, resulting in an insufficient milk supply.

6. 1. Clients are not recommended to pump their breasts after feedings unless there is a specific reason to do so.
   2. This statement is true. The best way to prevent engorgement is to feed the baby every 2 to 3 hours.
   3. Clients should not restrict babies' feeding times. Babies feed at different rates. Babies themselves, therefore, should regulate the amount of time they need to complete their feeds.
   4. Clients are not recommended to supplement with formula unless there is a specific reason to do so.

TEST-TAKING TIP: This question is similar to the preceding question except that this question tests the nurse's ability to evaluate a client's response rather than to perform a nursing action.

7. 1. It is not recommended that breastfeeding mothers go on weight-reduction diets. In addition, it is not necessary for mothers to drink milk to make breast milk.
   2. When a breastfeeding woman has a poor diet, the quality of her breast milk changes very little. In fact, if a mother consumes a poor diet, it is her own body that will suffer.
   3. Mothers do not need to eat 3,000 calories a day while breastfeeding.
   4. Many mothers who consume approximately the same number of calories while breastfeeding as they did when they were pregnant do lose weight while breastfeeding.

TEST-TAKING TIP: Mothers should be advised to eat a well-balanced diet and drink sufficient quantities of fluids while breastfeeding. There is no absolute number of calories that the mother should consume, but if she does go on a restrictive diet, it is likely that her milk

supply may dwindle. Babies do take in about 600 calories a day at the breast; therefore, mothers can be advised that breastfeeding alone is a form of dieting.

8. 1. Heavy lochia is not a normal finding. Moderate lochia, which is similar in quantity to a heavy menstrual period, is a normal finding.
   2. The woman's fundus is firm. There is no need to massage the fundus.
   3. The fundus is at the umbilicus and it is firm. It is unlikely that her bladder is full.
   4. Because of the heavy lochia, the nurse should notify the woman's health care provider.

TEST-TAKING TIP: The nurse must do some detective work when observing unexpected signs/symptoms. This client is bleeding more heavily than the nurse would expect. When the nurse assesses the two most likely sources of the bleeding—the fundus and the perineal sutures—normal findings are noted. The next most likely source of the bleeding —a laceration in the birth canal—is unobservable to the nurse because performing a postpartum internal examination is not a nursing function. The nurse, therefore, must notify the health care practitioner of the problem.

9. 4 and 5 are correct.
   1. It is unnecessary for a bottle-feeding mother to increase her fluid intake.
   2. It is inadvisable for a bottle-feeding mother to massage her breasts.
   3. It is inadvisable for a bottle-feeding mother to apply heat to her breasts.
   4. The mother should be advised to wear a supportive bra 24 hours a day for a week or so.
   5. The mother should be advised to stand with her back toward the warm shower water.

TEST-TAKING TIP: The postpartum body naturally prepares to breastfeed a baby. To suppress the milk production, the mother should refrain from stimulating her breasts. Both massage and heat stimulate the breasts to produce milk. Mothers, therefore, should be encouraged to refrain from touching their breasts and when showering to direct the warm water toward their backs rather than toward their breasts. A supportive bra will help to minimize any engorgement that the client may experience.

10. 1. The client should apply ice packs to her axillae and breasts.
    2. Engorgement will not be relieved by applying lanolin to the breasts. And the act of applying the lanolin may actually stimulate milk production.
    3. If the woman expresses milk from her breasts, she will stimulate the breasts to produce more milk.
    4. The Food and Drug Administration (FDA) recommends that milk suppressants not be administered because of the serious side effects of the medications.

TEST-TAKING TIP: Breast milk is produced in the glandular tissue of the breast. An adequate blood supply to the area is required for the milk production. When cold is applied to the breast, the blood vessels constrict, decreasing the blood supply to the area. This is a relatively easy, nonhazardous action that helps to suppress breast milk production.

11. 1. It is inappropriate to advise a breastfeeding mother to switch to the bottle unless there is a specific medical reason for her to do so.
    2. Massaging the fundus will not relieve the client's discomfort.
    3. An alternate position will not relieve the client's discomfort.
    4. The nurse should discuss the action of oxytocin.

TEST-TAKING TIP: Oxytocin, the hormone of labor, also stimulates the uterus to contract in the postpartum period to reduce blood loss at the placental site. Oxytocin is the same hormone that regulates the milk ejection reflex. Whenever a mother breastfeeds, therefore, oxytocin stimulates her uterus to contract. In essence, therefore, breastfeeding naturally benefits the mother by contracting the uterus and preventing excessive bleeding.

12. 1. Celery is especially high in vitamin K, but it contains very little iron or vitamin A. Cream cheese is very high in fat.
    2. Yogurt is high in calcium but is not high in either iron or vitamin A. Bananas are high in vitamin B_6, potassium, and vitamin C, but they are not high in either iron or vitamin A.
    3. Strawberries are very high in vitamin C, but they are not high in either iron or vitamin A.
    4. Broccoli is very high in vitamin A and also contains iron.

TEST-TAKING TIP: Breastfeeding clients should be advised to consume a well-balanced diet high in vitamins and minerals. As a result, nurses must be prepared to suggest foods that meet those needs.

13. 1. Nipple shields should be used sparingly. Other interventions should be tried first.
    2. Soap will deplete the breast of its natural lanolin. It is recommended that women wash their breasts with warm water only while breastfeeding.
    3. **Rotating positions at feedings is one action that can help to minimize the severity of sore nipples.**
    4. It is inappropriate to recommend that the woman switch to formula at this time.

TEST-TAKING TIP: If a mother rotates positions at each breastfeeding, the baby is likely to put pressure on varying points on the nipple. A good, deep latch, however, is the most important way to prevent nipple soreness and cracking. The mother could also apply lanolin to her breasts after each feeding.

14. 1. Although breastfeeding does have a protective effect on postpartum blood loss, involution can take up to 6 weeks in breastfeeding women as well as bottle-feeding women.
    2. There is evidence to show that women who breastfeed their babies are less likely to develop type 2 diabetes later in life.
    3. Women who breastfeed have not been shown to have higher levels of bone density later in life.
    4. Breastfed babies are less likely to develop infections than are bottle-fed babies. The mothers, however, have not been shown to have the same protection.

TEST-TAKING TIP: Breastfeeding has many beneficial properties for both mothers and babies. It is a nursing responsibility to provide couples with the knowledge so that they can make fact-based decisions about how they will feed their babies.

15. 1. The woman is not exhibiting symptoms of galactorrhea, which occurs when a woman produces breast milk even though she has not delivered a baby.
    2. **This is true. Oxytocin stimulates sexual orgasms and is also the hormone that stimulates the milk ejection reflex.**
    3. This is incorrect. Galactosemia is a genetic disease. Babies who have the disease are

unable to digest galactose, the predominant sugar in breast milk.

4. This is an unlikely explanation of the problem.

TEST-TAKING TIP: It is important for the nurse in the obstetrician's office to warn breastfeeding clients of this situation. Because clients are strongly encouraged to refrain from having intercourse until they are 6 weeks postpartum, the postpartum nurse may not include this information in the client's discharge instructions. When the client is seen for her postpartum check, however, the information should be included.

16. 1. This response is correct. The couple is encouraged to wait until after involution is complete.
2. Although some clients do begin having intercourse once the episiotomy is healed and lochia stops, it is recommended that clients wait the full 6 weeks.
3. The couple is encouraged to wait until after involution is complete.
4. The couple is encouraged to wait until after involution is complete.

TEST-TAKING TIP: There have been some cases, albeit rare, of women dying from air emboli when they had intercourse early in the puerperium. It is recommended that couples wait 6 weeks before resuming intercourse.

17. 1. This response is inappropriate. It is likely that as long as the woman breastfeeds she will experience vaginal dryness.
2. This is an inappropriate response. It is unlikely that a proliferation of *Candida* is the problem.
3. This response is correct. The woman should be encouraged to use a lubricating jelly or oil.
4. It is unlikely that the problem is related to the episiotomy repair.

TEST-TAKING TIP: When women breastfeed, their estrogen levels remain low. As a result, they often complain of vaginal dryness and dyspareunia. The woman should be advised to try an over-the-counter lubricant. If that is not helpful, the woman may be prescribed an estrogen-based vaginal cream by her health care practitioner.

18. 1. The urinary output increases during the early postpartum period.
2. The blood pressure should remain stable during the postpartum.
3. The blood volume does drop precipitously during the early postpartum period.
4. The estrogen levels drop during the early postpartum period.

TEST-TAKING TIP: During pregnancy, the blood volume increased by almost 50%. Once the placenta is delivered, the client no longer needs the added blood volume. Immediately after delivery, therefore, the woman experiences marked diuresis and diaphoresis as the blood volume drops.

19. 1. It is unlikely that the woman is febrile.
2. The woman should maintain an adequate fluid intake.
3. Diaphoresis is normal during the postpartum period.
4. There is no need to report the diaphoresis to the baby's pediatrician.

TEST-TAKING TIP: Because the client's blood volume is returning to its nonpregnant level, the client loses fluids via both the kidneys and through insensible loss. As a result, postpartum women often awake from sleep with their nightwear saturated with perspiration.

20. 1. The hematocrit is often low in postpartum clients.
2. The nurse would expect to see an elevated white cell count.
3. The red blood cell count is often low in postpartum clients.
4. The hemoglobin is often low in postpartum clients.

TEST-TAKING TIP: If the test taker is familiar with normal lab values, he or she could easily deduce the answer to this question by comparing the values. Three of the values—hematocrit, hemoglobin, and red blood cell count—relate to the oxygen-carrying properties of the blood, and all of these values are on the upper end of normal. Only one answer, white blood cell count, is different from the others. The white blood cell count elevates late in the third trimester and stays elevated during labor and the early postpartum period to protect the mother from infection during the delivery and puerperium.

21. The pad with the moderate amount of lochia flow would be marked with an "X."

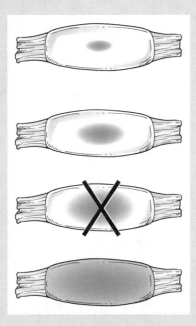

TEST-TAKING TIP: Determining the amount of lochia flow does include some subjectivity. The best guidelines to follow for a 1-hour time frame are up to 1 inch of lochia on the peripad—a scanty amount; less than 4 inches on the pad—light amount; 4 to 6 inches on the pad—moderate amount; and saturated pad—heavy amount.

22. 1. To perform Kegel exercises, the client should be advised to contract and relax the muscles that stop the urine flow.
    2. This is a correct statement.
    3. Kegel exercises can be performed in any position.
    4. Lochia flow is unaffected by contracting the pubococcygeal muscles.

    TEST-TAKING TIP: Doing Kegel exercises during the postpartum period helps clients to regain the muscle tone in the pubococcygeal muscles that may have been affected during pregnancy and labor and delivery. Clients should be advised to perform them periodically throughout the day. They can be performed in any position and in any location.

23. 1. The fundus should have descended below the umbilicus and there is no such lochia as "lochia rosa."
    2. The fundus should have descended below the umbilicus and the lochia does not turn to alba until about 10 days postpartum.

3. The fundus is usually 3 cm below the umbilicus on day 3 and the lochia usually has turned to serosa by day 3.
4. The fundus is usually 3 cm below the umbilicus on day 3 and the lochia usually has turned to serosa by day 3.

TEST-TAKING TIP: Although each client's postpartum course is slightly different, on day 3 postpartum, the nurse would expect the fundus of most clients to be 3 cm below the umbilicus and the lochia to have become serosa.

24. 1. Diaphoresis has usually subsided by this time.
    2. The nurse would expect that the client would have lochia alba.
    3. The nurse would not expect the client's nipples to be cracked.
    4. The nurse would not expect the client to be hypertensive.

    TEST-TAKING TIP: The normal progression of lochial change is as follows: lochia rubra, days 1 to 3; lochia serosa, days 3 to 10; and lochia alba, days 10 until discharge stops. There is some variation in the exact timing of the lochial change, but it is important for the client to know that the lochia should not revert backward. In other words, if a client whose lochia is alba again begins to have bright red discharge, she should notify her health care practitioner.

25. 1. It is unlikely that this client needs to be catheterized.
    2. It is unnecessary to measure this client's output.
    3. This response is correct. Polyuria is normal.
    4. It is unnecessary to do a specific gravity on the client's output.

    TEST-TAKING TIP: This client's physical assessment is normal. If the client's bladder were distended, the client's fundus would be elevated in the abdomen and the client would have excess blood loss. It is unnecessary, therefore, either to catheterize the woman or to measure her output. Polyuria is normal because the client no longer needs the large blood volume she produced during her pregnancy.

26. 1. An assessment of the woman's pulse rate is important, but it is not the most important assessment.
    2. An assessment of the woman's fundus is the most important assessment to perform on this client.

3. An assessment of the woman's bladder is important, but it is not the most important assessment.
4. An assessment of the woman's breasts is important, but is not the most important assessment.

TEST-TAKING TIP: This client's gravidity and parity indicate that she is a grand multipara. She has been pregnant 10 times, carrying 6 babies to term and 4 babies preterm. Because her uterus has been stretched so many times, she is at high risk for uterine atony during the postpartum period. The nurse must, therefore, monitor the postpartum contraction of her uterus very carefully.

27. 1. This response is incorrect. Clients who have had spinal anesthesia are at high risk for spinal headaches when they are elevated soon after surgery.
2. It is unnecessary to report absent bowel sounds to the client's physician.
3. The woman should turn, cough, and deep breathe every 2 hours.
4. There is no indication in the scenario that this client needs patellar reflex assessments every 2 hours.

TEST-TAKING TIP: Spinal anesthesia is administered directly into the spinal column. As a result, spinal fluid is able to escape through the puncture wound. When there is a drop in the amount of spinal fluid, clients often develop severe headaches. It is recommended that clients who have had spinals be elevated only slightly during the early postoperative period. To maintain pulmonary health, however, it is essential that clients perform respiratory exercises frequently during the postoperative period.

28. 1. It is appropriate to apply an ice pack to the area.
2. The sitz bath is an appropriate intervention beginning on the second postpartum day, not 2 hours after delivery. Sitz baths are usually performed 2 to 3 times a day.
3. It is not necessary for the client to sit on a pillow.
4. It is unnecessary for the client to be advised to put nothing in her rectum. Second-degree lacerations do not reach the rectum.

TEST-TAKING TIP: A second-degree laceration affects the skin, vaginal mucosa, and underlying muscles. (It does not affect the rectum or rectal sphincter.) Because of the injury, the area often swells, causing

pain. Ice packs help to reduce the inflammatory response and numb the area.

29. 1. This response is accurate, but the nurse is exhibiting a lack of caring.
2. This response is inappropriate. Even if the lung fields are clear, the client should perform respiratory exercises.
3. This response is inappropriate. Simply breathing deeply may not be as effective as coughing.
4. This is the appropriate response. The nurse is providing the client with a means of reducing the discomfort of post-surgical coughing.

TEST-TAKING TIP: Clients with abdominal incisions experience significant postoperative pain. And because their abdominal muscles have been incised, the pain is increased when the clients breathe in and cough. Bracing the abdominal muscles with a pillow or a blanket helps to reduce the discomfort.

30. 1. This is unnecessary. PCA pumps monitor the number of attempts patients make.
2. This information is correct. Clients often experience nausea and/or itching when PCA narcotics are administered.
3. This is a false statement. Family members should not press the button for the client.
4. This information is untrue. It is unnecessary for family members to inform the nurse. It is not unusual for clients to fall asleep when receiving PCA.

TEST-TAKING TIP: It is important for the nurse to teach a client's family members not to touch the PCA pump. Even though the pump is programmed with a minimum time between medication attempts, there is a possibility that the client could receive an overdose of medication if someone else controls the administrations. If a client is able to push the button herself she is, by definition, awake and alert.

31. 1. This comment is inappropriate. It does not acknowledge the client's likely disappointment about having to have a cesarean section.
2. This comment conveys sensitivity and understanding to the client.
3. This comment may be true, but it does not acknowledge the client's likely disappointment about having to have a cesarean section.

4. This comment may be true, but it does not acknowledge the client's likely disappointment about having to have a cesarean section.

TEST-TAKING TIP: Clients who must have cesarean sections when they had developed birth plans for vaginal deliveries are often very disappointed. They may express regret and/or anger over the experience. The nurse must realize that such clients are not angry with the nurse, but rather at the situation. It is essential for the nurse to accept the clients' feelings with understanding and caring.

32. 0.6 mL.
The formula to use is:

$$\frac{\text{Known dosage}}{\text{Known volume}} = \frac{\text{Desired dosage}}{\text{Desired volume}}$$

$$\frac{10 \text{ mg}}{1 \text{ mL}} = \frac{6 \text{ mg}}{x \text{ mL}}$$

$$10 \ x = 6$$

$$x = 0.6 \text{ mL}$$

TEST-TAKING TIP: Since the medication on hand is 10 mg and the nurse is to give 4 mg, the nurse must waste 6 mg. The nurse, therefore, must determine the volume that is equivalent to 6 mg.

33. 1. This answer is correct. Because the medication in a PCA pump is controlled by law, the medication must be wasted in the presence of another nurse.
2. This answer is inappropriate. A pain level of 0 is unrealistic after abdominal surgery. The nurse, however, should request that the doctor order one of the many oral analgesics to control the woman's discomfort.
3. This answer is inappropriate. Unless the nurse has a rationale to question the order, he or she should discontinue the medication as soon as the order has been received.
4. This answer is inappropriate. Once the intravenous has been punctured and used for one client, the bag cannot be reused.

TEST-TAKING TIP: There are a number of considerations that the nurse must make when giving medications, especially when administering controlled substances. The nurse is legally bound to account for the administration of or the disposal of narcotic medications. If any narcotic is wasted, a second nurse must cosign the disposal.

34. 1. This action is appropriate. This client's respiratory rate is below normal.
2. A complaint of thirst is within normal. There is no need to notify the physician.
3. This urinary output is normal for a postpartum client. There is no need to notify the physician.
4. Clients who have received epidurals will have numbness of their feet and ankles until the medication has metabolized. There is no need to notify the physician.

TEST-TAKING TIP: One of the serious complications of narcotic administration is respiratory depression. This client's respiratory rate is well below expected. The nurse should continue to monitor the client carefully and notify the anesthesiologist of the complication.

35. 1. It is not unusual for post–cesarean section clients to have had no bowel movements. The client should be advised to drink fluids and to ambulate to stimulate peristalsis.
2. This response is inappropriate. This client is obviously very concerned about her bowel pattern.
3. This response is inaccurate. Clients who have received antibiotics often complain of diarrhea as a result of the change in their intestinal flora.
4. Consuming fluids and fiber and exercising all help clients to reestablish normal bowel function.

TEST-TAKING TIP: This client is 2 days postoperative. She may not be consuming a normal diet as yet, but she will be able to ambulate and to drink fluids. Once she is able to consume foods, she should be encouraged to eat nutritious, high-fiber foods like fresh fruits and vegetables.

36. 1. The client's subjective pain level is 2/5. It is unlikely that she needs stronger medication.
2. This statement is correct. One of the common side effects of narcotics is constipation.
3. This statement is incorrect. As long as the client feeds her baby frequently, the use of narcotics should not affect her milk production.
4. This statement is incorrect. This client's narcotic use is short term. Postoperative narcotic medications are considered safe for the breastfeeding baby. If the mother were a chronic narcotic user, the baby's response would be a concern.

TEST-TAKING TIP: Because clients who take narcotics are high risk for constipation,

the nurse should inform clients of the potential and advise them to take necessary precautions. For example, the clients should be advised to drink fluids, eat high-fiber foods, and ambulate regularly.

37. 1. This fundal height is within normal limits. Clients who have had cesarean sections often involute at a slightly slower pace than clients who have had vaginal deliveries.
    2. This finding is normal. Pregnant clients and clients in the early postpartum period have nodular breasts in preparation for lactation.
    3. This pulse rate is normal. Once the placenta is delivered, the reservoir for the large blood volume is gone. Clients often develop bradycardia as a result.
    4. This blood loss is excessive, especially for a postoperative cesarean section client. The surgeon should be notified.

    TEST-TAKING TIP: Because the placenta is manually removed and the uterine cavity is manually scraped during cesarean deliveries, it is common for postoperative clients to have a scanty lochial flow. This client is having a heavy loss. After the fundal assessment is complete, the observations should be reported to the surgeon.

38. 1. The nurse would not expect to see any drainage.
    2. **The nurse would expect to see well-approximated edges.**
    3. The nurse would not expect to see ecchymosis.
    4. The nurse would not expect to see redness.

    TEST-TAKING TIP: The best tool to use when assessing any incision is the REEDA scale. The nurse assesses for: R—redness, E—edema, E—ecchymosis, D—drainage, and A—poor approximation. If there is evidence of any of the findings, they should be documented and monitored and reported.

39. 1. Even though this response may be true, the client's feelings are being ignored by the nurse.
    2. This response is inappropriate. Even though the baby is well, the client feels disappointed with her performance.
    3. Even though this response may be true, the client's feelings are being ignored by the nurse.

4. This response shows that the nurse has an understanding of the client's feelings.

TEST-TAKING TIP: When clients express their feelings, nurses must provide acceptance and implicit approval to encourage the clients to continue to express those feelings. Comments like "Don't say that. There are many women who would be ecstatic to have that baby" close down conversation and communicate disapproval.

40. 1. Episiotomy sutures are not removed.
    2. Clients who have had episiotomies may or may not require pain medication. The medicine should be offered throughout the day since it is usually ordered prn.
    3. **This statement is correct. When clients contract their buttocks before sitting, they usually feel less pain than when they sit directly on the suture line.**
    4. It is not recommended to irrigate episiotomy incisions.

    TEST-TAKING TIP: Clients who have had episiotomies often avoid sitting normally. Nurses should encourage them to take medications as needed, to contract their buttocks before sitting, and to sit normally rather than trying to favor one buttock over the other. Mediolateral incisions do tend to be more painful than midline incisions.

41. 1. The client should ambulate. There is nothing in the scenario indicating that the client must use a bedpan.
    2. It is likely that the client needs to urinate.
    3. In-dwelling catheters are rarely inserted for vaginal deliveries.
    4. **This is the appropriate action by the nurse.**

    TEST-TAKING TIP: Because they have elevated clotting factors, postpartum clients are at high risk for thrombus formation. When they need to urinate, they should be encouraged to ambulate to the bathroom to prevent pooling of blood. Clients should be accompanied to the bathroom, however, because they may be light-headed from the stress and work of labor and delivery.

42. 1. Fundal height is measured using a centimeter tape during pregnancy, not in the postpartum period.
    2. **The nurse should stabilize the base of the uterus with his or her dependent hand.**

3. The fundus should be palpated using the flat surface of the fingers.
4. No vaginal examination should be performed by the nurse.

TEST-TAKING TIP: If the base of the uterus is not stabilized during the assessment, there is a possibility that the uterus may invert or prolapse. While stabilizing the base, the nurse should gently assess for the fundus by palpating the abdomen with the flat part of the fingers until the fundus is felt.

43. 1. This response is correct. Reassuring the client is appropriate.
2. It is unlikely that the client has a urinary tract infection.
3. The urine will be blood tinged from the lochia.
4. This question is unnecessary. It is unlikely that the client has a urinary tract infection.

TEST-TAKING TIP: Frequent urination is normal after a delivery. The urine of a postpartum client will be blood tinged. This does not mean that the client has red blood cells in her urine, but rather that the lochia from the vagina has contaminated the sample. Unless a catheterized sample is obtained, it is virtually impossible to obtain an uncontaminated urine sample in the postpartum period.

44. 1. The white blood cell count is within normal limits for a postpartum client.
2. The red blood cell count is within normal limits for a postpartum client.
3. **The client's hematocrit is well below normal. This value should be reported to the client's health care provider.**
4. The hemoglobin is within normal limits for a postpartum client.

TEST-TAKING TIP: The hematocrit of a postpartum woman is likely to be below the "normal" of 35% to 45%, but a hematocrit of 30% or lower is considered abnormal and should be reported to the client's health care provider. It is likely that the client will be prescribed iron supplements.

45. 1. This response is not appropriate. This client is bleeding heavily and she is not breastfeeding.
2. It is unlikely that this client is menstruating since she is only 11/2 weeks postpartum.
3. This response is not appropriate. The client should not bleed heavily, especially so long after delivery.

4. This response is appropriate. The client should be examined to assess her involution.

TEST-TAKING TIP: One important piece of information in this question is the fact that the client is bottle feeding her baby. If she were breastfeeding, she could be encouraged to put the baby to breast and see if the bleeding subsided. Since oxytocin is released when babies suckle at the breast, this is a noninvasive method of promoting uterine contraction.

46. 1. This response is not accurate. Clients can begin to perform some exercises during the postpartum period.
2. The client can begin Kegel exercises, and little by little she can add other muscle-toning exercises during the postpartum period.
3. It is inappropriate to make this statement to a client. Her prepregnancy exercise schedule may be beyond her physical abilities at this time.
4. **This statement is correct. The client should begin with Kegel exercises shortly after delivery, move to abdominal tightening exercises in the next couple of days, and then slowly progress to stomach crunches, and so on.**

TEST-TAKING TIP: It is important for the postpartum client to begin muscle toning early in the postpartum period. However, she should not do any weight lifting or high-impact or stressful aerobic exercising until after her 6-week postpartum check.

47. 1. The involution is normal.
2. The involution is normal and the lochia is rubra.
3. **This response is correct. The involution is normal and the lochia is rubra.**
4. The lochia is moderate rubra.

TEST-TAKING TIP: Lochia rubra is bright red, lochia serosa is pinkish to brownish, and lochia alba is whitish. The nurse would expect the fundus to descend below the umbilicus approximately 1 cm per postpartum day. In other words, 1 day postpartum, the fundus is usually felt 1 cm below the umbilicus; 2 days postpartum, it is usually felt 2 cm below the umbilicus, and so on.

48. 1. This is an incorrect statement.
2. **This statement is accurate. Mothers often do not feel bladder pressure after delivery.**

3. Local anesthesia does not affect a client's ability to feel bladder distension.

4. This statement is inappropriate. The nurse should escort the woman to the bathroom to urinate.

TEST-TAKING TIP: During pregnancy, the bladder loses its muscle tone because of the pressure exerted on it by the gravid uterus. As a result, after delivery mothers often fail to feel when their bladders become distended.

49. 1. This action may be needed, but it is not the first action that should be taken.
2. This action is the first that the nurse should take.
3. This action may be needed, but it is not the first action that should be taken.
4. This action is needed, but it is not the first action that should be taken.

TEST-TAKING TIP: When a postpartum client's bladder is distended, the uterus becomes displaced and boggy. The client should be escorted to the bathroom to void; the lochia flow should also be assessed. However, before escorting the client to urinate, the nurse should gently massage the uterus.

50. 2 and 4 are correct.
1. The client should perform pericare at each toileting and whenever she changes her peripad.
2. This statement is correct. The woman should wash her hands before and after performing pericare care.
3. When a client sits in a warm water bath, she is taking a sitz bath.
4. This statement is accurate.
5. Hydrogen peroxide is not added to a perineal irrigation bottle (peri bottle).

TEST-TAKING TIP: A postpartum client is taught to spray warm tap water with nothing added on the perineum, from front to back, after each toileting and whenever she changes her peripads. She should also be taught to wash her hands before and after the procedure.

51. 1. Ibuprofen is usually administered every 4 to 6 hours.
2. This statement is correct. Ibuprofen has an antiprostaglandin effect.
3. Ibuprofen is administered orally.
4. This is not the reason ibuprofen is especially effective for postpartum cramping.

TEST-TAKING TIP: Prostaglandins are produced as part of the inflammatory

response. When ibuprofen is administered, the client receives the pain-reducing action of the medication as well as its anti-inflammatory properties.

52. An "X" should be placed on the line drawing at the level of the umbilicus.

TEST-TAKING TIP: By 12 hours after delivery, the fundus is usually felt at the level of the umbilicus. Every postpartum day thereafter, the fundus will descend about 1 cm.

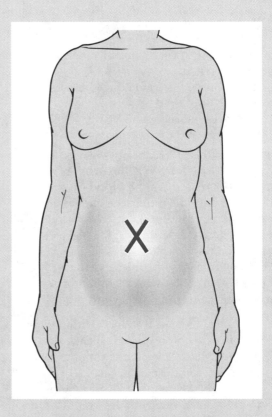

53. 1. Milk inhibits the absorption of iron. Milk and iron should not be consumed at the same time.
2. There is no recommendation that iron be taken with ginger ale.
3. The nurse would recommend that the iron be taken with orange juice because ascorbic acid, which is in orange juice, promotes the absorption of iron into the body.
4. There is no recommendation that iron be taken with chamomile tea.

TEST-TAKING TIP: Since ascorbic acid promotes the absorption of iron into the body, it is appropriate for the nurse to recommend that the client take her iron supplement with a food source high in ascorbic acid, like orange juice.

54. 1. The nurse would not expect the values to rise. These results may indicate that the client is dehydrated or third spacing fluids (i.e., fluid is shifting into her interstitial spaces).
    2. The nurse would not expect the values to remain the same. On average, clients lose about 500 mL of blood during spontaneous vaginal deliveries.
    3. The nurse would expect these values—a slight decrease in both hemoglobin and hematocrit values.
    4. The nurse would not expect the values to drop to these levels.

    TEST-TAKING TIP: Because clients do lose blood during their deliveries, the nurse would expect to see approximately a 2% drop in the hematocrit and about a 0.5 gm/dL drop in the hemoglobin. If the hematocrit drops below 30%, the nurse should notify the health care practitioner.

55. 1, 2, and 5 are correct.
    1. Sitz baths do have a soothing affect for clients with hemorrhoids.
    2. Clients often feel some relief when external hemorrhoids are reinserted into the rectum.
    3. Oxytocin will have no effect on the hemorrhoids.
    4. It is impossible to tell whether or not the hemorrhoids will change with subsequent pregnancies.
    5. Topical anesthetics can provide relief from the discomfort of hemorrhoids.

    TEST-TAKING TIP: Hemorrhoids are varicose veins of the rectum. They develop as a result of the weight of the gravid uterus on the client's dependent blood vessels. In addition to the actions noted above, the client should be advised to eat high-fiber foods and drink to prevent constipation.

56. 1. Fundal assessment is the priority nursing action.
    2. Pain level assessment is important, but it is not the priority nursing action.
    3. Performing pericare is important, but it is not the priority nursing action.
    4. Breast assessment is important, but it is not the priority nursing action.

    TEST-TAKING TIP: Hemorrhage is one of the primary causes of morbidity and mortality in postpartum women. It is essential, therefore, that nurses repeatedly assess a client's postpartum uterine contraction.

When the uterus is well contracted, a woman is unlikely to bleed heavily after delivery.

57. 1. The appropriate action is to provide the client with warm blankets.
    2. Postpartum shaking is very common. It is unnecessary to place the client in the Trendelenburg position.
    3. Postpartum shaking is very common. It is unnecessary to notify the client's health care provider.
    4. Postpartum shaking is very common. It is unnecessary to increase the client's intravenous fluid rate.

    TEST-TAKING TIP: Postpartum shaking is thought to be caused by nervous responses and/or vasomotor changes. The shaking is very common and, unless accompanied by a fever, is of no physiological concern. The best action by the nurse is supportive—providing the client with a warm blanket and reassuring her that the response is within normal limits.

58. 2, 3, and 4 are correct.
    1. Although clients should drink fluids, this is not a goal related to the identified nursing diagnosis.
    2. An important goal is that the woman's WBC will remain stable.
    3. An important goal is that the woman's temperature will remain normal.
    4. An important goal is that the woman's lochia will smell normal.
    5. Sitz baths are not given to prevent infections. They do help to soothe the pain and/or the inflammation associated with episiotomies and hemorrhoids.

    TEST-TAKING TIP: The WBC is elevated during late pregnancy, delivery, and early postpartum, but if it rises very rapidly, the rise is often associated with a bacterial infection. The lochia usually smells "musty." When a client has endometritis, however, the lochia smells "foul." A temperature above 100.4°F after the first 24 hours postpartum is indicative of a puerperal infection.

59. 1. Early ambulation does help to prevent thrombophlebitis.
    2. Oral fluid intake does not directly prevent thrombophlebitis.
    3. Massaging of the legs is not helpful and in some situations can actually be harmful. If there is a clot in one of a client's lower

extremity blood vessels, it can be dislodged when the leg is vigorously massaged.

4. High-fiber foods will prevent constipation, not thrombophlebitis.

TEST-TAKING TIP: Postpartum clients are at high risk for thrombophlebitis because of an increase in the quantity of circulating clotting factors. To prevent clot formation, clients should ambulate as soon as possible after delivery. If they must be bed bound because of complications, the nurse should contact the physician for an order for antiembolic stockings and/or antiembolic pressure boots and have the client perform active range-of-motion exercises.

60. 1. Clients in the taking in phase are not receptive to teaching.
2. During the taking in phase, clients need to internalize their labor experiences. Discussing the labor process is appropriate for this postpartum phase.
3. Clients in the taking in phase do not focus on future issues or needs.
4. Clients in the taking in phase are not receptive to teaching.

TEST-TAKING TIP: The taking in postpartum phase is the first phase that clients pass through after they deliver their baby. During this time they are especially "me oriented." They wish and need to be cared for. This is a time when they should be given a bed bath and allowed to rest. They take in nourishment and take in the experience that they have just been through. Primigravid and cesarean section clients often proceed more slowly through this phase than do other clients.

61. 1. Nourishment is a need of the client in the taking in phase.
2. Rest is a need of the client in the taking in phase.
3. Assistance with self-care is a need of the client in the taking in phase.
4. Clients in the taking hold phase need assurance that they are learning the skills they will need to care for their new baby.

TEST-TAKING TIP: During the taking hold phase, clients regain their independence. They care for their own bodies and are very receptive to learning about child care as well as self-care. Primigravidas are especially open to learning about caring for their baby during this phase and are

especially vulnerable if they feel incompetent when performing baby-care tasks.

62. 1. Although the client is showing signs of positive bonding, she definitely needs a great deal of teaching.
2. This response is correct. The client is showing signs of positive bonding—en face positioning and stroking of the baby's cheeks—and is in need of information on child care.
3. This action is absolutely inappropriate at this time. There are no signs of poor bonding or of abuse.
4. There are no signs of poor bonding.

TEST-TAKING TIP: This client has never held a newborn before. The nurse, therefore, should be prepared to provide the client with information on newborn care. Two signs of positive bonding are holding a baby in the en face position—so that the mother is looking directly into the baby's eyes—and stroking the baby's cheeks.

63. 1. The client is not exhibiting signs of social isolation.
2. The client is not exhibiting signs of child neglect.
3. The client is exhibiting normal postpartum behavior.
4. The client is not exhibiting signs of postpartum depression.

TEST-TAKING TIP: This client is exhibiting signs of the postpartum taking in phase. She is a primigravida who delivered only 2 hours earlier. Her comments are well within those expected of a client at this point during her postpartum period.

64. 1. Fathers have not been shown to experience postpartum blues.
2. This information is correct. The blues usually resolve within 2 weeks of delivery.
3. Medications are usually not administered to relieve postpartum blues. Medications can be prescribed for clients who experience postpartum depression or postpartum psychosis.
4. This information is incorrect. The majority of women will experience postpartum blues during the first week or two postpartum.

TEST-TAKING TIP: The test taker must not confuse the three psychological changes that mothers may experience postpartum: postpartum blues, postpartum depression, and postpartum psychosis. Postpartum blues is a normal phenomenon related to fatigue, hormonal shifts, and the enormous responsibility of becoming a mother. Postpartum depression and postpartum psychosis are pathological conditions that only some women experience.

65. 1. This is not the best response by the nurse.
    2. This is not the best response by the nurse.
    3. **The nurse should forewarn the mother about the likelihood of the 2-year-old's jealousy.**
    4. This is not the best response by the nurse.

TEST-TAKING TIP: The test taker must be familiar with the growth and development of children at all ages and be prepared to convey this information to new parents. Older siblings, especially toddlers, often express jealousy when a new baby enters the home. This is normal, but the parents must be aware of the potential for toddlers to inadvertently injure the baby.

66. 1. This diagnosis is inappropriate. There is no indication that this client is suicidal or psychotic.
    2. This diagnosis is inappropriate. There is no indication in the scenario that the client had a traumatic delivery.
    3. **This diagnosis is appropriate. This client is showing signs of postpartum blues; one of the main reasons for this problem is related to the hormonal changes that occur after delivery.**
    4. This diagnosis is inappropriate. Nothing in the scenario implies that the client is in spiritual difficulties.

TEST-TAKING TIP: It is essential that nurses discuss postpartum blues with clients. When clients are unfamiliar with the phenomenon, they often feel like they are going crazy or that there is something very wrong with them. Other members of the family, especially the woman's partner, should also be forewarned.

67. 1. This is inappropriate. Pork products are prohibited foods for Muslims.
    2. This is inappropriate. Pork products are prohibited foods for Muslims.
    3. This is inappropriate. Pork products are prohibited foods for Muslims.
    4. **Although this is not a traditional Muslim dish, the foods are allowable by Muslim tradition.**

TEST-TAKING TIP: Clients in the immediate postdelivery period are in need of nourishment. It is very important that the

nurse be aware of cultural differences and provide foods that are acceptable to the clients. Most Muslim clients adhere to religious dietary restrictions, called *halal.*

68. 1. **This question is appropriate. Seventh Day Adventists usually follow vegetarian diets.**
    2. This question is inappropriate. The Seventh Day Adventist Sabbath is on Saturday, not on Sunday.
    3. This question is inappropriate. Baptism in the Seventh Day Adventist tradition is performed after the child reaches the age of accountability.
    4. This question is inappropriate. Rabbis are the leaders of people of the Jewish faith. And *mohels*, who are not necessarily rabbis, perform ritual Jewish circumcisions.

TEST-TAKING TIP: There are a number of religious traditions. The nurse should be familiar with the major precepts of each religion to provide clients with holistic care.

69. 1. **This action is appropriate. Asians, many of whom believe in the hot-cold theory of disease, will often not drink cold fluids or eat cold foods during the postpartum period.**
    2. This action is not necessary at this time.
    3. It is unlikely that the temperature will change significantly in 30 minutes.
    4. This information is correct but it does not take into consideration the client's beliefs and traditions.

TEST-TAKING TIP: The knowledge that consuming fluids is important is not in conflict with this client's traditions. There is no reason the client must consume cold fluids. The nurse should provide the client with the warm fluids required by her beliefs.

70. 1. The apical pulse need not be assessed before Methergine is administered.
    2. The vaginal discharge need not be assessed before Methergine is administered.
    3. **The blood pressure should be assessed before administering Methergine.**
    4. The episiotomy need not be assessed before Methergine is administered.

TEST-TAKING TIP: Methergine is an oxytoxic agent that works directly on the myofibrils of the uterus. The smooth muscle of the vascular tree is also affected. The blood pressure may elevate, therefore, to dangerous levels. The medication should be held if the blood pressure is 130/90 or higher

and the woman's health care practitioner should be notified if appropriate.

71. 1. Lying prone on a pillow helps to relieve some women's afterbirth pains.
     2. Contracting the abdominal muscles has not been shown to alleviate afterbirth pains.
     3. Ambulation has not been shown to alleviate afterbirth pains.
     4. Drinking ice tea has not been shown to alleviate afterbirth pains.

TEST-TAKING TIP: Afterbirth pains can be quite uncomfortable, especially for multiparas. The nurse should suggest that the clients take prn medications—ibuprofen is especially helpful—and try complementary therapies like lying on a small pillow and placing a hot water bottle on the abdomen.

72. 1. The client should not develop a headache from Methergine.
     2. The client should not become nauseated from Methergine.
     3. Cramping is an expected outcome of the administration of Methergine.
     4. The client should not become fatigued from Methergine.

TEST-TAKING TIP: Methergine is administered to postpartum clients to stimulate their uterus to contract. As a consequence, clients frequently complain of cramping after taking the medication. The nurse can administer the prn pain medication to the client at the same time the Methergine is administered to help to mitigate the client's discomfort.

73. 1. Estrogen drops precipitously after the placenta is delivered.
     2. Prolactin will elevate sharply in the client's bloodstream.
     3. Human placental lactogen drops precipitously after the placenta is delivered.
     4. Human chorionic gonadotropin is produced by the fertilized ovum.

TEST-TAKING TIP: To answer this question correctly, it is important for the test taker to know what happens at the end of the third stage of labor—that is, the delivery of the placenta. Because the hormones of pregnancy produced by the placenta—progesterone and estrogen—drop precipitously at this time, prolactin is no longer inhibited and, therefore, rises. The way the woman intends to feed her baby is irrelevant.

74. 1. Colace capsules should not be crushed, broken, or chewed.
     2. The capsule should be taken with juice or food to minimize the bitter taste.
     3. Headache is not a side effect of Colace.
     4. The medication does not change the color of a client's urine.

TEST-TAKING TIP: The medication, a stool softener, is contained in a capsule that must be swallowed whole. Many physicians order Colace for postoperative cesarean section clients until their bowel patterns return to normal.

75. 1. This client's lochia flow and vital signs are normal. She is exhibiting no signs of fluid volume deficit.
     2. This client has had no episiotomy or perineal laceration. She is exhibiting no signs of impaired skin integrity.
     3. This client is voiding as expected—approximately every 2 hours. She is exhibiting no signs of impaired urinary elimination.
     4. This client is a primigravida. The nurse would anticipate that she is in need of teaching regarding newborn care as well as self-care.

TEST-TAKING TIP: This is a difficult analysis level question. The test taker must determine, based on the facts given, which nursing diagnosis is appropriate. This question, however, should be approached the same way that all other questions are approached: (1) determine what is being asked; (2) develop possible answers to the question BEFORE reading the given responses; (3) read the responses and compare them with the list of possible answers; and (4) choose the one response that best compares with the list of possible answers.

76. 1. This is not the best response because the answer implies that the stitches are near the rectum. The stitches are not near the rectal area.
     2. This is the best response. A right mediolateral episiotomy is angled away from the perineum and rectum.
     3. This is not the best response because the answer implies that the stitches are near the rectum. The stitches are not near the rectal area.
     4. This is not the best response because the answer implies that the stitches are near

the rectum. The stitches are not near the rectal area.

TEST-TAKING TIP: Women often are fearful of having a bowel movement when they have had an episiotomy or a laceration. Unless they have a third- or fourth-degree laceration, they should be assured that the stitches are a distance away from the rectal area.

77. 42 gtt/min

The formula to calculate an intravenous drip rate is:

$$\frac{\text{Volume} \times \text{Drop factor}}{\text{Time in minutes}}$$

$$\frac{250 \text{ mL} \times 10 \text{ gtt/mL}}{60 \text{ min}} = \frac{2,500}{60} = 42 \text{ gtt/min}$$

TEST-TAKING TIP: The test taker should remember three things when calculating the answer to this question: (1) the quantity of fluid left in the IV is irrelevant because the physician has ordered the rate per hour; (2) the dosage of the medication is irrelevant because the volume of the fluid is not related to the medication dosage; and (3) time is always converted to minutes when a drip rate is calculated. (When a pump is being calibrated, on the other hand, the drip rate is programmed in mL/hr.)

78. 1. Although this is an important goal, it is not the most important.
2. Although this is an important goal, it is not the most important.
3. This is the most important goal during the immediate postdelivery period.
4. Although this is an important goal, it is not the most important.

TEST-TAKING TIP: When establishing priorities, the test taker should consider the client's most important physiological functions—that is, the C-A-B —circulation, airway, and breathing. If the client were to bleed heavily, her circulation would be compromised. None of the other goals is directly related to the C-A-Bs.

79. 1. It is inappropriate for the nurse to delegate this action. Physical assessment is a skill that requires professional nursing judgment.
2. It is inappropriate for the nurse to delegate this action. Teaching is a skill that requires professional nursing knowledge.
3. This action can be delegated to a nursing assistant. Once the vital signs are checked, the nursing assistant can

report the results to the nurse for his or her interpretation.
4. It is inappropriate for the nurse to delegate this action. The chart is a legal document and documentation is a skill that requires professional nursing knowledge.

TEST-TAKING TIP: Delegation is an important skill. Nurses are unable to meet all the needs of all of their patients. They must ask other health care workers, e.g., licensed practical nurses and nursing assistants, to meet some of the clients' needs. It is essential, however, that the nurse delegate appropriately. Assessment, teaching, and documentation are tasks that should not be delegated to nursing assistants.

80. 1. There is nothing in the scenario that indicates that the client's feet and ankles need to be assessed.
2. This is unnecessary. The blood pressure can be assessed while a client is breastfeeding.
3. This action is very important. If the legs are removed from the stirrups one at a time then the woman is at high risk for back and abdominal injuries.
4. It is unnecessary to measure the episiotomy. It is sufficient to document the type of episiotomy that was performed.

TEST-TAKING TIP: Stirrups may not be used during normal spontaneous deliveries; however, when forceps or vacuum-extractors are used, physicians often request that the client's legs be placed in stirrups. The nurse should raise the woman's legs simultaneously when placing her legs in stirrups and lower her legs simultaneously when the delivery is complete to prevent injury. The nurse should also position the legs with care. Pressure on the popliteal space can lead to thrombus formation.

81. 1. Although the weight does drop precipitously when the baby is born, this is not the primary reason for the client's cardiovascular compromise.
2. This response is true. Once the placenta is birthed, the reservoir for the mother's large blood volume is gone.
3. This response is not accurate. The cervix begins to contract shortly after delivery and the lochial flow is not related to the cardiovascular compromise that affects all postpartum patients.

4. This is a false statement. Maternal blood pressure does not drop precipitously when the baby's head emerges.

TEST-TAKING TIP: It is essential that the nurse closely monitor the vital signs of a newly delivered gravida. Because of the surge in blood volume resulting from the delivery of the placenta, the woman is high risk for cardiovascular compromise. Women frequently develop bradycardia, a normal finding, as a result of the increased peripheral blood volume.

82. 1. **Discharge teaching should be initiated at the time of admission. This nurse is correct in initiating the process in the labor room.**
    2. Discharge teaching should be initiated at the time of admission. This nurse is correct in initiating the process in the labor room.
    3. Discharge teaching should be initiated at the time of admission. This nurse is correct in initiating the process in the labor room.
    4. Discharge teaching should be initiated at the time of admission. This nurse is correct in initiating the process in the labor room.

TEST-TAKING TIP: It is essential that nurses begin discharge teaching upon entry to the hospital. If nurses wait until the time of discharge, clients are expected to process a large amount of information during a very stressful time. Even when initiated early in the hospital stay, the nurse will likely need to repeat his or her instructions many times before the client is fully prepared to leave the hospital.

83. 1. This action is unsafe. It is unsafe to place anything in the vagina before involution is complete.
    2. This response is inappropriate. The amount of discharge does not determine the type of pad that can be used.
    3. This response is inappropriate. The client's pain does not determine the type of pad that can be used.
    4. **This response is correct. It is unsafe to place anything in the vagina before involution is complete.**

TEST-TAKING TIP: This question examines whether or not the test taker is aware of changes in care that are determined by the situation. Because the cervix is still dilated

and the uterine body is high risk for infection, it is unsafe to insert anything into the vagina until involution is complete.

84. 1. **This answer is correct. The nurse should assess the level of anesthesia every 15 minutes while in the postanesthesia care unit.**
    2. This answer is inappropriate. The client had an indwelling catheter inserted for the surgery. And even if the catheter were removed immediately after the operation, she is paralyzed from the spinal anesthesia and unable to void.
    3. This answer is inappropriate. The client has had major surgery. She will be consuming clear fluids, at the most, immediately after the cesarean section.
    4. This answer is inappropriate. Immediately after surgery, the incision is covered by a dressing. Plus, it is too early for an infection to have appeared.

TEST-TAKING TIP: The key to answering this question is the fact that the client has just moved from the operating room. The nurse in the postanesthesia care unit (PACU) is concerned with monitoring for immediate postoperative and postpartum complications and the client's recovery from the anesthesia.

85. 1. Cesarean section incisions do not routinely need to be irrigated.
    2. **This is appropriate. The nurse should assess for all signs on the REEDA scale.**
    3. The incision is held together with sutures or staples. It is unnecessary to apply steristrips at this time.
    4. It is inappropriate for the nurse to palpate the suture line.

TEST-TAKING TIP: Once the dressing has been removed, the nurse on each shift should monitor the incision line for all signs on the REEDA scale—redness, edema, ecchymosis, discharge, and approximation.

86. **1, 3, 4, and 5 are correct.**
    1. **The nurse should palpate the breasts to assess for fullness and/or engorgement.**
    2. The postpartum assessment does not include carotid auscultation.
    3. **The nurse should check the client's vaginal discharge.**
    4. **The nurse should assess the client's extremities.**

5. The nurse should inspect the client's perineum.

TEST-TAKING TIP: The best way to remember the items in the postpartum assessment is to remember the acronym **BUBBLEHE**. The letters stand for: B—breasts; U—uterus; B—bladder; B—bowels and rectum (for hemorrhoids); L—lochia; E—episiotomy; H—Homan's sign; and E—emotional status. But it is important to note that Homan's sign is no longer recommended. Rather, careful inspection of the calves for signs of DVT should be performed.

87. 1, 2, and 5 are correct.
    1. The nurse would assess for pain.
    2. The nurse would assess for warmth.
    3. The nurse would not be assessing for discharge.
    4. The nurse would not be assessing for ecchymosis.
    5. The nurse would assess for redness.

TEST-TAKING TIP: Postpartum clients are high risk for deep vein thrombosis (DVT). At each postpartum assessment the nurse assesses the calves for signs of the complication, i.e., those seen in any inflammatory response: pain, warmth, redness, and edema. If the signs/symptoms are noted, the nurse should request an order from the primary healthcare practitioner for diagnostic tests to be performed, like a Doppler series. Homan's sign is no longer recommended to assess for DVT.

High-Risk Antepartum

Although pregnancy should be considered a healthy state, there are many complications that may occur during the antepartum period, some of which result from preexisting conditions and some of which develop during the pregnancy. Any of these can affect the mother and/or the developing fetus. Questions in this chapter are concerned with a number of topics, from spontaneous abortion to gestational diabetes to infectious diseases to third-trimester bleeding. To answer the questions, the nurse must be familiar not only with the pathology of the conditions but also with the impact that the complications may have on the pregnancy.

KEYWORDS

The following words include English vocabulary, nursing/medical terminology, concepts, principles, or information relevant to content specifically addressed in the chapter or associated with topics presented in it. English dictionaries, your nursing textbooks, and medical dictionaries such as *Taber's Cyclopedic Medical Dictionary* are resources that can be used to expand your knowledge and understanding of these words and related information.

ABO incompatibility
adolescent pregnancy
amniocentesis
biophysical profile
caudal agenesis
cervical cerclage
cervical insufficiency
clonus
complementary therapy
contraction stress test
Coombs' testing
dilation and curettage (D&C)
dizygotic twins
eclampsia
ectopic pregnancy
erythroblastosis fetalis
fern test
fetal kick count
gestational diabetes mellitus (GDM)
gestational trophoblastic disease
glucose challenge test (GCT)
glucose tolerance test (GTT)
glycosylated hemoglobin (HbA$_{1c}$)
hemoglobin A$_{1c}$ (HbA$_{1c}$)

HELLP syndrome (hemolysis, elevated liver enzymes, low platelet count)
human placental lactogen (hPL)
hydatidiform mole
hydramnios (polyhydramnios)
hyperemesis gravidarum
hypertensive illnesses of pregnancy
incompetent cervix
lecithin/sphingomyelin ratio (L/S ratio)
listeriosis
monozygotic twins
nipple stimulation test
nonstress test (NST)
oligohydramnios
placental abruption
placenta previa
preeclampsia
pregnancy-induced hypertension (PIH)
preterm labor
preterm premature rupture of the membranes (PPROM)
pseudocyesis
reflex assessment
Rh incompatibility

RhoGAM   spontaneous abortion
rubella   teratogen
shake test (foam test)   third-trimester bleed
sickle cell disease   toxemia
spina bifida   toxoplasmosis

QUESTIONS

1. During a prenatal interview, a client tells the nurse, "My mother told me she had toxemia during her pregnancy and almost died!" Which of the following questions should the nurse ask in response to this statement?
   1. "Does your mother have a cardiac condition?"
   2. "Did your mother tell you what she was toxic from?"
   3. "Does your mother have diabetes now?"
   4. "Did your mother say whether she had a seizure or not?"

2. A patient, 32 weeks pregnant with severe headache, is admitted to the hospital with preeclampsia. In addition to obtaining baseline vital signs and placing the client on bed rest, the physician ordered the following four items. Which of the orders should the nurse perform first?
   1. Assess deep tendon reflexes.
   2. Obtain complete blood count.
   3. Assess baseline weight.
   4. Obtain routine urinalysis.

3. A nurse is counseling a preeclamptic client about her diet. Which should the nurse encourage the woman to do?
   1. Restrict sodium intake.
   2. Increase intake of fluids.
   3. Eat a well-balanced diet.
   4. Avoid simple sugars.

4. The nurse is evaluating the effectiveness of bed rest for a client with mild preeclampsia. Which of the following signs/symptoms would the nurse determine is a positive finding?
   1. Weight loss.
   2. 2+ proteinuria.
   3. Decrease in plasma protein.
   4. 3+ patellar reflexes.

5. A 32-week-gestation client was last seen in the prenatal client at 28 weeks' gestation. Which of the following changes should the nurse bring to the attention of the certified nurse midwife?
   1. Weight change from 128 pounds to 138 pounds.
   2. Pulse rate change from 88 bpm to 92 bpm.
   3. Blood pressure change from 120/80 to 118/78.
   4. Respiratory rate change from 16 rpm to 20 rpm.

6. A 24-week-gravid client is being seen in the prenatal clinic. She states, "I have had a terrible headache for the past 2 days." Which of the following is the most appropriate action for the nurse to perform next?
   1. Inquire whether or not the client has allergies.
   2. Take the woman's blood pressure.
   3. Assess the woman's fundal height.
   4. Ask the woman about stressors at work.

7. A nurse remarks to a 38-week-gravid client, "It looks like your face and hands are swollen." The client responds, "Yes, you're right. Why do you ask?" The nurse's response is based on the fact that the changes may be caused by which of the following?
   1. Altered glomerular filtration.
   2. Cardiac failure.
   3. Hepatic insufficiency.
   4. Altered splenic circulation.

8. A client has severe preeclampsia. The nurse would expect the primary health care practitioner to order tests to assess the fetus for which of the following?
   1. Severe anemia.
   2. Hypoprothrombinemia.
   3. Craniosynostosis.
   4. Intrauterine growth restriction.

9. A gravid client with 4+ proteinuria and 4+ reflexes is admitted to the hospital. The nurse must closely monitor the woman for which of the following?
   1. Grand mal seizure.
   2. High platelet count.
   3. Explosive diarrhea.
   4. Fractured pelvis.

10. A client is admitted to the hospital with severe preeclampsia. The nurse is assessing for clonus. Which of the following actions should the nurse perform?
    1. Strike the woman's patellar tendon.
    2. Palpate the woman's ankle.
    3. Dorsiflex the woman's foot.
    4. Position the woman's feet flat on the floor.

11. The nurse is grading a woman's reflexes. Which of the following grades would indicate reflexes that are slightly brisker than normal?
    1. +1.
    2. +2.
    3. +3.
    4. +4.

12. A 26-week-gestation woman is diagnosed with severe preeclampsia with HELLP syndrome. The nurse will assess for which of the following signs/symptoms?
    1. Low serum creatinine.
    2. High serum protein.
    3. Bloody stools.
    4. Epigastric pain.

13. A 29-week-gestation woman diagnosed with severe preeclampsia is noted to have blood pressure of 170/112, 4+ proteinuria, and a weight gain of 10 pounds over the past 2 days. Which of the following signs/symptoms would the nurse also expect to see?
    1. Fundal height of 32 cm.
    2. Papilledema.
    3. Patellar reflexes of +2.
    4. Nystagmus.

14. A client with mild preeclampsia who has been advised to be on bed rest at home asks why doing so is necessary. Which of the following is the best response for the nurse to give the client?
    1. "Bed rest will help you to conserve energy for your labor."
    2. "Bed rest will help to relieve your nausea and anorexia."
    3. "Reclining will increase the amount of oxygen that your baby gets."
    4. "The position change will prevent the placenta from separating."

15. In anticipation of a complication that may develop in the second half of pregnancy, the nurse teaches an 18-week-gravid client to call the office if she experiences which of the following?
    1. Headache and decreased output.
    2. Puffy feet.
    3. Hemorrhoids and vaginal discharge.
    4. Backache.

16. Which of the following clients is at highest risk for developing a hypertensive illness of pregnancy?
    1. G1 P0000, age 44 with history of diabetes mellitus.
    2. G2 P0101, age 27 with history of rheumatic fever.
    3. G3 P1102, age 25 with history of scoliosis.
    4. G3 P1011, age 20 with history of celiac disease.

17. The nurse has assessed four primigravid clients in the prenatal clinic. Which of the women would the nurse refer to the nurse midwife for further assessment?
    1. 10 weeks' gestation, complains of fatigue with nausea and vomiting.
    2. 26 weeks' gestation, complains of ankle edema and chloasma.
    3. 32 weeks' gestation, complains of epigastric pain and facial edema.
    4. 37 weeks' gestation, complains of bleeding gums and urinary frequency.

18. A client's 32-week clinic assessment was: BP 90/60; TPR 98.6°F, P 92, R 20; weight 145 lb; and urine negative for protein. Which of the following findings at the 34-week appointment should the nurse highlight for the certified nurse midwife?
    1. BP 110/70; TPR 99.2°F, 88, 20.
    2. Weight 155 lb; urine protein +2.
    3. Urine protein trace; BP 88/56.
    4. Weight 147 lb; TPR 99.0°F, 76, 18.

19. A nurse is caring for a 25-year-old client who has just had a spontaneous first trimester abortion. Which of the following comments by the nurse is appropriate?
    1. "You can try again very soon."
    2. "It is probably better this way."
    3. "At least you weren't very far along."
    4. "I'm here to talk if you would like."

20. A hospitalized gravida's blood work is: hematocrit 30% and hemoglobin 10 gm/dL. In light of the laboratory data, which of the following meal choices should the nurse recommend to this patient?
    1. Chicken livers, sliced tomatoes, and dried apricots.
    2. Cheese sandwich, tossed salad, and rice pudding.
    3. Veggie burger, cucumber salad, and wedge of cantaloupe.
    4. Bagel with cream cheese, pear, and hearts of lettuce.

21. A woman has just been admitted to the emergency department subsequent to a head-on automobile accident. Her body appears to be uninjured. The nurse carefully monitors the woman for which of the following complications of pregnancy? **Select all that apply.**
    1. Placenta previa.
    2. Transverse fetal lie.
    3. Placental abruption.
    4. Severe preeclampsia.
    5. Preterm labor

22. A 25-year-old client is admitted with the following history: 12 weeks pregnant, vaginal bleeding, no fetal heartbeat seen on ultrasound. The nurse would expect the doctor to write an order to prepare the client for which of the following?
    1. Cervical cerclage.
    2. Amniocentesis.
    3. Nonstress testing.
    4. Dilation and curettage.

23. A client being seen in the ED has an admitting medical diagnosis of: third-trimester bleeding: rule out placenta previa. Each time a nurse passes by the client's room, the woman asks, "Please tell me, do you think the baby will be all right?" Which of the following is an appropriate nursing diagnosis for this client?
    1. Hopelessness related to possible fetal loss.
    2. Anxiety related to inconclusive diagnosis.
    3. Situational low self-esteem related to blood loss.
    4. Potential for altered parenting related to inexperience.

24. Which of the following long-term goals is appropriate for a client, 10 weeks' gestation, who is diagnosed with gestational trophoblastic disease (hydatidiform mole)?
    1. Client will be cancer free 1 year from diagnosis.
    2. Client will deliver her baby at full term without complications.
    3. Client will be pain free 3 months after diagnosis.
    4. Client will have normal hemoglobin and hematocrit at delivery.

25. Which of the following findings should the nurse expect when assessing a client, 8 weeks' gestation, with gestational trophoblastic disease (hydatidiform mole)?
    1. Protracted pain.
    2. Variable fetal heart decelerations.
    3. Dark brown vaginal bleeding.
    4. Suicidal ideations.

26. Which of the following findings would the nurse expect to see when assessing a first-trimester gravida suspected of having gestational trophoblastic disease (hydatidiform mole) that the nurse would not expect to see when assessing a first-trimester gravida with a normal pregnancy? **Select all that apply.**
    1. Hematocrit 39%.
    2. Grape-like clusters passed from the vagina.
    3. Markedly elevated blood pressure.
    4. White blood cell count 8,000/mm^3.
    5. Hypertrophied breast tissue.

27. Which finding should the nurse expect when assessing a client with placenta previa?
    1. Severe occipital headache.
    2. History of thyroid cancer.
    3. Previous premature delivery.
    4. Painless vaginal bleeding.

28. A nurse is caring for four prenatal clients in the clinic. Which of the clients is high risk for placenta previa? **Select all that apply.**
    1. Jogger with low body mass index.
    2. Primigravida who smokes 1 pack of cigarettes per day.
    3. Infertility client who is carrying in vitro triplets.
    4. Registered professional nurse who works 12-hour shifts.
    5. Police officer on foot patrol.

29. A woman has been diagnosed with a ruptured ectopic pregnancy. Which of the following signs/symptoms is characteristic of this diagnosis?
    1. Dark brown rectal bleeding.
    2. Severe nausea and vomiting.
    3. Sharp unilateral pain.
    4. Marked hyperthermia.

30. A client, G2 P1001, telephones the gynecology office complaining of left-sided pain. Which of the following questions by the triage nurse would help to determine whether the one-sided pain is due to an ectopic pregnancy?
    1. "When did you have your pregnancy test done?"
    2. "When was the first day of your last menstrual period?"
    3. "Did you have any complications with your first pregnancy?"
    4. "How old were you when you first got your period?"

31. Please place an "X" on the picture of the abdominal ectopic pregnancy.

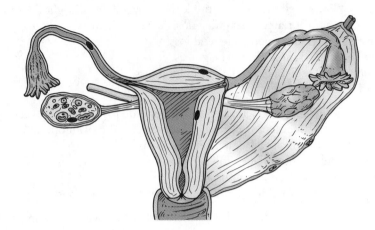

32. A woman, 8 weeks pregnant, is admitted to the obstetric unit with a diagnosis of threatened abortion. Which of the following tests would help to determine whether the woman is carrying a viable or a nonviable pregnancy?
    1. Luteinizing hormone level.
    2. Endometrial biopsy.
    3. Hysterosalpinogram.
    4. Serum progesterone level.

33. A woman with a diagnosis of ectopic pregnancy is to receive medical intervention rather than a surgical interruption. Which of the following intramuscular medications would the nurse expect to administer?
    1. Decadron (dexamethasone).
    2. Amethopterin (methotrexate).
    3. Pergonal (metotropin).
    4. Prometrium (progesterone).

34. A woman who has been diagnosed with an ectopic pregnancy is to receive methotrexate 50 mg/m² IM. The woman weighs 136 lb and is 5 ft 4 in tall. What is the maximum safe dose, in mg, of methotrexate that this woman can receive? **(If rounding is needed, please round to the nearest tenth.)**
    _____ mg

35. A woman is to receive methotrexate IM for an ectopic pregnancy. The drug reference states that the recommended safe dose of the medicine is 50 mg/m². She weighs 52 kg and is 148 cm tall. What is the maximum safe dose, in mg, of methotrexate that this woman can receive? **(If rounding is needed, please round to the nearest tenth.)**
    _____ mg

36. A woman is to receive methotrexate IM for an ectopic pregnancy. The nurse should teach the woman about which of the following common side effects of the therapy? **Select all that apply.**
    1. Nausea and vomiting.
    2. Abdominal pain.
    3. Fatigue.
    4. Light-headedness.
    5. Breast tenderness.

37. The nurse is caring for a client who was just admitted to the hospital to rule out ectopic pregnancy. Which of the following orders is the most important for the nurse to perform?
    1. Take the client's temperature.
    2. Document the time of the client's last meal.
    3. Obtain urine for urinalysis and culture.
    4. Assess for complaint of dizziness or weakness.

38. A gravid client is admitted with a diagnosis of third-trimester bleeding. It is priority for the nurse to assess for a change in which of the following vital signs?
    1. Temperature.
    2. Pulse.
    3. Respirations.
    4. Blood pressure.

39. A gravid client, G6 P5005, 24 weeks' gestation, has been admitted to the hospital for placenta previa. Which of the following is an appropriate long-term goal for this client?
    1. The client will state an understanding of need for complete bed rest.
    2. The client will have a reactive nonstress test on day 2 of hospitalization.
    3. The client will be symptom free until at least 37 weeks' gestation.
    4. The client will call her children shortly after admission.

40. Which of the following statements is appropriate for the nurse to say to a patient with a complete placenta previa?
    1. "During the first phase of labor you will do slow chest breathing."
    2. "You should ambulate in the halls at least two times each day."
    3. "The doctor will deliver you once you reach 25 weeks' gestation."
    4. "It is important that you inform me if you become constipated."

41. A 12-week-gravid client presents in the emergency department with abdominal cramps and scant dark red bleeding. Which of the following signs/symptoms should the nurse assess this client for? **Select all that apply.**
    1. Tachycardia.
    2. Referred shoulder pain.
    3. Headache.
    4. Fetal heart dysrhythmias.
    5. Hypertension.

42. A client, 32 weeks' gestation with placenta previa, is on total bed rest. The physician expects her to be hospitalized on bed rest until her cesarean section, which is scheduled for 38 weeks' gestation. To prevent complications while in the hospital, the nurse should do which of the following? **Select all that apply.**
    1. Perform passive range-of-motion exercises.
    2. Restrict the fluid intake of the client.
    3. Decorate the room with pictures of family.
    4. Encourage the client to eat a high-fiber diet.
    5. Teach the client deep-breathing exercises.

43. A gravid woman is carrying monochorionic twins. For which of the following complications should this pregnancy be monitored?
    1. Oligohydramnios.
    2. Placenta previa.
    3. Cephalopelvic disproportion.
    4. Twin-to-twin transfusion.

44. On ultrasound, it is noted that the pregnancy of a hospitalized woman who is carrying monochorionic twins is complicated by twin-to-twin transfusion. The nurse should carefully monitor this client for which of the following?
    1. Rapid fundal growth.
    2. Vaginal bleeding.
    3. Projectile vomiting.
    4. Congestive heart failure.

45. A nurse is performing an assessment on four 22-week-pregnant clients. The nurse reports to the obstetrician that which of the clients may be carrying twins?
    1. The client who states that she feels huge.
    2. The client with a weight gain of 13 pounds.
    3. The client whose fundal height measurement is 26 cm.
    4. The client whose alpha-fetoprotein level is one-half normal.

46. Which of the following pregnant clients is most high risk for preterm premature rupture of the membranes (PPROM)? **Select all that apply.**
    1. 31 weeks' gestation with prolapsed mitral valve (PMV).
    2. 32 weeks' gestation with urinary tract infection (UTI).
    3. 33 weeks' gestation with twins post–in vitro fertilization (IVF).
    4. 34 weeks' gestation with gestational diabetes (GDM).
    4. 35 weeks' gestation with deep vein thrombosis (DVT).

47. A client, G8 P3406, 14 weeks' gestation, is being seen in the prenatal clinic. During the nurse's prenatal teaching session, the nurse will emphasize that the woman should notify the obstetric office immediately if she notes which of the following?
    1. Change in fetal movement.
    2. Signs and symptoms of labor.
    3. Swelling of feet and ankles.
    4. Appearance of spider veins.

48. A woman, G4 P0210 and 12 weeks' gestation, has been admitted to the labor and delivery suite for a cerclage procedure. Which of the following long-term outcomes is appropriate for this client?
    1. The client will gain less than 25 pounds during the pregnancy.
    2. The client will deliver after 38 weeks' gestation.
    3. The client will have a normal blood glucose throughout the pregnancy.
    4. The client will deliver a baby that is appropriate for gestational age.

49. A woman, G5 P0401, is in the post-anesthesia care unit (PACU) after a cervical cerclage procedure. During the immediate postprocedure period, what should the nurse carefully monitor this client for?
    1. Hyperthermia.
    2. Hypotension.
    3. Uterine contractions.
    4. Fetal heart dysrhythmias.

50. A 30-week-gestation multigravida, G3 P1011, is admitted to the labor suite. She is contracting every 5 minutes × 40 seconds. Which of the comments by the client would be most informative regarding the etiology of the client's present condition?
    1. "For the past day I have felt burning when I urinate."
    2. "I have a daughter who is 2 years old."
    3. "I jogged 1½ miles this morning."
    4. "My miscarriage happened a year ago today."

51. A client who works as a waitress and is 35 weeks' gestation telephones the labor suite after getting home from work and states, "I am feeling tightening in my groin about every 5 to 6 minutes." Which of the following comments by the nurse is appropriate at this time?
    1. "Please lie down and drink about four full glasses of water or juice."
    2. "You are having false labor pains so you need not worry about them."
    3. "It is essential that you get to the hospital immediately."
    4. "That is very normal for someone who is on her feet all day."

52. A type 1 diabetic gravida has developed polyhydramnios. The client should be taught to report which of the following?
    1. Uterine contractions.
    2. Reduced urinary output.
    3. Marked fatigue.
    4. Puerperal rash.

53. A pregnant diabetic has been diagnosed with hydramnios. Which of the following would explain this finding?
    1. Excessive fetal urination.
    2. Recurring hypoglycemic episodes.
    3. Fetal sacral agenesis.
    4. Placental vascular damage.

54. A type 1 diabetic is being seen for preconception counseling. The nurse should emphasize that during the first trimester the woman may experience which of the following?
    1. Need for less insulin than she normally injects.
    2. An increased risk for hyperglycemic episodes.
    3. Signs and symptoms of hydramnios.
    4. A need to be hospitalized for fetal testing.

55. A woman's glucose challenge test (GCT) results are 155 mg/dL at 1 hour post–glucose ingestion. Which of the following actions, as ordered by the physician, is appropriate?
    1. Send the woman for a glucose tolerance test.
    2. Teach the woman how to inject herself with insulin.
    3. Notify the woman of the normal results.
    4. Provide the woman with oral hypoglycemic agents.

56. A 25-week-pregnant client, who had eaten a small breakfast, has been notified that her glucose challenge test results were 142 mg/dL 1 hour after ingesting the glucose. Which of the following is appropriate for the nurse to say at this time?
    1. "Because you ate before the test, the results are invalid and will need to be repeated."
    2. "Because your test results are higher than normal, you will have to have another, more specific test."
    3. "Because of the results you will have to have weekly glycohemoglobin testing done."
    4. "Because your results are within normal limits you need not worry about gestational diabetes."

57. In analyzing the need for health teaching in a client, G5 P4004 with gestational diabetes, the nurse should ask which of the following questions?
    1. "How old were you at your first pregnancy?"
    2. "Do you exercise regularly?"
    3. "Is your partner diabetic?"
    4. "Do you work outside of the home?"

58. A gravid woman, 36 weeks' gestation with type 1 diabetes, has just had a biophysical profile (BPP). Which of the following results should be reported to the obstetrician?
    1. One fetal heart acceleration in 20 minutes.
    2. Three episodes of fetal rhythmic breathing in 30 minutes.
    3. Two episodes of fetal extension and flexion of 1 arm.
    4. One amniotic fluid pocket measuring 3 cm.

59. A gravid client, 27 weeks' gestation, has been diagnosed with gestational diabetes. Which of the following therapies will most likely be ordered for this client?
    1. Oral hypoglycemic agents.
    2. Diet control with exercise.
    3. Regular insulin injections.
    4. Inhaled insulin.

60. A client has just done a fetal kick count assessment. She noted 6 movements during the past hour. If taught correctly, what should her next action be?
    1. Nothing, because further action is not warranted.
    2. Call the doctor to set up a nonstress test.
    3. Redo the test during the next half hour.
    4. Drink a glass of orange juice and redo the test.

61. A nurse who is caring for a pregnant diabetic should carefully monitor the client for which of the following? **Select all that apply.**
    1. Urinary tract infection.
    2. Multiple gestation.
    3. Metabolic acidosis.
    4. Pathological hypotension.
    5. Hypolipidemia

62. A gestational diabetic, who requires insulin therapy to control her blood glucose levels, telephones the triage nurse complaining of dizziness and headache. Which of the following actions should the nurse take at this time?
    1. Have the client proceed to the office to see her physician.
    2. Advise the client to drink a glass of juice and then call back.
    3. Instruct the client to inject herself with regular insulin.
    4. Tell the client immediately to telephone her medical doctor.

63. A diabetic client is to receive 5 units regular and 15 units NPH insulin at 0800. To administer the medication appropriately, what should the nurse do?
    1. Draw 5 units regular in one syringe and 15 units NPH in a second syringe and inject in different locations.
    2. Draw 5 units regular first and 15 units NPH second into the same syringe and inject.
    3. Draw 15 units NPH first and 5 units regular second into the same syringe and inject.
    4. Mix 5 units regular and 15 units NPH in a vial before drawing the full 20 units into a syringe and inject.

64. The nurse caring for a type 1 diabetic client who wishes to become pregnant notes that the client's glycohemoglobin, or glycosylated hemoglobin ($HgbA_{1c}$), result was 15% today and the fasting blood glucose result was 100 mg/dL. Which of the following interpretations by the nurse is correct in relation to these data?
    1. The client has been hyperglycemic for the past 3 months and is hyperglycemic today.
    2. The client has been normoglycemic for the past 3 months and is normoglycemic today.
    3. The client has been hyperglycemic for the past 3 months and is normoglycemic today.
    4. The client has been normoglycemic for the past 3 months and is hyperglycemic today.

65. An insulin-dependent diabetic woman will require higher doses of insulin as which of the following pregnancy hormones increases in her body?
    1. Estrogen.
    2. Progesterone.
    3. Human chorionic gonadotropin.
    4. Human placental lactogen.

66. A client has just been diagnosed with gestational diabetes. She cries, "Oh no! I will never be able to give myself shots!!" Which of the following responses by the nurse is appropriate at this time?
    1. "I am sure you can learn for your baby."
    2. "I will work with you until you feel comfortable giving yourself the insulin."
    3. "We will be giving you pills for the diabetes."
    4. "If you follow your diet and exercise you will probably need no insulin."

67. An insulin-dependent diabetic, G3 P0200, 38 weeks' gestation, is being seen in the labor and delivery suite in metabolic disequilibrium. The nurse knows that which of the following maternal blood values is most high risk to her unborn baby?
    1. Glucose 150 mg/dL.
    2. pH 7.25.
    3. pCO_2 34 mm Hg.
    4. Hemoglobin A_{1c} 10%.

68. A 30-year-old gravida, G3 P1101, 6 weeks' gestation, states that her premature baby boy, born 8 years ago, died shortly after delivery from an infection secondary to spina bifida. Which of the following interventions is most important for this client?
    1. Grief counseling.
    2. Nutrition counseling.
    3. Infection control counseling.
    4. Genetic counseling.

69. A gravid woman, who is 42 weeks' gestation, has just had a 20-minute nonstress test (NST). Which of the following results would the nurse interpret as a reactive test?
    1. Moderate fetal heart baseline variability.
    2. Maternal heart rate accelerations to 140 bpm lasting at least 20 seconds.
    3. Two fetal heart accelerations of 15 bpm lasting at least 15 seconds.
    4. Absence of maternal premature ventricular contractions.

70. A woman, G1 P0000, is 40 weeks' gestation. Her Bishop score is 4. Which of the following complementary therapies do midwives frequently recommend to clients in similar situations? **Select all that apply.**
    1. Sexual intercourse.
    2. Aromatherapy.
    3. Breast stimulation.
    4. Ingestion of castor oil.
    5. Aerobic exercise.

71. A pregnant woman, 24 weeks' gestation, who has been diagnosed with severe choledocholithiasis is scheduled for a cholecystectomy. In addition to routine surgical and post-surgical care, the nurses should pay special attention to which of the following? **Select all that apply.**
    1. The baby will be delivered by cesarean section at the same time as the cholescystectomy surgery.
    2. The woman should be placed in the lateral recumbent position during the surgical procedure.
    3. The post-anesthesia care nurse should monitor the woman carefully for nausea and vomiting.
    4. The post-anesthesia care nurse should monitor the woman carefully for hemorrhage at the surgical site.
    5. Antiembolic stockings should be placed on the woman's legs in the post-anesthesia care unit.

72. A gravid woman has sickle cell anemia. Which of the following situations could precipitate a vaso-occlusive crisis in this woman?
    1. Hypoxia.
    2. Alkalosis.
    3. Fluid overload.
    4. Hyperglycemia.

73. A gravid woman with sickle cell anemia is admitted in vaso-occlusive crisis. Which of the following is the priority intervention that the nurse must perform?
    1. Administer narcotic analgesics.
    2. Apply heat to swollen joints.
    3. Place on strict bed rest.
    4. Infuse intravenous solution.

74. An obese gravid woman is being seen in the prenatal clinic. The nurse will monitor this client carefully throughout her pregnancy because she is high risk for which of the following complications of pregnancy? **Select all that apply.**
    1. Placenta previa.
    2. Gestational diabetes.
    3. Abruptio placentae.
    4. Preeclampsia.
    5. Chromosomal defects.

75. An obese client is being seen by the nurse during her prenatal visit. Which of the following comments by the nurse is appropriate at this time?
    1. "We will want you to gain the same amount of weight we would encourage any pregnant woman to gain."
    2. "To have a healthy baby we suggest that you go on a weight reduction diet right away."
    3. "To prevent birth defects we suggest that you gain weight during the first trimester and then maintain your weight for the rest of the pregnancy."
    4. "We suggest that you gain weight throughout your pregnancy but not quite as much as other women."

76. The physician has ordered a nonstress test (NST) to be done on a 41-week-gestation client. During the half-hour test, the nurse observed three periods of fetal heart accelerations that were 15 beats per minute above the baseline and that lasted 15 seconds each. No contractions were observed. Based on these results, what should the nurse do next?
    1. Send the client home and report positive results to the MD.
    2. Perform a nipple stimulation test to assess the fetal heart in response to contractions.
    3. Prepare the client for induction with IV oxytocin or endocervical prostaglandins.
    4. Place the client on her side with oxygen via face mask.

77. A 39-year-old, 16-week-gravid woman has had an amniocentesis. Before discharge, the nurse teaches the woman to call her doctor if she experiences any of the following side effects? **Select all that apply.**
    1. Fever or chills.
    2. Lack of fetal movement.
    3. Abdominal pain.
    4. Rash or pruritus.
    5. Vaginal bleeding.

78. Which of the following would indicate that a nipple stimulation test is creating the desired effect?
    1. The woman's inverted nipples become erect.
    2. The woman's nipple and breast tissue hypertrophy.
    3. The woman's uterus contracts 3 times in 10 minutes.
    4. The woman's cervix dilates 2 centimeters in 3 hours.

79. The nurse notes that the results of a gravid woman's contraction stress test are equivocal. How should the nurse interpret the findings?
    1. Baby is acidotic and should be delivered.
    2. Fetal heart rate accelerated once during the test.
    3. Baby is preterm but the heart rate is normal.
    4. Additional data are needed to make a diagnosis.

80. A lecithin:sphingomyelin (L/S) ratio has been ordered by a pregnant woman's obstetrician. Which of the following data will the nurse learn from this test?
    1. Coagulability of maternal blood.
    2. Maturation of the fetal lungs.
    3. Potential for fetal development of erythroblastosis fetalis.
    4. Potential for maternal development of gestational diabetes.

81. The laboratory reported the L/S ratio results from an amniocentesis as 1:1. How should the nurse interpret the result?
    1. The baby is premature.
    2. The mother is high risk for hemorrhage.
    3. The infant has kernicterus.
    4. The mother is high risk for eclampsia.

82. A client is being taught fetal kick counting. Which of the following should be included in the patient teaching?
    1. The woman should choose a time when her baby is least active.
    2. The woman should lie on her side with her head elevated about 30°.
    3. The woman should report fetal kick counts of greater than 10 in an hour.
    4. The woman should refrain from eating immediately before counting.

83. An ultrasound is being done on an Rh-negative woman. Which of the following pregnancy findings would indicate that the baby has developed erythroblastosis fetalis?
    1. Caudal agenesis.
    2. Cardiomegaly.
    3. Oligohydramnios.
    4. Hyperemia.

84. A woman is to receive RhoGAM at 28 weeks' gestation. Which of the following actions must the nurse perform before giving the injection?
    1. Validate that the baby is Rh-negative.
    2. Assess that the direct Coombs' test is positive.
    3. Verify the identity of the woman.
    4. Reconstitute the globulin with sterile water.

85. A nurse is about to inject RhoGAM into an Rh-negative mother. Which of the following is the preferred site for the injection?
    1. Deltoid.
    2. Dorsogluteal.
    3. Vastus lateralis.
    4. Ventrogluteal.

86. A woman is recovering at the gynecologist's office following a late first-trimester spontaneous abortion. At this time, it is essential for the nurse to check which of the following?
    1. Maternal rubella titer.
    2. Past obstetric history.
    3. Maternal blood type.
    4. Cervical patency.

87. At 28 weeks' gestation, an Rh-negative woman receives RhoGAM. Which of the following would indicate that the medication is effective?
    1. The baby's Rh status changes to Rh-negative.
    2. The mother produces no Rh antibodies.
    3. The baby produces no Rh antibodies.
    4. The mother's Rh status changes to Rh-positive.

88. It is discovered that a 28-week-gestation gravid is leaking amniotic fluid. Before the client is sent home on bed rest, the nurse teaches her which of the following?
    1. Perform a nitrazine test every morning upon awakening.
    2. Immediately report any breast tenderness to the primary health care practitioner.
    3. Abstain from engaging in vaginal intercourse for the rest of the pregnancy.
    4. Carefully weigh all of her saturated peripads.

89. A 32-week-gestation client states that she "thinks" she is leaking amniotic fluid. Which of the following tests could be performed to determine whether the membranes had ruptured?
    1. Fern test.
    2. Biophysical profile.
    3. Amniocentesis.
    4. Kernig assessment.

90. A nurse is interviewing a prenatal client. Which of the following factors in the client's history should the nurse highlight for the health care practitioner?
    1. That she is eighteen years old.
    2. That she owns a cat and a dog.
    3. That she eats peanut butter daily.
    4. That she works as a surgeon.

91. A pregnant Latina is being seen in the prenatal clinic with diarrhea, fever, stiff neck, and headache. Upon inquiry, the nurse learns that the woman drinks unpasteurized milk and eats soft cheese daily. For which of the following bacterial infections should this woman be assessed?
    1. *Staphylococcus aureus.*
    2. *Streptococcus albicans.*
    3. *Pseudomonas aeruginosa.*
    4. *Listeria monocytogenes.*

92. A gravid woman has been diagnosed with listeriosis. She eats rare meat and raw smoked seafood. Which of the following signs/symptoms would this woman exhibit?
    1. Fever and muscle aches.
    2. Rash and thrombocytopenia.
    3. Petechiae and anemia.
    4. Amnionitis and epistaxis.

93. A patient who is 24 weeks pregnant has been diagnosed with syphilis. She asks the nurse how the infection will affect the baby. The nurse's response should be based on which of the following?
    1. She is high risk for premature rupture of the membranes.
    2. The baby will be born with congenital syphilis.
    3. Penicillin therapy will reduce the risk to the fetus.
    4. The fetus will likely be born with a cardiac defect.

94. Prenatal teaching for a pregnant woman should include instructions to do which of the following?
    1. Refrain from touching her pet bird.
    2. Wear gloves when gardening.
    3. Cook pork until medium well done.
    4. Avoid sleeping with the dog.

95. A child has been diagnosed with rubella. What must the pediatric nurse teach the child's parents to do?
    1. Notify any exposed pregnant friends.
    2. Give penicillin po every 6 hours for 10 full days.
    3. Observe the child for signs of respiratory distress.
    4. Administer diphenhydramine every 4 hours as needed.

96. A client, 37 weeks' gestation, has been advised that she is positive for group B streptococci. Which of the following comments by the nurse is appropriate at this time?
    1. "The doctor will prescribe intravenous antibiotics for you. A visiting nurse will administer them to you in your home."
    2. "You are very high risk for an intrauterine infection. It is important for you to check your temperature every day."
    3. "The bacteria are living in your vagina. They will not hurt you but we will give you medicine in labor to protect your baby from getting sick."
    4. "This bacteria causes scarlet fever. If you notice that your tongue becomes very red and that you feel feverish you should call the doctor immediately."

97. Which of the following nursing diagnoses would be most appropriate for a 15-year-old woman who is in her first trimester of pregnancy?
    1. Sleep pattern disturbance related to discomforts of pregnancy.
    2. Knowledge deficit related to care of infants.
    3. Anxiety related to fear of labor and delivery.
    4. Ineffective individual coping related to developmental level.

98. Nurses working in obstetric clinics know that, in general, teen pregnancies are high risk because of which of the following?
    1. High probability of chromosomal anomalies.
    2. High oral intake of manganese and zinc.
    3. High numbers of post-term deliveries.
    4. High incidence of late prenatal care registration.

99. A 14-year-old woman is seeking obstetric care. Which of the following vital signs must be monitored very carefully during this woman's pregnancy?
    1. Heart rate.
    2. Respiratory rate.
    3. Blood pressure.
    4. Temperature.

100. A 16-year-old woman is being seen for the first time in the obstetric office. Which of the following comments by the young woman is highest priority for the nurse to respond to?
    1. "My favorite lunch is a burger with fries."
    2. "I've been dating my new boyfriend for 2 weeks."
    3. "On weekends we go out and drink a few beers."
    4. "I dropped out of school about 3 months ago."

101. A 14-year-old woman is seeking obstetric care. Which of the following is an appropriate nursing care goal for this young woman? The young woman will:
    1. Bring her partner to all prenatal visits.
    2. Terminate the pregnancy.
    3. Continue her education.
    4. Undergo prenatal chromosomal analysis.

102. A nurse works in a clinic with a high adolescent pregnancy population. The nurse provides teaching to the young women to prevent which of the following high-risk complications of pregnancy?
    1. Preterm birth.
    2. Gestational diabetes.
    3. Macrosomic babies.
    4. Polycythemia.

103. Which of the following would be the best approach to take with an unmarried 14-year-old girl who tells the nurse that she is undecided whether or not to maintain an unplanned pregnancy?
    1. "You should consider an abortion since you are so young."
    2. "It is a difficult decision. What have you thought about so far?"
    3. "Studies show that babies living with teen mothers often become teen parents."
    4. "Why don't you keep the pregnancy? You could always opt for adoption later."

104. A 15-year-old client is being seen for her first prenatal visit. Because of this client's special nutritional needs, the nurse evaluates the client's intake of:
    1. Protein and magnesium.
    2. Calcium and iron.
    3. Carbohydrates and zinc.
    4. Pyroxidine and thiamine.

105. A woman with a history of congestive heart disease is 36 weeks pregnant. Which of the following findings should the nurse report to the primary health care practitioner?
    1. Presence of striae gravidarum.
    2. Dyspnea on exertion.
    3. 4-pound weight gain in a month.
    4. Patellar reflexes +2.

106. During a prenatal examination, the nurse notes scarring on and around the woman's genitalia. Which of the following questions is most important for the nurse to ask in relation to this observation?
    1. "Have you ever had surgery on your genital area?"
    2. "Have you worn any piercings in your genital area?"
    3. "Have you had a tattoo removed from your genital area?"
    4. "Have you ever been forced to have sex without your permission?"

107. A woman enters the prenatal clinic accompanied by her partner. When she is asked by the nurse about her reason for seeking care, the woman looks down as her partner states, "She says she thinks she's pregnant. She constantly complains of feeling tired. And her vomiting is disgusting!" Which of the following is the priority action for the nurse to perform?
    1. Ask the woman what times of the day her fatigue seems to be most severe.
    2. Recommend to the couple that they have a pregnancy test done as soon as possible.
    3. Continue the interview of the woman in private.
    4. Offer suggestions on ways to decrease the vomiting.

108. The nurse is providing health teaching to a group of women of childbearing age. One woman, who states that she is a smoker, asks about smoking's impact on the pregnancy. The nurse responds that which of the following fetal complications can develop if the mother smokes?
    1. Genetic changes in the fetal reproductive system.
    2. Extensive central nervous system damage.
    3. Addiction to the nicotine inhaled from the cigarette.
    4. Fetal intrauterine growth restriction.

109. A pregnant woman mentions to the clinic nurse that she and her husband enjoy working together on projects around the house and says, "I always wear protective gloves when I work." The nurse should advise the woman that even when she wears gloves, which of the following projects could be high risk to the baby's health?
    1. Replacing a light fixture in the nursery.
    2. Sanding the paint from an antique crib.
    3. Planting tulip bulbs in the side garden.
    4. Shoveling snow from the driveway.

110. A gravid client, 25 years old, is diagnosed with gallstones. She asks her nurse, "Aren't I too young to get gallstones?" The nurse bases her response on which of the following?
    1. Progesterone slows emptying of the gallbladder, making gravid women high risk for the disease.
    2. Gallbladder disease has a strong genetic component, so the woman should be advised to see a genetic counselor.
    3. Older women are no more prone to gallstones than are younger women.
    4. Gallbladder disease is related to a high dietary intake of carbohydrates.

111. A client has been diagnosed with pseudocyesis. Which of the following signs/symptoms would the nurse expect to see?
    1. 4+ pedal edema.
    2. No fetal heartbeat.
    3. Hematocrit above 40%.
    4. Denial of quickening.

112. Which of the following clients is highest risk for pseudocyesis?
    1. The client with lymphatic cancer.
    2. The client with celiac disease.
    3. The client with multiple miscarriages.
    4. The client with grand multiparity.

113. The nurse is caring for a 32-week G8 P7007 with placenta previa. Which of the following interventions would the nurse expect to perform? **Select all that apply.**
    1. Daily contraction stress tests.
    2. Blood type and cross match.
    3. Bed rest with passive range-of-motion exercises.
    4. Daily serum electrolyte assessments.
    5. Weekly biophysical profiles.

114. A client has been admitted with a diagnosis of hyperemesis gravidarum. Which of the following lab values would be consistent with this diagnosis?
    1. pO_2 90, pCO_2 35, HCO_3 19 mEq/L, pH 7.30.
    2. pO_2 100, pCO_2 30, HCO_3 21 mEq/L, pH 7.50.
    3. pO_2 60, pCO_2 50, HCO_3 28 mEq/L, pH 7.30.
    4. pO_2 90, pCO_2 45, HCO_3 30 mEq/L, pH 7.50.

115. A client has been admitted with a diagnosis of hyperemesis gravidarum. Which of the following orders written by the primary health care provider is highest priority for the nurse to complete?
    1. Obtain complete blood count.
    2. Start intravenous with multivitamins.
    3. Check admission weight.
    4. Obtain urine for urinalysis.

116. An ultrasound has identified that a client's pregnancy is complicated by oligohydramnios. The nurse would expect that an ultrasound may show that the baby has which of the following structural defects?
    1. Dysplastic kidneys.
    2. Coarctation of the aorta.
    3. Hydrocephalus.
    4. Hepatic cirrhosis.

117. An ultrasound has identified that a client's pregnancy is complicated by hydramnios. The nurse would expect that an ultrasound may show that the baby has which of the following structural defects?
    1. Pulmonic stenosis.
    2. Tracheoesophageal fistula.
    3. Ventriculoseptal defect.
    4. Developmental hip dysplasia.

118. A client, 8 weeks pregnant, has been diagnosed with a bicornuate uterus. Which of the following signs should the nurse teach the client to carefully monitor for?
    1. Hyperthermia.
    2. Palpitations.
    3. Cramping.
    4. Oliguria.

119. The nurse suspects that a client is third spacing fluid. Which of the following signs will provide the nurse with the best evidence of this fact?
    1. Client's blood pressure.
    2. Client's appearance.
    3. Client's weight.
    4. Client's pulse rate.

120. A client is being admitted to the labor suite with a diagnosis of eclampsia. The fetal heart rate tracing shows moderate variability with early decelerations. Which of the following actions by the nurse is appropriate at this time?
    1. Tape a tongue blade to the head of the bed.
    2. Pad the side rails and head of the bed.
    3. Provide the client with needed stimulation.
    4. Provide the client with grief counseling.

The correct answer number and rationale for why it is the correct answer are given in boldface blue type. Rationales for why the other possible answer options are incorrect also are given, but they are not in boldface type.

1. 1. Toxemia is not related to a cardiac condition.
   2. Toxemia is not related to a toxic substance.
   3. Toxemia is not directly related to diabetes mellitus.
   4. **This is the appropriate question. The nurse is asking whether or not the client's mother developed eclampsia.**

   TEST-TAKING TIP: **The hypertensive illnesses of pregnancy used to be called toxemia of pregnancy as well as pregnancy-induced hypertension. That term is still heard in the community because the mothers and grandmothers of clients were told that they had toxemia of pregnancy. Because daughters of clients who have had preeclampsia are high risk for hypertensive illness, it is important to find out whether or not the client's mother had developed eclampsia.**

2. 1. **The nurse should check the client's patellar reflexes. The most common way to assess the deep tendon reflexes is to assess the patellar reflexes.**
   2. The blood count is important, but the nurse should first assess patellar reflexes.
   3. The baseline weight is important, but the nurse should first assess patellar reflexes.
   4. The urinalysis should be obtained, but the nurse should first assess patellar reflexes.

   TEST-TAKING TIP: **Preeclampsia is a very serious complication of pregnancy. The nurse must assess for changes in the blood count, for evidence of marked weight gain, and for changes in the urinalysis. By assessing the patellar reflexes first, however, the nurse can make a preliminary assessment of the severity of the preeclampsia. For example, if the reflexes are +2, the client would be much less likely to become eclamptic than a client who has +4 reflexes with clonus.**

3. 1. Sodium restriction is not recommended.
   2. There is no need to increase fluid intake.
   3. **It is important for the client to eat a well-balanced diet.**
   4. Although not the most nutritious of foods, there is no need to restrict the intake of simple sugars.

   TEST-TAKING TIP: **Clients with preeclampsia are losing albumin through their urine. They should eat a well-balanced diet with sufficient protein to replace the lost protein. Even though preeclamptic clients are hypertensive, it is not recommended that they restrict salt—they should have a normal salt intake—because during pregnancy the kidney is salt sparing. When salt is restricted, the kidneys become stressed.**

4. 1. Weight loss is a positive sign.
   2. **This client is losing protein. The nurse would evaluate a 0-to-trace amount of protein as a positive sign.**
   3. A decrease in serum protein is a sign of pathology. An increase in serum protein would be a positive sign.
   4. 3+ reflexes are pathological. Normal reflexes are 2+.

   TEST-TAKING TIP: **The key to answering this question is the test taker's ability to interpret the meaning of mild preeclampsia and to realize that this is an evaluation question. There are two levels of preeclampsia. Mild preeclampsia is characterized by the following signs/symptoms: blood pressure 140/90, urine protein +2, patellar reflexes +3, and weight gain. As can be seen, the values included in answers 2 and 4 are the same as those in the diagnosis. They, therefore, are not signs that the preeclampsia is resolving. Similarly, loss of protein is not a sign of resolution of the disease.**

5. 1. **A weight gain of 10 pounds in a 4-week period is worrisome. The recommended weight gain during the second and third trimesters is approximately 1 pound per week.**
   2. The pulse rate normally increases slightly during pregnancy.
   3. A slight drop in BP is normal during pregnancy.
   4. The respiratory rate normally increases during pregnancy.

   TEST-TAKING TIP: **A weight gain above that which is recommended can be related to a few things, including preeclampsia, excessive food intake, or multiple gestations. The midwife should be advised of the weight gain to identify the reason for the increase and to intervene accordingly.**

6. 1. Discovering whether or not the client has allergies is important for the nurse to learn if medications are to be ordered, but that is not the most important information the nurse needs to learn.
   2. **The nurse should assess the client's blood pressure.**
   3. Fundal height assessment is important, but not the most important information the nurse needs to learn at this time.
   4. Discovering whether or not the client has stressors at work is important, but it is not the most important information the nurse needs to learn about.

TEST-TAKING TIP: Headache is a symptom of preeclampsia. Preeclampsia, a serious complication, is a hypertensive disease of pregnancy. To determine whether or not the client is preeclamptic, the next action by the nurse would be to assess the woman's blood pressure.

7. 1. Altered glomerular filtration leads to protein loss and, subsequently, to fluid retention, which can lead to swelling in the face and hands.
   2. Monitoring women for the appearance of swollen hands and puffy face is related to the development of preeclampsia, not of cardiac failure.
   3. Monitoring women for the appearance of swollen hands and puffy face is related to the development of preeclampsia, not of hepatic insufficiency.
   4. Monitoring women for the appearance of swollen hands and puffy face is related to the development of preeclampsia, not of altered splenic circulation.

TEST-TAKING TIP: The hypertension associated with preeclampsia results in poor perfusion of the kidneys. When the kidneys are poorly perfused, the glomerlular filtration is altered, allowing large molecules, most notably the protein albumin, to be lost through the urine. With the loss of protein, the colloidal pressure drops in the vascular tree, allowing fluid to third space. The body gets the message to retain fluids, exacerbating the problem. One of the early signs of the third spacing is the swelling of a client's hands and face.

8. 1. The fetus will not be assessed for signs of severe anemia.
   2. The fetus will not be assessed for signs of hypoprothrombinemia.
   3. The fetus will not be assessed for signs of craniosynostosis.

4. The fetus should be assessed for intrauterine growth restriction.

TEST-TAKING TIP: Perfusion to the placenta drops when clients are preeclamptic because the client's hypertension impairs adequate blood flow. When the placenta is poorly perfused, the baby is poorly nourished. Without the nourishment provided by the mother through the umbilical vein, the fetus's growth is affected.

9. 1. Clients with severe preeclampsia are high risk for seizure.
   2. Clients with severe preeclampsia should be monitored for a drop in platelets.
   3. Clients with severe preeclampsia are not at risk for explosive diarrhea.
   4. Clients with severe preeclampsia are not at risk for fractured pelvis.

TEST-TAKING TIP: A client who is diagnosed with 4+ proteinuria and 4+reflexes is severely preeclampsia and, therefore, at high risk for becoming eclamptic. Preeclamptic clients are diagnosed with eclampsia once they have had a seizure.

10. 1. Patellar reflexes are assessed by striking the patellar tendon.
    2. Clonus is not assessed by palpating the woman's ankle.
    3. **To assess clonus, the nurse should dorsiflex the woman's foot.**
    4. Clonus is not assessed by positioning the woman's feet flat on the floor.

TEST-TAKING TIP: When clients have severe preeclampsia, they are often hyperreflexic and develop clonus. To assess for clonus, the nurse should dorsiflex the foot and then let the foot go. The nurse should observe for and count any pulsations of the foot. The number of pulsations is documented. The higher the number of pulsations there are, the more irritable the woman's central nervous system is.

11. 1. +1 reflexes are defined as hyporeflexic.
    2. +2 reflexes are defined as normal.
    3. +3 reflexes are defined as slightly brisker than normal or slightly hyperreflexic.
    4. +4 reflexes are defined as much brisker than normal or markedly hyperreflexic.

TEST-TAKING TIP: Although, as seen above, a clear categorization of reflex assessment exists, the value assigned to a reflex by a clinician does have a subjective component. Therefore, it is recommended that at the

change of shift both the new and departing nurses together assess the reflexes of a client who has suspected abnormal reflexes. A common understanding of the reflex assessment can then be determined.

12. 1. The nurse would expect to see high serum creatinine levels associated with severe preeclampsia.
    2. The nurse would expect to see low serum protein levels with severe preeclampsia.
    3. Bloody stools are never associated with severe preeclampsia.
    4. Epigastric pain is associated with the liver involvement of HELLP syndrome.

TEST-TAKING TIP: When the liver is deprived of sufficient blood supply, as can occur with severe preeclampsia, the organ becomes ischemic. The client experiences pain at the site of the liver as a result of the hypoxia in the liver.

13. 1. At 29 weeks' gestation, the normal fundal height should be 29 cm. With severe preeclampsia, the nurse may see poor growth—that is, a fundal height below 29 cm.
    2. The nurse would expect to see papilledema.
    3. The nurse would expect to see hyperreflexia—that is, patellar reflexes higher than +2.
    4. The nurse would not expect to see nystagmus.

TEST-TAKING TIP: Intracranial pressure (ICP) is present in a client with severe preeclampsia because she is third spacing large quantities of fluid. As a result of the ICP, the optic disk swells and papilledema is seen when the disk is viewed through an ophthalmoscope.

14. 1. Bed rest for the preeclamptic client is not ordered so that she may conserve energy.
    2. Preeclamptic clients rarely complain of nausea or anorexia.
    3. Bed rest, especially side-lying, helps to improve perfusion to the placenta.
    4. Although indirectly this response may be accurate, that is not the primary reason for the positioning.

TEST-TAKING TIP: This question requires the nurse to have a clear understanding of the pathology of preeclampsia. Only with an understanding of the underlying disease can the test taker be able to remember the rationale for many aspects of client care. The vital organs of preeclamptic clients are being poorly perfused as a result of the abnormally high blood pressure. When a woman lies on her side, blood return to the heart is improved and the cardiac output is also improved. With improved cardiac output, perfusion to the placenta and other organs is improved.

15. 1. Headache and decreased output are signs of preeclampsia.
    2. Dependent edema is seen in most pregnant women. It is related to the weight of the uterine body on the femoral vessels.
    3. Hemorrhoids and vaginal discharge are experienced by many pregnant women. Hemorrhoids are varicose veins of the rectum. They develop as a result of chronic constipation and the weight of the uterine body on the hemorrhoidal veins. An increase in vaginal discharge results from elevated estrogen levels in the body.
    4. Backache is seen in most pregnant women. It develops as a result of the weight of the uterine body and the resultant physiological lordosis.

TEST-TAKING TIP: It is important for the test taker to realize that although some symptoms like puffy feet may seem significant, they are normal in pregnancy, while other symptoms like headache, which in a nonpregnant woman would be considered benign, may be potentially very important in a pregnant woman.

16. 1. This primigravid client—age 44 and with a history of diabetes—is very high risk for preeclampsia.
    2. Multigravid clients with a history of rheumatic fever are not significantly at high risk for preeclampsia, unless they have a history of preeclampsia with their preceding pregnancies, or have developed a vascular or hypertensive disease since their last pregnancy.
    3. Multigravid clients with scoliosis are not significantly at high risk for preeclampsia, unless they have a history of preeclampsia with their preceding pregnancies, or have developed a vascular or hypertensive disease since their last pregnancy.
    4. Multigravid clients with celiac disease are not significantly at high risk for preeclampsia, unless they have a history of preeclampsia with their preceding pregnancies, or have developed a vascular or hypertensive disease since their last pregnancy.

TEST-TAKING TIP: Preeclampsia is a vascular disease of pregnancy. Although any woman can develop the syndrome, women who are highest risk for the disease are primigravidas, those with multiple gestations, women who are younger than 17 or older than 34, those who had preeclampsia with their first pregnancy, and women who have been diagnosed with a vascular disease like diabetes mellitus or chronic hypertension.

17. 1. Fatigue and nausea and vomiting are normal in clients at 10 weeks' gestation.
    2. Ankle edema and chloasma are normal in clients at 26 weeks' gestation.
    3. Epigastric pain and facial edema are not normal. This client should be referred to the nurse midwife.
    4. Bleeding gums and urinary frequency are normal in clients at 37 weeks' gestation.

TEST-TAKING TIP: The nurse must be prepared to identify clients with symptoms that are unexpected. This question requires the test taker to differentiate between normal signs and symptoms of pregnancy at a variety of gestational ages and those that could indicate a serious complication of pregnancy.

18. 1. The vital signs are within normal limits.
    2. There has been a 10-lb weight gain in 2 weeks and a significant amount of protein is being spilled in the urine. This client should be brought to the attention of the primary caregiver.
    3. Trace urine protein is considered normal in pregnancy. The blood pressure is within normal limits.
    4. The client has had a normal 2-lb weight gain in the past 2 weeks and her vital signs are within normal limits.

TEST-TAKING TIP: There is a great deal of information included in this question. The test taker must methodically assess each of the pieces of data. Important things to attend to are the timing of the appointments—2 weeks apart; changes in vital signs—it is normal for pulse and respiratory rates to increase slightly and BP to drop slightly; changes in urinary protein—trace is normal, +2 is not normal; and changes in weight—2-lb increase over 2 weeks is normal, a 10-lb increase is not normal.

19. 1. It is inappropriate for the nurse to make this statement.

2. It is inappropriate for the nurse to make this statement.
3. It is inappropriate for the nurse to make this statement.
4. This statement is appropriate. The nurse is offering his or her assistance to the client.

TEST-TAKING TIP: Clients during the first trimester are often ambivalent about pregnancy. Those who abort at this time express a variety of feelings from intense sorrow to joy. The nurse should offer assistance to the client without making any assumptions about the client's feelings toward the pregnancy loss. Speaking platitudes is completely inappropriate.

20. 1. This meal choice is high in iron and ascorbic acid. It would be an excellent lunch choice for this client who has a below normal hematocrit and hemoglobin.
    2. Although high in calcium, this lunch choice will not help to change the client's lab values.
    3. Although nutritious, this lunch choice will not help to change the client's lab values.
    4. Cream cheese has little to no nutritional value. This meal choice would provide a large number of calories and is not the most nutritious choice.

TEST-TAKING TIP: The client in the scenario is anemic. Although a hematocrit of 32% in pregnancy is acceptable, it is recommended that the value not drop below that level. The nurse, having evaluated the lab statement, should choose foods that are high in iron. Liver and dried fruits are good iron sources. Tomatoes are high in vitamin C, which promotes the absorption of iron.

21. 3 and 5 are correct.
    1. Placenta previa is not an acute problem. It is related to the site of placental implantation.
    2. Transverse fetal lie is a malpresentation. It would not be related to the auto accident.
    3. Placental abruption may develop as a result of the auto accident.
    4. Preeclampsia does not occur as a result of an auto accident.
    5. The woman may go into preterm labor after an auto accident.

TEST-TAKING TIP: The fetus is well protected within the uterine body. The musculature of the uterus and the amniotic fluid provide the baby with enough cushioning

to withstand minor bumps and falls. A major automobile accident, however, can cause anything from preterm premature rupture of the membranes, to preterm labor, to a ruptured uterus, to placental abruption. The nurse should especially monitor the fetal heartbeat for any variations.

22. 1. Cervical cerclage is performed on clients with cervical insufficiency.
    2. Amniocentesis is performed to obtain fetal cells to assess genetic information.
    3. Nonstress testing is performed during the third trimester to monitor the well-being of the fetus.
    4. Dilation and curettage (D&C) is performed on a client with an incomplete abortion.

    TEST-TAKING TIP: This client is experiencing an incomplete abortion. The baby has died—there is no fetal heartbeat—and she has expelled some of the products of conception, as evidenced by frank vaginal bleeding. It is important for the remaining products of conception to be removed to prevent hemorrhage and infection. A D&C in which the physician dilates the cervix and scrapes the lining of the uterus with a curette is one means of completing the abortion. Another method of completing the abortion is by administering an abortifacient medication.

23. 1. This client is not exhibiting signs of hopelessness.
    2. This client is very anxious.
    3. This client is not exhibiting signs of low self-esteem.
    4. This client is not showing signs that she will be a poor parent.

    TEST-TAKING TIP: Situational crises arise when problems occur unexpectedly. And crises are often intensified when information is lacking. In this situation, the exact diagnosis is unknown. The client is exhibiting her fright and concern by repeatedly asking the nurse his or her opinion of the baby's health.

24. 1. This long-term goal is appropriate.
    2. This client is not pregnant. She will not deliver a baby.
    3. This client is not in intense pain. This long-term goal is not appropriate.
    4. This client is not pregnant. She will not deliver a baby.

    TEST-TAKING TIP: When nurses plan care, they have in mind short-term and long-term goals that their clients will achieve. Short-term goals usually have a time frame of a week or two and often are specific to the client's current hospitalization. Long-term goals are expectations of client achievement over extended periods of time. It is important for nurses to develop goals to implement appropriate nursing interventions.

25. 1. Pain is not associated with this condition.
    2. There is no fetus; therefore, there will be no fetal heart.
    3. The condition is usually diagnosed after a client complains of brown vaginal discharge early in the "pregnancy."
    4. Suicidal ideations are not associated with this condition.

    TEST-TAKING TIP: The most important thing to remember when answering questions about hydatidiform mole is the fact that, even though a positive pregnancy test has been reported, there is no "pregnancy." The normal conceptus develops into two portions—a blastocyst, which includes the fetus and amnion, and a trophoblast, which includes the fetal portion of the placenta and the chorion. In gestational trophoblastic disease (hydatidiform mole), only the trophoblastic layer develops; no fetus develops. With the proliferation of the chorionic layer, the client is high risk for gynecological cancer.

26. 2 and 3 are correct.
    1. A hematocrit of 39% is well within normal limits.
    2. Women with hydatidiform mole often expel grape-like clusters from the vagina.
    3. Although signs and symptoms of preeclampsia usually appear only after a pregnancy has reached 20 weeks or later, preeclampsia is seen in the first trimester of pregnancy in women with hydatidiform mole
    4. A WBC of 8,000/mm³ is well within normal limits.
    5. Hypertrophied breast tissue is expected early in pregnancy.

    TEST-TAKING TIP: It is very important that the test taker know the normal values of common laboratory values, especially the complete blood count, and that the test taker be familiar with deviations from normal diagnostic signs and symptoms.

27.
1. Headaches are not associated with the diagnosis of placenta previa.
2. A history of thyroid cancer is rarely associated with a diagnosis of placenta previa.
3. Previous preterm deliveries are not associated with a diagnosis of placenta previa.
4. **Painless vaginal bleeding is often the only symptom of placenta previa.**

TEST-TAKING TIP: There are three different forms of placenta previa: low-lying placenta—one that lies adjacent to, but not over, the internal cervical os; partial—one that partially covers the internal cervical os; and complete—a placenta that completely covers the internal cervical os. There is no way to deliver a live baby vaginally when a client has a complete previa, although there are cases when live babies have been delivered when the clients had low-lying or partial previas.

28. **2 and 3 are correct.**
1. A jogger with low body mass index is not necessarily high risk for placenta previa.
2. **A smoker is high risk for placenta previa.**
3. **A woman carrying triplets is high risk for placenta previa.**
4. Registered professional nurses are not high risk for placenta previa.
5. Police officers are not high risk for placenta previa.

TEST-TAKING TIP: The placenta usually implants at a vascular site on the posterior portion of the uterine wall. Two of the women are at high risk for placenta previa. There are 3 placentas nourishing fraternal triplets. Because of the amount of space needed for the placentas, it is not unusual for one to implant near or over the cervical os. The uterine lining of women who smoke is often not well perfused, sometimes resulting in the placenta implanting on or near the cervical os. Women with vascular disease and grand multigravidas are also high risk for placenta previa.

29.
1. After the embryo dies, the nurse would expect to see vaginal bleeding. Rectal bleeding would not be expected.
2. Nausea and vomiting are not characteristic of a ruptured ectopic.
3. **Sharp unilateral pain is a common symptom of a ruptured ectopic.**
4. Hyperthermia is not characteristic of a ruptured ectopic.

TEST-TAKING TIP: The most common location for an ectopic pregnancy to implant is in a fallopian tube. Because the tubes are nonelastic, when the pregnancy becomes too big, the tube ruptures. Unilateral pain can develop because only one tube is being affected by the condition, but some women complain of generalized abdominal pain.

30.
1. The timing of the pregnancy test is irrelevant.
2. **The date of the last menstrual period will assist the nurse in determining how many weeks pregnant the client is.**
3. The woman's previous complications are irrelevant at this time.
4. The age of the woman's menarche is irrelevant.

TEST-TAKING TIP: The date of the last menstrual period is important for the nurse to know. Ectopic pregnancies are usually diagnosed between the 8th and the 9th week of gestation because, at that gestational age, the conceptus has reached a size that is too large for the fallopian tube to hold.

31. **An "X" will be placed on the picture of the abdominal ectopic pregnancy.**

TEST-TAKING TIP: Ectopic pregnancies rarely develop to full term. It is possible, however, for a placenta to attach to the outside of the uterus and to provide enough nutrition and oxygen to a fetus for the fetus to come to term. In that case, the baby would have to be birthed via an abdominal incision.

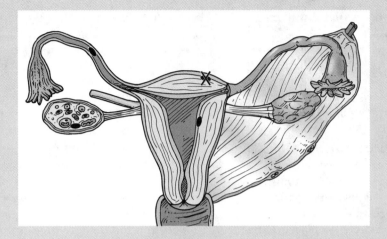

32.
1. A luteinizing hormone level will not provide information on the viability of a pregnancy.
2. Endometrial biopsy will not provide information on the viability of a pregnancy.
3. Hysterosalpingogram is not indicated in this situation.
4. Serum progesterone will provide information on the viability of a pregnancy.

TEST-TAKING TIP: When a previously gravid client is seen by her health care practitioner with a complaint of vaginal bleeding, it is very important to determine the viability of the pregnancy as soon as possible. Situational crises are often exacerbated when clients face the unknown. One relatively easy way to determine the viability of the conceptus is by performing a serum progesterone test; high levels indicate a viable baby whereas low levels indicate a pregnancy loss. Ultrasonography to assess for a beating heart may also be performed.

33.
1. Decadron is a steroid. It is not an appropriate therapy for this situation.
2. Methotrexate is the likely medication.
3. Pergonal is an infertility medication. It is not an appropriate therapy for this situation.
4. Progesterone injections are administered to clients who have a history of preterm labor. It is not an appropriate therapy for this situation.

TEST-TAKING TIP: Methotrexate is an antineoplastic agent. Even if the test taker were unfamiliar with its use in ectopic pregnancy but was aware of the action of methotrexate, he or she could deduce its efficacy here. Methotrexate is a folic acid antagonist that interferes with DNA synthesis and cell multiplication. The conceptus is a ball of rapidly multiplying cells. Methotrexate interferes with that multiplication, killing the conceptus and, therefore, precluding the need for the client to undergo surgery.

34. 83.5 mg
Because the recommended dosage is written per square meters, the nurse must calculate a safe dosage level for this medication using a body surface area formula. The formula for determining the body surface area (BSA) of a client, using the English system, is:

$$BSA = \frac{\sqrt{weight\ (lb) \times height\ (in.)}}{3,131}$$

The nurse first calculates the BSA. (The test taker must remember that there are 12 inches in 1 foot.)
The calculation in this situation is:

$$\sqrt{\frac{136 \times 64}{3,131}}$$

$$\sqrt{\frac{8,704}{3,131}}$$

$$\sqrt{2.779}$$

$$BSA = \sqrt{2.78}$$

$$BSA = 1.67\ m^2$$

Second, a ratio and proportion equation must be created and solved:

$$\frac{Recommended\ dosage}{1\ m^2} = \frac{Safe\ dosage}{Client's\ BSA}$$

$$\frac{50}{1} = \frac{x}{1.67}$$

$$x = 83.5\ mg$$

The nurse now knows that the maximum dosage of methotrexate that this client can safely receive is 83.5 mg.

35. 73 mg

    This question resembles the preceding question, except the weight and height are written in the metric system rather than the English system. The formula for BSA using the metric system is:

    $$BSA = \sqrt{\frac{weight\ (kg) \times height\ (cm)}{3,600}}$$

    The solution in this situation is:

    $$BSA = \sqrt{\frac{52\ kg \times 148\ cm}{3,600}}$$

    $$BSA = \sqrt{\frac{7,696}{3,600}}$$

    $$BSA = \sqrt{2.14}$$

    $$BSA = 1.46\ m^2$$

    Then, a ratio and proportion equation must be created:

    $$\frac{Recommended\ dosage}{1\ m^2} = \frac{Safe\ dosage}{Client's\ BSA}$$

    $$\frac{50}{1} = \frac{x}{1.46}$$

    $$x = 73\ mg$$

    The maximum dosage of methotrexate that this client can safely receive is 73 mg. Note that no decimal point or zero is seen after the 73, even though the stem stated "if rounding is needed, please round to the nearest tenth." The Joint Commission states that trailing zeroes should never be used.

36. 1, 2, 3, and 4 are correct.
    1. Nausea and vomiting are common side effects.
    2. Abdominal pain is a common side effect. The pain associated with the medication needs to be carefully monitored to differentiate it from the pain caused by the ectopic pregnancy itself.
    3. Fatigue is a common side effect.
    4. Light-headedness is a common side effect.
    5. Breast tenderness is not seen with this medication.

    TEST-TAKING TIP: Because methotrexate is an antineoplastic agent, the nurse would expect to see the same types of complaints that he or she would see in a patient receiving chemotherapy for cancer. It is very important that the abdominal pain seen with the medication not be dismissed because the most common complaint of women with ectopic pregnancies is pain. The source of the pain, therefore, must be clearly identified.

37. 1. Taking the client's temperature is important, but assessing for dizziness and weakness is more important.
    2. Documenting the contents and timing of the client's last meal is not the most important action.
    3. Obtaining urine for urinalysis and culture is not the most important action.
    4. It is most important for the nurse to assess for complaints of dizziness or weakness.

    TEST-TAKING TIP: The nurse must prioritize care. When the question asks the test taker to decide which action is most important, all four possible responses are plausible actions. The test taker must determine which is the one action that cannot be delayed. In this situation, the most important action for the nurse to perform is to assess for complaints of dizziness or weakness. These symptoms are seen when clients develop hypovolemia from internal bleeding.

38. 1. Temperature is not the highest priority in this situation.
    2. The pulse is the highest priority in this situation.
    3. The respiratory rate is not the highest priority in this situation.
    4. The blood pressure is not the highest priority in this situation.

    TEST-TAKING TIP: The key to answering this question is the fact that the nursing care plan is for a client with third-trimester bleeding. By the end of the second trimester, pregnant women have almost doubled their blood volume. Because of this, if they bleed, they are able to maintain their blood pressure for a relatively long period of time. Their pulse rate, however, does rise. Nurses, therefore, must carefully attend to the pulse rate of pregnant women who have been injured or who are being observed for third-trimester bleeding. A drop in blood pressure is a very late and ominous sign.

39. 1. Women with placenta previa are often on bed rest. This is, however, a short-term goal.
    2. Another short-term goal is that the baby would have a reactive NST on day 2 of hospitalization.
    3. That the client be symptom-free until at least 37 weeks' gestation is a long-term goal.

4. Another short-term goal is that the woman would call her children shortly after admission.

TEST-TAKING TIP: Each and every one of the goals is appropriate for a client with placenta previa. Only the statement that projects the client's response into the future is, however, a long-term goal.

40. 1. This is inappropriate. The client will have to have a cesarean section.
    2. Clients with complete placenta previa are discouraged from ambulating extensively. Usually they are placed on bed rest only, although they may have bathroom privileges.
    3. This is inappropriate. A 25-week-gestation baby is very preterm. The pregnancy will be maintained as long as possible, at least until 37 weeks.
    4. Straining at stool can result in enough pressure to result in placental bleeding.

TEST-TAKING TIP: Clients diagnosed with complete placenta previa are usually maintained on bed rest. Because one of the many complications of bed rest is constipation, these clients must be monitored carefully. Many physicians order Colace (docusate sodium), a stool softener, to prevent this complication.

41. **1, 3, 4, and 5 are correct.**
    1. The client should be assessed for tachycardia, which could indicate that the client is bleeding internally.
    2. Referred shoulder pain is a symptom seen in clients with ruptured ectopic pregnancies. It is unlikely that this client has an ectopic pregnancy because the signs and symptoms of that complication appear earlier in pregnancy, usually at 8 to 9 weeks' gestation.
    3. This client's signs and symptoms are consistent with both spontaneous abortion and hydatidiform mole. Although this client is only at 12 weeks' gestation, if she has a hydatidiform mole, she may be exhibiting signs of preeclampsia, including headache and hypertension.
    4. This client's signs and symptoms are consistent with both spontaneous abortion and hydatidiform mole. To determine whether or not the patient is carrying a viable fetus, the nurse should check the fetal heart rate.
    5. This client's signs and symptoms are consistent with both spontaneous abortion and hydatidiform mole. Although this client is only 12 weeks' gestation,

if she has a hydatidiform mole, she may be exhibiting signs of preeclampia, including headache and hypertension.

TEST-TAKING TIP: It is essential that the test taker carefully read the weeks of gestation when answering pregnancy-related questions. If the client had been earlier in the first trimester of her pregnancy, the signs and symptoms would also have been consistent with an ectopic pregnancy. It would then have been appropriate to assess for referred shoulder pain as well.

42. **1, 3, 4, and 5 are correct.**
    1. Passive range-of-motion will help to decrease the potential for muscle atrophy and thrombus formation.
    2. Fluid restriction is inappropriate. To maintain healthy bowel and bladder function the client should drink large quantities of fluids.
    3. This client is separated from family. The separation can lead to depression. Decorating the room and enabling family to visit freely is very important.
    4. A high-fiber diet will help to maintain normal bowel function.
    5. Deep breathing exercises are important to maintain the client's respiratory function.

TEST-TAKING TIP: Although bed rest is often used as therapy for antenatal clients, it does not come without its complications—constipation, depression, respiratory compromise, muscle atrophy, to name but a few. The nurse must provide preventive care to maintain the health and well-being of the client as much as possible.

43. 1. The client is not at high risk for oligohydramnios but rather for polyhydramnios.
    2. Because there are two placentas, placenta previa is more common in dizygotic twins. There is only one placenta in a monozygotic twin pregnancy, however.
    3. Twins are usually smaller than singletons. Although malpresentation may occur, it is unlikely that cephalopelvic disproportion will occur.
    4. Twin-to-twin transfusion is a relatively common complication of monozygotic twin pregnancies.

TEST-TAKING TIP: The key to answering this question is the fact that the twins originate from the same egg—that is, they are monozygotic twins. They share a placenta and a chorion. Because their blood supply

is originating from the same source, the twins' circulations are connected. As a result, one twin may become the donor twin while the second twin may become the recipient. The donor grows poorly and develops severe anemia. The recipient becomes polycythemic and large.

44. 1. Fundal growth is often accelerated.
    2. Vaginal bleeding is not related to twin-to-twin transfusion.
    3. Vomiting is not related to twin-to-twin transfusion.
    4. Congestive heart failure is not related to twin-to-twin transfusion.

    TEST-TAKING TIP: Fundal growth is accelerated for two reasons: (a) With two babies in utero, uterine growth is increased and (b) the recipient twin—the twin receiving blood from the other twin—often produces large quantities of urine, resulting in polyhydramnios.

45. 1. Many pregnant women, whether carrying a single baby or twins, feel big.
    2. This is an appropriate weight increase: approximately 3 lb during the entire first trimester and approximately 1 lb per week after that—3 (first trimester) + 10 (1 lb per week for 10 weeks) = 13 pounds.
    3. It is possible that this client is carrying twins.
    4. Low alpha-fetoprotein levels are associated with Down syndrome pregnancies.

    TEST-TAKING TIP: After 20 weeks' gestation, the nurse would expect the fundal height to be equal to the number of weeks of the woman's gestation. Because the fundal height is 4 cm above the expected 22 cm, it is likely that the woman is either having twins or has polyhydramnios.

46. 2 and 3 are correct.
    1. Clients who have a history of prolapsed mitral valve are not at high risk for PPROM.
    2. Clients with UTIs are high risk for PPROM.
    3. Clients carrying twins, whether spontaneous or post-IVF, are at high risk for PPROM.
    4. Clients with gestational diabetes are not high risk for PPROM.
    5. Clients with deep vein thrombosis are not high risk for PPROM.

    TEST-TAKING TIP: Although the exact mechanism is not well understood, clients

who have urinary tract infections are high risk for PPROM. This is particularly important as pregnant clients often have urinary tract infections that present either with no symptoms at all or only with urinary frequency, a complaint of many pregnant clients. Also, clients carrying twins are at high risk for PPROM.

47. 1. The obstetric history is high risk for preterm delivery, not of fetal death.
    2. The nurse should emphasize the need for the client to notify the office of signs of preterm labor.
    3. Dependent edema is a normal complication of pregnancy.
    4. The appearance of spider veins is a normal complication of pregnancy.

    TEST-TAKING TIP: The test taker must be able to interpret a client's gravidity and parity. The letter "G" stands for gravid, or the number of pregnancies. The letter "P" stands for para, or the number of deliveries. The delivery information is further distinguished by 4 separate numbers: the first refers to the number of full-term pregnancies the client has had, the second refers to the number of preterm pregnancies the client has had, the third refers to the number of abortions the client has had (any pregnancy loss before 20 weeks' gestation), and the fourth refers to the number of living children that the client currently has. The client in the scenario, therefore, has had 8 pregnancies (she is currently pregnant) with 3 full-term deliveries, 4 preterm deliveries, and no abortions, and she currently has 6 living children.

48. 1. There is nothing in this scenario that implies that this client is overweight or has gained too much weight during the pregnancy.
    2. This client is at high risk for pregnancy loss. This is an appropriate long-term goal.
    3. There is nothing in this scenario that implies that this client is at high risk for gestational diabetes.
    4. There is nothing in this scenario that implies that this client is at high risk for delivering babies that are either small-for-gestational or large-for-gestational age.

    TEST-TAKING TIP: This question requires the test taker to know why a client may have cervical cerclage placed—namely,

because of multiple pregnancy losses from cervical insufficiency (incompetent cervix). The gravidity and parity information provides an important clue to the question. The client has had four pregnancies—with two preterm births and one abortion, but she has no living children. The goal for the therapy, therefore, is that the pregnancy will go to term.

49. 1. Clients who have cerclages placed are not high risk for hyperthermia in the immediate postprocedure period.
2. Hypotension is not a major complication of clients who have had a cerclage placed.
3. Preterm labor is a complication in the immediate postprocedure period.
4. A fetal heart dysrhythmia is not a complication related to the placement of the cerclage.

TEST-TAKING TIP: Cerclages are inserted when clients have a history of recurring pregnancy loss related to a cervical insufficiency. This client has had 5 pregnancies but only one living child. Unfortunately, with the manipulation of the cervix at the time of the cerclage, the clients may develop preterm labor. The clients should be monitored carefully with a tocometer to assess for labor contractions.

50. 1. This is the most important statement made by the client.
2. The age of her first child is not relevant.
3. Her exercise regimen is not relevant.
4. The date of her miscarriage is not relevant.

TEST-TAKING TIP: Preterm labor is strongly associated with the presence of a urinary tract infection. Whenever an infection is present in the body, the body produces prostaglandins. Prostaglandins ripen the cervix and the number of oxytocin receptor sites on the uterine body increase. Preterm labor can then develop.

51. 1. The first intervention for preterm labor is hydration. Clients who are dehydrated are at high risk for preterm labor.
2. This statement is inappropriate. The client may actually be in true labor.
3. After being hydrated it is possible that the client's cramping will stop.
4. It is not normal for a client to have rhythmic cramping even if she works on her feet.

TEST-TAKING TIP: Preterm cramping should never be ignored. To assess

whether or not a client is in true labor, clients are encouraged to improve their hydration. The client is encouraged to drink about 1 quart of fluid and to lie on her side. If the contractions do not stop, she should proceed to the hospital to have her cervix assessed. If the cervix begins to dilate or efface, a diagnosis of preterm labor would be made. If the contractions stop, clients are usually allowed to begin light exercise. But if the contractions restart, the woman should proceed to the hospital to be assessed.

52. 1. The client should be taught to observe for signs of preterm labor.
2. The client is not at high risk for decreased urinary output.
3. The client is not at high risk for marked fatigue.
4. Puerperal complications occur postpartum.

TEST-TAKING TIP: Clients with hydramnios have excessive quantities of amniotic fluid in their uterine cavities. The excessive quantities likely result from increased fetal urine production, caused by the mother's having periods of hyperglycemia. When the uterus is overextended from the large quantities of fluid, these women are at high risk for preterm labor.

53. 1. The hydramnios is likely a result of excessive fetal urination.
2. The hydramnios is unlikely related to hypoglycemic episodes.
3. Fetal sacral agenesis can result from maternal hyperglycemic episodes during the fetal organogenic period.
4. The hydramnios is unlikely related to impaired placental function.

TEST-TAKING TIP: The majority of amniotic fluid is created as urine by the fetal kidneys. Fetuses of diabetic mothers often experience polyuria as a result of hyperglycemia. If the mother's diabetes is out of control, excess glucose diffuses across the placental membrane, resulting in the fetus becoming hyperglycemic. As a result, the fetus exhibits the classic sign of diabetes—polyuria. If the mother's serum glucose levels are very high during the first trimester, it is likely that the fetus will develop structural congenital defects. Sacral agenesis is one of the most severe of these defects.

54. 1. Type 1 diabetics often need less insulin during the first trimester than they did preconception.
    2. The client will be at high risk for hypoglycemic episodes.
    3. Hydramnios does not develop until the 2nd or 3rd trimester.
    4. The client will likely be hospitalized during the 2nd and/or 3rd trimesters for fetal testing.

    TEST-TAKING TIP: Nausea and vomiting are common complaints of gravid clients during the first trimester. As a result, women, including diabetic women, consume fewer calories than they did before becoming pregnant. Their need for insulin drops commensurately. Therefore, it is very important that the women monitor their blood glucose regularly upon awakening and throughout the day.

55. 1. The 1-hour GCT results are above normal. She needs a 3-hour glucose tolerance test (GTT).
    2. The 1-hour GCT results are above normal. She needs a 3-hour GTT.
    3. The 1-hour GCT results are above normal. She needs a 3-hour GTT.
    4. The 1-hout GCT results are above normal. She needs a 3-hour GTT.

    TEST-TAKING TIP: The glucose challenge test (GCT) is a nonfasting test performed on the vast majority of pregnant clients at or about 24 weeks' gestation. The test is performed to assess for gestational diabetes. Clients with test results of 130 mg/dL or higher (Some physicians use 140 mg/dL as the cutoff.) are referred for a 3-hour glucose tolerance test to make a definitive diagnosis.

56. 1. This comment is inappropriate. The GCT is a nonfasting test.
    2. This comment is appropriate. The client will be referred for a 3-hour glucose tolerance test.
    3. This comment is inappropriate. Glycohemoglobin levels are assessed about once a month, not once a week.
    4. The results are not normal. This client will be referred for a GTT.

    TEST-TAKING TIP: The GCT is merely a screening test. The vast majority of women are sent for the test at about 24 weeks' gestation when their human placental lactogen (a placental hormone that is an insulin antagonist) levels reach a specific point. If

the GCT results are 130 mg/dL or higher (or 140 mg/dL or higher), the client is referred for a 3-hour glucose tolerance test.

57. 1. This question is not related to the client's need for health teaching.
    2. The likelihood of developing either gestational or type 2 diabetes is reduced when clients exercise regularly.
    3. This question is not related to the client's need for health teaching.
    4. This question is not related to the client's need for health teaching.

    TEST-TAKING TIP: There are a number of issues that the nurse should discuss with a client who has been diagnosed with gestational diabetes. The need for exercise is one of those topics. Other topics are diet, blood glucose testing, treatment for hypoglycemic episodes, and the like.

58. 1. There should be a minimum of 2 fetal heart accelerations in 20 minutes (approximately 1 every 10 minutes).
    2. This result is acceptable. There should be a minimum of 1 episode of fetal rhythmic breathing in 30 minutes.
    3. This result is acceptable. There should be a minimum of 1 fetal limb extension and flexion.
    4. This result is acceptable. There should be a minimum of 1 amniotic fluid pocket measuring 2 cm.

    TEST-TAKING TIP: The BPP is a comprehensive assessment geared to evaluate fetal health. In addition to the four items mentioned above, the fetus should exhibit 3 or more discrete body or limb movements in 30 minutes.

59. 1. About 95% of gestational diabetic clients are managed with diet and exercise alone.
    2. About 95% of gestational diabetic clients are managed with diet and exercise alone.
    3. About 95% of gestational diabetic clients are managed with diet and exercise alone.
    4. About 95% of gestational diabetic clients are managed with diet and exercise alone.

    TEST-TAKING TIP: Gestational diabetic clients are first counseled regarding proper diet and exercise as well as blood glucose assessments. The vast majority of women are able to regulate their glucose levels with this intervention. If the glucose levels do not stabilize, the obstetrician will determine whether to order oral hypoglycemics or injectable insulin.

60. 1. She should do nothing because the woman should feel 3 or more counts in 1 hour.
    2. A nonstress test is warranted if the woman feels fewer than 3 counts in an hour.
    3. There is no need to redo the test.
    4. There is no need for the client to redo the test.

TEST-TAKING TIP: Fetal kick counting is a valuable, noninvasive means of monitoring fetal well-being. Mothers are taught to consciously count the numbers of times they feel their baby kick during one or more 60-minute periods during the day. If the baby kicks 3 or more times, the woman can be reassured that the baby is healthy. If the baby kicks fewer times, the woman should notify her health care practitioner, who will likely perform either a nonstress test or, in some situations, a more sophisticated fetal assessment test.

61. 1 and 3 are correct.
    1. Pregnant diabetic clients are particularly at high risk for urinary tract infections.
    2. Pregnant diabetic clients are not at high risk for twinning.
    3. Pregnant diabetic clients are at high risk for acidosis.
    4. Pregnant diabetic clients are at high risk for hypertension, not hypotension.
    5. Pregnant diabetic clients are at high risk for hyperlipidemia, not hypolipidemia.

TEST-TAKING TIP: It is very important for the test taker to read each response carefully. If the test taker were to read the responses to the preceding question very quickly, he or she might choose incorrect answers. For example, the test taker might pick pathological hypotension, assuming that it says "hypertension." Pregnant diabetics are high risk for UTIs because they often excrete glucose in their urine. The glucose is an excellent medium for bacterial growth. They also should be assessed carefully for acidosis because an acidotic environment can be life threatening to a fetus.

62. 1. The client may need to be seen, but this is not the appropriate response by the nurse at this time.
    2. The client should drink a 4-ounce glass of juice.
    3. It is contraindicated to have the client inject herself with insulin.

4. The client may need to speak with her medical doctor, but that is not the appropriate response by the nurse at this time.

TEST-TAKING TIP: Because the signs and symptoms of hyperglycemia and hypoglycemia are very similar, it is important for the nurse to err on the side of caution. If the client should be hypoglycemic, this is a medical emergency. Drinking a glass of orange juice will stabilize the glucose in the woman's body. If she is hyperglycemic, the juice may increase the glucose levels, but not significantly. A blood glucose assessment can be done and insulin can be administered, if needed, shortly after consuming the juice.

63. 1. The regular and NPH can be administered in one syringe.
    2. This is the appropriate method. The regular insulin should be drawn up first and then the NPH insulin in the same syringe.
    3. Regular insulin should be drawn up first.
    4. The insulins should not be mixed together in a vial.

TEST-TAKING TIP: The nurse must be familiar with the appropriate method for administering medications. Insulin must be drawn up in the correct sequence: regular insulin first and NPH insulin second.

64. 1. The client has been hyperglycemic for 3 months but is normoglycemic today.
    2. The client has been hyperglycemic for 3 months but is normoglycemic today.
    3. The client has been hyperglycemic for 3 months but is normoglycemic today.
    4. The client has been hyperglycemic for 3 months but is normoglycemic today.

TEST-TAKING TIP: It is very important for a glycohemoglobin test to be performed at the same time that a fasting glucose is done to have an idea of a diabetic client's glucose control over the past 3 months in comparison to the results of the fasting test. When in a hyperglycemic environment, the red blood cell (RBC) becomes a compound molecule with a glucose group attached to it. Because the RBC lives for approximately 120 days, the health care practitioner can estimate the glucose control of the client over the preceding 3 months time by analyzing the glycohemoglobin. Up to 5% glycohemoglobin is considered normal. An $HgbA_{1c}$ level of

15%, therefore, indicates that the client has been hyperglycemic for the past 3 months. Because her fasting blood glucose level of 100 mg/dL is normal, however, she is normoglycemic today.

65. 1. Estrogen does not compete with insulin.
2. Progesterone does not compete with insulin.
3. Human chorionic gonadotropin does not compete with insulin.
4. Human placental lactogen is an insulin antagonist, so the client will require higher doses of insulin as the level of placental lactogen increases.

TEST-TAKING TIP: During the first trimester, the insulin needs of a woman with type 1 diabetes are usually low. Once the diabetic client enters the second trimester, however, insulin demands increase. One of the most important reasons that insulin demands increase is the increasingly higher levels of human placental lactogen that are found in the mother's bloodstream.

66. 1. It is unlikely that this client will need any medication.
2. It is unlikely that this client will need any medication.
3. It is unlikely that this client will need any medication.
4. It is unlikely that this client will need any medication. Diet and exercise will probably control the diabetes.

TEST-TAKING TIP: The client should be reminded that if she follows her diet and exercises regularly that she will likely be able to manage her diabetes without medication. She should also be encouraged to continue the diet and exercise after delivery to prevent the development of type 2 diabetes later in life.

67. 1. Hyperglycemia is most damaging to the fetus during the first trimester of pregnancy. Although it is abnormal at 38 weeks' gestation, it is not the most important finding.
2. Acidosis is fatal to the fetus. This is the most important finding.
3. Hypocapnia is abnormal, but it is not the most important finding.
4. A high glycohemoglobin is abnormal, but it is not the most important finding.

TEST-TAKING TIP: Acidosis is life threatening to the fetus. It is essential that the nurse monitor clients for situations that would put the fetus in jeopardy of being in an acidotic environment, including maternal hypoxia and diabetic ketoacidosis.

68. 1. This client is many years past her baby's death. Grief counseling is probably not needed at this time.
2. This client is in need of nutrition counseling.
3. The woman is not in need of infection control counseling at this time.
4. Although there may be some genetic basis to spina bifida, about 95% of affected babies are born to parents with no family history of the disease.

TEST-TAKING TIP: There is a strong association between low folic acid intake during the first trimester of pregnancy and spina bifida, a neural tube defect. It is very important that all clients, and especially clients with a family or personal history of a neural tube defect, consume adequate amounts of folic acid during their pregnancies. It is recommended that all women consume at least 600 micrograms of the vitamin per day. To that end, to prevent neural tube defects, it is recommended that pregnant women with no family history take a supplement of 400 micrograms per day, while pregnant women with a family history take a supplement that is 10 times the standard dose, or 4 mg per day.

69. 1. During a reactive nonstress test, the practitioner would expect to see moderate baseline variability in the FH but, according to the definition of a reactive NST, the nurse should see two fetal heart accelerations of 15 bpm lasting 15 or more seconds during a 20-minute period.
2. The maternal heart rate is not evaluated during an NST.
3. This is the definition of a reactive nonstress test—there are two fetal heart accelerations of 15 bpm lasting 15 or more seconds during a 20-minute period.
4. The maternal heart rate is not evaluated during an NST.

TEST-TAKING TIP: When a practitioner notes a reactive nonstress test, he or she can be fairly confident that the fetus is well and will probably remain well for at least 3 to 4 days. NSTs, therefore, are usually performed twice weekly. A nonreactive nonstress test, when the fetal heart fails to show 2 accelerations of 15 bpm lasting 15 or more seconds during a 20-minute period, is very hard to interpret. Usually practitioners order more extensive testing to determine the well-being of the baby after a nonreactive NST.

70. 1, 3, and 4 are correct.
    1. Sexual intercourse has been recommended to women as a means of increasing their Bishop score.
    2. Aromatherapy is not recommended to women as a means of increasing their Bishop score.
    3. Midwives have recommended that women employ breast stimulation as a means of stimulating labor.
    4. Midwives have recommended that women ingest castor oil as a means of increasing their Bishop score.
    5. Aerobic exercise is not recommended to women as a means of increasing their Bishop score.

    TEST-TAKING TIP: There are many interventions that have been used to increase women's Bishop scores and/or to stimulate labor. Because oxytocin is produced during orgasm and when the breasts are stimulated, intercourse and breast stimulation both can be used as complementary methods of stimulating labor. Castor oil stimulates the bowels. Prostaglandins, which ripen the cervix, are produced as a result of gastrointestinal stimulation. In addition, when ingested, primrose oil converts to prostaglandin in the body. If there is any indication that the baby may be unable to withstand labor, however, these means should not be employed.

71. 2, 3, and 5 are correct.
    1. Although there is an increased risk of the woman going into preterm labor, the goal will be to maintain the pregnancy.
    2. This response is correct. The woman should be maintained in the lateral recumbent position during the surgery because, if laid flat, the gravid uterus would compress the great vessels and impede the return of blood to the heart.
    3. This response is correct. The woman would be at high risk for postoperative vomiting and for postoperative gas pains for 2 reasons: progesterone slows gastric motility and the stomach and intestines are displaced by the gravid uterus.
    4. Pregnant clients are at no higher risk of hemorrhaging post-surgery than nonpregnant clients are.

5. This response is correct. After the surgery antiembolic stockings should be placed on the client for the entire time that she is immobile.

TEST-TAKING TIP: Surgery is performed on a pregnant woman only when absolutely necessary. When it is performed, however, the client's pregnancy hormone levels, the cardiovascular changes of pregnancy, and the size of the gravid uterus all place the client at risk of complications. In addition, of course, the maintenance of the pregnancy itself is at risk because of the surgery.

72. 1. Vaso-occlusive crises are precipitated by hypoxia in pregnant as well as nonpregnant sickle cell clients.
    2. Acidosis, not alkalosis, precipitates vaso-occlusive crises.
    3. Dehydration, not fluid overload, precipitates vaso-occlusive crises.
    4. A hyperglycemic state does not precipitate vaso-occlusive crises.

TEST-TAKING TIP: Sickle cell anemia is an autosomal recessive disease. The hemoglobin in the red blood cells of sickle cell clients becomes misshapen when the clients are hypoxic, acidotic, and/or dehydrated. This is a very serious state for the pregnant woman and her fetus. These clients must be cared for immediately with intravenous fluids and methods to reverse the hypoxia and acidosis.

73. 1. Although narcotic medications must be administered to relieve the pain of the crisis, this is not the priority action.
    2. Although heat to the joints must be applied to dilate the blood vessels, this is not the priority action.
    3. Although the client should be kept on bed rest to protect the joints and to prevent further sickling, this is not the priority action.
    4. Administering intravenous fluids is the priority action.

TEST-TAKING TIP: Although this question is not directly related to pregnancy, the nurse must be able to translate information from another medical discipline into the obstetric area. The priority action is to improve perfusion to the client's organs. By providing intravenous fluids, the blood can flow through the vessels and perfuse the organs, including the placenta. When the client is dehydrated, the sickled red blood cells clump together, inhibiting perfusion.

74. 2 and 4 are correct.
   1. Obese clients are not especially at high risk for placenta previa.
   2. Obese clients are at high risk for gestational diabetes.
   3. Obese clients are not especially at high risk for placental abruption.
   4. Obese clients are at high risk for preeclampsia.
   5. Obese clients are not especially at high risk for chromosomal defects.

   TEST-TAKING TIP: Because clients who enter pregnancy obese are at such high risk for gestational diabetes, many obstetricians skip the glucose challenge test and automatically schedule a glucose tolerance test at approximately 24 weeks' gestation. As a result, the complication is discovered much earlier and intervention can begin much earlier. The patients are also carefully monitored for signs and symptoms of preeclampsia.

75. 1. This statement is not true. Obese clients are encouraged to gain about 15 to 25 lb during their pregnancies.
   2. This statement is not true. Although obese clients are encouraged to eat fewer calories than are nonobese clients, they are still encouraged to gain weight during their pregnancies.
   3. This statement is not true. Obese clients are expected to gain 0.5–0.7 pounds per week during the second and third trimesters, or a total of 15 to 25 pounds during their pregnancies.
   4. This statement is true. Normal weight clients are encouraged to gain between 25 and 35 pounds.

   TEST-TAKING TIP: It is not appropriate for an obese client to lose weight or to refrain from gaining weight during her pregnancy. When clients lose weight, they begin to break down fats and ketones develop. An acidic environment is unsafe for the unborn baby (see http://www.iom.edu/~/media/Files/Report%20Files/2009/Weight-Gain-During-Pregnancy-Reexamining-the-Guidelines/Report%20Brief%20-%20Weight%20Gain%20During%20Pregnancy.pdf).

76. 1. The nurse should report the positive results to the doctor.

2. There is no need to perform the nipple stimulation test.
3. There is no need to induce the client.
4. There is no need to administer oxygen to the client.

TEST-TAKING TIP: This client is postdates. The NST is being performed to assess the well-being of the fetus. The results of the test—reactive NST results—are evidence that the fetus is well and will likely be well for another few days. There is no need to provide emergent care.

77. 1, 2, 3, and 5 are correct.
   1. The client should call her practitioner if she experiences fever or chills.
   2. Because the fetus can be injured during an amniocentesis, the client should report either a decrease or an increase in fetal movement.
   3. The client should report abdominal pain or cramping. An amniocentesis can precipitate preterm labor.
   4. Neither rash nor pruritus is associated with amniocentesis.
   5. The client should report any vaginal loss—blood or amniotic fluid. The placenta may become injured or the membranes may rupture during an amniocentesis.

   TEST-TAKING TIP: During an amniocentesis, the amniotic sac is entered with a large needle. As a result of the procedure, a number of complications can develop, including infection, preterm labor, rupture of the membranes, and/or fetal injury. Although the incidence of complications is small, it is very important for the nurse to advise the client of the signs of each of these problems.

78. 1. A nipple stimulation test is performed to assess the baby's response to contractions.
   2. A nipple stimulation test is performed to assess the baby's response to contractions.
   3. The nipples are stimulated with the goal of achieving a q 3-minute contraction pattern.
   4. The nipple stimulation test is not performed to induce labor.

   TEST-TAKING TIP: If the primary health care practitioner is questioning the well-being of the fetus, he or she may order a nipple stimulation test. One nipple is stimulated for 2 minutes followed by a 5-minute rest period. The process is repeated with the other nipple until the uterus begins to contract approximately every 3 minutes. The fetal heart is then assessed in relation to the contraction pattern. A negative test result—which is a positive finding—occurs when there are no fetal heart decelerations noted. A positive test result—which is a negative finding—is the presence of fetal heart decelerations.

79. 1. Equivocal results are difficult to interpret. Additional information is needed.
    2. Fetal heart accelerations are not evaluated during contraction stress tests.
    3. Contraction stress tests are not performed on preterm clients.
    4. Equivocal results are difficult to interpret. Additional information is needed.

    TEST-TAKING TIP: When a test is equivocal, the results can be interpreted both positively and negatively. When contraction stress test results are equivocal, one of two things has usually happened: (a) either there are late decelerations noted, but they are not consistent or (b) the client has developed a hyperstimulated contraction pattern. In either case, the results of the test are uninterpretable and, therefore, additional testing is usually ordered.

80. 1. The L/S ratio indicates the maturity of the fetal lungs, not the coagulability of maternal blood.
    2. The L/S ratio indicates the maturity of the fetal lungs.
    3. The L/S ratio indicates the maturity of the fetal lungs, not the potential for erythroblastosis fetalis.
    4. The L/S ratio indicates the maturity of the fetal lungs, not the potential for gestational diabetes.

    TEST-TAKING TIP: Lecithin and sphingomyelin are two components of surfactant, the slippery substance that lines the alveoli. The fetal lungs have usually reached maturation when the ratio of the substances is 2:1 or higher. To perform the test, the obstetrician must obtain amniotic fluid during an amniocentesis. A quick test, called a shake or foam test, can also be performed on the amniotic fluid to assess fetal lung maturation. (It is important to note that even with an L/S ratio above 2:1, the lungs of fetuses of diabetic mothers are often immature.)

81. 1. The baby is preterm.
    2. The L/S ratio is not related to blood loss.

3. The L/S ratio is not related to hyperbilirubinemia.
4. The L/S ratio is not related to preeclampsia.

TEST-TAKING TIP: The amount of lecithin must be 2 times the amount of sphingomyelin before the practitioner can be assured that the fetal lungs are mature. The ratio in the scenario—1:1—indicates that the surfactant is insufficient for extrauterine respirations.

82. 1. It would be best to choose a time when the fetus is most active.
    2. This is the best position for perfusing the placenta.
    3. Fewer than 3 counts in 1 hour should be reported.
    4. It is unnecessary to refrain from eating prior to the test.

    TEST-TAKING TIP: Because the goal of fetal kick counting is to monitor fetal well-being, it is best to do the test when the baby is most active and is most likely to be well nourished and well oxygenated. Many women find that the best time for the assessment is immediately after a meal.

83. 1. Caudal agenesis is a severe birth defect that can result from maternal hyperglycemia in early pregnancy.
    2. Cardiomegaly is one of the common signs of erythroblastosis fetalis.
    3. The nurse would expect to see polyhydramnios, not oligohydramnios.
    4. Hyperemia is not related to erythroblastosis fetalis or Rh incompatibility.

    TEST-TAKING TIP: Erythroblastosis fetalis is the fetal condition that results when an Rh– mother who is sensitized to Rh+ blood is pregnant with an Rh+ baby. Maternal antibodies cross the placenta and destroy the fetal red blood cells. As a result, the baby becomes severely anemic. Cardiomegaly is one of the complications that occurs as a result of the severe anemia.

84. 1. RhoGAM is administered to Rh– mothers only.
    2. Although in rare instances the Coombs' test may be positive, the direct Coombs' test is usually negative.
    3. Although this is an important action that must be taken before the administration of any medication, it is especially critical in this situation.
    4. RhoGAM is not reconstituted.

TEST-TAKING TIP: When RhoGAM is given, the nurse is administering Rh antibodies to Rh– mothers. If the nurse should make a mistake and administer the dosage to an Rh+ mother, the client would then have been injected with antibodies that would act to destroy her own blood.

85. 1. Although the dosage can be administered in the gluteal muscles, the deltoid is the preferred site of the RhoGAM injection.
2. Although the dosage can be administered in the gluteal muscles, the deltoid is the preferred site of the RhoGAM injection.
3. Although the dosage can be administered in the vastus lateralis, the deltoid is the preferred site of the RhoGAM injection.
4. Although the dosage can be administered in the gluteal muscles, the deltoid is the preferred site of the RhoGAM injection.

TEST-TAKING TIP: Whenever possible, it is preferable to inject the antibodies into the recommended injection site. The antibodies are absorbed optimally from that site and, therefore, are more apt to suppress the mother's immune response.

86. 1. Although the woman's rubella titer is important, it is not essential that it be assessed at this time.
2. Although the woman's obstetric history is important, it is not essential that it be assessed at this time.
3. It is essential that the woman's blood type be assessed.
4. It is not appropriate to assess the woman's cervical patency.

TEST-TAKING TIP: If the woman is found to be Rh–, even though the fetal blood type is unknown, the woman must receive a dose of RhoGAM within 72 hours of the abortion. If the fetus were Rh+ and the woman were not to receive RhoGAM, the woman's immune system might be stimulated to produce antibodies against Rh+ blood. Any future Rh+ fetus would be in danger of developing erythroblastosis fetalis.

87. 1. The baby's Rh status cannot change.
2. That the mother produces no Rh antibodies is the goal of RhoGAM administration.
3. The baby will not produce antibodies.
4. The mother's Rh status cannot change.

TEST-TAKING TIP: The test taker should review the immune response to an antigen. In this situation, the antigen is the baby's Rh+ blood. It can leak into the maternal bloodstream from the fetal bloodstream at various times during the pregnancy. Most commonly it happens at the time of placental delivery. Because the mother is antigen negative—that is, Rh–, when exposed to Rh+ blood, her immune system develops antibodies. RhoGAM is composed of Rh+ antibodies. It acts as passive immunity. Because antibodies are already present in the mother's bloodstream, her immune system is suppressed and fails to develop antibodies via the active immune response.

88. 1. It is unnecessary to perform a daily nitrazine assessment
2. Breast tenderness is unrelated to PPROM.
3. This client must abstain from vaginal intercourse for the remainder of the pregnancy.
4. It is unnecessary for the client to weigh her saturated pads.

TEST-TAKING TIP: Once the membranes are ruptured, the barrier between the vagina and the uterus is broken. As a result, the pathogens in the vagina and the external environment are potentially able to ascend into the sterile uterine body. In addition, once the membranes are ruptured, the client is at high risk for preterm labor. Intercourse must be curtailed for both of these reasons.

89. 1. A fern test is performed to assess for the presence of amniotic fluid.
2. A biophysical profile assessment is performed to assess fetal well-being, not for the presence of amniotic fluid.
3. During amniocentesis, amniotic fluid is extracted from the uterine body to perform genetic analyses or fetal lung maturation assessments as well as other analyses. It is not done to assess for rupture of the membranes.
4. The Kernig assessment is performed on clients who are suspected of having meningeal irritation. It is unrelated to pregnancy.

TEST-TAKING TIP: The fern test was so named because when amniotic fluid is viewed under a microscope, it appears as a fern-like image. The image is a reflection of the high estrogen levels in the fluid that create a crystalline pattern. When the fern appears, the nurse can be assured that amniotic fluid is leaking from the amniotic sac.

90. 1. It is not unsafe for women 18 years of age to become pregnant.
    2. Cat feces are a potential source of toxoplasmosis.
    3. Peanut butter is an excellent source of protein.
    4. Women who work as surgeons are not especially at high risk.

TEST-TAKING TIP: The nurse must be familiar with any possible circumstances that place antepartal clients and their fetuses at high risk. Toxoplasmosis is an illness caused by a protozoan. The organism can be contracted in a number of ways, including eating rare or raw meat, drinking unpasteurized goat milk, and coming in contact with cat feces. When contracted by the mother during pregnancy, it can cause serious fetal and neonatal disease.

91. 1. The symptoms are not likely caused by *Staphylococcus aureus*.
    2. The symptoms are not likely caused by *Streptococcus albicans*.
    3. The symptoms are not likely caused by *Pseudomonas aeruginosa*.
    4. The client is likely suffering from listeriosis, an infection caused by *Listeria monocytogenes* bacteria.

TEST-TAKING TIP: Latin women are especially at high risk for listeriosis because of their dietary patterns. They often eat soft cheeses and are unlikely to fear drinking unpasteurized milk. It is important that the nurse communicate to all pregnant women the need to refrain from consuming those substances with a clear rationale for the warning.

92. 1. The symptoms of listeriosis are similar to symptoms of the flu and include fever and muscle aches.
    2. Neither rash nor thrombocytopenia is related to listeriosis.
    3. Neither petechiae nor anemia is related to listeriosis.
    4. Neither amnionitis nor epistaxis is related to listeriosis.

TEST-TAKING TIP: Even though the adult disease is relatively mild, if listeriosis is contracted during pregnancy, it can lead

to serious fetal and neonatal complications. It is important for the nurse to provide the client with needed dietary education to prevent antepartal disease.

93. 1. If treated early, there likely will be no pregnancy or fetal damage noted.
    2. If treated, the baby will not be born with congenital syphilis.
    3. Usually a single shot of penicillin, administered to the mother, will cure her and protect the baby.
    4. The woman is past the first trimester when the major organ systems are developed.

TEST-TAKING TIP: Clients are assessed for sexually transmitted infections during the pregnancy—usually at the first prenatal visit and shortly before the expected date of delivery. It is important to test all women, even those who have an apparently low probability of diseases like married women and women from the upper socioeconomic strata. Infections, including those that are sexually transmitted, can be contracted by anyone.

94. 1. Domestic birds rarely carry serious disease.
    2. The client should be advised to wear gloves when gardening.
    3. All meat should be cooked until well done to prevent contracting toxoplasmosis.
    4. Dogs rarely carry serious disease.

TEST-TAKING TIP: Clients should be advised to wear gloves when gardening because cat feces can carry the toxoplasmosis protozoa. Feral and outdoor domestic cats are nondiscriminating about where they urinate and defecate. They easily could be using the vegetable garden for a cat box. As such, it is also very important for everyone, and especially pregnant women, to wash fresh fruits and vegetables before eating them.

95. 1. Rubella is a teratogenic disease. The parents should notify any pregnant friends.
    2. Rubella is a virus. Penicillin will not treat it.
    3. Rubella is a relatively benign illness when contracted in childhood.
    4. Rubella is not a pruritic illness. Diphenhydramine is not needed.

TEST-TAKING TIP: Of all of the communicable illnesses, rubella is the most potentially teratogenic. If mothers contract the disease during the first trimester, up to 50% of the fetuses will develop congenital defects. The incidence of disease does drop with each successive week, but babies are still at high risk for injury. The most common defects from rubella are deafness, cataracts, and cardiovascular disease.

96. 1. This answer is incorrect. Antibiotics, if given prenatally, are administered orally.
2. This answer is incorrect. Group B strep bacteria are normal flora for this client. She need not take her temperature.
3. **This answer is correct. Exposure to group B strep is very dangerous for neonates.**
4. Group B strep does not cause scarlet fever. Group A strep causes scarlet fever and strep pharyngitis.

TEST-TAKING TIP: Group B strep can cause serious neonatal disease. Babies are at high risk for meningitis, sepsis, pneumonia, and even death. IV antibiotics are administered to the laboring mother every 4 hours to decrease the colonization in the mother's vagina and rectum. In addition, the antibiotics cross the placenta and act as a prophylaxis for the baby.

97. 1. Pregnant women are often fatigued and it is not uncommon for adolescents to sleep long hours. This is not the best nursing diagnosis.
2. The teen is likely to need teaching regarding the care of infants, but it is too early in the pregnancy for this diagnosis to take precedence.
3. The teen is likely to be anxious regarding labor and delivery, but it is too early in the pregnancy for this diagnosis to take precedence.
4. **The developmental tasks of adolescence are often in conflict with the tasks of pregnancy. This nursing diagnosis is the most appropriate.**

TEST-TAKING TIP: The major developmental tasks of adolescence—completing her education, developing abstract thinking, and developing skills that foster independence—can be in conflict with those of pregnancy. Adolescents often test rules, use drugs, and drink alcohol, all of which are detrimental to the developing fetus. At the very least, teens socialize with friends, often eating at fast-food restaurants where a well-balanced high-calcium, high-iron diet is hard to obtain.

98. 1. There is not a high incidence of chromosomal defects in babies born to teen mothers.
2. Teens do not have an inordinately high intake of manganese and zinc.
3. **Teens are prone to having preterm deliveries rather than post-term deliveries.**
4. Teens are likely to delay entry into the health care system.

TEST-TAKING TIP: Late entry into prenatal care is particularly problematic for teen pregnancies. Because organogenesis occurs during the first trimester, by the time many teens acknowledge that they are pregnant and seek care they are already past this critical period. They are likely to have consumed damaging substances or, at the very least, consumed inadequate quantities of essential nutrients, like folic acid.

99. 1. The client's heart rate is important but it is not the most important vital sign.
2. The client's respiratory rate is important but it is not the most important vital sign.
3. **The client's blood pressure is the most important vital sign.**
4. The client's temperature is important but it is not the most important vital sign.

TEST-TAKING TIP: Adolescents who are 16 years old or younger are particularly high risk for hypertensive illnesses of pregnancy. It is especially important for the nurse and the client's primary health care practitioner to determine the client's baseline blood pressure to identify any elevations as early as possible.

100. 1. Although eating burgers with fries is not the best choice for the young woman to make, it is not the most important comment for the nurse to respond to at this time.
2. This comment is informative because the nurse learns that this client has multiple sex partners. It is not the most important comment, however.
3. **The nurse must respond to this comment. This young woman is repeatedly exposing her fetus to alcohol.**
4. This comment is important because this young woman is not completing her education but it is not the most important comment for the nurse to respond to at this time.

TEST-TAKING TIP: The nurse must prioritize her care with teen clients as well as with mature clients. This young woman will eventually need to be counseled regarding diet, infection control, and her education, but the fetus is at highest risk at the present time from repeated alcohol exposure. Indeed, alcohol exposure is injurious for the unborn child throughout the entire pregnancy. The nurse must discuss this with the young woman at this time.

101. 1. The teen's partner may or may not be actively engaged in the pregnancy process. If he is interested in attending prenatal appointments, he should be welcomed. If not, the nurse should help the young woman to identify other important support people.
      2. The pregnant teen has the same choices that the pregnant adult has. She can decide to terminate the pregnancy, maintain the pregnancy and give the child up for adoption, or maintain the pregnancy and retain custody of the child. It is not the nurse's choice to make, although the nurse should provide the young woman with all of her options.
      3. It is important for the young woman to work toward completing the tasks of adolescence at the same time that she is engaged in maintaining a healthy pregnancy. She should continue her education.
      4. It is unnecessary, unless a chromosomal anomaly is in the young woman's medical history, for the client to undergo chromosomal analysis.

TEST-TAKING TIP: Working with adolescents can be exciting as well as challenging. The nurse is likely to be the young woman's most important support system during the early weeks of the pregnancy. Slowly, with the nurse's help, it is hoped that the young woman will make healthy choices, including eating well, refraining from drinking alcohol and using drugs, and staying in school.

102. 1. Adolescents are at high risk for preterm labor.
      2. Lifestyle issues and ethnicity are more important high-risk predictors of GDM than is age.
      3. Pregnant teens are high risk for delivering babies that are small-for-gestational age rather than macrosomic babies.

      4. Pregnant teens are high risk for anemia rather than for polycythemia.

TEST-TAKING TIP: It is very important that pregnant teens learn the telltale signs of preterm labor, such as intermittent backache, cramping, discomfort low in the pelvic area, and the like. Because of their lifestyle choices, pregnant teens are at high risk for low-birth-weight, preterm births.

103. 1. This is an inappropriate statement. The nurse should act as a counselor, not as a decision maker.
      2. **This is an excellent response. The question opens the door for the teenager to discuss her feelings and thoughts.**
      3. This is a true statement, but it is inappropriate to say to a young woman who is ambivalent about her pregnancy.
      4. This is an inappropriate statement. The nurse should act as a counselor, not as a decision maker.

TEST-TAKING TIP: It is very important that nurses working in the obstetric area come to terms with their role and with their own beliefs and biases. One's personal belief system should not influence the nurse's teaching and counseling roles. The nurse must be truthful and unbiased when counseling any prenatal client, including the pregnant teen.

104. 1. Pregnant adolescents usually have an excellent protein intake, although they may or may not have an adequate magnesium intake.
      2. **Pregnant adolescents' diets are often deficient in calcium and iron.**
      3. Pregnant adolescents usually have an excellent carbohydrate intake and zinc intake.
      4. Cereals and grains are enriched with the B vitamins, and most adolescents do eat these foods.

TEST-TAKING TIP: Adolescents are in need of higher levels of both calcium and iron during their pregnancies than are adult women. These nutrients are needed because many of the teens who become pregnant have not completed their own growth. Calcium is, of course, needed for the teen's own bone growth as well as for the bone growth of the fetus. Similarly, iron is needed for the teen's hematological function as well as the baby's blood supply.

105. 1. Striae gravidarum, stretch marks, are a normal pregnancy finding.
2. A client who is complaining of dyspnea on exertion is likely going into left-sided congestive heart failure.
3. It is expected for a client in the third trimester to gain approximately 1 pound per week, or 4 pounds per month.
4. Patellar reflexes of +2 is a normal finding.

TEST-TAKING TIP: It is important for the test taker to know that pregnancy is a significant stressor on the cardiac system. Women who enter the pregnancy with a history of cardiac problems must be monitored very carefully not only by the obstetric practitioner but also by an internist or cardiologist. The nurse must be vigilant in observing for signs of cardiac failure, including respiratory and systemic congestion.

106. 1. This is a possible follow-up question that may be asked, but it is not the most important question that the nurse should ask.
2. This is a possible follow-up question that may be asked, but it is not the most important question that the nurse should ask.
3. This is a possible follow-up question that may be asked, but it is not the most important question that the nurse should ask.
4. This is an essential question for the nurse to ask.

TEST-TAKING TIP: The nurse should question all obstetric clients about a possible history of physical abuse and/or sexual abuse. Women are especially high risk for abusive injuries during the pregnancy period. Any gravida who exhibits trauma to the genital area, therefore, must be viewed as a possible victim of sexual abuse.

107. 1. This is not a priority action.
2. This is not a priority action.
3. This is the priority action. The nurse should escort the client to a location where the partner cannot follow.
4. This is not a priority action.

TEST-TAKING TIP: This couple is exhibiting classic signs of an abusive relationship. The woman is subjective, looking down and allowing her partner to respond to questions. The partner is dominant and demeaning in his description of his

partner. To question the woman regarding her relationship, it is important for the nurse to interview the client in private. The women's bathroom is an excellent location for the interview.

108. 1. Genetic changes in the fetal reproductive system have not been associated with smoking during pregnancy.
2. Extensive central nervous system damage has not been associated with smoking during pregnancy.
3. There is no direct evidence that prenatal smoking causes fetal nicotine addiction.
4. Smoking in pregnancy does cause fetal intrauterine growth restriction.

TEST-TAKING TIP: When someone smokes, there is a vasoconstrictive effect that occurs in the body. This vasoconstrictive effect is also seen at the placental site. Placentas of women who smoke are much smaller than those of nonsmoking women; because of this, babies receive less oxygen and nutrients via the placenta. As a result, their growth is restricted.

109. 1. This project should not adversely affect the pregnancy.
2. Antique cribs are often painted with lead-based paint. This is a dangerous activity.
3. As long as she wears gloves, this activity should be safe.
4. As long as she does not become dyspneic, this activity should be safe.

TEST-TAKING TIP: It is very important that clients stay away from aerosolized lead that can develop when lead paint is being sanded. Lead can enter the body through the respiratory tract as well as through the gastrointestinal tract. Once it is ingested, the lead enters the vascular tree and is transported across the placenta to the unborn baby. The baby, especially the baby's central nervous system, can be severely adversely affected by the lead.

110. 1. Progesterone is a hormone that relaxes smooth muscle. This action leads to the delayed emptying of the gallbladder during pregnancy.
2. Although there is a genetic tendency for people of some ethnic groups to excrete large quantities of cholesterol, a contributing factor in gallbladder disease,

there is not a direct genetic link to the problem.

3. Women are more likely to have gallbladder disease than are men and older women are more prone to the disease than are younger women.

4. Gallbladder disease is related to high levels of cholesterol in the diet and in the bloodstream.

TEST-TAKING TIP: The hormones of pregnancy not only maintain the pregnancy but also affect all parts of the body. High estrogen levels can lead to nosebleeds and gingivitis and high progesterone levels can lead to constipation and gallbladder disease.

111. 1. Pedal edema is not related to pseudocyesis.
2. There will be no fetal heartbeat when a client has pseudocyesis.
3. Polycythemia (hematocrit above 40%) is not related to pseudocyesis.
4. Clients who have pseudocyesis state that they do feel their babies move.

TEST-TAKING TIP: Although rare, there are some women who develop pregnancy symptoms and believe themselves pregnant but who are not actually pregnant. This is a psychiatric illness. The women may develop many of the presumptive signs of pregnancy but there will be few, if any, probable signs and no positive signs of pregnancy.

112. 1. Although women who have had gynecological cancer and who are unable to conceive may be at high risk, those with cancers in other systems are not at high risk.
2. Women with celiac disease are not at high risk for pseudocyesis.
3. Women who have had a number of miscarriages are at high risk for pseudocyesis.
4. Grand multiparas are not at high risk for pseudocyesis.

TEST-TAKING TIP: The prefix "pseudo" means "false" and "cyesis" means "pregnancy." Women who develop pseudocyesis are women who have an overwhelming desire to become pregnant. Those who have had multiple miscarriages may be so desperate they develop signs of pregnancy but are not really pregnant.

113. 2, 3, and 5 are correct.
1. It would be inappropriate to perform contraction stress tests.

2. There should be blood available in the blood bank in case the woman begins to bleed.
3. The nurse would expect to keep the woman on bed rest with bathroom privileges only.
4. Although important to monitor, it would be unnecessary to assess the electrolytes daily. The client is able to eat a normal diet.
5. The nurse would expect that weekly biophysical profiles would be done to assess fetal well-being.

TEST-TAKING TIP: Because clients with placenta previa are at high risk for bleeding from the placental site, it is essential that they be limited in their activity and have blood on hand in case of hemorrhage. In addition, their babies must be monitored carefully for signs of fetal well-being. It would be inappropriate to stimulate contractions because dilation of the cervix would stimulate bleeding.

114. 1. This client is in metabolic acidosis. This is consistent with a diagnosis of diarrhea.
2. This client is in respiratory alkalosis. This is consistent with a diagnosis of hyperventilation.
3. This client is in respiratory acidosis. This is consistent with a diagnosis of respiratory distress.
4. This client is in metabolic alkalosis. This is consistent with a diagnosis of hyperemesis gravidarum.

TEST-TAKING TIP: The test taker must not panic when confronted with blood gas data. If assessed methodically, the test taker should have little trouble determining the correct answer. The first action is to determine what the results should show. If a woman is vomiting repeatedly, one would expect her to have lost acid from the stomach. She would, therefore, be in metabolic alkalosis. The test taker should then look at the pH levels—they should be elevated—and the O_2 levels— they should be normal—to begin to determine which response is correct.

115. 1. The blood count is important but it is not highest priority.
2. Starting an intravenous with multivitamins takes priority.
3. An admission weight is important but is not highest priority.

4. The urinalysis is important but is not highest priority.

TEST-TAKING TIP: Clients who are vomiting repeatedly are energy depleted, vitamin depleted, electrolyte depleted, and often dehydrated. It is essential that the client receive her IV therapy as quickly as possible. The other orders should be completed soon after the IV is started.

116. 1. The nurse would expect that the baby has dysplastic kidneys.
2. The nurse would not expect to find that the baby has coarctation of the aorta.
3. The nurse would not expect to find that the baby has hydrocephalus.
4. The nurse would not expect to find that the baby has hepatic cirrhosis.

TEST-TAKING TIP: The majority of amniotic fluid is produced by the fetal kidneys. When a pregnancy is complicated by oligohydramnios, ultrasounds may be performed to check for defects in the fetal renal system.

117. 1. The nurse would not expect to find that the baby has pulmonic stenosis.
2. The nurse would expect to find that the baby has tracheoesophageal fistula.
3. The nurse would not expect to find that the baby has ventriculoseptal defect.
4. The nurse would not expect to find that the baby has developmental hip dysplasia.

TEST-TAKING TIP: Babies swallow the amniotic fluid while in utero. When there is a surplus of fluid, ultrasounds may be performed to check for defects in the fetal gastrointestinal system.

118. 1. A bicornuate uterus will not predispose a client to infection.
2. A bicornuate uterus will not predispose a client to palpitations.
3. A bicornuate uterus will predispose a client to cramping and preterm labor.
4. A bicornuate uterus will not predispose a client to oliguria.

TEST-TAKING TIP: If the test taker is unfamiliar with the term *bicornuate*, he or she could break down the word into its parts to determine its meaning: "bi" means "2" and "cornuate" means "horn." A bicornuate uterus, therefore, is a uterus that has a septum down the center, creating a 2-horned fundus.

Sometimes the uterus is heart-shaped and sometimes the uterus is divided in half. Because of its shape, there is often less room for the fetus to grow. The uterus becomes irritable and predisposes the client to preterm labor.

119. 1. Clients who are third spacing are often preeclamptic. The blood pressure, therefore, may be elevated. This is not, however, the most important sign for the nurse to assess.
2. The faces and hands of clients who are third spacing often appear puffy. The appearance, however, is not the most important sign for the nurse to assess.
3. Weight is the most important sign for the nurse to assess.
4. The client's pulse rate may change, but it is not the most important sign for the nurse to assess.

TEST-TAKING TIP: When clients third space, they are retaining fluids. Fluid is very heavy. A sudden weight increase is, therefore, the most important assessment the nurse can make to determine whether or not a client is third spacing. Clients who are being assessed for preeclampsia, therefore, should be weighed daily.

120. 1. This is not appropriate. Because it is dangerous for tongue blades to be inserted into the mouths of seizing clients, the nurse should not place a tongue blade in the client's room.
2. This is appropriate. The side rails and the headboard should be padded.
3. The room of an eclamptic client should be quiet. Excess stimulation can precipitate a seizure.
4. There is no reason to provide grief counseling to this client.

TEST-TAKING TIP: When a client has been diagnosed with eclampsia, she has already had at least one seizure. The nurse, therefore, must be prepared to care for the client during another seizure. The most important action during the seizure is to protect the client from injury. Padding the side rails and headboard will provide that protection. This client's fetus is exhibiting a normal heart rate pattern.

High-Risk Intrapartum

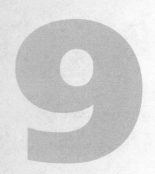

Both the mother and the fetus are at risk during the intrapartum period—that is, during labor and delivery. As labor progresses, the risk increases. There are a variety of obstetric emergencies as well as medical problems that can adversely impact both the mother and the fetus during labor and delivery. For example, hypertensive illnesses, diabetes mellitus, dystocias, and placental dysfunction as well as induced labors and operative deliveries are potentially harmful to both mother and baby. In addition, labors that begin preterm or post-term can markedly impact fetal well-being. For the nurse to provide quality care, he or she must be familiar with the medical monitoring required to identify the complications and be able to provide the appropriate interventions. At the same time, the nurse must provide supportive care to the laboring couple to foster trust and calm.

KEYWORDS

The following words include English vocabulary, nursing/medical terminology, concepts, principles, or information relevant to content specifically addressed in the chapter or associated with topics presented in it. English dictionaries, your nursing textbooks, and medical dictionaries such as *Taber's Cyclopedic Medical Dictionary* are resources that can be used to expand your knowledge and understanding of these words and related information.

abruptio placentae (placental abruption)

betamethasone (Celestone)

biophysical profile

Bishop score

calcium gluconate

cesarean section

cord compression

dexamethasone (Decadron)

dinoprostone (Cervidil, Prepidil)

disseminated intravascular coagulation (DIC)

eclampsia

external version

fetal heart decelerations (late and variable)

forceps

general anesthesia

grief and mourning

group B streptococcus

head compression

HELLP syndrome

hepatitis B

herpes simplex type 2

HIV/AIDS

hyperstimulation

hypertensive illnesses of pregnancy

induction

magnesium sulfate

McRoberts' maneuver

misoprostol (Cytotec)

multigravida

multipara

naloxone (Narcan)

nifedipine (Procardia)

oxytocin (Pitocin)

placenta previa

post-term labor

preeclampsia

preterm labor

primigravida

primipara

prolapsed cord

prostaglandins

regional anesthesia (epidural and spinal)

terbutaline (Brethine)

tocolytic   uteroplacental insufficiency
uterine rupture   vacuum extraction

QUESTIONS

1. A client has been diagnosed with water intoxication after having received IV oxytocin (Pitocin) for over 24 hours. Which of the following signs/symptoms would the nurse expect to see?
   1. Confusion, drowsiness, and vomiting.
   2. Hypernatremia and hyperkalemia.
   3. Thrombocytopenia and neutropenia.
   4. Paresthesias, myalgias, and anemia.

2. The physician has ordered oxytocin (Pitocin) for induction for 4 gravidas. In which of the following situations should the nurse refuse to comply with the order?
   1. Primigravida with a transverse lie.
   2. Multigravida with cerebral palsy.
   3. Primigravida who is 14 years old.
   4. Multigravida who has type 1 diabetes.

3. A client, 38 weeks' gestation, is being induced with IV oxytocin (Pitocin) for hypertension and oligohydramnios. She is contracting q 3 min × 60 to 90 seconds. She suddenly complains of abdominal pain accompanied by significant fetal heart bradycardia. Which of the following interventions should the nurse perform first?
   1. Turn off the oxytocin infusion.
   2. Administer oxygen via face mask.
   3. Reposition the patient.
   4. Call the obstetrician.

4. An induction of a 42-week gravida with IV oxytocin (Pitocin) is begun at 0900 at a rate of 0.5 milliunits per minute. The woman's primary physician orders: Increase the oxytocin drip by 0.5 milliunits per minute every 10 minutes until contractions are every 3 minutes × 60 seconds. The nurse refuses to comply with the order. Which of the following is the rationale for the nurse's action?
   1. Fetal distress has been noted in labors when oxytocin dosages greater than 2 milliunits per minute are administered.
   2. The relatively long half-life of oxytocin can result in unsafe intravascular concentrations of the drug.
   3. It is unsafe practice to administer oxytocin intravenously to a woman who is carrying a postdates fetus.
   4. A contraction duration of 60 seconds can lead to fetal compromise in a baby that is postmature.

5. A 40-week-gestation woman has received Cytotec (misoprostol) for cervical ripening. For which of the following signs/symptoms should the nurse carefully monitor the client?
   1. Diarrhea and back pain.
   2. Hypothermia and rectal pressure.
   3. Urinary retention and rash.
   4. Tinnitus and respiratory distress.

6. A woman, G3 P1010, is receiving oxytocin (Pitocin) via IV pump at 3 milliunits/min. Her current contraction pattern is every 3 minutes × 45 seconds with moderate intensity. The fetal heart rate is 150 to 160 bpm with moderate variability. Which of the following interventions should the nurse take at this time?
   1. Stop her infusion.
   2. Give her oxygen.
   3. Change her position.
   4. Monitor her labor.

7. A woman is to receive Prepidil (dinoprostone gel) for labor induction. The nurse should be prepared to administer the medication via which of the following routes?
   1. Intravenously.
   2. Orally.
   3. Endocervically.
   4. Intrathecally.

8. A woman, 40²/₇ weeks' gestation, has had ruptured membranes for 15 hours with no labor contractions. Her obstetrician has ordered 10 units oxytocin (Pitocin) to be diluted in 1,000 mL D5½ NS. The order reads: Administer oxytocin IV at 0.5 milliunits per min. Calculate the drip rate for the infusion pump to be programmed. **Please calculate to the nearest whole number.**
   _____ mL/hr.

9. The nurse turns off the oxytocin (Pitocin) infusion after a period of hyperstimulation. Which of the following outcomes indicates that the nurse's action was effective?
   1. Intensity moderate.
   2. Frequency every 3 minutes.
   3. Duration 130 seconds.
   4. Attitude flexed.

10. A nurse is monitoring the labor of a client who is receiving IV oxytocin (Pitocin) at 6 mL per hour. Which of the following clinical signs would lead the nurse to stop the infusion?
   1. Change in maternal pulse rate from 76 to 98 bpm.
   2. Change in fetal heart rate from 128 to 102 bpm.
   3. Maternal blood pressure of 150/100.
   4. Maternal temperature of 102.4°F.

11. A primigravid client received Cervidil (dinoprostone) for induction 8 hours ago. The Bishop score is now 10. Which of the following actions by the nurse is appropriate?
   1. Perform nitrazine analysis of amniotic fluid.
   2. Report abnormal findings to the obstetrician.
   3. Place woman on her side.
   4. Monitor for onset of labor.

12. The physician has ordered Prepidil (dinoprostone) for four gravidas at term. The nurse should question the order for which of the women?
   1. Primigravida with Bishop score of 4.
   2. Multigravida with late decelerations.
   3. G1 P0000 contracting every 20 minutes × 30 seconds.
   4. G6 P3202 with blood pressure 140/90 and pulse 92.

13. A client, G4 P1021, has been admitted to the labor and delivery suite for induction of labor. The following assessments have been made: Bishop score of 2, fetal heart rate of 156 with good variability and no decelerations, TPR 98.6°F, P 88, R 20, BP 120/80, negative obstetric history. Cervidil (dinoprostone) has been inserted. Which of the following findings would warrant the removal of the prostaglandin?
   1. Bishop score of 4.
   2. Fetal heart rate of 152.
   3. Respiratory rate of 24.
   4. Contraction frequency of 1 minute.

14. There are four clients in active labor in the labor suite. Which of the women should the nurse monitor carefully for the potential of uterine rupture?
    1. Age 15, G3 P0020, in active labor.
    2. Age 22, G1 P0000, eclampsia.
    3. Age 25, G4 P3003, last delivery by cesarean section.
    4. Age 32, G2 P0100, first baby died during labor.

15. A client is admitted in labor with spontaneous rupture of membranes 24 hours earlier. The fluid is clear and the fetal heart rate is 124 with moderate variability. Which assessment is most important for the nurse to make at this time?
    1. Contraction frequency and duration.
    2. Maternal temperature.
    3. Cervical dilation and effacement.
    4. Maternal pulse rate.

16. A client, 39 weeks' gestation, fetal heart baseline at 144 bpm, tells the admitting labor and delivery room nurse that she has had to wear a pad for the past 4 days "because I keep leaking urine." Which of the following is an appropriate action for the nurse to perform at this time?
    1. Palpate the woman's bladder to check for urinary retention.
    2. Obtain a urine culture to check for a urinary tract infection.
    3. Assess the fluid with nitrazine and see if the paper turns blue.
    4. Percuss the woman's uterus and monitor for ballottement.

17. The nurse is to intervene when caring for a laboring client whose baby is exhibiting signs of fetal distress. Which of the following actions should the nurse take?
    1. Administer oxygen via nasal cannula.
    2. Place the client in high Fowler's position.
    3. Remove the internal fetal monitor electrode.
    4. Increase the intravenous infusion rate.

18. Four women request to labor in the hospital bathtub. In which of the following situations is the procedure contraindicated? **Select all that apply.**
    1. Woman during transition.
    2. Woman during second stage of labor.
    3. Woman receiving oxytocin for induction.
    4. Woman with meconium-stained fluid.
    5. Woman with fetus in the occiput posterior position.

19. A full-term client, contracting every 15 min × 30 sec, has had ruptured membranes for 20 hours. Which of the following nursing interventions is contraindicated at this time?
    1. Intermittent fetal heart auscultation.
    2. Vaginal examination.
    3. Intravenous fluid administration.
    4. Nipple stimulation.

20. A woman, 39 weeks' gestation, is admitted to the delivery unit with vaginal warts from human papillomavirus. Which of the following actions by the nurse is appropriate?
    1. Notify the health care practitioner for a surgical delivery.
    2. Follow standard infectious disease precautions.
    3. Notify the nursery of the imminent delivery of an infected neonate.
    4. Wear a mask whenever the perineum is exposed.

21. A client telephones the labor and delivery suite and states, "My bag of waters just broke and it smells funny." Which of the following responses would be appropriate for the nurse make at this time?
    1. "Have you notified your doctor of the smell?"
    2. "The bag of waters always has an unusual odor."
    3. "Your labor should start very soon."
    4. "Have you felt the baby move since the membranes broke?"

22. A client, G3 P2002, 40 weeks' gestation, who has vaginal candidiasis, has just been admitted in early labor. Which of the following should the nurse advise the woman?
    1. She may need a cesarean delivery.
    2. She will be treated with antibiotics during labor.
    3. The baby may develop thrush after delivery.
    4. The baby will be isolated for at least one day.

23. A woman who is hepatitis B–surface antigen positive is in active labor. Which action by the nurse is appropriate at this time?
    1. Obtain an order from the obstetrician to prepare the client for cesarean delivery.
    2. Obtain an order from the obstetrician to administer intravenous ampicillin during labor and the immediate postpartum.
    3. Obtain an order from the pediatrician to administer hepatitis B immune globulin and hepatitis B vaccine to the baby after birth.
    4. Obtain an order from the pediatrician to place the baby in isolation after delivery.

24. A client has just entered the labor and delivery suite with ruptured membranes for 2 hours, fetal heart rate of 146, contractions every 5 minutes × 60 seconds, and a history of herpes simplex type 2. She has no observable lesions. After notifying the doctor of the admission, which of the following is the appropriate action for the nurse to take?
    1. Check dilation and effacement.
    2. Prepare the client for surgery.
    3. Place the bed in Trendelenburg position.
    4. Check the biophysical profile results.

25. Immediately prior to an amniotomy, the external fetal heart monitor tracing shows 145 bpm with early decelerations. Immediately following the procedure, an internal tracing shows a fetal heart rate of 120 with variable decelerations. A moderate amount of clear, amniotic fluid is seen on the bed linens. The nurse concludes that which of the following has occurred?
    1. Placental abruption.
    2. Eclampsia.
    3. Prolapsed cord.
    4. Succenturiate placenta.

26. Immediately after a woman spontaneously ruptures her membranes, the nurse notes a loop of the umbilical cord protruding from the woman's vagina. Which of the following actions should the nurse perform first?
    1. Put the client in the knee-chest position.
    2. Assess the fetal heart rate.
    3. Administer oxygen by tight face mask.
    4. Telephone the obstetrician with the findings.

27. A client just spontaneously ruptured membranes. Which of the following factors makes her especially at high risk for having a prolapsed cord? **Select all that apply.**
    1. Breech presentation.
    2. Station –3.
    3. Oligohydramnios.
    4. Dilation 2 cm.
    5. Transverse lie.

28. A nurse is caring for four clients on the labor and delivery unit. Which of the following actions should the nurse take first?
    1. Check the blood sugar of a gestational diabetic.
    2. Assess the vaginal blood loss of a client who is post–spontaneous abortion.
    3. Assess the patellar reflexes of a client with mild preeclampsia.
    4. Check the fetal heart rate of a client who just ruptured membranes.

29. A delirious patient is admitted to the hospital in labor. She has had no prenatal care and vials of crack cocaine are found in her pockets. The nurse monitors this client carefully for which of the following intrapartal complications?
    1. Prolonged labor.
    2. Prolapsed cord.
    3. Abruptio placentae.
    4. Retained placenta.

30. A known drug addict is in active labor. She requests pain medication. Which of the following actions by the nurse is appropriate?
    1. Encourage the woman to refrain from taking medication to protect the fetus.
    2. Notify the physician of her request.
    3. Advise the woman that she can receive only an epidural because of her history.
    4. Assist the woman to do labor breathing.

31. The nurse is caring for a laboring gravida who is 43 weeks pregnant. For which of the following should the nurse carefully monitor this client and fetus?
    1. Late decelerations.
    2. Hyperthermia.
    3. Hypotension.
    4. Early decelerations.

32. A woman, G3 P2002, is 6 cm dilated. The fetal monitor tracing shows recurring deep late decelerations. The woman's doctor informs her that the baby must be delivered by cesarean section. The woman refuses to sign the informed consent. Which of the following actions by the nurse is appropriate?
    1. Strongly encourage the woman to sign the informed consent.
    2. Prepare the woman for the cesarean section.
    3. Inform the woman that the baby will likely die without the surgery.
    4. Provide the woman with ongoing labor support.

33. Given the fetal heart rate pattern shown below, which of the following interventions should the nurse perform first?

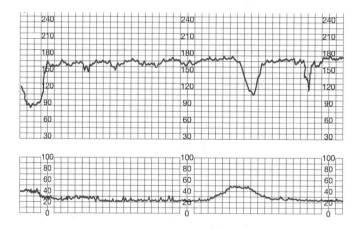

    1. Increase the intravenous drip rate.
    2. Apply oxygen by face mask.
    3. Turn the woman on her side.
    4. Report the tracing to the obstetrician.

34. Which of the tracings shown below would the nurse interpret as indicative of uteroplacental insufficiency?

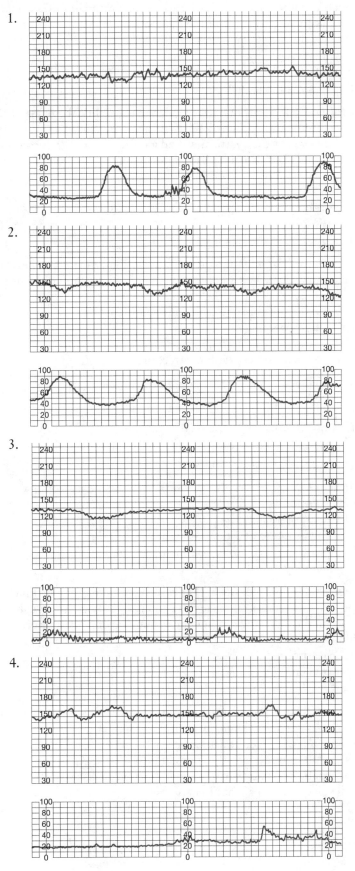

35. A client's assessments reveal that she is 4 cm dilated and 80% effaced with a fetal heart tracing showing frequent late decelerations and strong contractions every 3 minutes, each lasting 90 seconds. The nursing management of the client should be directed toward which of the following goals?
    1. Completion of the first stage of labor.
    2. Delivery of a healthy baby.
    3. Safe pain medication management.
    4. Prevention of a vaginal laceration.

36. When monitoring a fetal heart rate with moderate variability, the nurse notes V-shaped decelerations to 80 from a baseline of 120. One occurred during a contraction, another occurred 10 seconds after the contraction, and a third occurred 40 seconds after yet another contraction. The nurse interprets these findings as resulting from which of the following?
    1. Metabolic acidosis.
    2. Head compression.
    3. Cord compression.
    4. Insufficient uteroplacental blood flow.

37. A nurse notes a sinusoidal fetal heart pattern while analyzing a fetal heart tracing of a newly admitted client. Which of the following actions should the nurse take at this time?
    1. Encourage the client to breathe with contractions.
    2. Notify the practitioner.
    3. Increase the intravenous infusion.
    4. Encourage the client to push with contractions.

38. The results from a fetal blood sampling test are reported as pH 7.22. The nurse interprets the results as:
    1. The baby is severely acidotic.
    2. The baby must be delivered as soon as possible.
    3. The results are equivocal, warranting further sampling.
    4. The results are within normal limits.

39. A client is in active labor. Which of the following assessments would warrant immediate intervention?
    1. Maternal $PaCO_2$ of 40 mm Hg.
    2. Alpha-fetoprotein values of 2 times normal.
    3. 3 fetal heart accelerations during contractions.
    4. Fetal scalp sampling pH of 7.19.

40. A woman being induced with oxytocin (Pitocin) is contracting every 3 min × 30 seconds. Suddenly the woman becomes dypsneic and cyanotic, and begins to cough up bloody sputum. Which of the following nursing interventions is of highest priority?
    1. Check blood pressure.
    2. Assess fetal heart rate.
    3. Administer oxygen.
    4. Stop oxytocin infusion.

41. Which of the following is the appropriate nursing care outcome for a woman who suddenly develops an amniotic fluid embolism during her labor?
    1. Client will be infection free at discharge.
    2. Client will exhibit normal breathing function at discharge.
    3. Client will exhibit normal gastrointestinal function at discharge.
    4. Client will void without pain at discharge.

42. A laboring woman, who has developed an apparent amniotic fluid embolism, is not breathing and has no pulse. In addition to calling for assistance, which of the following actions by the nurse, who is alone with the patient, is appropriate at this time?
    1. Perform cardiac compressions and breaths in a 15 to 2 ratio.
    2. Provide chest compressions at a depth of at least 2 inches.
    3. Compress the chest at the lower ½ of the sternum.
    4. Provide rescue breaths over a 10-second time frame.

43. A 38-week-gestation woman is in labor and delivery with a painful, board-like abdomen and progressively larger serial girth measurements. Which of the following assessments is appropriate at this time?
    1. Fetal heart rate.
    2. Cervical dilation.
    3. White blood cell count.
    4. Maternal lung sounds.

44. The labor nurse has just received a shift report on four gravid patients. Which of the patients should the nurse assess first?
    1. G5 P2202, 32 weeks, placenta previa, today's hemoglobin 11.6 g/dL.
    2. G2 P0101, 39 weeks, type 2 diabetic, blood glucose (15 minutes ago) 85 mg/dL.
    3. G1 P0000, 32 weeks, placental abruption, fetal heart (15 minutes ago) 120 bpm.
    4. G2 P1001, 39 weeks, Rh-negative, today's hematocrit 31%.

45. Which of the following signs/symptoms would the nurse expect to see in a woman with abruptio placentae?
    1. Increasing fundal height measurements.
    2. Pain-free vaginal bleeding.
    3. Fetal heart accelerations.
    4. Hyperthermia with leukocytosis.

46. A nurse is caring for four laboring women. Which of the women will the nurse carefully monitor for signs of abruptio placentae?
    1. G2 P0010, 27 weeks' gestation.
    2. G3 P1101, 17 years of age.
    3. G4 P2101, cancer survivor.
    4. G5 P1211, cocaine abuser.

47. A labor nurse is caring for a client, 38 weeks' gestation, who has been diagnosed with symptomatic placenta previa. Which of the following physician orders should the nurse question?
    1. Begin oxytocin drip rate at 0.5 milliunits/min.
    2. Assess fetal heart rate every 10 minutes.
    3. Weigh all vaginal pads.
    4. Assess hematocrit and hemoglobin.

48. The doctor writes the following order for a 31-week-gravid client with symptomatic placenta previa: Weigh all vaginal pads and estimate blood loss. The nurse weighs one of the client's saturated pads at 24 grams and a dry pad at 4 grams. How many milliliters (mL) of blood can the nurse estimate the client has bled? **Calculate to the nearest whole number.**
    _____ mL.

49. A 29-week-gravid client is admitted to the labor and delivery unit with vaginal bleeding. To differentiate between placenta previa and abruptio placentae, the nurse should assess which of the following?
    1. Leopold's maneuver results.
    2. Quantity of vaginal bleeding.
    3. Presence of abdominal pain.
    4. Maternal blood pressure.

50. A client with a complete placenta previa is on the antepartum clinical unit in preparation for delivery. Which of the following should the nurse include in a teaching session for this client?
    1. Coughing and deep breathing.
    2. Phases of the first stage of labor.
    3. Lamaze labor techniques.
    4. Leboyer hydrobirthing.

51. An obstetrician declares at the conclusion of the third stage of labor that a woman is diagnosed with placenta accreta. The nurse would expect to see which of the following signs/symptoms?
    1. Hypertension.
    2. Hemorrhage.
    3. Bradycardia.
    4. Hyperthermia.

52. A labor nurse is caring for a client, 30 weeks' gestation, who is symptomatic from a complete placenta previa. Which of the following physician orders should the nurse question?
    1. Administer betamethasone (Celestone) 12 mg IM daily times 2.
    2. Maintain strict bed rest.
    3. Assess cervical dilation.
    4. Regulate intravenous (Ringer's lactate: drip rate to 150 mL/hr).

53. The nurse is monitoring a woman, G2 P1001, 41 weeks' gestation, in labor. A 12 p.m. assessment revealed: cervix, 4 cm; 80% effaced; −3 station; and FH 124 with moderate variability. A 5 p.m. assessment: cervix, 6 cm; 90% effaced; −3 station; and FH 120 with moderate variability. A 10 p.m. assessment: cervix, 8 cm; 100% effaced; −3 station; and FH 124 with moderate variability. Based on the assessments, which of the following should the nurse conclude?
    1. Labor is progressing well.
    2. The woman is likely carrying a macrosomic fetus.
    3. The baby is in fetal distress.
    4. The woman will be in second stage in about five hours.

54. After a multiparous woman has been in active labor for 15 hours, an ultrasound is done. The results state that the obstetric conjugate is 10 cm and the suboccipitobregmatic diameter is 10.5 cm. Which of the following labor findings is related to these results?
    1. Full dilation of the cervix.
    2. Full effacement of the cervix.
    3. Station of −3.
    4. Frequency every 5 minutes.

55. Which of the following situations is considered a vaginal delivery emergency?
    1. Third stage of labor lasting 20 minutes.
    2. Fetal heart dropping during contractions.
    3. Three-vessel cord.
    4. Shoulder dystocia.

56. During a vaginal delivery, the obstetrician declares that a shoulder dystocia has occurred. Which of the following actions by the nurse is appropriate at this time?
    1. Administer oxytocin intravenously per doctor's orders.
    2. Flex the woman's thighs sharply toward her abdomen.
    3. Apply oxygen using a tight-fitting face mask.
    4. Apply downward pressure on the woman's fundus.

57. The fetal monitor tracing of a laboring woman who is 9 cm dilated shows recurring late decelerations to 100 bpm. The nurse notes a moderate amount of greenish-colored amniotic fluid gush from the vagina after a practitioner performs an amniotomy. Which of the following nursing diagnoses is appropriate at this time?
    1. Risk for infection related to rupture of membranes.
    2. Risk for fetal injury related to possible intrauterine hypoxia.
    3. Risk for impaired tissue integrity related to vaginal irritation.
    4. Risk for maternal injury related to possible uterine rupture.

58. In which of the following clinical situations would it be appropriate for an obstetrician to order a labor nurse to perform amnioinfusion?
    1. Placental abruption.
    2. Meconium-stained fluid.
    3. Polyhydramnios.
    4. Late decelerations.

59. A nurse is monitoring a client who is receiving an amnioinfusion. Which of the following assessments is critical for the nurse to make to prevent a serious complication related to the procedure?
    1. Color of the amniotic fluid.
    2. Maternal blood pressure.
    3. Cervical effacement.
    4. Uterine resting tone.

60. During the delivery of a macrosomic baby, the woman develops a fourth-degree laceration. How should the nurse document the extent of the laceration in the woman's medical record?
    1. Into the musculature of the buttock.
    2. Through the urinary meatus.
    3. Through the rectal sphincter.
    4. Into the head of the clitoris.

61. Which of the following lab values should the nurse report to the physician as being consistent with the diagnosis of HELLP syndrome?
    1. Hematocrit 48%.
    2. Potassium 5.5 mEq/L.
    3. Platelets 75,000.
    4. Sodium 130 mEq/L.

62. A client who has been diagnosed with severe preeclampsia is being administered magnesium sulfate via IV pump. Which of the following medications must the nurse have immediately available in the client's room?
    1. Calcium gluconate.
    2. Morphine sulfate.
    3. Naloxone (Narcan).
    4. Meperidine (Demerol).

63. Which of the following physical findings would lead the nurse to suspect that a client with severe preeclampsia has developed HELLP syndrome? **Select all that apply.**
    1. +3 pitting edema.
    2. Petechiae.
    3. Jaundice.
    4. +4 deep tendon reflexes.
    5. Elevated specific gravity.

64. A client is on magnesium sulfate for severe preeclampsia. The nurse must notify the attending physician regarding which of the following findings?
    1. Patellar and biceps reflexes of +3.
    2. Urinary output of 30 mL/hr.
    3. Respiratory rate of 16 rpm.
    4. Serum magnesium level of 9 g/dL.

65. A woman with severe preeclampsia, 38 weeks' gestation, is being induced with IV oxytocin (Pitocin). Which of the following would warrant the nurse to stop the infusion?
    1. Blood pressure 160/110.
    2. Frequency of contractions every 3 minutes.
    3. Duration of contractions of 130 seconds.
    4. Fetal heart rate 156 with early decelerations.

66. A client is in labor and delivery with a diagnosis of HELLP syndrome. The nurse notes the following blood values:
    PT (prothrombin time)   99 sec (normal 60 to 85 sec).
    PTT (partial thromboplastin time)   30 sec (normal 11 to 15 sec).
    For which of the following signs/symptoms would the nurse monitor the client?
    1. Pink-tinged urine.
    2. Early decelerations.
    3. Patellar reflexes +1.
    4. Blood pressure 140/90.

67. The nurse is caring for an eclamptic client. Which of the following is an important action for the nurse to perform?
    1. Check each urine for presence of ketones.
    2. Pad the client's bed rails and headboard.
    3. Provide visual and auditory stimulation.
    4. Place the bed in the high Fowler's position.

68. A 40-week-gestation client has an admitting platelet count of 90,000 cells/mm^3 and a hematocrit of 29%. Her lab values 1 week earlier were platelet count 200,000 cells/mm^3 and hematocrit 37%. Which additional abnormal lab value would the nurse expect to see?
    1. Decreased serum creatinine level.
    2. Elevated red blood count (RBC).
    3. Decreased alkaline phosphatase.
    4. Elevated alanine transaminase (ALT).

69. A nurse administers magnesium sulfate via infusion pump to an eclamptic woman in labor. Which of the following outcomes indicates that the medication is effective?
    1. Client has no patellar reflex response.
    2. Urinary output is 30 mL/hr.
    3. Respiratory rate is 16 rpm.
    4. Client has no grand mal seizures.

70. A doctor orders a narcotic analgesic for a laboring client. Which of the following situations would lead a nurse to hold the medication?
    1. Contraction pattern is every 3 min × 60 sec.
    2. Fetal monitor tracing shows late decelerations.
    3. Client sleeps between contractions.
    4. The blood pressure is 150/90.

71. A client with an internal fetal monitor catheter in place has just received IV butorphanol (Stadol) for pain relief. Which of the following monitor tracing changes should the nurse anticipate?
    1. Early decelerations.
    2. Late decelerations.
    3. Diminished short- and long-term variability.
    4. Accelerations after contractions.

72. The nurse is caring for two post–cesarean section clients in the postanesthesia suite. One of the clients had her surgery under spinal anesthesia, while the other client had her surgery under epidural anesthesia. Which of the following is an important difference between the two types of anesthesia that the nurse should be aware of?
    1. The level of the pain relief is lower in spinals.
    2. Placement of the needle is higher in epidurals.
    3. Epidurals do not fully sedate motor nerves.
    4. Spinal clients complain of nausea and vomiting.

73. To reduce possible side effects from a cesarean section under general anesthesia, clients are routinely given which of the following medications?
    1. Antacids.
    2. Tranquilizers.
    3. Antihypertensives.
    4. Anticonvulsants.

74. During intubation, the anesthesiologist asks the nurse to apply cricoid pressure. Place an "X" on the location where the nurse should apply the pressure.

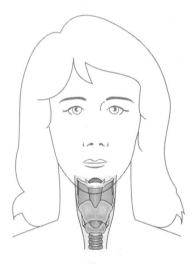

75. A physician has given a nurse a verbal order to apply cricoid pressure. Which of the following is the likely indication for the action?
    1. Forceps delivery.
    2. Endotracheal tube insertion.
    3. Epidural insertion.
    4. Third stage of labor.

76. The nurse identifies the following nursing diagnosis for a client undergoing an emergency cesarean section: Risk for ineffective individual coping related to emergency procedure. Which of the following nursing interventions would be appropriate in relation to this diagnosis?
    1. Apply antiembolic boots bilaterally.
    2. Explain all procedures slowly and carefully.
    3. Administer an antacid per MD orders.
    4. Monitor the FH and maternal vital signs.

77. A pregnant woman, G3 P2002, had her two other children by cesarean section. Which of the following situations would mandate that this delivery also be by cesarean?
    1. The woman refuses to have a regional anesthesia.
    2. The woman is postdates with intact membranes.
    3. The baby is in the occiput posterior position.
    4. The previous uterine incisions were vertical.

78. A woman in active labor received Nubain (nalbuphine hydrochloride) 14 mg IV for pain relief. One half hour later her respirations are 8 rpm. The nurse reports the respiratory rate to the physician. Which of the following medications would be appropriate for the physician to order at this time?
    1. Narcan (naloxone).
    2. Reglan (metoclopramide).
    3. Benadryl (diphenhydramine).
    4. Vistaril (hydroxyzine).

79. The nurse is assisting in the delivery of a baby via vacuum extraction. Which of the following nursing diagnoses for the gravida is appropriate at this time?
    1. Risk for impaired skin integrity.
    2. Risk for body image disturbance.
    3. Risk for impaired parenting.
    4. Risk for ineffective sexuality pattern.

80. An anesthesiologist informs the nurse that a woman scheduled for cesarean section will have the procedure under general anesthesia with postoperative patient-controlled analgesia rather than under continuous epidural infusion. Which of the following would warrant this decision?
    1. The woman has a history of drug addiction.
    2. The woman is allergic to morphine sulfate.
    3. The woman is a thirteen-year-old adolescent.
    4. The woman has had surgery for scoliosis.

81. A woman is delivering a macrosomic baby. The midwife is performing a mediolateral episiotomy. Draw a line where the episiotomy is being performed.

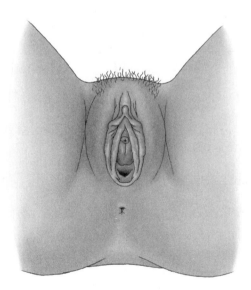

82. The nurse is admitting four full-term primigravid clients to the labor and delivery unit. The nurse requests pre–cesarean section orders from the health care practitioner for which of the clients? The client who has: **Select all that apply.**
    1. Cervical cerclage.
    2. FH 156 with beat-to-beat variability.
    3. Maternal blood pressure of 90/60.
    4. Full effacement.
    5. Active herpes simplex 2

83. A woman has been in the second stage of labor for 2½ hours. The fetal head is at +4 station and the fetal heart is showing mild late decelerations. The obstetrician advises the woman that the baby will be delivered with forceps. Which of the following actions should the nurse take at this time?
    1. Obtain a consent for the use of forceps.
    2. Encourage the woman to push between contractions.
    3. Assess the fetal heart rate after each contraction.
    4. Advise the woman to refuse the use of forceps.

84. The nurse is caring for four women who are in labor. The nurse is aware that he or she will likely prepare which of the women for cesarean delivery? **Select all that apply.**
    1. Fetus is in the left sacral posterior position.
    2. Placenta is attached to the posterior portion of the uterine wall.
    3. Fetus has been diagnosed with meningomyelocele.
    4. Client is hepatitis B surface antigen positive.
    5. The lecithin/sphingomyelin ratio in the amniotic fluid is 1.5:1.

85. Which of the following situations in a fully dilated client is incompatible with a forceps delivery? **Select all that apply.**
    1. Maternal history of asthma.
    2. Right occiput posterior position at +4 station.
    3. Transverse fetal lie.
    4. Fetal heart rate of 60 beats per minute at –1 station.
    5. Maternal history of cerebral palsy.

86. A client had an epidural inserted 2 hours ago. It is functioning well, the client is hemodynamically stable, and the client's labor is progressing as expected. Which of the following assessments is highest priority at this time?
    1. Assess blood pressure every 15 minutes.
    2. Assess pulse rate every 1 hour.
    3. Palpate bladder.
    4. Auscultate lungs.

87. A baby is entering the pelvis in the vertex presentation and in the extended attitude. The nurse determines that which of the following positions is consistent with this situation?
    1. LMA (left mentum anterior).
    2. LSP (left sacral posterior).
    3. RScT (right scapular transverse).
    4. ROP (right occiput posterior).

88. A woman is scheduled to have an external version for a breech presentation. The nurse carefully assesses the client's chart knowing that which of the following is a contraindication to this procedure?
    1. Station –2.
    2. 38 weeks' gestation.
    3. Reactive NST.
    4. Previous cesarean section.

89. A client is scheduled for an external version. The nurse would expect to prepare which of the following medications to be administered prior to the procedure?
    1. Oxytocin (Pitocin).
    2. Ergonovine (Methergine).
    3. Betamethasone (Celestone).
    4. Terbutaline (Brethine).

90. A physician has notified the labor and delivery suite that four clients will be admitted to the unit. The client with which of the following clinical findings would be a candidate for an external version?
    1. +3 station.
    2. Left sacral posterior position.
    3. Flexed attitude.
    4. Rupture of membranes for 24 hours.

91. A client, G3 P2002, is immediately postexternal version. The nurse monitors this client carefully for which of the following?
    1. Decreased urinary output.
    2. Elevated blood pressure.
    3. Severe occipital headache.
    4. Variable fetal heart decelerations.

92. A woman, 32 weeks' gestation, contracting every 3 min × 60 sec, is receiving magnesium sulfate. For which of the following maternal assessments is it critical for the nurse to monitor the client?
    1. Low urinary output.
    2. Temperature elevation.
    3. Absent pedal pulses.
    4. Retinal edema.

93. A nurse is caring for a gravid client who is G1 P0000, 35 weeks' gestation. Which of the following would warrant the nurse to notify the woman's health care practitioner that the client is in preterm labor? **Select all that apply.**
    1. Contraction frequency every 15 minutes.
    2. Effacement 10%.
    3. Dilation 3 cm.
    4. Cervical length of 2 cm.
    5. Contraction duration of 30 seconds.

94. The nurse in the obstetrician's office is caring for four 25-week-gestation prenatal clients who are carrying singleton pregnancies. With which of the following clients should the nurse carefully review the signs and symptoms of preterm labor (PTL)? **Select all that apply.**
    1. 38-year-old in an abusive relationship.
    2. 34-year-old whose first child was born at 32 weeks' gestation.
    3. 30-year-old whose baby has a two-vessel cord.
    4. 26-year-old with a history of long menstrual periods.
    5. 22-year-old who smokes 2 packs of cigarettes every day.

95. The nurse is caring for a 30-week-gestation client whose fetal fibronectin (fFN) levels are positive. It is essential that she be taught about which of the following?
    1. How to use a blood glucose monitor.
    2. Signs of preterm labor.
    3. Signs of preeclampsia.
    4. How to do fetal kick count assessments.

96. A 28-week-gestation client with intact membranes is admitted with the following findings: Contractions every 5 min × 60 sec, 3 cm dilated, 80% effaced. Which of the following medications will the obstetrician likely order?
    1. Oxytocin (Pitocin).
    2. Ergonovine (Methergine).
    3. Magnesium sulfate.
    4. Morphine sulfate.

97. Three 30-week-gestation clients are on the labor and delivery unit in preterm labor. For which of the clients should the nurse question a doctor's order for beta agonist tocolytics?
    1. A client with hypothyroidism.
    2. A client with breast cancer.
    3. A client with cardiac disease.
    4. A client with asthma.

98. A client is receiving terbutaline (Brethine) for preterm labor. Which of the following findings would warrant stopping the infusion? **Select all that apply.**
    1. Change in contraction pattern from q 3 min × 90 sec to q 2 min × 60 sec.
    2. Change in fetal heart pattern from no decelerations to early decelerations.
    3. Change in beat-to-beat variability from minimal to moderate.
    4. Change in fetal heart rate from 160 bpm to 210 bpm.
    5. Change in the amniotic sac from intact to ruptured.

99. A client is on terbutaline (Brethine) via subcutaneous pump for preterm labor. The nurse auscultates the fetal heart rate at 100 beats per minute via Doppler. Which of the following actions should the nurse perform next?
    1. Assess the maternal pulse while listening to the fetal heart rate.
    2. Notify the health care provider.
    3. Stop the terbutaline infusion.
    4. Administer oxygen to the mother via face mask.

100. A preterm labor client, 30 weeks' gestation, who ruptured membranes 4 hours ago, is being given IM dexamethasone (Decadron). When she asks why she is receiving the drug, the nurse replies:
    1. "To help to stop your labor contractions."
    2. "To prevent an infection in your uterus."
    3. "To help to mature your baby's lungs."
    4. "To decrease the pain from the contractions."

101. An insulin-dependent diabetic is in active labor. The physician has written the following order: Administer regular insulin 5 units per hour via IV pump. The insulin has been diluted as follows: 50 units/500 mL normal saline. At what rate should the nurse set the pump? **Please calculate to the nearest whole number.**
    _____ mL/hr.

102. A 30-year-old G2 P0010 in preterm labor is receiving nifedipine (Procardia). Which of the following maternal assessments noted by the nurse must be reported to the health care practitioner immediately?
    1. Heart rate of 100 bpm.
    2. Wakefulness.
    3. Audible rales.
    4. Daily output of 2,000 mL.

103. A woman, G3 P2002, 42 weeks' gestation, is admitted to the labor suite for induction. A biophysical profile (BPP) report on the client's chart states BPP score of 6 of 10. The nurse should monitor this client carefully for which of the following?
    1. Maternal hypertension.
    2. Maternal hyperglycemia.
    3. Increased fetal heart variability.
    4. Late fetal heart decelerations.

104. The health care practitioner performed an amniotomy 5 minutes ago on a client, G3 P1011, 40 weeks' gestation, –4 station, and ROP position. The fetal heart rate is 140 with variable decelerations. The fluid is green tinged and smells musty. The nurse concludes that which of the following situations is present at this time?
    1. The fetus is post-term.
    2. The presentation is breech.
    3. The cord is prolapsed.
    4. The amniotic fluid is infected.

105. The nurse is assessing the Bishop score on a postdates client. Which of the following measurements will the nurse assess? **Select all that apply.**
    1. Gestational age.
    2. Rupture of membranes.
    3. Cervical dilation.
    4. Fetal station.
    5. Cervical position.

106. The nurse is admitting a 38-week-gestation client in labor. The nurse is unable to find the fetal heartbeat with a Doppler. Which of the following comments by the nurse would indicate that the nurse is in denial?
    1. "I'll keep trying until I find the heartbeat."
    2. "I am sure it is the machine. If I change the battery, I'm sure it will work."
    3. "I am so sorry. I am not able to find your baby's heartbeat."
    4. "Sometimes I really hate these machines."

107. A client with a fetal demise is admitted to labor and delivery in the latent phase of labor. Which of the following behaviors would the nurse expect this client to exhibit?
    1. Crying and sad.
    2. Talkative and excited.
    3. Quietly doing rapid breathing.
    4. Loudly chanting songs.

108. A physician writes the following order—Administer ampicillin 1 g IV q 4 h until delivery—for a newly admitted laboring client with ruptured membranes. The client had positive vaginal and rectal cultures for group B streptococcal bacteria at 36 weeks' gestation. Which of the following is a rationale for this order?
    1. The client is at high risk for chorioamnionitis.
    2. The baby is at high risk for neonatal sepsis.
    3. The bacterium is sexually transmitted.
    4. The bacterium causes puerperal sepsis.

109. A client, 42 weeks' gestation, is admitted to the labor and delivery suite with a diagnosis of acute oligohydramnios. The nurse must carefully observe this client for signs of which of the following?
    1. Fetal distress.
    2. Dehydration.
    3. Oliguria.
    4. Jaundice.

110. A nurse has been assigned to circulate during the cesarean section of triplets. Which of the following actions should the nurse take before the birth of the babies? **Select all that apply.**
    1. Count the number of sterile sponges.
    2. Document the time of the first incision.
    3. Notify the pediatric staff.
    4. Perform a sterile scrub.
    5. Assemble the sterile instruments.

111. A client enters the labor and delivery suite. It is essential that the nurse note the woman's status in relation to which of the following infectious diseases? **Select all that apply.**
    1. Hepatitis B.
    2. Rubeola.
    3. Varicella.
    4. Group B streptococcus.
    5. HIV/AIDS.

The correct answer number and rationale for why it is the correct answer are given in **boldface blue type**. Rationales for why the other possible answer options are incorrect also are given, but they are not in boldface type.

1. 1. **These are the classic signs of water intoxication.**
   2. With water intoxication, the woman would show signs of hyponatremia and hypokalemia.
   3. Thrombocytopenia and neutropenia are unrelated to water intoxication.
   4. Paresthesias, myalgias, and anemia are unrelated to water intoxication.

   TEST-TAKING TIP: Clients who receive oxytocin over a long period of time are at high risk for water intoxication. The oxytocin molecule is similar in structure to the antidiuretic hormone (ADH) molecule. The body retains fluids in response to the medication much the same way it would in response to ADH. The nurse, therefore, should carefully monitor intake and output when clients are induced with oxytocin.

2. 1. **Induction is contraindicated in transverse lie.**
   2. When indicated, it is safe to induce a woman with cerebral palsy.
   3. When indicated, it is safe to induce a pregnant adolescent.
   4. When indicated, it is safe to induce a woman with diabetes mellitus.

   TEST-TAKING TIP: A baby in the transverse lie is in a scapular presentation. The baby is incapable of being birthed vaginally. Whenever a vaginal birth is contraindicated, induction is also contraindicated.

3. 1. **Whenever there is marked fetal bradycardia and oxytocin is running, the nurse should immediately turn off the oxytocin drip.**
   2. Oxygen should be administered, but the mask should be put on after the oxytocin has been turned off.
   3. Repositioning is indicated, but should be performed after the oxytocin has been turned off.
   4. The obstetrician should be called, but after the oxytocin has been turned off.

   TEST-TAKING TIP: Oxytocin stimulates the contractility of the uterine muscle. When the muscle is contracted, the blood flow to

the placenta is reduced. Whenever there is evidence of fetal compromise and oxytocin is being infused, the intravenous should be stopped immediately to maximize placental perfusion.

4. 1. As long as oxytocin is increased slowly and the contraction pattern and fetal response are monitored carefully, there is no absolute, unsafe maximum dosage of oxytocin.
   2. **The practitioner should increase the dosage of oxytocin at a minimum time interval of every 30 minutes.**
   3. Although postdates babies are higher risk for fetal distress, it is not contraindicated to induce with oxytocin.
   4. A 60-second contraction duration is normal.

   TEST-TAKING TIP: The half-life (the time it takes half of a medication to be metabolized by the body) of oxytocin is relatively long—about 15 minutes. And at least 3 half-lives usually elapse before therapeutic responses are noted. Increasing the infusion rate too rapidly, therefore, can lead to hyperstimulation of the uterine muscle and consequent fetal distress.

5. 1. **A common side effect of Cytotec is diarrhea and labor contractions are often first felt in the back.**
   2. Hypothermia and rectal pain are not associated with Cytotec administration.
   3. Urinary retention and rash are not associated with Cytotec administration.
   4. Tinnitus and respiratory distress are not associated with Cytotec administration.

   TEST-TAKING TIP: Cytotec (misoprostol) is a synthetic prostaglandin medication used to ripen the cervix for induction. Gastrointestinal side effects are commonly seen when prostaglandin is used, because the gastrointestinal system is adjacent to the vagina where the medication is inserted. In addition, the nurse must be watchful for signs of labor.

6. 1. The infusion should be maintained.
   2. There is no indication for oxygen at this time.
   3. If she is comfortable, there is no need to change her position.
   4. **It is appropriate to monitor the woman's labor.**

   TEST-TAKING TIP: Even if the test taker were unfamiliar with a normal contraction pattern—as seen in the stem of the question—if he or she knew that the fetal heart pattern is normal, he or she could deduce the correct answer. Three of the responses infer that the nurse should take action because of a complication. Only response 4 indicates that the nurse should continue monitoring the labor. In this situation, the one response that is different from the others is the correct answer.

7. 1. Prepidil is not administered intravenously
   2. Prepidil is not administered orally.
   3. Prepidil is administered endocervically.
   4. Prepidil is not administered intrathecally.

   TEST-TAKING TIP: Prostaglandins, hormone-like substances that mediate a wide range of physiological functions, do so locally. Prepidil, therefore, is administered adjacent to the cervix where it acts to soften the cervix in preparation for dilation and effacement.

8. 3 mL/hr.

   TEST-TAKING TIP: The nurse must do a number of calculations to determine the pump drip rate in this client. First, the nurse must determine how many milliunits are in 1,000 mL of fluid:

   10 units in 1,000 mL

   = 10,000 milliunits in 1,000 mL

   Next, the nurse must determine how many milliunits are to be infused per hour (because pumps are always calibrated mL/hour):

   0.5 millliunits per minute

   = 30 milliunits per 60 minutes

   Finally, the nurse must do a ratio and proportion to determine the mL per hour:

   10,000 milliunits/1000 mL

   = 30 milliunits/x mL

   x = 3 mL/hr

9. 1. Uterine hyperstimulation can be seen with moderate intensities.
   2. A frequency pattern of every 3 minutes is ideal.
   3. A duration of 130 seconds is indicative of tachysystole.
   4. The attitude of the baby has nothing to do with hyperstimulation.

TEST-TAKING TIP: This question is asking the test taker to evaluate an expected outcome. When a nurse intervenes, he or she is expecting a positive outcome. In this situation, the nurse is determining whether or not the action has reversed the hyperstimulation that developed from oxytocin administration. The normal contraction frequency is evidence of a positive outcome.

10. 1. The pulse rate has likely increased because the woman is working with her labor. It is not an indication to turn off the oxytocin.
    2. The baseline fetal heart rate has dropped over 20 bpm. This finding warrants that the oxytocin be stopped.
    3. Hypertension is not an indication to stop oxytocin administration.
    4. Hyperthermia is not an indication to stop oxytocin administration.

    TEST-TAKING TIP: The test taker must determine which of the vital signs is unsafe in the presence of oxytocin. Oxytocin increases the contractility of the uterine muscle. When the muscle contracts, the blood supply to the fetus is diminished. A drop in fetal heart rate, therefore, is indicative of poor oxygenation to the fetus and is unsafe in the presence of oxytocin.

11. 1. There is no indication in the scenario that the membranes have ruptured.
    2. The Bishop score is expected to rise when Cervidil is administered.
    3. There is no sign of distress in the scenario; therefore, a change in position is unnecessary.
    4. The nurse should monitor this client for the onset of labor.

    TEST-TAKING TIP: The Bishop score indicates the inducibility of the cervix of a client. Five signs are assessed—cervical position, cervical dilation, cervical effacement, cervical station, and cervical consistency. A total score is calculated. A primigravid cervix is considered inducible when the Bishop score is 9 or higher. A multigravid cervix is considered inducible when the Bishop score is 5 or higher.

Prelabor Status Evaluation Scoring System

	Score			
	0	1	2	3
Cervical position	Posterior	Midposition	Anterior	—
Cervical consistency	Firm	Medium	Soft	—
Cervical effacement (%)	0–30	40–50	60–70	≥0
Cervical dilation (cm)	Closed	1–2	3–4	≥5
Fetal station	−3	−2	−1	+1/+2

Adapted from Bishop, E.H. (1964). Pelvic scoring for elective induction. *Obstetrics & Gynecology, 24*, 266.

12. 1. A primipara with a Bishop score of 4 is not inducible with oxytocin. Prepidil helps to improve cervical readiness for an oxytocin induction.
    2. This client's fetus is already showing signs of fetal distress. Induction increases the risk of fetal injury.
    3. This woman's contractions are not effective. The medicine may help to promote more effective labor.
    4. Neither a high gravidity nor an elevated blood pressure is a contraindication to Prepidil administration.

    TEST-TAKING TIP: It is important to remember that although the fetus of a pregnant woman may be at term, it is not always safe for labor contractions to be stimulated. Although Prepidil is not directly used for induction, it is an agent that promotes cervical ripening in preparation for labor. A baby who is exhibiting signs of poor uteroplacental blood flow is likely to be compromised further by the addition of the medication.

13. 1. The expected outcome from the administration of Cervidil is an increase in the Bishop score.
    2. A fetal heart rate of 152 is within normal limits and not significantly different from the original baseline of 156.
    3. A respiratory rate of 24 is not a contraindication to the administration of prostaglandins for cervical ripening.
    4. A contraction frequency of 1 minute, even with a short duration, would warrant the removal of the medication.

    TEST-TAKING TIP: A frequency of 1 minute, even if the duration were 30 seconds, would mean that there were only 30 seconds when the uterine muscle was relaxed. This short amount of time would not provide the placenta with enough time to be sufficiently perfused. Fetal bradycardia is a likely outcome to such a short frequency period.

14. 1. Although this teenager has had two abortions, she is not markedly at high risk for uterine rupture.
    2. A primigravida with eclampsia is not markedly at high risk for uterine rupture.
    3. A woman, no matter what her age, who has had a previous cesarean section is at risk for uterine rupture.
    4. A woman who has a history of fetal death is not markedly at high risk for uterine rupture.

    TEST-TAKING TIP: When babies are birthed via cesarean section, the surgeon must create an incision through the uterine body. The muscles of the uterus have, therefore, been ligated and a scar has formed at the incision site. Scars are not elastic and do not contract and relax the way muscle tissue does. A vaginal birth after cesarean (VBAC) section can be performed only if the woman had a low flap (Pfannenstiel) incision in the uterus during her previous cesarean section.

15. 1. Frequency and duration are important, but they are not the highest priority at this time.
    2. Maternal temperature is the highest priority.
    3. Cervical change is important, but it is not the highest priority at this time.
    4. Maternal pulse rate is important, but it is not the highest priority at this time.

    TEST-TAKING TIP: The test taker must remember that the uterine cavity is a sterile space and the vaginal vault is an unsterile space. When membranes have ruptured over 24 hours, there is potential for pathogens to ascend into the uterine cavity and infection to result. Elevated temperature is a sign of infection.

16. 1. It is unlikely that the woman has a distended bladder.
2. Although the woman may have a UTI, an order is needed for a urine culture. This is not the first action that the nurse should take.
3. The fluid should be assessed with nitrazine paper.
4. This action is not a priority at this time.

TEST-TAKING TIP: Nitrazine paper is another name for litmus paper. It detects the pH of fluid. Amniotic fluid is alkaline, whereas urine is acidic. If the paper turns a dark blue, the nurse can conclude that the membranes have ruptured and that the woman is leaking amniotic fluid.

17. 1. Oxygen administered during labor should be delivered via a tight-fitting mask at 8 to 10 liters per minute.
2. The client should be positioned on her side or in Trendelenburg position.
3. The best way to monitor the fetus is with an internal electrode.
4. Increasing the IV rate helps to improve perfusion to the placenta.

TEST-TAKING TIP: Because the fetus is being oxygenated via the placenta, it is essential that in cases of fetal distress, the amount of oxygen perfusing the placenta be maximized. That requires high concentrations of oxygen being administered via mask, blood volume being increased by increasing the IV drip rate, and cardiac blood return being maximized by positioning the client to remove pressure from the aorta and the vena cava.

18. 3 and 4 are correct.
1. The transition phase is an excellent time to use hydrotherapy.
2. Many women do push during second stage in the water bath.
3. Women undergoing induction should not labor in a water bath. During induction, the fetus should be monitored continually by electronic fetal monitoring.
4. Meconium-stained amniotic fluid may indicate fetal distress. Continuous electronic fetal monitoring would, therefore, be indicated.

5. A posterior fetal position is not a contraindication for the use of a water bath.

TEST-TAKING TIP: Hydrotherapy is an excellent complementary therapy for the laboring woman. The warm water is relaxing and many women find that their pain is minimized. Induction and continuous electronic fetal monitoring, however, are incompatible with the intervention.

19. 1. Intermittent fetal heart auscultation is appropriate at this time.
2. Vaginal examination is contraindicated.
3. Intravenous fluid administration is appropriate at this time.
4. Nipple stimulation is appropriate at this time.

TEST-TAKING TIP: The client in this scenario is at risk of an ascending infection from the vagina to the uterine body because she has prolonged rupture of membranes. Any time a vaginal examination is performed, the chance of infection rises. Nipple stimulation is appropriate because endogenous oxytocin will be released, which would augment the client's weak labor pattern.

20. 1. Human papillomavirus is not an indication for cesarean section.
2. Standard precautions are indicated in this situation.
3. A baby born to a woman with HPV receives standard care in the well-baby nursery.
4. HPV is not airborne. A mask is not required.

TEST-TAKING TIP: Although HPV is a sexually transmitted infection and it can in rare instances be contracted by the neonate from the mother, the Centers for Disease Control and Prevention do not recommend that cesarean section be performed merely to prevent vertical transmission of HPV (see http://www.cdc.gov/std/HPV/STD-Fact-HPV.htm).

21. 1. This comment is inappropriate. The nurse should ask the woman whether or not she has felt fetal movement.
2. The amniotic fluid smells musty but it does not naturally have an offensive smell.
3. This statement is likely true but the nurse should ask the woman whether or not she has felt fetal movement and the woman should be advised to go to the hospital for evaluation.
4. The most important information needed by the nurse should relate to

the health and well-being of the fetus. Fetal movement indicates that the baby is alive.

TEST-TAKING TIP: There are two concerns in this scenario: the fact that the membranes just ruptured and the smell of the fluid. The nurse should, therefore, consider two possible problems: possible prolapsed cord, which may occur as a result of the rupture of the amniotic sac, and possible infection, which may be indicated by the smell. Normal fetal movement will give the nurse some confidence that the cord is not prolapsed. This is the first question that should be asked. Then, the client should be encouraged to go to the hospital to be assessed for possible infection and signs of labor.

22. 1. Candidiasis is not an indication for cesarean section.
    2. *Candida* is a fungus. Antibiotics do not treat this problem.
    3. Thrush is the term given to oral candidiasis, which the baby may develop after delivery.
    4. There is no need to isolate a baby born to a woman with candidiasis.

TEST-TAKING TIP: *Candida* can be transmitted to a baby during delivery as well as postdelivery via the mother's hands. Initially, the baby will develop thrush, but eventually the mother may notice a bright pink diaper rash on the baby. Also, if she is breastfeeding her baby, she may develop a yeast infection of the breast that is very painful. The mother with candidiasis should be advised to wash her hands carefully after toileting.

23. 1. Cesarean delivery is not recommended for women who are hepatitis B positive.
    2. Ampicillin is ineffective against hepatitis B, which is a virus. Ampicillin may be administered to women who have group B strep vaginal or rectal cultures.
    3. Within 12 hours of birth, the baby should receive both the first injection of hepatitis B vaccine and HBIG.
    4. Babies born to women who are hepatitis B–surface antigen positive are cared for in the well-baby nursery. No isolation is needed.

TEST-TAKING TIP: Although this is a woman who is in labor, the nurse must anticipate the needs of the neonate after delivery. Because it is recommended that the baby

receive the medication within a restricted time frame, it is especially important for the nurse to be proactive and obtain the physician's order (see http://www.cdc.gov/hepatitis/HBV/PDFs/DeliveryHospitalPreventPerinatalHBVTransmission.pdf).

24. 1. It is appropriate for the nurse to assess the client's dilation and effacement.
    2. Surgical delivery is not indicated by the scenario.
    3. There is no reason to place the client in the Trendelenburg position.
    4. There is no indication that a BPP has been performed.

TEST-TAKING TIP: Although cesarean deliveries are recommended to be performed when a client has an active case of herpes simplex, surgical delivery is not indicated when no lesions are present. Clients who have histories of herpes with no current outbreak, therefore, are considered to be healthy laboring clients who may deliver vaginally (see http://www.cdc.gov/std/treatment/2006/specialpops.htm#specialpops1).

25. 1. There are no signs of placenta abruption in this scenario.
    2. The woman has not seized. She is not eclamptic.
    3. The drop in fetal heart rate with variable decelerations indicates that the cord has likely prolapsed.
    4. There are no signs that this client has a succenturiate placenta.

TEST-TAKING TIP: The test taker must remember that variable decelerations are caused by cord compression. The fact that variables are seen in the scenario as well as a precipitous drop in the fetal heart baseline is an indirect indication that the cord is being compressed, resulting in decreased oxygenation to the fetus.

26. 1. The first action the nurse should take is to place the woman in the knee-chest position.
    2. The nurse should assess the fetal heart rate, but this is not the first action.
    3. Oxygen should be administered, but this is not the first action.
    4. The physician should be advised, but this is not the first action.

TEST-TAKING TIP: The weight of the fetus on the prolapsed cord can rapidly result in fetal death. Therefore, the nurse must act quickly to relieve the pressure on the cord. Additional actions that can take pressure off the cord are placing the client in the Trendelenburg position and pushing the head off the cord with a gloved hand. This situation is an obstetric emergency.

27. 1, 2, and 5 are correct.
 1. When a baby is in the breech presentation, there is increased risk of prolapsed cord.
 2. The presenting part is floating, which increases the risk of prolapsed cord.
 3. With decreased quantity of amniotic fluid there is no increased risk of prolapsed cord.
 4. 2-cm dilation is not a situation that is at high risk for prolapsed cord.
 5. When a baby is in the transverse lie, there is increased risk for prolapsed cord.

TEST-TAKING TIP: Once the membranes have ruptured, there are several situations that can increase the possibility of the cord prolapsing, i.e., when the cord slips past the baby and becomes the presenting part. The baby then compresses the cord, preventing the baby from being oxygenated. The situations include malpresentations, like breech and shoulder presentations. A shoulder presentation is the same as a transverse lie. Additional situations that are at high risk for cord prolapse are hydramnios, premature rupture of membranes, and negative fetal station.

28. 1. Although the blood glucose of a client with diabetes is important, it can wait.
 2. Although the vaginal blood loss assessment of a client who has had a spontaneous abortion is important, it is usually minimal. This client can wait.
 3. It is important to assess the patellar reflexes of a client with preeclampsia, but with mild disease, that action can wait.
 4. The priority action for this nurse is to assess the fetal heart rate of a client who has just ruptured membranes. The nurse is assessing for prolapsed cord, which is an obstetric emergency.

TEST-TAKING TIP: Identifying the priority action is the most difficult thing that nurses must do. The nurse must determine which of the situations is most life threatening. Of the four choices above, prolapsed cord is life threatening to the fetus. None of the other situations, as stated in the question, is life threatening to either the mother or the fetus.

29. 1. Prolonged labor is not associated with maternal illicit drug use.
 2. Prolapsed cord is not associated with maternal illicit drug use.
 3. Placental abruption is associated with maternal illicit drug use.
 4. Retained placenta is not associated with maternal illicit drug use.

TEST-TAKING TIP: Crack cocaine is a powerful vasoconstrictive agent. The chorionic villi atrophy as a result of the vasoconstrictive effects of the drug. Placental abruption, when the placenta detaches from the decidual lining of the uterus, is therefore of particular concern.

30. 1. It is inappropriate to discourage a laboring client from taking pain medication simply because she has abused drugs.
 2. The nurse should notify the health care practitioner of the client's request.
 3. Substance abuse is not a contraindication for analgesic medication in labor.
 4. Although the client may benefit from labor breathing, she has requested pain medication and that request should be acted upon.

TEST-TAKING TIP: The test taker should be aware of two important facts: Pain is the fifth vital sign as identified by The Joint Commission, and actions must be taken to reduce drug abusers' pain in the same manner that non–drug abusers' pain is managed. Although it is strongly discouraged for women to take illicit drugs when pregnant, the nurse must maintain his or her caring philosophy and provide unbiased care to addicted clients.

31. 1. This baby is high risk for the development of late fetal heart decelerations.
 2. Based on the scenario, neither mother nor baby is at high risk for hyperthermia.
 3. Based on the scenario, neither mother nor baby is at high risk for hypertension.
 4. Early decelerations are normal. They are usually seen during transition and stage 2.

TEST-TAKING TIP: The test taker must attend to all important information in the question. The gestational age of this fetus is 43 weeks. The baby and placenta, therefore, are both postdates. Placental function usually deteriorates after 40 weeks' gestation. As late decelerations result from poor uteroplacental blood flow, the nurse should monitor this client carefully for late decelerations.

32. 1. The woman does have a legal right not to sign the form. To badger her about her decision is inappropriate.
    2. Practitioners who perform surgery on a client who has refused to sign a consent form can be arrested for assault and battery.
    3. It is inappropriate to scare a patient into submission.
    4. At this point the appropriate action for the nurse to take is to continue providing labor support. If accepted, emergency interventions, like providing oxygen by face mask and repositioning the client, would also be indicated.

TEST-TAKING TIP: If the client's practitioner is convinced that surgery is the only appropriate intervention, he or she could get a court order to mandate the woman to accept surgery. The nurse's role at this point, however, is to provide the client with care in a nonthreatening, compassionate manner. The nurse must acknowledge and accept the client's legal right to refuse the surgery.

33. 1. Increasing the IV rate is appropriate, but it is not the first action that should be taken.
    2. Applying oxygen via face mask is appropriate, but it is not the first action that should be taken.
    3. Repositioning the woman is the first action that should be taken.
    4. Although the decelerations should be reported to the health care practitioner, this is not the first action that should be taken.

TEST-TAKING TIP: To answer this question, the test taker must fully understand the etiology of the decelerations. Variable decelerations occur as a result of umbilical cord compression. It is possible, therefore, that if the mother is positioned differently, the pressure will be shifted and the decelerations will resolve. If the first position change does not resolve the problem, the nurse should try additional position changes. It is also important for the nurse to do all that he or she can to resolve the problem—by administering oxygen and increasing the IV drip rate—before calling the physician. To do otherwise could constitute patient abandonment.

34. 1. This monitor tracing shows a variable fetal heart baseline. This is a tracing of a well-oxygenated fetus.
    2. This monitor tracing shows a variable fetal heart baseline with early decelerations.

Early decelerations are related to head compression. This is a normal finding during transition and stage 2 of labor.
    3. This monitor tracing shows a fetal heart baseline with minimal variability and with late decelerations. These decelerations are related to uteroplacental insufficiency.
    4. This monitor tracing shows a variable fetal heart baseline with accelerations. This depicts a well-oxygenated fetus.

TEST-TAKING TIP: A tracing that depicts decelerations that begin late in a contraction and return to baseline well past the time that the contraction ends are called late decelerations. Late decelerations are related to poor uteroplacental blood flow.

35. 1. This client is only 4 cm dilated. Unless the late decelerations resolve, completion of stage 1 is not a priority.
    2. The nurse's goal at this point must be the delivery of a healthy baby.
    3. Because late decelerations are present, pain management is not a priority at this time.
    4. Unless the late decelerations resolve, this client may not deliver vaginally.

TEST-TAKING TIP: Nursing goals may change repeatedly during a client's labor. The nurse must assess the woman's progress in relation to the health and well-being of the fetus. As long as the baby is responding well, the nurse's focus should relate to maternal comfort and care. Once fetal compromise is noted, however, nursing actions often shift.

36. 1. Diminished variability is an indication of fetal acidosis.
    2. Decelerations related to head compression mirror contractions and occur at the same time as the contractions (early decelerations).
    3. The contractions described in the scenario result from cord compression (variable decelerations).
    4. Decelerations related to uteroplacental insufficiency mirror contractions but begin late in the contraction and return to baseline after the contraction ends (late decelerations).

TEST-TAKING TIP: First, the test taker should be able to interpret fetal heart tracings both visually and verbally. This includes baseline data as well as acceleration and deceleration changes. Second, the test taker should know the

etiology of each of the tracings. Third, the test taker should know the appropriate nursing intervention related to each tracing.

37. 1. Although breathing with contractions is important, the nurse must notify the practitioner as soon as possible.
2. Sinusoidal patterns are related to Rh isoimmunization, fetal anemia, severe fetal hypoxia, or a chronic fetal bleed. They also may occur transiently as a result of Demerol (meperidine) or Stadol (butorphanol) administration. As this client has just been admitted, medication administration is not a likely cause. The health care practitioner should be notified.
3. Increasing the intravenous fluid rate will not help to resolve any of these severe fetal problems.
4. There is no indication in the scenario that this client is fully dilated.

TEST-TAKING TIP: Sinusoidal fetal heart patterns exhibit no variability and have a uniform wave-like pattern (see below). The nurse would note no periods when the heart rate appears normal. The fetus is in imminent danger. The practitioner must be notified as soon as possible so that he or she can determine the appropriate intervention.

fetal pH is defined as 7.25 to 7.35. An acidotic fetus has a pH that is less than 7.20. When the pH is between 7.20 to 7.25, the value is considered to be equivocal with a need for further testing. Usually interventions are instituted—oxygen applied, position changed, IV fluid increased—and another sampling is done in 10 to 15 minutes.

39. 1. The normal $PaCO_2$ of an adult is 35 to 45 mm Hg. There is no need to intervene, therefore, if the $PaCO_2$ is 40 mm Hg.
2. Although the alpha-fetoprotein level is well above normal, high levels of AFP are indicative of spina bifida, not of an acute problem.
3. Fetal heart accelerations, especially when they occur during contractions, are indicative of fetal well-being.
4. A fetal scalp pH of 7.19 is indicative of an acidotic fetus.

TEST-TAKING TIP: The test taker must read all four responses before choosing the best one. Although answer 2 includes a value that is not normal, it does not describe a situation that requires the nurse to take immediate action. A fetal scalp sampling pH below 7.20, however, is of immediate concern.

40. 1. Blood pressure assessment is important, but it is not the priority action.

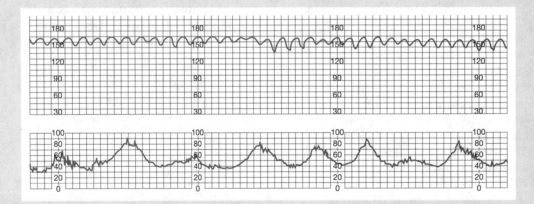

38. 1. The results are equivocal; therefore, the nurse cannot conclude that the baby is severely acidotic.
2. Practitioners usually will repeat the test a few minutes after an equivocal result.
3. Further testing is indicated.
4. The results are not within normal limits.

TEST-TAKING TIP: Some practitioners perform fetal scalp sampling when there is a decrease in fetal heart variability. A normal

2. FH assessment is important, but it is not the priority action.
3. The nurse's priority action is to administer oxygen.
4. It is appropriate to stop the infusion, but that is not the priority action.

TEST-TAKING TIP: This client is exhibiting the classic signs of an amniotic fluid embolism. At this point, the baby's health is secondary because the mother is in a life-threatening situation. The nurse must apply oxygen and call a code immediately.

41. 1. Infection is not directly related to the presence of amniotic fluid emboli.
2. The appropriate nursing care outcome is that the client survives and is breathing normally at discharge.
3. Gastrointestinal function is not related to the presence of amniotic fluid emboli.
4. Urinary function is not related to the presence of amniotic fluid emboli.

TEST-TAKING TIP: At the time of placental separation or during stage 1 of labor, a small amount of amniotic fluid sometimes seeps into the mother's bloodstream via the chorionic villi. With the contraction of the uterus, the fluid is shunted into the peripheral circulation and forced into the woman's lung fields. If there is meconium or other foreign material in the fluid, the woman's prognosis declines. Women who experience forceful, rapid labors are especially at risk for this life-threatening complication.

42. 1. The protocol for cardiac compression and breath ratio is 30 to 2.
2. Chest compressions should be delivered at a depth of at least 2 inches.
3. Because of the size of the gravid uterus, the hands should be placed slightly higher than the lower 1/2 of the sternum when delivering cardiac compressions. For a non-pregnant client, the hands are placed on the lower 1/2 of the sternum.
4. Each breath should be delivered over a 1-second time frame.

TEST-TAKING TIP: The American Heart Association frequently revises cardiopulmonary resuscitation (CPR) guidelines. The responses above reflect the 2010 guidelines. The test taker should make sure that he or she is familiar with current protocols. In addition to the responses above, it is important for the rescuer to tilt the woman slightly toward the left to decrease the compression of the gravid uterus on the aorta and vena cava (see http://circ.ahajournals.org/content/122/18_suppl_3/S685.full.pdf+html?sid=dac0e1cf-9ded-4c9e-a02d-1b31d84e37be).

43. 1. A fetal heart check is the appropriate assessment.
2. Cervical dilation is not important at this time.
3. The white blood cell count is unrelated to the clinical situation.

4. Maternal lung sounds are unrelated to the clinical situation.

TEST-TAKING TIP: The clinical scenario is indicative of a placental abruption. Because the only oxygenation available to the fetus is via the placenta, the appropriate action by the nurse at this time is to determine the well-being of the fetus.

44. 1. Although placenta previa is an obstetric complication, the hemoglobin is within normal limits.
2. Although diabetes mellitus is an obstetric complication, the blood glucose is within normal limits.
3. A placental abruption is a life-threatening situation for the fetus. It has been 15 minutes since the fetal heart was assessed. This is the nurse's priority.
4. A woman who is Rh-negative may or not may not be carrying a baby who is Rh-positive. Either way, a hematocrit of 31%, although low, is not an emergent value.

TEST-TAKING TIP: In this question, the test taker must discriminate among four situations to discern which is the highest priority. Although a client with placenta previa is at high risk for bleeding, it is very likely that if she did start to bleed spontaneously then she would notify the nurse. The fetus of a client who has a placental abruption, however, is already in a life-threatening situation.

45. 1. Fundal heights increase during pregnancy approximately 1 cm per week. When a placental abruption occurs, the height increases hour by hour.
2. Pain-free vaginal bleeding is consistent with a diagnosis of placenta previa.
3. The nurse would expect to see late fetal heart decelerations.
4. This is not an infectious state. The nurse would not expect to see hyperthermia.

TEST-TAKING TIP: When a placenta abrupts, it separates from the uterine wall. As a result, a pool of blood appears behind the placenta. The pool of blood takes up space leading to an increase in the size of the uterus. The fundal height increases as the uterine size increases.

46. 1. This client has had one abortion. Although it is not clear whether the abortion was spontaneous or induced, this client is not at high risk for placental abruption.
2. This client is an adolescent. She has delivered one full-term baby and one

preterm baby. Teens are at high risk for preterm deliveries but are not especially at high risk for placental abruption.

3. Cancer survivors are not especially high risk for placental abruption.
4. Cocaine is a powerful vasoconstrictive agent. It places pregnant clients at high risk for placental abruptions.

TEST-TAKING TIP: It is very important that the test taker not read into any question or response. In the preceding question, all four of the women have had complicated pregnancies. The test taker should not presume the cause of the complications when they are not stated but rather look for the answer that does absolutely place the client at high risk for the abruption.

47. 1. An order for oxytocin administration should be questioned.
2. The fetal heart should be assessed regularly.
3. Weighing the vaginal pads is appropriate at this time.
4. Assessing the hemoglobin and hematocrit is appropriate at this time.

TEST-TAKING TIP: Because the stem states that this woman has symptomatic placenta previa, the test taker can conclude that the woman is bleeding vaginally. It would be appropriate to monitor the fetal heart for any signs of distress, to weigh pads to determine the amount of blood loss, and to assess the hematocrit and hemoglobin to check for anemia. Labor, however, is contraindicated, because vaginal delivery is contraindicated.

48. 20 mL of blood

TEST-TAKING TIP: The nurse must remember that 1 mL of fluid weighs approximately 1 gram. The nurse can estimate, therefore, that the blood loss is:

$$24 - 4 = 20 \text{ mL of blood}$$

49. 1. Leopold's maneuvers assess for fetal positioning in utero. Placental placement cannot be assessed externally.
2. Although women can have completely concealed bleeding with an abruption, the quantity of blood loss will not differentiate between the two pathologies.
3. The most common difference between placenta previa and placenta abruption is the absence or presence of abdominal pain.
4. Maternal blood pressure is inconclusive. Women with chronic hypertension are at high risk for both problems.

TEST-TAKING TIP: Because at least some of the blood from a placental abruption is trapped behind the placenta, women with that complication usually complain of intense, unrelenting pain. But because the blood from a symptomatic placenta previa flows freely through the vagina, the bleeding from that complication is virtually pain free.

50. 1. Because the client will have a cesarean section with anesthesia, the woman should be taught coughing and deep-breathing exercises for the postoperative period.
2. Because the woman will not be going through labor, it is inappropriate to teach her about the phases of the first stage of labor.
3. Because the woman will not be going through labor, it is inappropriate to teach her about Lamaze breathing techniques.
4. Because the woman will not be going through labor, it is inappropriate to teach her about Leboyer hydrobirthing.

TEST-TAKING TIP: When a client has a complete placenta previa, the placenta has attached to the uterine lining so that it fully covers the internal cervical os. If the woman were to go through labor, during dilation and effacement the villi of the placenta would incrementally be exposed, leading the client to bleed profusely. The baby would exsanguinate and die. The only safe way to deliver the baby, therefore, is via cesarean section.

51. 1. Hypertension is not related to the diagnosis of placenta accreta.
2. The nurse would expect the woman to hemorrhage.
3. Bradycardia is not related to the diagnosis of placenta accreta.
4. Hyperthermia is not related to the diagnosis of placenta accreta.

TEST-TAKING TIP: A placenta accreta is present when the chorionic villi attach directly to or invade through the myometrium of the uterus. There is no way, therefore, for the placenta to separate from the uterine wall. Hemorrhage results. It is not uncommon for a hysterectomy to have to be performed to save the woman's life.

52. 1. The administration of betamethasone is appropriate.
2. Bed rest is appropriate.
3. An order to assess the woman's cervical dilation should be questioned.

4. An intravenous of Ringer's lactate is appropriate.

TEST-TAKING TIP: If the nurse were to assess the cervical dilation of a client with complete previa, he or she could puncture the placenta. Vaginal examinations are absolutely contraindicated with a diagnosis of complete placenta previa. Betamethasone is administered to promote maturation of the baby's lungs.

53. 1. Although dilation is progressing, the station is unchanged. The baby, therefore, is not descending into the birth canal. The nurse cannot conclude that the labor is progressing well.
2. **Because the presenting part is not descending into the birth canal, the nurse can logically conclude that the baby is macrosomic.**
3. There is no sign of fetal distress in this scenario.
4. This woman is a multigravida. The average length of the transition phase of labor for multiparas is 10 minutes.

TEST-TAKING TIP: The test taker must carefully analyze the results of the three vaginal examinations. The fetal heart is virtually unchanged: The rate is within normal limits and the variability is normal. There is no sign of fetal distress. The dilation and effacement are changing, but the lack of progressive descent of the presenting part is unexpected. When babies are too big to fit through a client's pelvis, they fail to descend. That is the conclusion that the nurse must make from the findings.

54. 1. Cervical dilation is not related to the data in the scenario.
2. Cervical effacement is not related to the data in the scenario.
3. **A high station is consistent with the data in the scenario.**
4. Contraction frequency is not related to the data in the scenario.

TEST-TAKING TIP: The dimensions noted in the stem are consistent with a diagnosis of cephalopelvic disproportion because the anterior-posterior diameter of the pelvis (obstetric conjugate) is smaller than the diameter of the baby's head (suboccipito-bregmatic). When the fetal head is larger than the maternal pelvis, the baby is unable to descend.

55. 1. The normal time frame for the third stage of labor is between 5 and 30 minutes.

2. This is a description of an early deceleration. Early decelerations are expected during the late first stage and the second stage of labor.
3. A three-vessel umbilical cord is normal.
4. **Shoulder dystocia is an obstetric emergency.**

TEST-TAKING TIP: "Dystocia" means "difficult delivery." A shoulder dystocia, therefore, refers to difficulty in delivering a baby's shoulders. This is an obstetric emergency because the dystocia occurs in the middle of the delivery when the head has been delivered but the shoulders remain wedged in the pelvis. The most common complications are related to nerve palsies from traction placed on the baby's head in attempts to deliver the shoulder. In addition, the baby's life is threatened because the baby is unable to breathe and umbilical cord flow is often dramatically reduced during this phase of the delivery.

56. 1. Intravenous oxytocin administration is inappropriate. This would cause the uterus to contract markedly but would not assist with the delivery of the fetal shoulders.
2. **Flexing the woman's hips sharply toward her abdomen, called McRoberts' maneuver, is appropriate.**
3. Oxygen administration will not assist with the delivery of the fetal shoulders.
4. Fundal pressure is inappropriate.

TEST-TAKING TIP: Flexing the woman's hips sharply toward her abdomen increases slightly the diameter of the pelvic outlet and straightens the pelvic curve, both of which often enable the practitioner to successfully deliver the baby. It is especially important to note that fundal pressure is contraindicated because it may actually magnify the problem by wedging the shoulders into the pelvis even more deeply. Suprapubic pressure, on the other hand, is often helpful in assisting with the delivery.

57. 1. Although infection can occur with prolonged rupture of the membranes, it is not a priority diagnosis at this time because the membranes were just ruptured.
2. **Green amniotic fluid in the presence of late decelerations is indicative of fetal distress.**
3. Vaginal irritation from meconium-stained fluid is not a relevant nursing diagnosis.

4. There is little to no risk to the mother from rupturing the membranes.

TEST-TAKING TIP: Late decelerations are related to poor uteroplacental blood flow. As a result of the poor blood flow, the fetus is being poorly oxygenated and nourished. Amniotic fluid becomes green tinged in the presence of meconium. Meconium is expelled in utero when the fetal anal sphincter relaxes. Sphincters relax when the body is hypoxic. The nurse, therefore, must conclude that the fetus is at high risk for injury related to intrauterine hypoxia.

58. 1. It is inappropriate to perform amnioinfusion when a placental abruption has occurred.
2. It would be appropriate for a health care practitioner to order an amnioinfusion when a client's amniotic fluid is meconium stained.
3. Amnioinfusion would increase the fluid volume even more if it were performed when polyhydramnios is evident.
4. Late decelerations, with no other finding, would not warrant amnioinfusion.

TEST-TAKING TIP: Amnioinfusion is the instillation of intravenous fluid into the uterine cavity through intravenous tubing inserted via the vagina. It may be ordered if the amniotic fluid is meconium stained. The infusion would dilute the concentration of meconium to decrease the potential of the baby aspirating large quantities of meconium at birth.

59. 1. The color of the amniotic fluid will change. This is not a critical assessment, however.
2. Maternal blood pressure should be monitored carefully throughout labor. The assessment is not directly related to the amnioinfusion, however.
3. The effacement of the cervix should be monitored carefully throughout labor. The assessment is not directly related to the amnioinfusion, however.
4. The uterine resting tone should be carefully monitored with an internal pressure electrode during amnioinfusion.

TEST-TAKING TIP: Because fluid is being instilled into the uterine cavity, there is potential for the fluid to overload the space. As a result, the uterine resting tone will increase dramatically with the potential that the uterus could rupture. It is critically important, therefore, that

the nurse monitor the resting tone frequently throughout the procedure.

60. 1. A laceration into the musculature of the buttocks is defined as a second-degree laceration.
2. A fourth-degree laceration extends through the rectal sphincter.
3. A fourth-degree laceration extends through the rectal sphincter.
4. A fourth-degree laceration extends through the rectal sphincter.

TEST-TAKING TIP: One of the many complications that can occur with the delivery of a macrosomic baby is a perineal laceration. If the laceration is extensive and it progresses through the rectal sphincter, it is defined as a fourth degree. As a result, this client is at high risk for the development of a vaginal-rectal fistula.

61. 1. A hematocrit of 48% is indicative of hemoconcentration, not of HELLP syndrome.
2. Abnormal potassium levels are not related to HELLP syndrome.
3. Low platelets are consistent with the diagnosis of HELLP syndrome.
4. Abnormal sodium levels are not related to HELLP syndrome.

TEST-TAKING TIP: HELLP is the acronym for a serious complication of pregnancy and labor and delivery. The letters represent the following information: H, hemolysis; EL, elevated liver enzymes; LP, low platelets. When a client has HELLP syndrome, the nurse would, therefore, expect to see low hemoglobin and hematocrit levels, high aspartate aminotransferase (AST) and alanine aminotransferase (ALT) levels, and low platelets, as seen in the scenario.

62. 1. The nurse must have calcium gluconate in the client's room.
2. Morphine sulfate should not be in the client's room. It is a controlled substance.
3. Narcan does not have to be in the client's room.
4. Demerol should not be in the client's room. It is a controlled substance.

TEST-TAKING TIP: Calcium gluconate is the antidote for magnesium sulfate toxicity. It is very important the test taker know that, if needed, calcium gluconate must be administered very slowly. If calcium gluconate is administered rapidly, the client may experience sudden convulsions.

63. 2 and 3 are correct.
    1. A client with severe preeclampsia could exhibit symptoms of +3 pitting edema without the addition of HELLP syndrome.
    2. Petechiae may develop when a client is thrombocytopenic, one of the signs of HELLP syndrome.
    3. Hyperbilirubinemia develops when red blood cells hemolyze, one of the changes that may develop as a result of liver necrosis. Jaundice is a manifestation of hyperbilirubinemia.
    4. +4 reflexes are consistent with a diagnosis of severe preeclampsia and may be present without the addition of HELLP syndrome.
    5. Elevated specific gravity is consistent with a diagnosis of severe preeclampsia and may be present without the addition of HELLP syndrome.

    TEST-TAKING TIP: The test taker must be able to discriminate between symptoms of severe preeclampsia and HELLP syndrome. If the nurse remembers what each of the letters in HELLP stands for, he or she can determine which of the responses is correct.

64. 1. Hyperreflexia is seen with severe preeclampsia. The magnesium sulfate is being administered to depress the hyperreflexia.
    2. 30 mL/hr is an acceptable urinary output.
    3. A respiratory rate of 16 rpm is within normal limits.
    4. A serum magnesium level of 9 g/dL is dangerously high. The health care practitioner should be notified.

    TEST-TAKING TIP: When magnesium sulfate is being administered, the nurse should monitor the client for adverse side effects including respiratory depression, oliguria, and depressed reflexes. When the magnesium level is above 7 g/dL, toxic effects can be seen.

65. 1. Oxytocin is safe to administer if a client has preeclampsia.
    2. The frequency is within normal limits.
    3. The duration of the contractions is prolonged. The baby will be deprived of oxygen.
    4. The FH is within normal limits.

    TEST-TAKING TIP: The test taker should consider that not only is this client receiving oxytocin, but she is also preeclamptic. Preeclampsia is a vasoconstrictive disease state. The likelihood of poor placental perfusion is already high. When the contraction duration is also prolonged,

the fetus is at high risk of becoming hypoxic.

66. 1. This client has likely developed disseminated intravascular coagulation (DIC). The nurse should watch for pink-tinged urine.
    2. Early decelerations are noted normally during late first stage as well as the second stage of labor. They are unrelated to deviations in PT and PTT.
    3. The reflex changes are unrelated to the lab deviations.
    4. The blood pressure is consistent with mild preeclampsia.

    TEST-TAKING TIP: The test taker must be familiar with the implications of standard blood tests like PT and PTT. Even if the nurse did not know that clients who are diagnosed with HELLP syndrome are at high risk for DIC, he or she should know that clients with prolonged PT and PTT times are at high risk for spontaneous bleeds.

67. 1. Eclamptic clients should be monitored for proteinuria, not for the presence of ketones.
    2. The side rails of an eclamptic client's bed should be padded.
    3. Eclamptic clients should be kept in a low-stimulation environment.
    4. There is no rationale for placing the head of an eclamptic patient's bed in high-Fowler's position.

    TEST-TAKING TIP: Eclamptic clients have had at least one seizure. To protect them from injury during any potential subsequent seizures, the nurse should pad the headboard and the side rails of the client's bed.

68. 1. The nurse would expect to see an elevated serum creatinine level, not a decreased level.
    2. The nurse would expect to see a low RBC count, not an elevated one.
    3. The nurse would expect to see an elevated alkaline phosphatase level, not a decreased one.
    4. The nurse would expect to see an elevated ALT.

    TEST-TAKING TIP: This is a difficult, critical thinking question. This client is exhibiting signs of HELLP syndrome (low platelets and hemolysis). Even though severe preeclampsia is not a part of the HELLP constellation, a client in severe preeclampsia would have poor renal function (elevated serum creatinine level). With hemolysis, the nurse would expect to see a drop in the RBC count,

and with a damaged liver, an elevated alkaline phosphatase level as well as an elevated ALT level.

69. 1. Completely depressed patellar reflexes are a sign of magnesium sulfate toxicity. This is not an expected outcome.
2. A normal urinary output is important, but it is not an expected outcome related to magnesium sulfate administration.
3. A normal respiratory rate is important, but it is not an expected outcome related to magnesium sulfate administration.
4. **The absence of seizures is an expected outcome related to magnesium sulfate administration.**

TEST-TAKING TIP: Eclamptic clients have seized. Magnesium sulfate is ordered and administered to these clients because it is an anticonvulsant. An expected outcome of its administration, therefore, is that the client will have no more seizures.

70. 1. This is a normal contraction pattern. It is not a contraindication to analgesic administration.
2. **Late decelerations are indicative of uteroplacental insufficiency and indicate fetal distress. It is inappropriate to administer a central nervous system (CNS) depressant to the mother at this time.**
3. Sleeping between contractions is a normal phenomenon. It is not a contraindication to analgesic administration.
4. Hypertension is not a contraindication to analgesic administration.

TEST-TAKING TIP: Analgesics are central nervous system (CNS) depressants. They not only depress the CNS of the mother, reducing her pain, but also depress the CNS of the baby. It is inappropriate to administer a depressant to a mother whose fetus is already exhibiting signs of distress. First, the variability of the baseline would be diminished, preventing the nurse from assessing that very important indicator of fetal well-being. And if the baby were to be delivered via cesarean section, the baby would likely be depressed and in need of resuscitation.

71. 1. Early decelerations are related to head compression. They would not be expected as a result of Stadol administration.
2. Late decelerations are related to uteroplacental insufficiency. They would not be expected as a result of Stadol administration.

3. Absent variability would be expected as a result of Stadol administration.
4. Postcontraction accelerations are seen in a well and fully alert fetus. The nurse would expect the incidence of accelerations to diminish as a result of Stadol administration.

TEST-TAKING TIP: Variability is an indicator of fetal well-being. It reflects the competition between the sympathetic and the parasympathetic nervous systems' effects on the fetal heart rate. When the CNS is depressed from the administration of a narcotic analgesic, therefore, the nurse should expect to see diminished variability.

72. 1. The level of pain relief is similar between the two types of anesthesia.
2. The level of placement of the needle is the same in the two types of anesthesia.
3. **Epidurals do not fully sedate the motor nerves of the client. Epidural clients are capable of moving their lower extremities even when fully pain free.**
4. Both epidural and spinal anesthesia clients have the potential of experiencing nausea and vomiting.

TEST-TAKING TIP: The single most important difference between epidural and spinal anesthesia is the depth of needle insertion. Epidural anesthesia is administered into the epidural space. This is outside of the spinal canal. The anesthesia, therefore, is not in direct contact with the spinal nerves. In contrast, spinal anesthesia, instilled into the spinal canal, is in direct contact with the spinal nerves. All of the spinal nerves of spinal anesthesia clients are anesthetized, including motor nerves. Spinal anesthesia clients are paralyzed until the anesthesia is metabolized by the body.

73. 1. **Antacids are routinely administered presurgically to cesarean section clients.**
2. Tranquilizers are not routinely administered presurgically to cesarean section clients.
3. Antihypertensives are not routinely administered presurgically to cesarean section clients.
4. Anticonvulsants are not routinely administered presurgically to cesarean section clients.

TEST-TAKING TIP: Progesterone is a muscle relaxant. Because pregnant women have elevated levels of progesterone, their cardiac sphincters are relaxed. They are at especially high risk, therefore, for

vomiting during surgery. To decrease the acidity of the vomitus in case of aspiration, gravid women are routinely given antacids presurgically.

74. An "X" will be placed on the cricoid cartilage.

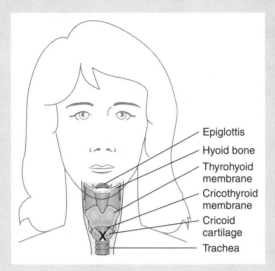

Epiglottis
Hyoid bone
Thyrohyoid membrane
Cricothyroid membrane
Cricoid cartilage
Trachea

TEST-TAKING TIP: To locate the cricoid cartilage, the nurse should find the thyroid prominence, which is the largest bulge in the middle of the front of the neck. The nurse should then, while staying in the midline, move the fingers lightly on the skin downward toward the chest until a gully or notch is felt. The next horizontal projection is the cricoid cartilage. With the thumb on one side of the cartilage and the index finger on the other side of the cartilage, the nurse should press firmly toward the client's back and keep pressing until the anesthesiologist advises him or her to let go. This action presses the cricoid against the esophagus, preventing regurgitation of the stomach contents.

75. 1. Cricoid pressure is not indicated during forceps deliveries.
    2. Cricoid pressure is indicated during endotracheal intubation.
    3. Cricoid pressure is not indicated during the administration of epidural anesthesia.
    4. Cricoid pressure is not indicated during the third stage of labor.

TEST-TAKING TIP: When a client is being intubated, there is a possibility that the stomach contents will be regurgitated. When the vomiting occurs, the client

may aspirate the contents. Because the contents are highly acidic, the trachea and lung fields can become damaged. Cricoid pressure helps to reduce the potential for respiratory aspiration of the stomach contents.

76. 1. Antiembolic stockings (sometimes called antiembolic boots) are often applied during and post–cesarean section. Their application is unrelated to the nursing diagnosis, however.
    2. **The nurse should explain all procedures slowly and carefully.**
    3. Antacid administration is warranted in this situation but is unrelated to the nursing diagnosis.
    4. The fetal heart and maternal vital signs should be carefully monitored, but they are unrelated to the nursing diagnosis.

TEST-TAKING TIP: Whenever a question is asked, the test taker must attend to the content of the question. All of the responses are appropriate in relation to cesarean deliveries, but only response 2 is related to the diagnosis of risk for ineffective individual coping.

77. 1. A vaginal delivery can be performed with no anesthesia.
    2. A postdates pregnancy is not an absolute indication for a cesarean delivery.
    3. An occiput posterior position is not an indication for a cesarean delivery.
    4. The presence of vertical incisions in the uterine wall is an absolute indication for a cesarean delivery.

TEST-TAKING TIP: The muscle tissue that contracts during labor is located in the fundal region of the uterus. A vertical incision into the uterus ligates fundal tissue. The scar that forms from the incision is nonelastic, putting the client at risk of uterine rupture. Having had a previous vertical uterine incision, therefore, is an absolute indicator for future cesarean delivery. In addition, some physicians also encourage clients who have had low-flap (Pfannenstiel) incisions into the uterus to have all subsequent children delivered via cesarean section. (It is important to note that the type of incision that the surgeon used to open the skin is not necessarily the type of incision used to open the uterus.)

78. 1. The nurse would expect to administer Narcan to the client.

2. There is no indication for the administration of Reglan (antiemetic agent) at this time.
3. There is no indication for the administration of Benadryl (antihistamine) at this time.
4. There is no indication for the administration of Vistaril (antihistamine) at this time.

TEST-TAKING TIP: Nubain is an opioid analgesia. It has markedly depressed the client's respiratory response. Narcan is an opioid antagonist. It is likely that the physician will order Narcan to be administered at this time.

79. 1. The woman is at risk of impaired skin integrity.
2. Risk for impaired body image is not appropriate at this time.
3. Risk for impaired parenting is not appropriate at this time.
4. Risk for ineffective sexuality pattern is not appropriate at this time.

TEST-TAKING TIP: Clients who are delivered by vacuum extraction are at high risk for lacerations. Their skin integrity, therefore, is at risk. The other nursing diagnoses are not applicable.

80. 1. A history of drug addiction is not a contraindication for epidural anesthesia.
2. An allergy to morphine is not a contraindication for epidural anesthesia.
3. Adolescence is not a contraindication for epidural anesthesia.
4. A history of scoliosis surgery is a contraindication for epidural anesthesia.

TEST-TAKING TIP: Scoliosis is a defect in the growth of the thoracic and lumbar spine. The surgery is, therefore, performed on the vertebrae of the spinal column. Any spinal surgery is a contraindication to the administration of regional anesthesia.

81. The test taker should have drawn an episiotomy that is about 45° from the midline. The direction in which the episiotomy is performed is usually dependent upon whether the practitioner is left-handed or right-handed.

TEST-TAKING TIP: Although the nurse does not perform the episiotomy, he or she is responsible for documenting the procedure in the medical record as well as for evaluating the incision postpartum. The mediolateral episiotomy is often performed when a macrosomic baby is being birthed. If a midline episiotomy were performed, and it were to extend, it could extend to, or even through, the rectal sphincter.

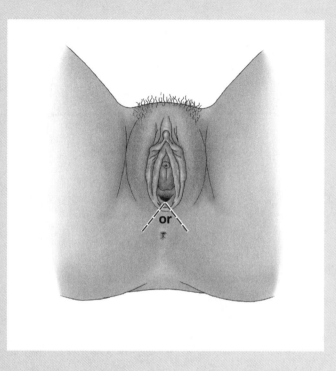

82. 1 and 5 are correct.
1. Cervical cerclage, a stitch encircling the cervix, is incompatible with vaginal delivery.
2. This FH is well within normal limits.
3. This BP is well within normal limits.
4. A fully effaced cervix is essential for a vaginal delivery. It is not an indication for a cesarean section.
5. Active herpes simplex 2 is an absolute indicator for a cesarean delivery.

TEST-TAKING TIP: The test taker must be able to differentiate in which circumstances a full-term, otherwise healthy woman, would be unable to deliver vaginally. There are a few absolute indicators for cesarean section: maternal infection with active herpes simplex 2 and HIV/AIDS (http://www.cdc.gov/hiv/topics/perinatal/overview_partner.htm#_strategies); malpresentation—for example, horizontal lie and breech; previous maternal surgery—e.g., myomectomy; a vertical cesarean scar; some congenital anomalies—e.g., hydrocephalus and meningomyelocele; and other physical conditions, including cervical cerclage in place, obstructive lesions in the lower gynecological system, and complete placenta previa. The test taker should become familiar with each of these.

83.   1. A consent for the use of forceps is not required. The general consent for vaginal delivery covers this possibility.
   2. Even when forceps are applied, the woman should push only during contractions.
   3. **The FH should always be assessed after each contraction during stage 2. Plus, this baby is especially at risk because the stage is prolonged and the physician is using forceps for delivery.**
   4. It is inappropriate for the nurse to advise the client to refuse the use of forceps.

TEST-TAKING TIP: This is an excellent example of a medically indicated use of forceps. The woman is likely fatigued from pushing for over 2 hours, the presenting part is at the pelvic floor, and the baby is showing signs of fetal distress. It would be advisable to deliver this baby in a timely fashion. The use of forceps should result in a speedy delivery.

84.   1 and 3 are correct.
   1. The baby in the LSP position is in a breech presentation. Most breech babies are delivered by cesarean section.
   2. The placenta usually attaches to the posterior portion of the uterine wall.
   3. The meningomyelocele sac could easily rupture during a vaginal delivery. When a fetus has been diagnosed with the defect, a cesarean is usually performed.
   4. Maternal hepatitis B antigen positive status is not an indication for cesarean delivery.
   5. The L/S ratio of 1.5:1 indicates that the baby's lung fields are not yet mature.

TEST-TAKING TIP: Although it is recommended that cesarean section be performed when a mother is affected by two viral illnesses—herpes simplex type 2 (only when active lesions are present) and HIV/AIDS—it is not recommended in the presence of other viral diseases. Hepatitis B is a very serious viral disease, but vertical transmission rates are not significantly different between those babies who are born vaginally and those babies who are born by cesarean section.

85.   3 and 4 are correct.
   1. Asthmatic clients, although needing careful monitoring, are able to deliver vaginally.
   2. It would be appropriate to deliver a baby whose position and station are ROP and +4 via forceps.
   3. A baby in transverse lie is physically incapable of delivering vaginally.

   4. It is not appropriate to deliver a baby vaginally who is at −1 station. The baby has yet to engage. This baby would likely be delivered by cesarean section for prolonged fetal distress.
   5. Clients with cerebral palsy may be delivered with forceps.

TEST-TAKING TIP: It is unsafe to use forceps to deliver a baby when the baby's station is above +2. When the baby is above that station, it is unknown whether or not there is sufficient room in the pelvis for the baby to pass. If there should be too little space, very serious fetal complications could arise, including fractured skull and subdural hematoma.

86.   1. The client is hemodynamically stable. Her blood pressure needs to be assessed about every 1 hour at this time.
   2. The client is hemodynamically stable. Her pulse needs to be assessed about every 4 hours at this time.
   3. **The client's bladder should be palpated.**
   4. There is nothing in the scenario that implies that the client's lung fields need to be assessed.

TEST-TAKING TIP: There are three very important reasons the client's bladder should be assessed. First, clients receive at least 1 liter of fluid immediately before the insertion of an epidural. Within a 2-hour period, it is likely that the woman's bladder has become full. Second, clients are unable to feel when they need to urinate with an epidural in place. Third, a full bladder can impede fetal descent.

87.   1. LMA position is consistent with that information.
   2. In the LSP position, the sacrum is presenting, not the vertex.
   3. In the RScT position, the fetus is in the transverse lie.
   4. In the ROP position, the occiput is presenting so the fetal attitude is flexed.

TEST-TAKING TIP: To conceptualize the relationship between attitude, presentation, and position, the test taker must first thoroughly understand the three concepts. The vertex presentation is a head-down presentation; both occipital and mentum presentations are vertex presentations. When the attitude is extended in a head-down presentation, the front of the head or the face is the presenting part, whereas when the

head is flexed, the back of the head, or occiput, is presenting. When the scapula is presenting, the baby is lying sideways in utero, called transverse lie.

88. 1. Station –2 is not a contraindication for external version.
2. Preterm gestational age is not a contraindication for external version.
3. Reactive NST is not a contraindication for external version.
4. Previous cesarean section is a contraindication for external version.

TEST-TAKING TIP: During external version, the health care practitioner moves the fetus from a malpresentation—usually breech—to a vertex presentation. To accomplish the movement, the physician manually palpates the fetus externally through the mother's abdominal and uterine walls. Because significant stress is placed on the uterine body, the presence of a cesarean scar is a contraindication to the procedure.

89. 1. Oxytocin (Pitocin) is a medication that contracts the uterus. It would not be administered prior to an external version.
2. Ergonovine (Methergine) is a medication that contracts the uterus. It should never be administered prior to the delivery of the placenta.
3. Betamethasone (Celestone) is a steroid that is administered to the mother of a preterm infant to stimulate the maturation of the fetus's lung fields. It would not be administered prior to an external version.
4. Terbutaline (Brethine) is a smooth, muscle-relaxing agent. It would be administered prior to an external version.

TEST-TAKING TIP: It is important that the uterine muscle not impede the physician's manipulations during an external version. To facilitate the movement, therefore, a muscle relaxant is administered. Terbutaline is one relaxing agent that is used by obstetricians.

90. 1. A fetus in +3 station is well below engagement. An external version would not be advisable.
2. LSP position is a breech presentation. It may be appropriate for a physician to perform an external version prior to this delivery.
3. There is no indication that the baby in the flexed attitude is in a malpresentation.
4. Prolonged rupture of membranes is not an indication for an external version.

TEST-TAKING TIP: If a baby is in the breech presentation, the version would have to be performed before the baby had engaged. Once the baby is well established in the true pelvis, it is at high risk for the baby to be moved.

91. 1. A change in urinary output postexternal version is unlikely.
2. An elevation in the maternal blood pressure postexternal version is unlikely.
3. The presence of severe occipital headache postexternal version is unlikely.
4. The nurse should monitor the client carefully for variable fetal heart decelerations.

TEST-TAKING TIP: The umbilical cord can become compressed during an external version. Variable decelerations are caused by umbilical cord compression. If the cord were to become compressed, the nurse would note variable decelerations on the fetal heart monitor tracing.

92. 1. The urinary output should be carefully monitored.
2. Magnesium sulfate administration does not place clients at high risk for a temperature elevation.
3. Magnesium sulfate administration does not place clients at high risk for cessation of peripheral circulation.
4. Magnesium sulfate administration does not place clients at high risk for retinal edema.

TEST-TAKING TIP: Even though this client is receiving magnesium sulfate to treat preterm labor and not preeclampsia, the medication still has the same side effects. Magnesium sulfate is excreted through the kidneys. If the urinary output drops, the concentration of magnesium sulfate can rise in the bloodstream. Because, at toxic levels, the client can experience respiratory depression and cardiac compromise, it is very important for the nurse carefully to monitor the client's urinary output.

93. 3 and 4 are correct.
1. The presence of contractions without cervical change is not diagnostic of preterm labor.
2. Preterm labor is defined as cervical effacement of greater than 80%. Although the client has effaced slightly, a diagnosis of preterm labor cannot as yet be made.
3. The dilation of 3 cm is indicative of preterm labor.
4. A cervical length of 2 cm is indicative of preterm labor.

5. The presence of 30-second–duration contractions is not diagnostic of preterm labor.

TEST-TAKING TIP: Preterm labor is defined as labor before 38 weeks' gestation with 3 or more contractions occurring within a 30-minute period PLUS cervical change of one of the following: cervical effacement greater than 80%, cervical dilation greater than 1 cm, or cervical length of less than 2.5 cm. The change in cervical length is diagnosed by transvaginal ultrasound.

94. 1, 2, and 5 are correct.
    1. This client is high risk for PTL because she is over 35 years of age and in an abusive relationship.
    2. A previous preterm delivery places a client at increased risk of preterm labor.
    3. The presence of a two-vessel cord does not place a client at increased risk of preterm labor.
    4. A history of long menstrual periods does not place a client at increased risk of preterm labor.
    5. A woman who smokes cigarettes is at high risk for preterm labor.

TEST-TAKING TIP: Even though medical and psychosocial histories are not absolute predictors of preterm labor, there are a number of factors that have been shown to place clients at risk, including pregnancy history of multiple gestations; previous preterm deliveries; cigarette smoking and/or illicit drug use; a number of medical histories like diabetes and hypertension; and social issues like adolescent pregnancy and domestic violence.

95. 1. Fetal fibronectin is not related to glucose metabolism.
    2. Positive fetal fibronectin levels are seen in clients who deliver preterm.
    3. Fetal fibronectin is not related to hypertensive conditions.
    4. Fetal fibronectin is not related to fetal distress.

TEST-TAKING TIP: Fetal fibronectin (fFN) is a substance that is metabolized by the chorion. Although positive during the first half of pregnancy, it is very rare to see positive results between 24 and 34 weeks' gestation unless the client's cervix begins to efface and dilate. It is an excellent predictor of preterm labor (PTL); therefore, many practitioners assess the cervical and vaginal secretions of women at high risk for PTL for the presence of fFN.

96. 1. Oxytocin will increase the client's contractions. The administration of this medication is inappropriate at this time.
    2. Methergine should never be administered unless the placenta is already delivered.
    3. Magnesium sulfate is a tocolytic agent. It would be appropriate for this medication to be administered at this time.
    4. Morphine sulfate is an opioid. There is no rationale for its administration in the scenario.

TEST-TAKING TIP: The client in the scenario is exhibiting signs that meet the criteria for preterm labor. The test taker should deduce, therefore, that a tocolytic agent may be ordered in this situation. The only tocolytic agent included in the choices is magnesium sulfate.

97. 1. A history of hypothyroidism does not place a client who is to receive a beta agonist medication at risk.
    2. A history of breast cancer does not place a client who is to receive a beta agonist medication at risk.
    3. A history of cardiac disease would place a client who is to receive a beta agonist medication at risk. The nurse should question this order.
    4. A history of asthma does not place a client who is to receive a beta agonist medication at risk.

TEST-TAKING TIP: The test taker should remember that beta agonists stimulate the "fight or flight" response. The client's heart rate will increase precipitously and there is a possibility that the potassium levels of the client may fall. These side effects place the client with heart disease at risk of heart failure and/or dysrhythmias. The client is also at high risk for pulmonary edema and congestive heart failure, so lung field assessments should be done regularly.

98. 4 and 5 are correct.
    1. A decrease in the frequency of the contractions from q 3 min × 90 sec to q 2 min × 60 is the expected, therapeutic response. This change does not warrant stopping the medication.
    2. A change in fetal heart rate pattern from no decelerations to early decelerations is a benign change. This change does not warrant stopping the medication.

3. Minimal variability is a sign of poor fetal oxygenation, whereas moderate variability is a sign of good fetal oxygenation. This change does not warrant stopping the medication.
4. When the fetal heart rate pattern is greater than 200 bpm, the medication should be stopped.
5. Terbutaline is contraindicated when the membranes have ruptured prematurely.

TEST-TAKING TIP: Terbutaline, a beta agonist, stimulates the "fight or flight" response in the mother and in the fetus. The fetal heart rate, therefore, increases in response to the medication. When the rate is too high, however, there is insufficient time for the blood to enter the heart, which leads to a drop in cardiac output.

99. 1. The nurse should assess the fetal heart and the maternal pulse simultaneously.
2. It is not necessary to notify the doctor at this time.
3. It is not necessary to stop the medication at this time.
4. It is not necessary to administer oxygen to the mother at this time.

TEST-TAKING TIP: Because the medication should increase both the mother's pulse and fetal heart rates, it is likely that the fetal monitor is mistakenly registering the maternal pulse rather than the fetal heart rate. If the pulsations are the same when the radial pulse of the mother and the fetal heart are monitored simultaneously, the nurse can determine that, indeed, the mother's pulse rate is being monitored.

100. 1. Decadron is not a tocolytic.
2. Decadron is not an anti-infective.
3. Decadron is a steroid that hastens the maturation of the fetal lung fields.
4. Decadron is not an analgesic.

TEST-TAKING TIP: Steroids (either IM betamethasone or IM dexamethasone) are given over a 2-day period to mothers in preterm labor. The medications have been shown to hasten the development of surfactant in the lung fields of fetuses. Babies whose mothers have received one of the medications experience fewer respiratory complications.

101. 50 mL/hr

$$50 \text{ units}/500 \text{ mL} = 5 \text{ units}/x \text{ mL}$$
$$50\,x = 5 \times 500$$
$$50\,x = 2,500$$
$$x = 50 \text{ mL/hr}$$

TEST-TAKING TIP: There are two important things for the test taker to remember in relation to this question. First, this is a ratio and proportion question. The known quantity, 50 units/500 mL, is placed on one side of the equation, and the unknown, 5 units/x mL, is placed on the other side of the equation. With cross multiplication, the correct answer is found. Second, IV pumps are always set at a mL/hr setting. There is, therefore, no need to know a drop factor. The test taker should also note that the term "units" is written out. The Joint Commission has identified a number of unacceptable abbreviations. U and mU are unacceptable; instead, "units" and "milliunits" must always be written out.

102. 1. Mild tachycardia is an expected, but benign, side effect.
2. Wakefulness is an expected, but benign side effect.
3. Audible rales should be reported to the health care practitioner.
4. Daily output of 2,000 mL is within normal.

TEST-TAKING TIP: The presence of audible rales is indicative of pulmonary edema, a serious side effect related to the medication. The pulmonary edema may be caused by the development of congestive heart failure. Whenever a client is on nifedipine, the nurse should regularly monitor the client's lung fields.

103. 1. There is nothing in the scenario that indicates that the woman is at high risk for hypertensive illness.
2. There is nothing in the scenario that indicates that the woman is at high risk for hyperglycemia.
3. Increased fetal heart variability is not expected in this situation.
4. The baby is at high risk for late fetal heart decelerations secondary to a postmature placenta.

TEST-TAKING TIP: A BPP of 8 or lower indicates that the fetus is in jeopardy. The five assessments that constitute the BPP are nonstress test (NST), fetal movement, fetal breathing, amniotic fluid volume, and fetal tone. Each assessment is given a score of 0 or 2.

104. 1. The fetus is full-term. Post-term is defined by most texts as 42 weeks' gestation or later and by some as 41 weeks' gestation or later.
    2. The fetus is not breech; it is vertex.
    3. It is likely that the cord is prolapsed because the amniotomy was performed when the presenting part was not yet engaged and because variable decelerations are seen on the FH monitor.
    4. If the client were infected, the amniotic fluid would be foul smelling.

TEST-TAKING TIP: The likelihood of a prolapsed cord occurring during an amniotomy increases when the fetal presenting part is in negative station. As the amniotic fluid is released from the uterus during the rupture of membranes, the cord can slip and precede the fetus. At that time, variable decelerations are seen on the electronic fetal monitor tracing because the cord is being compressed by the presenting part.

105. 3, 4, and 5 are correct.
    1. Gestational age is not part of the Bishop score.
    2. The status of the membranes is not part of the Bishop score.
    3. Cervical dilation is part of the Bishop score.
    4. Fetal station is part of the Bishop score.
    5. Cervical position is part of the Bishop score.

TEST-TAKING TIP: The Bishop score is calculated to determine the inducibility of the cervix. Although gestational age may be an indication for calculating the score, it does not have a direct impact on the status of the cervix. Similarly, although rupture of the membranes may be an indication for calculating the score, that fact does not have a direct impact on the status of the cervix.

106. 1. This is an example of the stage of denial.
    2. This is an example of the stage of bargaining.
    3. This is an example of the stage of acceptance.
    4. This is an example of the stage of anger.

TEST-TAKING TIP: It is essential that the test taker be familiar with the concepts of grief and mourning. Everyone who is caring for a couple who experiences a fetal or neonatal loss, as well as the couple themselves, will progress through the stages of grief. It is very important that the nurse realize that grieving is individual and that the stages of grief are never experienced in a linear fashion. Health care staff progress rapidly through the stages, whereas the couple's grief is likely to be delayed.

107. 1. The nurse would expect the client to be crying and sad.
    2. It is unlikely that the client would be talkative and excited.
    3. It is unlikely that the client would be quietly doing rapid breathing.
    4. It is unlikely that the client would be loudly chanting.

TEST-TAKING TIP: A client in the latent phase of labor who is carrying a healthy fetus is likely to be talkative and excited, but a woman whose fetus has died is likely to be crying and sad throughout her labor. Clients in the latent phase usually are performing slow chest breathing.

108. 1. Although the bacterium can cause chorioamnionitis, this is not the rationale for administering the antibiotic during labor.
    2. Babies are susceptible to neonatal sepsis from vertical transmission of the bacteria.
    3. The bacteria are not sexually transmitted. Approximately one third of all women carry group B strep as normal vaginal and/or rectal flora.
    4. Puerperal sepsis is usually caused by *Staphylococcus aureus* or group A strep.

TEST-TAKING TIP: At approximately 36 weeks' gestation, pregnant women are cultured for group B strep. If they culture positive, standard protocol is to administer a broad-spectrum antibiotic IV q 4 hours from the time her membranes rupture until delivery. That action markedly decreases the vertical transmission of the bacteria to neonates.

109. 1. The nurse should carefully monitor the client for fetal distress.
    2. It is unlikely that the client is dehydrated.

3. It is unlikely that the client will have oliguria.
4. It is unlikely that the client will develop jaundice.

TEST-TAKING TIP: Oligohydramnios is often seen in post-term pregnancies. When the placenta begins to deteriorate, the hydration of the baby drops. Because the predominant component of amniotic fluid is fetal urine, when the baby is dehydrated, the quantity of amniotic fluid drops. Fetal distress can occur because of two factors: cord compression, because there is insufficient fluid to cushion the umbilical cord, and uteroplacental insufficiency, because the placenta is functioning suboptimally.

110. 1, 2, and 3 are correct.
1. The circulating nurse should count the sterile sponges. This is done together with the scrub nurse.
2. The circulating nurse must document in the medical record all key events that occur during the surgery, including the time of the first incision.
3. The circulating nurse should notify the pediatric staff. There should be one resuscitation team assembled in the delivery room for each baby that will be delivered.
4. It is not necessary for the circulating nurse to perform a sterile scrub. He or she is a nonsterile member of the operative team.
5. It is not appropriate for the circulating nurse to assemble the sterile instruments because he or she is not sterile.

TEST-TAKING TIP: The circulating nurse is responsible for coordinating the activity in the operating room. He or she is the only member of the team who is able to move freely throughout the room to make telephone calls, obtain needed supplies, maintain the documentation record, and so on. When multiple babies are being birthed, he or she is especially important. The more babies who are birthed at once—e.g., twins, triplets—the more vulnerable the babies are at birth. Multiple-gestation babies are often born preterm and small-for-gestational age. There must be a resuscitation team available for each baby in case emergent care is needed.

111. 1, 4, and 5 are correct.
1. The client's hepatitis B status should be assessed.
2. The client's rubeola status is not immediately important.
3. The client's varicella status is not immediately important.
4. The client's group B streptococcus status should be assessed.
5. The client's HIV/AIDS status should be assessed.

TEST-TAKING TIP: There are several infectious diseases that affect care given during pregnancy, labor and delivery, postpartum, and in the newborn nursery. The hepatitis B status must be assessed to notify the nursery for care needed by the baby. Group B strep status must be assessed to administer needed antibiotics to the mother during labor and to monitor the baby's status in the newborn nursery. The HIV/AIDS status must be assessed to administer needed antiviral medications to the mother in labor and/or to the baby postdelivery. HIV/AIDS is also an indication for cesarean section delivery.

High-Risk Newborn

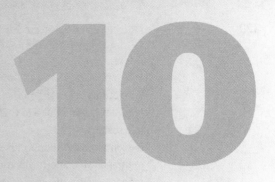

Although the vast majority of babies born in the United States are healthy and full-term, there are a number of neonates who need specialized care immediately after delivery. One out of every eight babies born today is premature. Even with the high-quality care that preterm babies receive, many of them will develop acute and chronic illnesses as sequelae to their immaturity. There are fewer postmature babies born today than in the past, but when a baby is born that is over 40 weeks' gestation, the nurse must be prepared to monitor the baby for potentially serious complications. Maternal diseases, such as diabetes mellitus and preeclampsia, often result in neonatal problems. And there are a number of congenital diseases that affect babies. In each and every one of these cases, the nurse must possess the knowledge and expertise to provide the babies with specialized care.

KEYWORDS

The following words include English vocabulary, nursing/medical terminology, concepts, principles, or information relevant to content specifically addressed in the chapter or associated with topics presented in it. English dictionaries, your nursing textbooks, and medical dictionaries such as *Taber's Cyclopedic Medical Dictionary* are resources that can be used to expand your knowledge and understanding of these words and related information.

ABO incompatibility

acyanotic heart defects (e.g., ventricular septal defect, atrial septal defect, patent ductus arteriosus)

appropriate-for-gestational age (AGA)

arm recoil sign

Babinski reflex

Ballard scale

beractant (Survanta)

bronchopulmonary dysplasia

café au lait spot

chignon

choanal atresia

cleft lip and palate

clubfoot

cold stress syndrome

conduction

convection

Coombs' test (direct and indirect)

continuous positive airway pressure (CPAP)

cyanotic heart defects (e.g., tetralogy of Fallot, transposition of the great vessels)

desquamation

developmental dysplasia of the hip

diaphragmatic hernia

digoxin (Lanoxin)

Down syndrome

dysmaturity

erythroblastosis fetalis

esophageal atresia/tracheoesophageal fistula

evaporation

fetal alcohol syndrome (FAS)

galactosemia

gastroschisis

gestational age assessment

group B streptococcus

hemangioma

hemolytic jaundice

Hirschsprung's disease

hydrocephalus

hyperbilirubinemia

hypoglycemia

infant of diabetic mother (IDM)

intracostal retractions

intrauterine growth restriction (IUGR)

jitters	popliteal angle
kangaroo care	port wine stain
kernicterus	positive end-expiratory pressure (PEEP)
large-for-gestational age (LGA)	postdates
macrosomia	postmaturity
meconium aspiration syndrome	prematurity
meningomyelocele (myelomeningocele)	radiation
monochorionic twins	respiratory distress syndrome
naloxone (Narcan)	Rh incompatibility
necrotizing enterocolitis	scarf sign
neonatal abstinence syndrome	small-for-gestational age (SGA)
oligohydramnios	square window sign
opisthotonus	tachycardia
Ortolani sign	tachypnea
paregoric	talipes equinovarus
phototherapy	thermoregulation
polyhydramnios	twin-to-twin transfusion

QUESTIONS

1. A 1-day-old neonate, 32 weeks' gestation, is in an overhead warmer. The nurse assesses the morning axillary temperature as 96.9°F. Which of the following could explain this assessment finding?
   1. This is a normal temperature for a preterm neonate.
   2. Axillary temperatures are not valid for preterm babies.
   3. The supply of brown adipose tissue is incomplete.
   4. Conduction heat loss is pronounced in the baby.

2. Which of the following neonates is at highest risk for cold stress syndrome?
   1. Infant of diabetic mother.
   2. Infant with Rh incompatibility.
   3. Postdates neonate.
   4. Down syndrome neonate.

3. Which of the following would lead the nurse to suspect cold stress syndrome in a newborn with a temperature of 96.5°F?
   1. Blood glucose of 50 mg/dL.
   2. Acrocyanosis.
   3. Tachypnea.
   4. Oxygen saturation of 96%.

4. Four babies are in the newborn nursery. The nurse pages the neonatologist to see the baby who exhibits which of the following?
   1. Intracostal retractions.
   2. Erythema toxicum.
   3. Pseudostrabismus.
   4. Vernix caseosa.

5. A baby is grunting in the neonatal nursery. Which of the following actions by the nurse is appropriate?
   1. Place a pacifier in the baby's mouth.
   2. Check the baby's diaper.
   3. Have the mother feed the baby.
   4. Assess the respiratory rate.

6. A 6-month-old child developed kernicterus immediately after birth. Which of the following tests should be done to determine whether or not this child has developed any sequelae to the illness?
   1. Blood urea nitrogen and serum creatinine.
   2. Alkaline phosphatase and bilirubin.
   3. Hearing testing and vision assessment.
   4. Peak expiratory flow and blood gas assessments.

7. A baby with hemolytic jaundice is being treated with fluorescent phototherapy. To provide safe newborn care, which of the following actions should the nurse perform?
   1. Cover the baby's eyes with eye pads.
   2. Turn the lights on for ten minutes every hour.
   3. Clothe the baby in a shirt and diaper only.
   4. Tightly swaddle the baby in a baby blanket.

8. A baby is born with erythroblastosis fetalis. Which of the following signs/symptoms would the nurse expect to see?
   1. Ruddy complexion.
   2. Anasarca.
   3. Alopecia.
   4. Erythema toxicum.

9. Which of the following laboratory findings would the nurse expect to see in a baby diagnosed with erythroblastosis fetalis?
   1. Hematocrit 24%.
   2. Leukocyte count 45,000 cells/mm^3.
   3. Sodium 125 mEq/L.
   4. Potassium 5.5 mEq/L.

10. A baby's blood type is B negative. The baby is at risk for hemolytic jaundice if the mother has which of the following blood types?
    1. Type O negative.
    2. Type A negative.
    3. Type B positive.
    4. Type AB positive.

11. A newborn admitted to the nursery has a positive direct Coombs' test. Which of the following is an appropriate action by the nurse?
    1. Monitor the baby for jitters.
    2. Assess the blood glucose level.
    3. Assess the rectal temperature.
    4. Monitor the baby for jaundice.

12. An 18-hour-old baby is placed under the bili-lights with an elevated bilirubin level. Which of the following is an expected nursing action in these circumstances?
    1. Give the baby oral rehydration therapy after all feedings.
    2. Rotate the baby from side to back to side to front every two hours.
    3. Apply restraints to keep the baby under the light source.
    4. Administer intravenous fluids via pump per doctor orders.

13. A jaundice neonate must have a heel stick to assess bilirubin levels. Which of the following actions should the nurse make during the procedure?
    1. Cover the foot with an iced wrap for one minute prior to the procedure.
    2. Avoid puncturing the lateral heel to prevent damaging sensitive structures.
    3. Blot the site with a dry gauze after rubbing it with an alcohol swab.
    4. Firmly grasp the calf of the baby during the procedure to prevent injury.

14. A newborn nursery nurse notes that a 36-hour-old baby's body is jaundiced. Which of the following nursing interventions will be most therapeutic?
    1. Maintain a warm ambient environment.
    2. Have the mother feed the baby frequently.
    3. Have the mother hold the baby skin to skin.
    4. Place the baby naked by a closed sunlit window.

15. A neonate is under phototherapy for elevated bilirubin levels. The baby's stools are now loose and green. Which of the following actions should the nurse take at this time?
    1. Discontinue the phototherapy.
    2. Notify the health care practitioner.
    3. Take the baby's temperature.
    4. Assess the baby's skin integrity.

16. A nursing diagnosis for a 5-day-old newborn under phototherapy is: Risk for fluid volume deficit. For which of the following client outcomes should the nurse plan to monitor the baby?
    1. 6 saturated diapers in 24 hours.
    2. Breastfeeds 6 times in 24 hours.
    3. 12% weight loss since birth.
    4. Apical heart rate of 176 bpm.

17. There is a baby in the neonatal intensive care unit (NICU) who is exhibiting signs of neonatal abstinence syndrome. Which of the following medications is contraindicated for this neonate?
    1. Morphine.
    2. Opium.
    3. Narcan.
    4. Phenobarbital.

18. A baby is in the NICU whose mother was addicted to heroin during the pregnancy. Which of the following nursing actions would be appropriate?
    1. Tightly swaddle the baby.
    2. Place the baby prone in the crib.
    3. Provide needed stimulation to the baby.
    4. Feed the baby half-strength formula.

19. A newborn in the nursery is exhibiting signs of neonatal abstinence syndrome. Which of the following signs/symptoms is the nurse observing? **Select all that apply.**
    1. Hyperphagia.
    2. Lethargy.
    3. Prolonged periods of sleep.
    4. Hyporeflexia.
    5. Persistent shrill cry.

20. Based on maternal history of alcohol addiction, a baby in the neonatal nursery is being monitored for signs of fetal alcohol syndrome (FAS). The nurse should assess this baby for which of the following?
    1. Poor suck reflex.
    2. Ambiguous genitalia.
    3. Webbed neck.
    4. Absent Moro reflex.

21. A baby born addicted to cocaine is being given paregoric. The nurse knows that which of the following is a rationale for its use?
    1. Paregoric is nonaddictive.
    2. Paregoric corrects diarrhea.
    3. Paregoric is nonsedating.
    4. Paregoric suppresses the cough reflex.

22. A baby was born 24 hours ago to a mother who received no prenatal care. The infant has tremors, sneezes excessively, constantly mouths for food, and has a shrill, high-pitched cry. The baby's serum glucose levels are normal. For which of the following should the nurse request an order from the pediatrician?
    1. Urine drug toxicology test.
    2. Biophysical profile test.
    3. Chest and abdominal ultrasound evaluations.
    4. Oxygen saturation and blood gas assessments.

23. A nurse makes the following observations when admitting a full-term, breastfeeding baby into the neonatal nursery: 9 lb 2 oz, 21 inches long, TPR: 96.6°F, 158, 62, jittery, pink body with bluish hands and feet, crying. Which of the following actions is of highest probability?
    1. Swaddle the baby to provide warmth.
    2. Assess the glucose level of the baby.
    3. Take the baby to the mother for feeding.
    4. Administer the neonatal medications.

24. An infant admitted to the newborn nursery has a blood glucose level of 35 mg/dL. The nurse should monitor this baby carefully for which of the following?
    1. Jaundice.
    2. Jitters.
    3. Erythema toxicum.
    4. Subconjunctival hemorrhages.

25. A full-term infant admitted to the newborn nursery has a blood glucose level of 35 mg/dL. Which of the following actions should the nurse perform at this time?
    1. Feed the baby formula or breast milk.
    2. Assess the baby's blood pressure.
    3. Tightly swaddle the baby.
    4. Monitor the baby's urinary output.

26. A nurse is inserting a gavage tube into a preterm baby who is unable to suck and swallow. Which of the following actions must the nurse take during the procedure?
    1. Measure the distance from the tip of the ear to the nose.
    2. Lubricate the tube with an oil-based solution.
    3. Insert the tube quickly if the baby becomes cyanotic.
    4. Inject a small amount of sterile water to check placement.

27. A neonate is in the warming crib for poor thermoregulation. Which of the following sites is appropriate for the placement of the skin thermal sensor?
    1. Xiphoid process.
    2. Forehead.
    3. Abdominal wall.
    4. Great toe.

28. The nurse must perform nasopharyngeal suctioning of a newborn with profuse secretions. Place the following nursing actions for nasopharyngeal suctioning in chronological order.
    1. Slowly rotate and remove the suction catheter.
    2. Place thumb over the suction control on the catheter.
    3. Assess type and amount of secretions.
    4. Insert free end of the tubing through the nose.

29. A neonate is being given intravenous fluids through the dorsal vein of the wrist. Which of the following actions by the nurse is essential?
    1. Tape the arm to an arm board.
    2. Change the tubing every 24 hours.
    3. Monitor the site every 5 minutes.
    4. Infuse the fluid intermittently.

30. A Roman Catholic couple has just delivered a baby with an Apgar score of 1 at 1 minute, 2 at 5 minutes, and 2 at 10 minutes. Which of the following interventions is appropriate at this time?
    1. Advise the parents that they should pray very hard so that everything turns out well.
    2. Ask the parents whether they would like the nurse to baptize the baby.
    3. Leave the parents alone to work through their thoughts and feelings.
    4. Inform the parents that a priest will listen to their confessions whenever they are ready.

31. The nurse assesses a newborn as follows:
    Heart rate: 70
    Respirations: weak and irregular
    Tone: flaccid
    Color: pale
    Baby grimaces when a pediatrician attempts to insert an endotracheal tube
    What should the nurse calculate the baby's Apgar score to be?

    _____

32. A neonate is in the neonatal intensive care nursery with a diagnosis of large-for-gestational age. The baby was born at 38 weeks' gestation and weighed 3,500 grams. Based on this information, which of the following responses is correct?

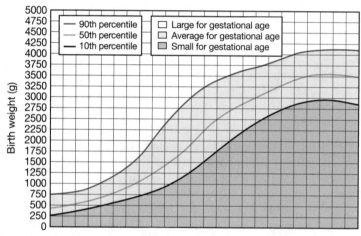

1. The diagnosis is accurate because the baby's weight is too high for a diagnosis of appropriate-for-gestational age.
2. The diagnosis is inaccurate because the baby's weight needs to be higher than 3,500 grams.
3. The diagnosis is inaccurate because the baby's weight needs to be lower than 3,500 grams.
4. The diagnosis is inaccurate because full-term babies are never large-for-gestational age.

33. A neonate has been admitted to the neonatal intensive care unit with the following findings:

Completely flaccid posturing
Square window sign of 60°
Arm recoil of 180°
Popliteal angle of 160°
Full scarf sign
Heel that touches the ear
Skin that is red and translucent
Sparse lanugo
Faint red marks on the plantar surface
Barely perceptible breast tissue
Eyelids that are open but flat ear pinnae
Prominent clitoris and small labia minora

Using the Ballard scale, what is the gestational age of this neonate estimated to be?
_____ weeks

Neuromuscular Maturity

	-1	0	1	2	3	4	5
Posture							
Square Window (Wrist)	-90°	90°	60°	45°	30°	0°	
Arm Recoil		180°	140°–180°	110°–140°	90°–110°	<90°	
Popliteal Angle	180°	160°	140°	120°	100°	90°	<90°
Scarf Sign							
Heel To Ear							

Physical Maturity

Skin	sticky; friable; transparent	gelatinous; red; translucent	smooth pink; visible veins	superficial peeling or rash, few veins	cracking; pale areas; rare veins	parchment; deep cracking; no vessels	leathery; cracked; wrinkled
Lanugo	none	sparse	abundant	thinning	bald areas	mostly bald	
Plantar Surface	heel-toe 40–50 mm:-1 <40 mm:-2	>50 mm no crease	faint red marks	anterior transverse crease only	creases ant. 2/3	creases over entire sole	
Breast	imperceptible	barely perceptible	flat areola; no bud	stippled areola; 1–2 mm bud	raised areola; 3–4 mm bud	full areola; 5–10 mm bud	
Eye/ear	lids fused; loosely:-1 tightly:-2	lids open; pinna flat; stays folded	sl. curved pinna; soft; slow recoil	well-curved pinna; soft but ready recoil	formed and firm; instant recoil	thick cartilage; ear stiff	
Genitals (Male)	scrotum flat, smooth	scrotum empty; faint rugae	testes in upper canal; rare rugae	testes descending; few rugae	testes down; good rugae	testes pendulous; deep rugae	
Genitals (Female)	clitoris prominent; labia flat	prominent clitoris; small labia minora	prominent clitoris; enlarging minora	majora and minora equally prominent	majora large; minora small	majora cover clitoris and minora	

Maturity Rating

Score	Weeks
-10	20
-5	22
0	24
5	26
10	28
15	30
20	32
25	34
30	36
35	38
40	40
45	42
50	44

From: Ballard, J. L., Khoury, L. C., Wedig, K., et al. (1991). New Ballard Score, expanded to include extremely premature infants. *Journal of Pediatrics*, 19 (3), 417-423. With permission.

34. A neonate is in the neonatal intensive care unit. The baby is 28 weeks' gestation and weighs 1,000 grams. Which of the following is correct in relation to this baby's growth?

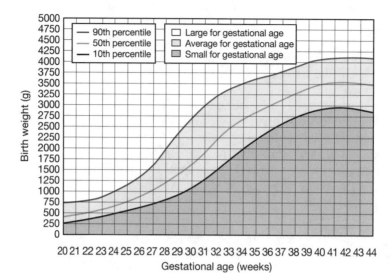

Gestational age (weeks)

1. Weight is appropriate-for-gestational age.
2. Weight is below average for gestational age.
3. Baby experienced intrauterine growth restriction.
4. Baby experienced congenital growth hypertrophy.

35. A neonate, 40 weeks by dates, has been admitted to the nursery. Place an "X" on the graph where the baby would be labeled large-for-gestational age.

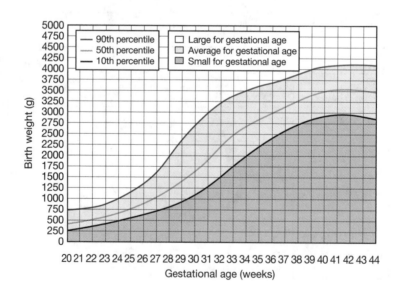

Gestational age (weeks)

36. A 42-week-gestation baby, 2,400 grams, whose mother had no prenatal care, is admitted into the NICU. The neonatologist orders blood work. Which of the following laboratory findings would the nurse expect to see?
1. Blood glucose 30 mg/dL.
2. Leukocyte count 1,000 cells/mm³.
3. Hematocrit 30%.
4. Serum pH 7.8.

37. A woman who received an intravenous analgesic 4 hours ago has had prolonged late decelerations in labor. She will deliver her baby shortly. Which of the following is the priority action for the delivery room nurse to take?
    1. Preheat the overhead warmer.
    2. Page the neonatologist on call.
    3. Draw up Narcan (naloxone) for injection.
    4. Assemble the neonatal eye prophylaxis.

38. A baby has been admitted to the neonatal intensive care unit with a diagnosis of postmaturity. The nurse expects to find which of the following during the initial newborn assessment?
    1. Abundant lanugo.
    2. Flat breast tissue.
    3. Prominent clitoris.
    4. Wrinkled skin.

39. A 42-week-gestation baby has been admitted to the neonatal intensive care unit. At delivery, thick green amniotic fluid was noted. Which of the following actions by the nurse is critical at this time?
    1. Bath to remove meconium-contaminated fluid from the skin.
    2. Ophthalmic assessment to check for conjunctival irritation.
    3. Rectal temperature to assess for septic hyperthermia.
    4. Respiratory evaluation to monitor for respiratory distress.

40. A 42-week gravida is delivering her baby. A nurse and pediatrician are present at the birth. The amniotic fluid is green and thick. The baby fails to breathe spontaneously. Which of the following actions should the nurse take next?
    1. Stimulate the baby to breathe.
    2. Assess neonatal heart rate.
    3. Assist with intubation.
    4. Place the baby in the prone position.

41. Thirty seconds after birth a baby, who appears preterm, has exhibited no effort to breathe even after being stimulated. The heart rate is assessed at 50 bpm. Which of the following actions should the nurse perform first?
    1. Perform a gestational age assessment.
    2. Inflate the lungs with positive pressure.
    3. Provide external chest compressions.
    4. Assess the oxygen saturation level.

42. A neonatologist requests Narcan (naloxone) during a neonatal resuscitation effort for a baby weighing 3 kg. Which of the following dosages would be within the range of safety for the nurse to prepare?
    1. 4 micrograms.
    2. 40 micrograms.
    3. 4 milligrams.
    4. 40 milligrams.

43. During neonatal cardiopulmonary resuscitation, which of the following actions should be performed?
    1. Provide assisted ventilation at 40 to 60 breaths per minute.
    2. Begin chest compressions when heart rate is 0 to 20 beats per minute.
    3. Compress the chest using the three-finger technique.
    4. Administer compressions and breaths in a 5:1 ratio.

44. The staff on the maternity unit is developing a protocol for nurses to follow after a baby is delivered who fails to breathe spontaneously. Which of the following should be included in the protocol as the first action for the nurse to take?
    1. Prepare epinephrine for administration.
    2. Provide positive pressure oxygen.
    3. Administer chest compressions.
    4. Rub the back and feet of the baby.

45. A nurse in the newborn nursery suspects that a new admission, 42 weeks' gestation, was exposed to meconium in utero. What would lead the nurse to suspect this?
    1. The baby is bradycardic.
    2. The baby's umbilical cord is green.
    3. The baby's anterior fontanel is sunken.
    4. The baby is desquamating.

46. The birth of a baby, weight 4,500 grams, was complicated by shoulder dystocia. Which of the following neonatal complications should the nursery nurse observe for?
    1. Leg deformities.
    2. Brachial palsy.
    3. Fractured radius.
    4. Buccal abrasions.

47. During a health maintenance visit at the pediatrician's office, the nurse notes that a breastfeeding baby has thrush. Which of the following actions should the nurse take?
    1. Nothing because thrush is a benign problem.
    2. Advise the mother to bottle feed until the thrush is cured.
    3. Obtain an order for antifungals for both mother and baby.
    4. Assess for other evidence of immunosuppression.

48. A neonate whose mother is HIV positive is admitted to the NICU. A nursing diagnosis: Risk for infection related to perinatal exposure to HIV/AIDS is made. Which of the following interventions should the nurse make in relation to the diagnosis?
    1. Monitor daily viral load laboratory reports.
    2. Check the baby's viral antibody status.
    3. Obtain an order for antiviral medication.
    4. Place the baby on strict precautions.

49. A baby was just born to a mother who had positive vaginal cultures for group B streptococcus. The mother was admitted to the labor room 2 hours before the birth. For which of the following should the nursery nurse closely observe this baby?
    1. Hypothermia.
    2. Mottling.
    3. Omphalocele.
    4. Stomatitis.

50. A baby in the newborn nursery was born to a mother with spontaneous rupture of membranes for 14 hours. The woman has *Candida* vaginitis. For which of the following should the baby be assessed?
    1. Papular facial rash.
    2. Thrush.
    3. Fungal conjunctivitis.
    4. Dehydration.

51. A baby has been admitted to the neonatal nursery whose mother is hepatitis B–surface antigen positive. Which of the following actions by the nurse should be taken at this time?
    1. Monitor the baby for signs of hepatitis B.
    2. Place the baby on contact isolation.
    3. Obtain an order for the hepatitis B vaccine and the immune globulin.
    4. Advise the mother that breastfeeding is absolutely contraindicated.

52. Four full-term babies were admitted to the neonatal nursery. The mothers of each of the babies had labors of 4 hours or less. The nursery nurse should carefully monitor which of the babies for hypothermia?
    1. The baby whose mother cultured positive for group B strep during her third trimester.
    2. The baby whose mother had gestational diabetes.
    3. The baby whose mother was hospitalized for 3 months with complete placenta previa.
    4. The baby whose mother previously had a stillbirth.

53. Four 38-week-gestation gravidas have just delivered. Which of the babies should be monitored closely by the nurse for respiratory distress?
    1. The baby whose mother has diabetes mellitus.
    2. The baby whose mother has lung cancer.
    3. The baby whose mother has hypothyroidism.
    4. The baby whose mother has asthma.

54. A client is seeking preconception counseling. She has type 1 diabetes mellitus and is found to have an elevated glycosylated hemoglobin (HgbA$_{1c}$) level. Before actively trying to become pregnant, she is strongly encouraged to stabilize her blood glucose to reduce the possibility of her baby developing which of the following?
    1. Port wine stain.
    2. Cardiac defect.
    3. Hip dysplasia.
    4. Intussusception.

55. A baby is born with caudal agenesis. Which of the following maternal complications is associated with this defect?
    1. Poorly controlled myasthenia gravis.
    2. Poorly controlled diabetes mellitus.
    3. Poorly controlled splenic syndrome.
    4. Poorly controlled hypothyroidism.

56. A macrosomic infant of a non–insulin dependent diabetic mother has been admitted to the neonatal nursery. The baby's glucose level on admission to the nursery is 25 mg/dL and after a feeding of mother's expressed breast milk is 35 mg/dL. Which of the following actions should the nurse take at this time?
    1. Nothing, because the glucose level is normal for an infant of a diabetic mother.
    2. Administer intravenous glucagon slowly over five minutes.
    3. Feed the baby a bottle of dextrose and water and reassess the glucose level.
    4. Notify the neonatologist of the abnormal glucose levels.

57. A baby has just been born to a type 1 diabetic mother with retinopathy and nephropathy. Which of the following neonatal findings would the nurse expect to see?
    1. Hyperalbuminemia.
    2. Polycythemia.
    3. Hypercalcemia.
    4. Hypoinsulinemia.

58. A baby is born to a type 1 diabetic mother. Which of the following lab values would the nurse expect the neonate to exhibit?
    1. Plasma glucose 30 mg/dL.
    2. Red blood cell count 1 million/mm^3.
    3. White blood cell count 2,000/mm^3.
    4. Hemoglobin 8 g/dL.

59. A baby has just been admitted into the neonatal intensive care unit with a diagnosis of intrauterine growth restriction (IUGR). Which of the following maternal factors would predispose the baby to this diagnosis? **Select all that apply.**
    1. Hyperopia.
    2. Gestational diabetes.
    3. Substance abuse.
    4. Chronic hypertension.
    5. Advanced maternal age.

60. A baby has been admitted to the neonatal intensive care unit with a diagnosis of symmetrical intrauterine growth restriction (IUGR). Which of the following pregnancy complications would be consistent with this diagnosis?
    1. Severe preeclampsia.
    2. Chromosomal defect.
    3. Infarcts in an aging placenta.
    4. Premature rupture of the membranes.

61. A neonate has intrauterine growth restriction secondary to placental insufficiency. Which of the following signs/symptoms should the nurse expect to observe at delivery? **Select all that apply.**
    1. Thrombocytopenia.
    2. Neutropenia.
    3. Polycythemia.
    4. Hypoglycemia.
    5. Hyperlipidemia.

62. A woman is visiting the NICU to see her 26-week-gestation baby for the first time. Which of the following methods would the nurse expect the mother to use when first making physical contact with her baby?
    1. Fingertip touch.
    2. Palmar touch.
    3. Kangaroo hold.
    4. Cradle hold.

63. A 6-month-old child is being seen in the pediatrician's office. The child was born preterm and remained in the neonatal intensive care unit for the first 5 months of life. The child is being monitored for 5 chronic problems. Which of the following problems are directly related to the prematurity? **Select all that apply.**
    1. Bronchopulmonary dysplasia.
    2. Cerebral palsy.
    3. Retinopathy.
    4. Hypothyroidism.
    5. Seizure disorders.

64. A neonatologist prescribes Garamycin (gentamicin) for a 2-day-old, septic preterm infant who weighs 1,653 grams and is 38 centimeters long. The drug reference states: Neonatal dosage of Garamycin for babies less than 1 week of age is 2.5 mg/kg q 12–24 hours. Calculate the safe daily dosage of this medication. (**Calculate to the nearest hundredth.**)
    _____ mg q 24 hours.

65. The neonatologist has ordered 12.5 micrograms of digoxin po for a neonate in congestive heart failure. The medication is available in the following elixir—0.05 mg/mL. How many milliliters (mL) should the nurse administer? (**Calculate to the nearest hundredth.**)
    _____ mL.

66. A neonatologist prescribes Platinol-AQ (cisplatin) for a neonate born with a neuroblastoma. The baby's current weight is 3,476 grams and the baby is 57 centimeters long. The drug reference states: Children: IV 30 mg/m² q week. Calculate the safe dosage of this medication. (**Calculate to the nearest tenth.**)
    _____ mg q week.

67. A preterm baby is to receive 4 mg Garamycin (gentamicin) IV every 24 hours. The medication is being injected into an IV soluset. A total of 5 mL is to be administered via IV pump over 90 minutes. The pump should be set at what rate? (**Calculate to the nearest hundredth.**)
    _____ mL/hr.

68. A mother of a preterm baby is performing kangaroo care in the neonatal nursery. Which of the following responses would the nurse evaluate as a positive neonatal outcome?
    1. Respiratory rate of 70.
    2. Temperature of 97.0°F.
    3. Licking of mother's nipples.
    4. Flaring of the baby's nares.

69. A neonate is being assessed for necrotizing enterocolitis (NEC). Which of the following actions by the nurse is appropriate? **Select all that apply.**
    1. Perform hemoccult test on stools.
    2. Monitor for an increase in abdominal girth.
    3. Measure gastric contents before each feed.
    4. Assess bowel sounds before each feed.
    5. Assess for anal fissures daily.

70. A woman whose 32-week-gestation neonate is to begin oral feedings is expressing breast milk (EBM) for the baby. The neonatologist is recommending that fortifier be added to the milk because which of the following needs of the baby are not met by the EBM?
    1. Need for iron and zinc.
    2. Need for calcium and phosphorus.
    3. Need for protein and fat.
    4. Need for sodium and potassium.

71. A 1,000-gram neonate is being admitted to the neonatal intensive care unit. The surfactant Survanta (beractant) has just been prescribed to prevent respiratory distress syndrome. Which of the following actions should the nurse take while administering this medication?
    1. Flush the intravenous line with normal saline solution.
    2. Assist the neonatologist during the intubation procedure.
    3. Inject the medication deep into the vastus lateralis muscle.
    4. Administer the reconstituted liquid via an oral syringe.

72. A 30-week-gestation neonate, 2 hours old, has received Survanta (beractant). Which of the following would indicate a positive response to the medication?
    1. Axillary temperature 98.0°F.
    2. Oxygen saturation 96%.
    3. Apical heart rate 154 bpm.
    4. Serum potassium 4.0 mEq/L.

73. For which of the following reasons would a nurse in the well-baby nursery report to the neonatologist that a newborn appears to be preterm?
    1. Baby has a square window angle of 90°.
    2. Baby has leathery and cracked skin.
    3. Baby has popliteal angle of 90°.
    4. Baby has pronounced plantar creases.

74. A full-term neonate in the NICU has been diagnosed with congestive heart failure secondary to a cyanotic heart defect. Which of the following activities is most likely to result in a cyanotic episode?
    1. Feeding.
    2. Sleeping in the supine position.
    3. Rocking in an infant swing.
    4. Swaddling.

75. The nurse is providing discharge teaching to the parents of a baby born with a cleft lip and palate. Which of the following should be included in the teaching?
    1. Correct technique for the administration of a gastrostomy feeding.
    2. Need to watch for the appearance of blood-stained mucus from the nose.
    3. Optimal position for burping after nasogastric feedings.
    4. Need to give the baby sufficient time to rest during each feeding.

76. A baby is suspected of having esophageal atresia. The nurse would expect to see which of the following signs/symptoms? **Select all that apply.**
    1. Frequent vomiting.
    2. Excessive mucus.
    3. Ruddy complexion.
    4. Abdominal distention.
    5. Pigeon chest.

77. The nurse is teaching a couple about the special health care needs of their newborn child with Down syndrome. The nurse knows that the teaching was successful when the parents state that the child will need which of the following?
    1. Yearly three-hour glucose tolerance testing.
    2. Immediate intervention during bleeding episodes.
    3. A formula that is low in lactose and phenylalanine.
    4. Prompt treatment of upper respiratory infections.

78. An infant in the neonatal nursery has low-set ears, Simian creases, and slanted eyes. The nurse should monitor this infant carefully for which of the following signs/symptoms?
    1. Blood-tinged urine.
    2. Hemispheric paralysis.
    3. Cardiac murmur.
    4. Hemolytic jaundice.

79. Which of the following actions would the NICU nurse expect to perform when caring for a neonate with esophageal atresia and tracheoesophageal fistula (TEF)?
    1. Position the baby flat on the left side.
    2. Maintain low nasogastric suction.
    3. Give small, frequent feedings.
    4. Place on hypothermia blanket.

80. A nurse is assisting a mother to feed a baby born with cleft lip and palate. Which of the following should the nurse teach the mother?
    1. The baby is likely to cry from pain during the feeding.
    2. The baby is likely to expel milk through the nose.
    3. The baby will feed more quickly than other babies.
    4. The baby will need to be fed high calorie formula.

81. A neonate that is admitted to the neonatal nursery is noted to have a 2-vessel cord. The nurse notifies the neonatologist to get an order for which of the following assessments?
    1. Renal function tests.
    2. Echocardiogram.
    3. Glucose tolerance test.
    4. Electroencephalogram.

82. In the delivery room, which of the following infant care interventions must a nurse perform when a neonate with a meningomyelocele is born?
    1. Perform nasogastric suctioning.
    2. Place baby in the prone position.
    3. Administer oxygen via face mask.
    4. Swaddle the baby in warmed blankets.

83. A baby in the NICU, who is exhibiting signs of congestive heart failure from an atrioventricular canal defect, is receiving a diuretic. In the plan of care, the nurse should include that the desired outcome for the child will be which of the following?
    1. Loss of body weight.
    2. Drop in serum sodium level.
    3. Rise in urine specific gravity.
    4. Increase in blood pressure.

84. The nurse caring for a neonate with congestive heart failure identifies which of the following nursing diagnoses as highest priority?
    1. Fatigue.
    2. Activity intolerance.
    3. Sleep pattern disturbance.
    4. Altered tissue perfusion.

85. The nurse administers Lanoxin (digoxin) to a baby in the NICU that has a cardiac defect. The baby vomits shortly after receiving the medication. Which of the following actions should the nurse perform next?
    1. Give a repeat dose.
    2. Notify the physician.
    3. Assess the apical and brachial pulses concurrently.
    4. Check the vomitus for streaks of blood.

86. A baby is born with a meningomyelocele at L2. In assessing the baby, which of the following would the nurse expect to see?
    1. Sensory loss in all four extremities.
    2. Tuft of hair over the lumbosacral region.
    3. Flaccid paralysis of the legs.
    4. Positive Moro reflex.

87. When examining a nenonate in the well-baby nursery, the nurse notes that the sclerae of the baby's eyes are visible above the iris of the eyes. Which of the following assessments is highest priority for the nurse to make next?
    1. Babinski and tonic neck reflexes.
    2. Evaluation of bilateral eye coordination.
    3. Blood type and Coombs' test results.
    4. Circumferences of the head and chest.

88. A baby is born with a suspected coarctation of the aorta. Which of the following assessments should be done by the nurse?
    1. Check blood pressures in all four limbs.
    2. Palpate the anterior fontanel for bulging.
    3. Assess hematocrit and hemoglobin values.
    4. Monitor for harlequin color changes.

89. The nurse is developing a teaching plan for parents of an infant with a tetralogy of Fallot. In which of the following positions should parents be taught to place the infant during a "blue," or "tet," spell?
    1. Supine.
    2. Prone.
    3. Knee-chest.
    4. Semi-Fowler's.

90. A child has been diagnosed with a small ventricular septal defect (VSD). Which of the following symptoms would the nurse expect to see?
    1. Cyanosis and clubbing of the fingers.
    2. Respiratory distress and extreme fatigue.
    3. Systolic murmur with no other obvious symptoms.
    4. Feeding difficulties with marked polycythemia.

91. A newborn in the NICU has just had a ventriculoperitoneal shunt inserted. Which of the following signs indicates that the shunt is functioning properly?
    1. Decrease of the baby's head circumference.
    2. Absence of cardiac arrhythmias.
    3. Rise of the baby's blood pressure.
    4. Appearance of setting sun sign.

92. A neonate has just been born with a meningomyelocele. Which of the following nursing diagnoses should the nurse identify as related to this medical diagnosis?
    1. Deficient fluid volume.
    2. High risk for infection.
    3. Ineffective breathing pattern.
    4. Imbalanced nutrition: less than body requirements.

93. The neonatologist assesses a newborn for Hirschsprung's disease after the baby exhibited which of the following signs/symptoms?
    1. Passed meconium at 50 hours of age.
    2. Apical heart rate of 200 beats per minute.
    3. Maculopapular rash.
    4. Asymmetrical leg folds.

94. The nurse assessed four newborns admitted to the neonatal nursery and called the neonatologist for a consult on the baby, who exhibited which of the following?
    1. Excessive amounts of frothy saliva from the mouth.
    2. Blood-tinged discharge from the vaginal canal.
    3. Secretion of a milk-like substance from both breasts.
    4. Heart rate that sped during inhalation and slowed with exhalation.

95. The nurse is caring for a baby diagnosed with developmental dysplasia of the hip (DDH). Which of the following therapeutic interventions should the nurse expect to perform?
    1. Place the baby's legs in abduction.
    2. Administer pain medication as needed.
    3. Assist with bilateral leg casting.
    4. Monitor pedal pulses bilaterally.

96. A baby has been diagnosed with developmental dysplasia of the hip (DDH). Which of the following findings would the nurse expect to see?
    1. Pronounced hip abduction.
    2. Swelling at the site.
    3. Asymmetrical leg folds.
    4. Weak femoral pulses.

97. The nurse suspects that a newborn in the nursery has a clubbed right foot because the foot is plantar flexed as well as which of the following?
    1. Inability to move the foot into alignment.
    2. Positive Ortolani sign on the right.
    3. Shortened right metatarsal arch.
    4. Positive Babinski reflex on the right.

98. The parents of a baby born with bilateral talipes equinovarus ask the nurse what medical care the baby will likely need. Which of the following should the nurse tell the parents? The baby will:
    1. Need a series of leg casts until the correction is accomplished.
    2. Have a Harrington rod inserted when the child is about three years old.
    3. Have a Pavlik harness fitted before discharge from the nursery.
    4. Need to wear braces on both legs until the child begins to walk.

99. The nurse caring for an infant with a congenital cardiac defect is monitoring the child for which of the following early signs of congestive heart failure? **Select all that apply.**
    1. Palpitations.
    2. Tachypnea.
    3. Tachycardia.
    4. Diaphoresis.
    5. Irritability

100. The nurse assessed four newborns in the neonatal nursery. The nurse called the neonatologist for a cardiology consult on the baby, who exhibited which of the following signs/symptoms?
    1. Setting sun sign.
    2. Anasarca.
    3. Flaccid extremities.
    4. Polydactyly.

101. A preterm infant has a patent ductus arteriosus (PDA). Which of the following explanations should the nurse give to the parents about the condition?
    1. Hole has developed between the left and right ventricles.
    2. Hypoxemia occurs as a result of the poor systemic circulation.
    3. Oxygenated blood is reentering the pulmonary system.
    4. Blood is shunting from the right side of the heart to the left.

102. A nurse hears a heart murmur on a full-term neonate in the well-baby nursery. The baby's color is pink while at rest and while feeding. Which of the following cardiac defects is consistent with the nurse's findings? **Select all that apply.**
    1. Transposition of the great vessels.
    2. Tetralogy of Fallot.
    3. Ventricular septal defect.
    4. Pulmonic stenosis.
    5. Patent ductus arteriosus.

103. Four babies are born with distinctive skin markings. Identify which marking matches its description:
    1. Café au lait spot   A. Raised, blood vessel–filled lesion.
    2. Hemangioma   B. Flat, sharply demarcated red-to-purple lesion.
    3. Mongolian spots   C. Multiple grayish-blue, hyperpigmented skin areas.
    4. Port wine stain   D. Pale tan- to coffee-colored marking.

104. A baby, admitted to the nursery, was diagnosed with galactosemia from an amniocentesis. Which of the following actions must the nurse take?
    1. Feed the baby a specialty formula.
    2. Monitor the baby for central cyanosis.
    3. Do hemoccult testing on every stool.
    4. Monitor the baby for signs of abdominal pain.

105. On admission to the nursery, a baby's head and chest circumferences are 39 cm and 32 cm, respectively. Which of the following actions should the nurse take next?
    1. Assess the anterior fontanel.
    2. Measure the abdominal girth.
    3. Check the apical pulse rate.
    4. Monitor the respiratory effort.

106. A neonate is found to have choanal atresia on admission to the nursery. Which of the following physiological actions will be hampered by this diagnosis?
    1. Feeding.
    2. Digestion.
    3. Immune response.
    4. Glomerular filtration.

107. A baby is born to a mother who was diagnosed with oligohydramnios during her pregnancy. The nurse notifies the neonatologist to order tests to assess the functioning of which of the following systems?
    1. Gastrointestinal.
    2. Hepatic.
    3. Endocrine.
    4. Renal.

108. A baby is born with esophageal atresia and tracheoesophageal fistula. Which of the following complications of pregnancy would the nurse expect to note in the mother's history?
    1. Preeclampsia.
    2. Idiopathic thrombocytopenia.
    3. Polyhydramnios.
    4. Severe iron deficiency anemia.

109. A baby is born with a diaphragmatic hernia. Which of the following signs/symptoms would the nurse observe in the delivery room?
    1. Projectile vomiting.
    2. High-pitched crying.
    3. Respiratory distress.
    4. Fecal incontinence.

110. A woman, who has recently received Demerol (meperidine) 100 mg IM for labor pain, is about to deliver. Which of the following medications is highest priority for the nurse to prepare in case it must be administered to the baby following the delivery?
    1. Oxytocin (Pitocin).
    2. Xylocaine (Lidocaine).
    3. Naloxone (Narcan).
    4. Butorphanol (Stadol).

111. A newborn in the well-baby nursery is noted to have a chignon. The nurse concludes that the baby was born via which of the following methods?
    1. Cesarean section.
    2. High forceps delivery.
    3. Low forceps delivery.
    4. Vacuum extraction.

112. A baby born by vacuum extraction has been admitted to the well-baby nursery. The nurse should assess this baby for which of the following?
    1. Pedal abrasions.
    2. Hypobilirubinemia.
    3. Hyperglycemia.
    4. Cephalhematoma.

113. A macrosomic baby in the nursery is suspected of having a fractured clavicle from a traumatic delivery. Which of the following signs/symptoms would the nurse expect to see? **Select all that apply.**
    1. Pain with movement.
    2. Hard lump at the fracture site.
    3. Malpositioning of the arm.
    4. Asymmetrical Moro reflex.
    5. Marked localized ecchymosis.

114. Four babies in the well-baby nursery were born with congenital defects. Which of the babies' complications developed as a result of the delivery method?
    1. Clubfoot.
    2. Brachial palsy.
    3. Gastroschisis.
    4. Hydrocele.

115. Monochorionic twins, whose gestation was complicated by twin-to-twin transfusion, are admitted to the neonatal intensive care unit. Which of the following characteristic findings would the nurse expect to see in the smaller twin?
    1. Pallor.
    2. Jaundice.
    3. Opisthotonus.
    4. Hydrocephalus.

116. Monochorionic twins, whose gestation was complicated by twin-to-twin transfusion, are admitted to the neonatal intensive care unit. Which of the following characteristic findings would the nurse expect to see?
    1. Recipient twin has petechial rash.
    2. Recipient twin is 20% larger than the donor twin.
    3. Donor twin has 30% higher hematocrit than recipient twin.
    4. Donor twin is ruddy and plethoric.

117. A nurse working with a 24-hour-old neonate in the well-baby nursery has made
the following nursing diagnosis: Risk for altered growth. Which of the following
assessments would warrant this diagnosis?
    1. The baby has lost 8% of weight since birth.
    2. The baby has not urinated since birth.
    3. The baby weighed 3,000 grams at birth.
    4. The baby exhibited signs of torticollis.

118. A baby exhibits weak rooting and sucking reflexes. Which of the following nursing
diagnoses would be appropriate?
    1. Risk for deficient fluid volume.
    2. Activity intolerance.
    3. Risk for aspiration.
    4. Feeding self-care deficit.

119. A baby, born at 3,199 grams, now weighs 2,746 grams. The baby is being monitored
for dehydration because of the following percent weight loss. **(Calculate to the
nearest hundredth.)**
    _____%

The correct answer number and rationale for why it is the correct answer are given in **boldface blue type**. Rationales for why the other possible answer options are incorrect also are given, but they are not in boldface type.

1. 1. The normal temperature of a premature baby is the same as a full-term baby.
   2. Axillary temperatures, when performed correctly, provide accurate information.
   3. **Preterm babies are born with an insufficient supply of brown adipose tissue that is needed for thermogenesis, or heat generation.**
   4. There is nothing in the question that would explain conduction heat loss.

   TEST-TAKING TIP: It is important for the test taker not to read into questions. Even though conduction can be a means of heat loss in the neonate and, more particularly, in the premature, there are three other means by which neonates lose heat—radiation, convection, and evaporation. Conduction could be singled out as a cause of the hypothermia only if it were clear from the question conduction was the cause of the problem.

2. 1. Infants of diabetic mothers are often large-for-gestational age, but they are not especially at high risk for cold stress syndrome.
   2. Infants born with Rh incompatibility are not especially at high risk for cold stress syndrome.
   3. **Postdate babies are at high risk for cold stress syndrome because while still in utero they often metabolize the brown adipose tissue for nourishment when the placental function deteriorates.**
   4. Down syndrome babies are hypotonic, but they are not especially at high risk for cold stress syndrome.

   TEST-TAKING TIP: The test taker must know that cold stress syndrome results from a neonate's inability to create heat through metabolic means. In lieu of food intake, brown adipose tissue (BAT) and glycogen stores in the liver are the primary substances used for thermogenesis. The test taker must then deduce that the infant most likely to have poor supplies of BAT and glycogen is the postdates infant.

3. 1. Infants with cold stress exhibit hypoglycemia. A neonatal blood glucose of 50 mg/dL is normal.
   2. Acrocyanosis—bluish hands and feet—is normal for the neonate during the first day or two.
   3. **Babies who have cold stress syndrome will develop respiratory distress. One symptom of the distress is tachypnea.**
   4. The oxygen saturation is within normal limits.

   TEST-TAKING TIP: It is important for the test taker to know the normal variations seen in the neonate—for example, normal blood glucoses are lower in neonates than in the older child and adult and acrocyanosis is normal for a neonate's first day or two.

4. 1. **Intracostal retractions are symptomatic of respiratory distress syndrome.**
   2. Erythema toxicum is the normal newborn rash.
   3. Pseudostrabismus is a normal newborn finding.
   4. Vernix caseosa is the cheesy material that covers many babies at birth.

   TEST-TAKING TIP: It is important for the test taker to be familiar with the signs of respiratory distress in the neonate. Babies who are stressed by, for example, cold, sepsis, or prematurity will often exhibit signs of respiratory distress. The neonatologist should be called promptly.

5. 1. Grunting is a sign of respiratory distress. Offering a pacifier is an inappropriate intervention.
   2. Diapering is an inappropriate intervention.
   3. The baby is not hungry. Rather, the baby is in respiratory distress.
   4. **Grunting is often accompanied by tachypnea, another sign of respiratory distress.**

   TEST-TAKING TIP: If the test taker were to attempt to grunt, he or she would feel the respiratory effort that the baby is creating. Essentially, the baby is producing his or her own positive end-expiratory pressure (PEEP) to maximize his or her respiratory function.

6. 1. Blood urea nitrogen and serum creatinine tests are done to assess the renal system. Kernicterus does not affect the renal system. It results from an infiltration of bilirubin into the central nervous system.
2. Although alkaline phosphatase and bilirubin would be evaluated when a child is jaundiced, they are not appropriate as assessment tests for the child who has developed kernicterus.
3. **Because the central nervous system (CNS) may have been damaged by the high bilirubin levels, testing of the senses as well as motor and cognitive assessments are appropriate.**
4. The respiratory system is unaffected by high bilirubin levels.

TEST-TAKING TIP: The test taker must be aware that kernicterus is the syndrome that develops when a neonate is exposed to high levels of bilirubin over time. The bilirubin crosses the blood-brain barrier, often leading to toxic changes in the CNS.

7. 1. When phototherapy is administered, the baby's eyes must be protected from the light source.
2. Although the lights should be turned off and the pads removed periodically during the therapy, the lights should be on whenever the baby is in his or her crib.
3. The therapy is most effective when the skin surface exposed to the light is maximized. The shirt should be removed while the baby is under the lights.
4. The blanket should be removed while the baby is under the lights.

TEST-TAKING TIP: There is a difference between phototherapy administered by fluorescent light and phototherapy administered via fiber optic tubing to a bili-blanket. When a bili-blanket is used, the baby can be clothed and the baby's eyes do not need to be protected.

8. 1. Babies born with erythroblastosis fetalis are markedly anemic. They are not ruddy in appearance.
2. **Babies born with erythroblastosis fetalis often are in severe congestive heart failure and, therefore, exhibit anasarca.**
3. Babies with erythroblastosis fetalis are not at high risk for alopecia.
4. Erythema toxicum is a normal newborn rash that many healthy newborns have.

TEST-TAKING TIP: A baby with erythroblastosis fetalis has marked red blood cell destruction in utero secondary to the presence of maternal antibodies against the baby's blood. The severe anemia that results often leads to congestive heart failure of the fetus in utero.

9. 1. **The baby with erythroblastosis fetalis would exhibit signs of severe anemia, which a hematocrit of 24% reflects.**
2. Erythroblastosis fetalis is not an infectious condition. Leukocytosis is not a part of the clinical picture.
3. Hyponatremia is not part of the disorder.
4. Hyperkalemia is not part of the disorder.

TEST-TAKING TIP: The test taker must be familiar with the pathophysiology of Rh incompatibility. If a mother who is Rh-negative has been sensitized to Rh-positive blood, she will produce antibodies against the Rh-positive blood. If she then becomes pregnant with an Rh-positive baby, her anti-Rh antibodies will pass directly through the placenta into the fetal system. Hemolysis of fetal red blood cells results, leading to severe fetal anemia.

10. 1. **ABO incompatibility can arise when the mother is type O and the baby is either type A or type B.**
2. Hemolytic jaundice from ABO incompatibility is rarely seen when the maternal blood type is anything other than type O. Rh incompatibility can occur only if the mother is Rh-negative and the baby is Rh-positive.
3. Hemolytic jaundice from ABO incompatibility is rarely seen when the maternal blood type is anything other than type O. Rh incompatibility can only occur if the mother is Rh-negative and the baby is Rh-positive.
4. Hemolytic jaundice from ABO incompatibility is rarely seen when the maternal blood type is anything other than type O. Rh incompatibility can only occur if the mother is Rh-negative and the baby is Rh-positive.

TEST-TAKING TIP: A mother whose blood type is O, the blood type that is antigen negative, will produce anti-A and/or anti-B antibodies against blood types A and/or B, respectively. The anti-A (and/or anti-B) that passes into the baby's bloodstream via the placenta can attack the baby's red blood cells if he or she is type A or B. As a result of the blood cell destruction, the baby becomes jaundiced.

11. 1. The Coombs' test assesses for the presence of antibodies in the blood. The test will not predict or explain jitters in the neonate.
2. The Coombs' test will not predict or explain hypoglycemia in the neonate.
3. The Coombs' test will not predict or explain a change in temperature in the neonate.
4. **When the neonatal bloodstream contains antibodies, hemolysis of the red blood cells occurs and jaundice develops.**

TEST-TAKING TIP: **The indirect Coombs' test is performed on the pregnant woman to detect whether or not she carries antibodies against her fetus's red blood cells. The direct Coombs' test is performed on the newborn to detect whether or not he or she carries maternal antibodies against his or her blood.**

12. 1. The neonate needs nourishment with formula and/or breast milk.
2. **Rotating the baby's position maximizes the therapeutic response because the more skin surface that is exposed to the light source, the better the results are.**
3. It is unnecessary to restrain the baby while under the bili-lights.
4. Intravenous fluids would be administered only under extreme circumstances.

TEST-TAKING TIP: **Bilirubin levels decrease with exposure to a light source. The more skin surface that is exposed, the more efficient the therapy is. Although fluids are needed to maintain hydration and to foster stooling, oral rehydration therapy is nutritionally insufficient.**

13. 1. The foot should be covered with a warm wrap to draw blood to the area for the heel stick.
2. **The lateral heel is the site of choice because it contains no major nerves or blood vessels.**
3. Alcohol can irritate the punctured skin and can cause hemolysis.
4. The ankle and foot should be firmly grasped during the procedure.

TEST-TAKING TIP: **The test taker must be aware of the physiological structures in the body. In the case of a heel stick, if the posterior surface of the heel is punctured, the posterior tibial nerve and artery could be injured.**

14. 1. The ambient temperature will affect the baby's temperature, but it will not affect the bilirubin level.
2. **Bilirubin is excreted through the bowel. The more the baby consumes, the more stools she or he will produce; in other words, the more feces the baby excretes, the more bilirubin the baby will expel.**
3. Holding the baby skin to skin has no direct affect on the bilirubin level.
4. The bilirubin levels of babies exposed to direct sunlight will drop. It is unsafe, however, to expose a baby's skin to direct sunlight.

TEST-TAKING TIP: **This is one example of a change in practice that has occurred because of updated knowledge. In the past, babies have been placed in sunlight to reduce their bilirubin levels, but that practice is no longer considered to be safe. It is important, therefore, for the test taker to be up to date on current practice.**

15. 1. The stools are green from the increase in excreted bilirubin.
2. There is no need to inform the health care practitioner. Green stools are an expected finding.
3. Although green stools can be seen with diarrheal illnesses, in this situation, the green stools are expected and not related to an infectious state.
4. **The stools can be very caustic to the baby's delicate skin. The nurse should cleanse the area well and inspect the skin for any sign that the skin is breaking down.**

TEST-TAKING TIP: **The test taker must know the difference between signs that are normal and those that reflect a possible illness. Although green stools can be seen with diarrheal illnesses, in this situation, the green stools are expected. The green stools are due to the increased bilirubin excreted and not related to an infectious state.**

16. 1. Healthy, hydrated neonates saturate their diapers a minimum of 6 times in 24 hours.
2. To consume enough fluid and nutrients for growth and hydration, babies should breastfeed at least 8 times in 24 hours.
3. A weight loss of over 10% is indicative of dehydration.
4. Tachycardia can indicate dehydration.

TEST-TAKING TIP: This is an evaluation question. The test taker is being asked to identify signs that would indicate a baby that is fully hydrated. It is important for the test taker to know the expected intake and output of the neonate and to understand the evaluation phase of the nursing process.

17. 1. Morphine is an opiate narcotic. It may be administered to an addicted baby to control diarrhea associated with neonatal abstinence syndrome.
    2. Opium is administered to neonates who are exhibiting signs of severe neonatal abstinence syndrome.
    3. Narcan is an opiate. If it were to be given to the neonate with neonatal abstinence syndrome, the baby would go into a traumatic withdrawal.
    4. Phenobarbital is sometimes administered to drug-exposed neonates to control seizures.

TEST-TAKING TIP: "Neonatal abstinence syndrome" is the term used to describe the many behaviors exhibited by neonates who are born drug addicted. The behaviors range from hyperreflexia to excessive sneezing and yawning to loose diarrheal stools. Medications may or may not be administered to control the many signs/symptoms of the syndrome.

18. 1. Tightly swaddling drug-addicted babies often helps to control the hyperreflexia that they may exhibit.
    2. Placing hyperactive babies on their abdomens can result in skin abrasions on the face and knees from rubbing against the linens. And, like all babies, drug-addicted babies should be placed supine during all unsupervised time periods.
    3. Drug-exposed babies should be placed in a low-stimulation environment.
    4. The babies should be given small, frequent feedings either of full-strength formula or of breast milk.

TEST-TAKING TIP: Drug-exposed babies exhibit signs of neonatal abstinence syndrome: hyperactivity, hyperreflexia, and the like. The test taker should look for a nursing intervention that would minimize those behaviors. Tightly swaddling the baby would help to reduce the baby's behavioral responses.

19. 1 and 5 are correct.
    1. Babies with signs of neonatal abstinence syndrome repeatedly exhibit signs of hunger.
    2. Babies with neonatal abstinence syndrome are hyperactive, not lethargic.
    3. Babies with neonatal abstinence syndrome often exhibit sleep disturbances rather than prolonged periods of sleep.
    4. Babies with signs of neonatal abstinence syndrome are hyperreflexic, not hyporeflexic.
    5. Babies with signs of neonatal abstinence syndrome often have a shrill cry that may continue for prolonged periods.

TEST-TAKING TIP: The baby who is exhibiting signs of neonatal abstinence syndrome is craving an addicted drug. The baby's body is agitated because the illicit narcotics he or she has been exposed to are central nervous system depressants and their removal has agitated him or her. The test taker, therefore, should consider symptoms that reflect central nervous system stimulation as correct responses.

20. 1. FAS babies usually have a very weak suck.
    2. Ambiguous genitalia is not a characteristic anomaly seen in FAS.
    3. A webbed neck is not a characteristic anomaly seen in FAS.
    4. FAS babies usually have an intact CNS system with a positive Moro reflex.

TEST-TAKING TIP: The characteristic facial signs of fetal alcohol syndrome—shortened palpebral (eyelid) fissures, thin upper lip, and hypoplastic philtrum (median groove on the external surface of the upper lip)—are rarely evident in the neonatal period. They typically appear later in the child's life. Rather, the behavioral characteristics of the FAS baby, such as weak suck, irritability, tremulousness, and seizures, are present at birth.

21. 1. Paregoric contains morphine. It is addictive.
    2. Paregoric does help to control the diarrhea seen in drug-addicted neonates.
    3. Paregoric does cause drowsiness.
    4. Sneezing is a symptom seen in drug-addicted neonates, not coughing.

TEST-TAKING TIP: Paregoric, a liquid form of morphine, is an especially effective therapy for a baby who is experiencing severe neonatal abstinence syndrome. The narcotic relieves the cravings that the baby has for the addicted drug; in addition, paregoric is effective against the diarrhea that many addicted babies experience.

22. 1. The symptoms are characteristic of neonatal abstinence syndrome. A urine toxicology would provide evidence of drug exposure.
2. Biophysical profiles are done during pregnancy to assess the well-being of the fetus.
3. There is no indication from the question that this child has any chest or abdominal abnormalities.
4. This child is not exhibiting signs of respiratory distress.

TEST-TAKING TIP: It is important for the test taker to attend to the fact that this child has normal serum glucose levels. When babies exhibit tremors, the first thing the nurse should consider is hypoglycemia. Once that has been ruled out, and as the baby is exhibiting other signs of drug withdrawal, the nurse should consider drug exposure.

23. 1. This baby is hypothermic, but the best intervention would be to place the baby under a warmer rather than to swaddle the baby. Plus, the baby's glucose levels must be assessed to determine whether or not this baby is hypoglycemic. The glucose can be evaluated while the baby is under the warmer.
2. The glucose level should be assessed to determine whether or not this baby is hypoglycemic.
3. A feeding will elevate the glucose level if it is below normal. The nurse does need to assess the level, however, to make a clear determination of the problem.
4. The administration of the neonatal medicines is not a priority at this time.

TEST-TAKING TIP: The test taker should note that this baby is macrosomic and hypothermic, both of which make the baby at high risk for hypoglycemia. Plus, jitters are a classic symptom in hypoglycemic babies. To make an accurate assessment of the problem, the baby's glucose level must be assessed.

24. 1. Jaundice is not related to blood glucose levels.
2. Babies who are hypoglycemic will often develop jitters (tremors).

3. Erythema toxicum is the newborn rash. It is unrelated to blood glucose levels.
4. Subconjunctival hemorrhages are often evident in neonates. They are related to the trauma of delivery, not to blood glucose levels.

TEST-TAKING TIP: The test taker should remember that the normal glucose level for neonates in the immediate postdelivery period—approximately 45 to 90 mg/dL—is less than that seen in older babies and children.

25. 1. A baby with a blood glucose of 35 mg/dL is hypoglycemic. The action of choice is to feed the baby either formula or breast milk.
2. The baby's blood pressure is not a relevant factor at this time.
3. Tightly swaddling the baby may disguise a common finding, jitters or tremors, seen in babies who are hypoglycemic.
4. The baby's urinary output is not a relevant factor at this time.

TEST-TAKING TIP: Although the test taker may believe that glucose water should be fed to the baby at this time, the substance of choice is either formula or breast milk. The sugars in the milk will elevate the baby's blood values in the short term and the proteins and fats in the milk will help to maintain the glucose values in the normal range.

26. 1. The gavage tubing must be measured to approximate the length of the insertion.
2. The tubing should be lubricated with sterile water or a water-soluble lubricant, not an oil-based solution.
3. If the child becomes cyanotic, the tubing should be removed immediately.
4. A small amount of air should be injected into the tubing while the nurse listens with a stethoscope over the baby's stomach area.

TEST-TAKING TIP: The placement of gavage tubing is potentially dangerous. Not only must the distance between the nose and the ear be measured, but also the length from the ear to the point midway between the ear and the xiphoid process. This entire distance is the tubing insertion length. To assess placement, air should be injected into the tubing rather than water because the tubing may mistakenly have been inserted into the trachea.

27. 1. The appropriate placement for the skin thermal sensor is the abdominal wall, not the xiphoid process.
    2. The appropriate placement for the skin thermal sensor is the abdominal wall, not the forehead.
    3. The abdominal wall is the appropriate placement for the skin thermal sensor.
    4. The appropriate placement for the skin thermal sensor is the abdominal wall, not the great toe.

    TEST-TAKING TIP: It is essential that the test taker be prepared to perform relatively simple procedures for the premature infant. To monitor the temperature of the premature, the probes should be placed on a nonbony and well-perfused tissue site. The abdominal wall is the site of choice.

28. 4, 2, 1, and 3 is the correct order.
    1. Rotation and removal of the suction catheter should be done after the tubing has been inserted through the nose and a thumb placed over the suction control on the catheter.
    2. The nurse should place a thumb over the suction control on the catheter after inserting the free end of the tubing through the nose—and before the other two steps are taken.
    3. Assessing the type and amount of secretions is the last step in the process.
    4. Inserting the free end of the tubing through the nose is the first step in nasopharyngeal suctioning process.

    TEST-TAKING TIP: It is important for the test taker to remember that once the suction control is covered, the baby is unable to take in air. It is important, therefore, not to cover the suction control until the catheter is being removed.

29. 1. Neonates are incapable of controlling their movements. To maintain a safe IV site, it is essential to tape the baby's arm to an arm board.
    2. IV tubing is usually changed every 72 hours, not every 24 hours.
    3. The IV site should be assessed regularly, at least once an hour, but it is not necessary to check it every 5 minutes.
    4. IV infusions are usually continuous, unless a medication, like an antibiotic, is being administered.

TEST-TAKING TIP: Although restraints and arm boards are often unnecessary when caring for older children and adults, to be assured that the intravenous remains intact, the use of restraints and/or arm boards is often necessary when caring for infants, toddlers, and other young children.

30. 1. It is inappropriate to imply that, if a couple were to pray, their sick child will be "all right." The baby may be seriously ill and even may die.
    2. This baby's Apgar score is very low. There is a chance that the baby will not survive. It is appropriate to ask the parents, as they are known to be Roman Catholic, if they would like their baby baptized.
    3. Although it is often easier for the nurse to leave parents alone whose babies are doing poorly, it is rarely therapeutic.
    4. It is inappropriate to assume that the parents wish to give confession, although it may be appropriate to offer to have the priest visit them.

    TEST-TAKING TIP: When a baby is doing very poorly during the first minutes after delivery, there is a possibility that the baby may not survive. Couples who are Roman Catholic often wish to have their babies baptized in such situations. Because a priest is not present, it is appropriate for a nurse, of any religious faith, to perform the baptism at that time.

31. The baby's Apgar score is 3.

    TEST-TAKING TIP: Assessing the Apgar score is often a nursing function. The test taker, therefore, should know the criteria for the Apgar score (see table next page).

    The score is traditionally performed at 1 and 5 minutes after birth. A total score of 7 to 10 means that the baby is having little to no difficulty transitioning to extrauterine life. With a total score of 4 to 6, the baby is having moderate difficulty transitioning to extrauterine life. Resuscitative measures may need to be instituted. With a total score of 0 to 3, the baby is in severe distress. Resuscitative measures must be instituted.

Apgar Score

Sign	Score of 0	Score of 1	Score of 2
HEART RATE	Absent	Below 100 bpm	100 bpm and above
RESPIRATORY EFFORT	Absent	Slow and irregular	Lusty (vigorous) cry
MUSCLE TONE	Flaccid	Some flexion of the extremities	Active motion or well flexed extremities
REFLEX IRRITABILITY	Absent	Grimace	Lusty (vigorous) cry
COLOR	Completely cyanotic or very pale baby	Pink body with cyanotic extremities (acrocyanosis)	Pink body and extremities

32. 1. According to the graph, at 38 weeks' gestation, a 3,500-gram baby is between the 10th and the 90th percentiles for weight. The baby, therefore, is appropriate-for-gestation age.
    2. A baby who is large-for-gestational age is defined as a baby whose weight is above the 90th percentile. According to the graph, at 38 weeks' gestation, a 3,500-gram baby is below the 90th percentile for weight. Therefore, the diagnosis is inaccurate.
    3. A baby who is large-for-gestational age is defined as a baby whose weight is above the 90th percentile. According to the graph, at 38 weeks' gestation, a 3,500-gram baby is below the 90th percentile for weight.
    4. Any baby, born at any gestational age, can be found to be large for that gestational age.

TEST-TAKING TIP: It is important for the test taker to become comfortable with reading and interpreting graphs. The gestational age graph—weight in grams on the y-axis and weeks of gestation on the x-axis—is cut by 3 curves. The upper curve shows the weight at the 90th percentile for babies at differing gestational ages, whereas the lower curve shows the weight at the 10th percentile for babies of differing gestational ages. Those babies who fall above the upper curve—that is, whose weights are above the 90th percentile— are defined as large-for-gestational age (LGA). Those babies who fall below the lower curve—those with weights that are below the 10th percentile—are defined as small-for-gestational age (SGA). Those babies who fall between the upper and lower curves are defined as appropriate-for-gestational age (AGA). The middle curve shows the weights of babies at the 50th percentile.

33. 24 weeks

TEST-TAKING TIP: There are six characteristics on the neuromuscular maturity chart and six characteristics on the physical maturity chart (see the following charts). The baby is given a score for each characteristic and the scores are added together to get a total score. The total score is compared to the maturity rating chart. The baby in the question had a total score of 0, which relates to a gestational age score of 24 weeks.

34. 1. The baby's weight is appropriate-for-gestational age. The baby's weight of 1,000 grams falls between the 10th and 90th percentile curves for 28 weeks' gestation.
    2. The baby's weight is appropriate-for-gestational age.
    3. Babies who are intrauterine growth restricted would show weights that are below the 10th percentile for gestational age. 1,000 grams is not below the 10th percentile for a 28-week-gestation neonate.
    4. Babies who are hypertrophied would show weights that are above the 90th percentile for the gestational age.

TEST-TAKING TIP: Even if the test taker did not know the definitions of "intrauterine growth restriction" and "congenital growth hypertrophy," if the individual words are understood, the test taker would be able to deduce the meanings of the terms by defining each word in the terms and then putting the definitions together. "Intrauterine" means "in the uterus" and "restriction" is a "limitation." Intrauterine growth restriction, therefore, means limited growth in the uterus. The term "congenital" refers to conditions that are present at or before birth and "hypertrophy" means "enlargement" or "overgrowth." Congenital growth hypertrophy, therefore, refers to a baby that is larger than expected.

Neuromuscular Maturity

	–1	0	1	2	3	4	5
Posture							
Square Window (Wrist)	–90°	90°	60°	45°	30°	0°	
Arm Recoil		180°	140°–180°	110°–140°	90°–110°	<90°	
Popliteal Angle	180°	160°	140°	120°	100°	90°	<90°
Scarf Sign							
Heel To Ear							

Physical Maturity

Skin	sticky; friable; transparent	gelatinous; red; translucent	smooth pink; visible veins	superficial peeling or rash, few veins	cracking; pale areas; rare veins	parchment; deep cracking; no vessels	leathery; cracked; wrinkled
Lanugo	none	sparse	abundant	thinning	bald areas	mostly bald	
Plantar Surface	heel-toe 40–50 mm:–1 <40 mm:–2	>50 mm no crease	faint red marks	anterior transverse crease only	creases ant. 2/3	creases over entire sole	
Breast	imperceptible	barely perceptible	flat areola; no bud	stippled areola; 1–2 mm bud	raised areola; 3–4 mm bud	full areola; 5–10 mm bud	
Eye/ear	lids fused; loosely:–1 tightly:–2	lids open; pinna flat; stays folded	sl. curved pinna; soft; slow recoil	well-curved pinna; soft but ready recoil	formed and firm; instant recoil	thick cartilage; ear stiff	
Genitals (Male)	scrotum flat, smooth	scrotum empty; faint rugae	testes in upper canal; rare rugae	testes descending; few rugae	testes down; good rugae	testes pendulous; deep rugae	
Genitals (Female)	clitoris prominent; labia flat	prominent clitoris; small labia minora	prominent clitoris; enlarging minora	majora and minora equally prominent	majora large; minora small	majora cover clitoris and minora	

Maturity Rating

Score	Weeks
–10	20
–5	22
0	24
5	26
10	28
15	30
20	32
25	34
30	36
35	38
40	40
45	42
50	44

From: Ballard, J. L., Khoury, L. C., Wedig, K., et al. (1991). New Ballard Score, expanded to include extremely premature infants. *Journal of Pediatrics,* 19 (3), 417-423. With permission.

35. **TEST-TAKING TIP: The test taker should locate the 40-week-gestation line on the x-axis and follow it up to the 90th percentile curve. Babies whose weights are above the 90th percentile are labeled large-for-gestational age (see figure below).**

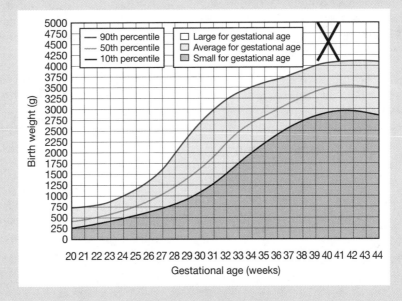

36. 1. This baby is small-for-gestational age. Full-term babies (40 weeks' gestation) should weigh between 2,500 and 4,000 grams. It is very likely that this baby used up his glycogen stores in utero because of an aging placenta. An aging placenta is unable to deliver sufficient nutrients to the fetus. As a result the fetus must use its glycogen stores to sustain life and, therefore, is high risk for hypoglycemia after birth.
2. There is no indication from this scenario that this baby is leukopenic.
3. Rather than being anemic, it is likely that this baby is polycythemic to compensate for the poor oxygenation from a poorly functioning placenta. In addition, it is likely that this baby is hemoconcentrated as a result of poor hydration.
4. It is unlikely that this baby would be alkalotic. Rather he may be acidotic from chronic hypoxemia and the metabolism of brown adipose tissue.

TEST-TAKING TIP: The test taker must attend carefully to the gestational age in any question relating to neonates. Post-term and preterm babies are at high risk for certain problems. Post-term babies are especially at high risk for hypoglycemia and chronic hypoxia because the aging placenta has not supplied sufficient quantities of oxygen and nutrients.

37. 1. The warmer must be preheated, but that is not the priority at this time.
2. The neonatologist must be called to the delivery room so that he or she arrives before the baby is delivered.
3. The woman did receive a narcotic analgesic 4 hours ago. Although Narcan may be needed, she has likely metabolized most of the medication by this time. The medication is not a priority at this time.
4. The eye prophylaxis can wait until this baby is at least 1 hour old. It is not a priority at this time.

TEST-TAKING TIP: This is a prioritizing question. Although all of these actions may be performed by the nurse, only one is a priority. This baby is showing signs of fetal distress—prolonged late decelerations. The baby may need to be resuscitated. The nurse must, therefore, page the neonatologist so that he or she is present for the birth of the baby.

38. 1. Abundant lanugo is seen in the preterm baby, not the post-term baby.
2. Absence of breast tissue is seen in the preterm baby, not the post-term baby.
3. Prominent clitoris is seen in the preterm baby, not the post-term baby.
4. The post-term baby does have dry, wrinkled, and often desquamating skin. The baby's dehydration is secondary to a placenta that progressively deteriorates after 40 weeks' gestation.

TEST-TAKING TIP: The test taker should be familiar with the characteristic presentations of preterm and postmature neonates. Studying the items on the New Ballard Scale and the corresponding gestational ages when the items are seen is an excellent way to associate certain characteristics with dysmature babies.

39. 1. Although the fluid is green tinged because the baby expelled meconium in utero, the baby's skin is not at high risk for injury.
2. The conjunctivae are not at high risk for irritation from the meconium-stained fluid.
3. There is nothing in the scenario that suggests that this baby is currently septic.
4. Meconium aspiration syndrome (MAS) is a serious complication seen in post-term neonates who are exposed to meconium-stained fluid. Respiratory distress would indicate that the baby has likely developed MAS.

TEST-TAKING TIP: Although meconium appears black in a newborn's diaper, it is actually a very dark green color. When diluted in the amniotic fluid, therefore, the fluid takes on a greenish tinge. Because meconium is a foreign substance, when aspirated by the baby, a chemical and, secondarily, a bacterial pneumonia often develop.

40. 1. Because meconium is present in the amniotic fluid, the baby should not be stimulated to breathe.
2. Although the heart rate is important, cardiac function is secondary to respiratory function.
3. Before breathing, the baby must be intubated so that the meconium-contaminated fluid can be aspirated from the baby's airway (See http://pediatrics.aappublications.org/content/126/5/e1400.full).

4. The baby is kept in a head-down, supine position.

TEST-TAKING TIP: The nurse, once the fluid was seen, should have paged the appropriate health care professional who would perform the intubation. The nurse would then assist with the procedure. Intubation is recommended for those babies who are not vigorous and who have yet to breathe. If a baby is breathing and active, however, intubation is not currently recommended.

41. 1. The gestational age assessment should be performed only after resuscitation efforts have been performed.
    2. **The baby's airway should be established by inflating the lungs with an ambu bag.**
    3. Chest compressions are begun after an airway is established and the heart rate has been assessed.
    4. Immediately after positive pressure ventilation (PPV) has been started, an oxygen saturation electrode should be placed on the baby's foot and the values should be monitored continuously

TEST-TAKING TIP: The steps of a neonatal resuscitation are slightly different from those for an older baby, child, or adult. Because the baby's survival is contingent upon the establishment of respiratory function, respiratory resuscitation must be instituted in a timely manner. If there is no spontaneous breathing and the heart rate is less than 100 bpm at 30 seconds after birth, PPV should be begun followed immediately by continuous O$_2$ saturation assessments. Cardiac compressions are started if the heart rate falls below 60 bpm (see http://pediatrics.aappublications.org/content/126/5/e1400.full).

42. 1. The 4 microgram dose is too low
    2. **The 40 microgram dose is within the range of safety**
    3. The 4 milligram dose is too high
    4. The 40 milligram dose is too high.

TEST-TAKING TIP: The recommended dosage for the administration of Narcan (naloxone) to a neonate has been cited as 0.01 mg/kg to 0.1 mg/kg. Because there are 1000 micrograms per mg, if the dosage were written in micrograms, the dosage for a 3-kg neonate would be: 30 micrograms to 300 micrograms. If the dosage were written in mg, the dosage for a 3-kg neonate would be: 0.03 mg to 0.3 mg.

The only choice that lies within the range of safety is 40 micrograms.

43. 1. Assisted ventilations should be administered at a rate of 40 to 60 per minute.
    2. Chest compressions should be begun when the heart rate is below 60 beats per minute.
    3. The chest should be compressed using either the "2-thumb" or the "2-finger" technique.
    4. **The compressions and ventilations should be administered in a 3:1 ratio.**

TEST-TAKING TIP: The correct answer could be deduced by the test taker by remembering the normal respiratory rate of the neonate (30 to 60 breaths per minute). During a resuscitation, the nurses and other health care practitioners would be attempting to simulate normal functioning (see http://pediatrics.aappublications.org/content/126/5/e1400.full).

44. 1. Epinephrine is administered only after other resuscitation measures have been instituted.
    2. Positive pressure oxygen is administered only after initial interventions of tactile stimulation and warmth have failed.
    3. Chest compressions are administered only after initial interventions have failed.
    4. **The first interventions when a neonate fails to breathe include providing tactile stimulation.**

TEST-TAKING TIP: When a neonate fails to breathe, the nurse should: dry the baby and provide tactile stimulation, place the child in the "sniff" position under a radiant warmer, and suction the mouth and nose of any mucus. Only after these initial actions fail—as the vast majority of the time the baby will respond—should further intervention be begun (see http://pediatrics.aappublications.org/content/126/5/e1400.full).

45. 1. Bradycardia is a sign of neonatal distress but it is not related to meconium exposure.
    2. **Because meconium is a dark green color, when it is expelled in utero, the baby can be stained green.**
    3. A sunken fontanel is an indication of dehydration, not of meconium exposure.
    4. A baby's skin often desquamates when he or she is post-term. Although meconium may be expelled by a post-term baby, desquamation is not related to the meconium.

TEST-TAKING TIP: The test taker may choose response 4 because he or she remembers that there is a relationship between babies who expel meconium and those who desquamate. That is true, but it is not a direct relationship. The fact that the baby is postdates is the common denominator between the two. The test taker should choose the response that is clearly correct: Because meconium is green it can stain the baby's tissues green. "Desquamation" is merely a fancy term for "skin peeling."

46. 1. Limb deformities develop during pregnancy. They are not related to dystocia.
    2. During a difficult delivery with shoulder dystocia, the brachial nerve can become stretched and may even be severed. The nurse should, therefore, observe the baby for signs of palsy.
    3. A fracture of the radius is an unlikely injury to occur even during a shoulder dystocia.
    4. Buccal surfaces lie inside the cheeks. Buccal abrasions are highly unlikely injuries for the baby to sustain during a shoulder dystocia.

TEST-TAKING TIP: The key to answering this question is understanding the terminology. A shoulder dystocia is a difficult delivery when the shoulder fails to pass easily through the pelvis. Deformities are disfigurements or malformations. Although the arm and shoulder may be injured, the baby is not disfigured. A buccal abrasion would occur on the inside of the cheek.

47. 1. *Candida* will infect both mother and baby.
    2. Only under very special circumstances should a mother be advised not to breastfeed. And it is safe to breastfeed when the baby has thrush.
    3. *Candida* is a fungal infection, and it is important to treat both the mother's breasts and the baby's mouth to prevent the infection from being transmitted back and forth between the two.
    4. Although immunosuppressed patients often do develop thrush, that is an unlikely cause of thrush in this situation.

TEST-TAKING TIP: It is important to keep from confusing pathology with the normal processes of birth and growth and development. Thrush, which is often seen in the mouth of immunosuppressed patients, is also a normal flora in the vagina of women. The baby may have contracted the fungus in his or her mouth during delivery or from his or her mother's poorly washed hands.

48. 1. The baby will have a positive antibody titer, as a result of passive immunity through the placenta, but there will be no evidence of active viral production that early in the newborn's life.
    2. There is no need to assess the antibody titer. It will definitely be positive because the mother has HIV/AIDS.
    3. The standard of care for neonates born to mothers with HIV/AIDS is to begin them on anti-AIDS medication in the nursery. The mother will be advised to continue to give the baby the medication after discharge.
    4. There is no need to place the baby on strict precautions. The institution of standard precautions in the well-baby nursery is sufficient.

TEST-TAKING TIP: The test taker should be aware that neonates must be followed after delivery because of the viral exposure in utero. The best way to prevent vertical transmission from the mother to the newborn is to administer antiviral medications to the mother during pregnancy and delivery and for 6 weeks to the newborn following delivery.

49. 1. Hypothermia in a neonate may be indicative of sepsis.
    2. Mottling is commonly seen in neonates shortly after birth. It is considered a normal finding.
    3. Omphalocele is not related to group B strep exposure.
    4. Stomatitis is not a sign associated with group B strep exposure.

TEST-TAKING TIP: Group B streptococci can seriously adversely affect neonates. In fact, group B strep has been called the "baby killer." To prevent a severe infection from the bacteria, mothers are given intravenous antibiotics every 4 hours from admission, or from rupture of membranes, until delivery. A minimum of 2 doses is considered essential to protect the baby. As this woman arrived only 2 hours prior to the delivery, there was not enough time for 2 doses to be administered.

50. 1. Although *Candida* can eventually lead to a maculopapular diaper rash, no facial rash is associated with a candidal infection.

2. Thrush is commonly seen in babies whose mothers have *Candida* vaginitis.

3. A neonatal fungal conjunctivitis is not associated with this problem.

4. Dehydration is not associated with this problem.

TEST-TAKING TIP: The test taker should be familiar with the various presentations of common fungi and bacteria. *Candida* is a fungus that is a normal vaginal flora. During pregnancy, it is not uncommon for the vaginal flora to shift and the woman to develop *Candida* vaginitis.

51. 1. Vertical transmission of hepatitis B does occur. Symptoms of the disease would not be evident during the neonatal period, however.

2. Standard precautions are sufficient for the care of the baby exposed to hepatitis B in utero.

3. Babies exposed to hepatitis B in utero should receive the first dose of hepatitis B vaccine as well as hepatitis B immune globulin (HBIG) within 12 hours of delivery to reduce transmission of the virus (see http://cdc.gov/hepatitis/ HBV/PDFs/DeliveryHospitalPrevent-PerinatalHBVTransmission.pdf).

4. Breastfeeding is not contraindicated when the mother is hepatitis B positive.

TEST-TAKING TIP: Although breastfeeding is contraindicated when a mother is HIV positive, hepatitis B transmission rates do not change significantly when a mother breastfeeds. The mother should, however, take care to prevent any cracking and bleeding from her breasts because the virus is bloodborne.

52. 1. Group B streptococcus causes severe infections in the newborn. A sign of neonatal sepsis is hypothermia.

2. Babies whose mothers had gestational diabetes (GDM) should be carefully monitored for hypoglycemia rather than for hypothermia.

3. There is no relationship between placenta previa and neonatal hypothermia.

4. There is no evidence from the question that the stillbirth was related to a gestational infection.

TEST-TAKING TIP: It is important for the test taker not to confuse terms. Babies with neonatal sepsis often become hypothermic, whereas babies born to mothers with GDM become hypoglycemic. The two

conditions are very different, although the prefix—"hypo"—is the same.

53. 1. The lung maturation of infants of diabetic mothers is often delayed. These babies must be monitored at birth for respiratory distress.

2. A maternal diagnosis of lung cancer will not affect her neonate's pulmonary function.

3. A maternal diagnosis of hypothyroidism does not put the baby at high risk for respiratory distress.

4. A maternal diagnosis of asthma does not put the baby at high risk for respiratory distress.

TEST-TAKING TIP: Two answers to this question relate to maternal pulmonary diagnoses, i.e., lung cancer and asthma. Simply because a mother has a pulmonary problem does not mean, however, that her neonate will have a similar problem. Even if the neonate has respiratory distress, it may not be related to the mother's problem. The test taker should not be swayed by this association. Babies born to diabetic mothers, however, are at risk for delayed lung maturation and should be monitored for respiratory distress.

54. 1. Although the etiology of port wine stain is unknown, it is unrelated to a maternal diagnosis of diabetes.

2. The incidence of cardiac defects and neural tube defects is high in infants born to diabetic mothers.

3. The incidence of hip dysplasia is not significantly higher in infants born to diabetic mothers.

4. Intussusception is an invagination of the small intestine. It is unrelated to a maternal diagnosis of diabetes.

TEST-TAKING TIP: The test taker should be familiar with maternal diseases that can seriously affect pregnancy. One of the most significant of the chronic diseases is diabetes. When a woman is in poor diabetic control during the first trimester, the incidence of birth defects is quite high.

55. 1. Myasthenia gravis is not associated with caudal agenesis in the fetus.

2. **Poorly controlled maternal diabetes mellitus is one of the most important predisposing factors for caudal agenesis in the fetus.**

3. Splenic syndrome is sometimes seen in patients with sickle cell disease. It is not related to caudal agenesis in the fetus.

4. Hypothyroidism is not related to caudal agenesis in the fetus.

TEST-TAKING TIP: Women with diabetes must be in excellent glucose control before becoming pregnant. Because fetal deformities develop during the organogenic period in the first trimester, it is too late to educate diabetic women to control their disease when they are already pregnant.

56. 1. Hypoglycemia in the neonate is defined as a glucose level less than 40 mg/dL. A level of 35 mg/dL, therefore, is not normal.
2. Glucagon may be ordered as a remedy for severe hypoglycemia. Although the glucose level is low, it is unlikely that glucagon is indicated. Plus, the nurse would not administer the medication without an order.
3. Both breast milk and formula contain lactose. If the glucose level has not risen to normal as a result of the feeding, the nurse must notify the physician.
4. If the glucose level has not risen to normal as a result of the feeding, the nurse should notify the physician and anticipate that the doctor will order an intravenous of dextrose and water.

TEST-TAKING TIP: The test taker should be aware that the normal glucose level of a neonate after delivery—40 mg/dL to 90 mg/L—is much lower than the adult normal of 60 to 110 mg/dL. Hypoglycemia is a common problem seen in infants, especially macrosomic infants and infants of diabetic mothers. Protocols to monitor for hypoglycemia in infants of diabetic mothers exist in all well-baby nurseries and NICUs.

57. 1. The baby's serum protein levels should be normal.
2. Because the placenta is likely to be functioning less than optimally, it is highly likely that the baby will be polycythemic. The increase in red blood cells would improve the baby's oxygenation in utero.
3. Rather than hypercalcemia, the nurse would expect to see hypocalcemia.
4. Rather than hypoinsulinemia, if the maternal glucose levels are higher than normal, the nurse would expect to see hyperinsulinemia in the neonate.

TEST-TAKING TIP: The test taker must be familiar with the pathology of diabetes and its effect on pregnancy. Although

infants of diabetic mothers (IDMs) are usually macrosomic as a result of increased plasma glucose levels, when mothers have vascular damage, the placenta functions poorly. The IDM consequently may be small-for-gestational age with intrauterine growth restriction and polycythemia from the poor nourishment and oxygenation.

58. 1. The nurse should anticipate that the plasma glucose levels would be low.
2. The nurse would expect to see elevated red blood cell counts rather than low red blood cell counts.
3. The white blood cell count should be within normal limits.
4. The nurse would expect to see elevated hemoglobin levels rather than low levels of hemoglobin.

TEST-TAKING TIP: The fetus, responding to elevated glucose levels from the mother, produces large quantities of insulin. After the birth, however, the placenta no longer is providing the baby with the mother's glucose. It takes the baby some time to adjust his or her extrauterine insulin production to be in synchrony with the sugars provided by the breast milk or formula feedings. Until the baby makes the adjustment, he or she will exhibit hypoglycemia (less than 40 mg/dL).

59. 3, 4, and 5 are correct.
1. Hyperopia, another name for farsightedness, is unrelated to placental function.
2. If the mother had gestational diabetes, the nurse would expect the baby to be macrosomic, not to have IUGR.
3. Placental function is affected by the vasoconstrictive properties of many illicit drugs, as well as by cigarette smoke.
4. Placental function is diminished in women who have chronic hypertension.
5. Placental function has been found to be diminished in women of advanced maternal age.

TEST-TAKING TIP: The test taker should be reminded that any condition that inhibits the flow of blood, including illicit drug use, hypertension, cigarette smoking, and the like, can lead to fetal IUGR—that is, a fetus smaller than expected for the gestational period.

60. 1. Severe preeclampsia is associated with asymmetrical IUGR.

2. Chromosomal abnormalities are associated with symmetrical IUGR.
3. An aging placenta is associated with asymmetrical IUGR.
4. PPROM is associated with asymmetrical IUGR.

TEST-TAKING TIP: There is a distinct difference between symmetrical and asymmetrical IUGR. Babies with chromosomal defects often grow poorly from the time of conception. Their entire bodies, therefore, will grow poorly and will be small. Babies that are exposed to complications like preeclampsia or an aging placenta during the pregnancy will grow normally during the beginning of the pregnancy but start to grow poorly at the time of the insult. Their growth, therefore, will be disproportionally affected.

61. 3 and 4 are correct.
    1. The baby will likely be born with a normal platelet count.
    2. The baby will likely be born with a normal white blood cell count.
    3. Babies who have lived in utero with an aging placenta usually are born with polycythemia.
    4. Babies who have lived in utero with an aging placenta usually are born with hypoglycemia.
    5. Rather than hyperlipidemia, babies who have lived in utero with an aging placenta may be born with hypolipidemia.

TEST-TAKING TIP: Even if the test taker were unfamiliar with the expected lab findings of a neonate that had been born after living with an aging placenta, deductive reasoning could assist the test taker to choose the correct response. Aging placentas function poorly, and therefore the fetuses receive less nutrition and oxygenation. The baby's body, therefore, must compensate for the losses by metabolizing glycogen and lipid stores and by producing increased numbers of red blood cells. The neonate, therefore, is often polycythemic, hypoglycemic, and hypolipidemic.

62. 1. Most mothers, even those of full-term babies, usually use fingertip touch during their first physical contact with their babies.
    2. Palmar touch usually follows fingertip touch.
    3. Kangaroo hold is used in NICUs as a means of facilitating parent-infant bonding

as well as promoting growth and development of the neonate.
4. Cradle hold is the classic hold of a mother with her baby. This hold follows other touch contact.

TEST-TAKING TIP: The delivery of a preterm infant is very stressful and frightening. In fact, the appearance of the premature can be overwhelming to new parents. To become familiar with their baby, all parents proceed through a pattern of touch behaviors. When the baby is preterm, the procession through touch responses is often slowed.

63. 1, 2, 3, and 5 are correct.
    1. Bronchopulmonary dysplasia often is a consequence of the respiratory therapy that preemies receive in the NICU.
    2. Cerebral palsy results from a hypoxic insult that likely occurred as a result of the baby's prematurity.
    3. Retinopathy of the premature is a disease resulting from the immaturity of the vascular system of the eye.
    4. Hypothyroidism is one of the diseases assessed for in the neonatal screen. It is very unlikely that this problem resulted from the baby's stay in the NICU.
    5. Seizure disorders can result either from a hypoxic insult to the brain or from a ventricular bleed. Both of these conditions likely occurred as a result of the prematurity.

TEST-TAKING TIP: Many parents are of the opinion that babies, even when born many weeks prematurely, will be healthy as they mature because there are so many machines and medications that can be given to the babies. Unfortunately, many babies suffer chronic problems as a result of their prematurity even when they receive excellent medical and nursing care.

64. 4.13 mg q 24 hours.
    The formula for calculating the safe dosage (per weight) is:

$$\frac{\text{Known dosage}}{1 \text{ kg}} = \frac{\text{Needed dosage}}{\text{Weight of the child in kg}}$$

$$\frac{2.5 \text{ mg}}{1 \text{ kg}} = \frac{x \text{ mg}}{1.653 \text{ kg}}$$

$$x = 4.13 \text{ mg q 24 hours}$$

TEST-TAKING TIP: When calculating the safe dosage of a medication for a child, the test taker must first note whether the

recommended dosage for the medication is written per kg or per meters squared. If the dosage is written per kg, then the denominator of the ratio and proportion equation is in kg. If the dosage is written per m², the denominator of the ratio and proportion equation is in m².

65. **0.25 mL.**

$$0.05 \text{ mg/mL} = 12.5 \text{ microgram}/x \text{ mL}$$
$$(0.05 \text{ mg} = 50 \text{ microgram})$$
$$50/1 = 12.5/x$$
$$50\,x = 12.5$$
$$x = 0.25 \text{ mL}$$

TEST-TAKING TIP: Digoxin is administered in very small dosages to infants and neonates. If the nurse calculates a quantity that is larger than 1 mL, it is very likely that the calculation is incorrect. The nurse should recalculate the quantity and, for safety's safe, ask another nurse to check the arithmetic.

66. **6.9 mg q week.**
The formula for calculating the safe dosage per body surface area in meters squared is:

$$\frac{\text{Known dosage}}{1 \text{ m}^2} = \frac{\text{Needed dosage}}{\text{Body surface area of the child}}$$

To calculate the body surface area for this baby the test taker must take the square root of the product of the baby's weight times its length.

$$\sqrt{\frac{3.476 \times 57}{3600}} = 0.23 \text{ m}^2$$

Then, to calculate the safe dosage, a ratio and proportion equation must be solved.

$$\frac{30 \text{ mg}}{1 \text{ m}^2} = \frac{x \text{ mg}}{0.23 \text{ m}^2}$$

$$x = 6.9 \text{ mg q week}$$

TEST-TAKING TIP: When calculating a safe dosage for a child using the body surface area formula, it is important for the test taker to note whether the child's statistics are written in the metric system or the English system. If in the metric system, the divisor for the formula is 3,600. If the statistics are in the English system, however, the divisor is 3,131. And it is important for the test taker to remember to take the square root of the calculation. It is very easy to forget that step.

67. **3.33 mL/hr.**
5 mL/90 min = 5 mL/1.5 hours = 3.33 mL/hr

TEST-TAKING TIP: Whenever a pump is used to deliver intravenous fluids, the rate should be set in mL/hr units. Pumps should always be used to deliver IV fluids to preterm neonates as, because of their small size, they can so easily become fluid overloaded.

68. 1. Respiratory rate of 70 is above normal. The rate should be between 30 and 60 breaths per minute.
2. Temperature of 97.0°F is below normal. The temperature should be between 97.6°F and 99°F.
3. The baby is showing signs of interest in breastfeeding. This is a positive sign.
4. Nasal flaring is an indication of respiratory distress, which is abnormal.

TEST-TAKING TIP: Kangaroo care, when mothers hold their babies skin-to-skin, is a technique that has been shown to benefit preterm infants. The vital signs of babies who kangaroo with their mothers have been shown to stabilize more quickly. The babies also have been shown to nipple feed earlier and to have shorter lengths of stay in the NICU.

69. **1, 2, 3, and 4 are correct.**
1. Babies with NEC have blood in their stools.
2. The abdominal girth measurements of babies with NEC increase.
3. When babies have NEC, they have increasingly larger undigested gastric contents after feeds.
4. The neonates' bowel sounds are diminished with NEC.
5. The presence of anal fissures is unrelated to NEC.

TEST-TAKING TIP: NEC is an acute inflammatory disorder seen in preterm babies. It appears to be related to the shunting of blood from the gastrointestinal tract, which is not a vital organ system, to the vital organs. The baby's bowel necroses with the shunting and the baby's once normal flora become pathological. Resection of the bowel is often necessary.

70. 1. EBM is sufficient in iron and zinc.
2. Calcium and phosphorus in EBM are in quantities that are less than body

requirements for the very low birth weight baby. Therefore, a fortifier may need to be added to the EBM.

3. Protein and fat are sufficient in EBM.
4. Sodium and potassium are sufficient in EBM.

TEST-TAKING TIP: Premature babies who are breastfed have fewer complications than bottle-fed babies, especially necrotizing enterocolitis. Unfortunately, very low birth weight babies do not receive sufficient quantities of calcium and phosphorus from the EBM. The breast milk, then, is enriched with a milk fortifier that contains the needed elements.

71. 1. Surfactant is not administered intravenously.
    2. **Surfactant is administered intratracheally. The baby must first be intubated. The nurse would assist the doctor with the procedure.**
    3. Surfactant is not administered parenterally.
    4. Surfactant is not administered orally.

TEST-TAKING TIP: Surfactant is a slippery substance that is needed to prevent the alveoli from collapsing during expiration. It is prescribed for preterm babies who are so immature that they do not produce sufficient quantities of the substance in their lung fields. The medication is used to prevent and/or to treat respiratory distress syndrome (RDS).

72. 1. Temperature is not related to the action of the medication.
    2. **A normal oxygen saturation level would be considered a positive result of the medication.**
    3. Heart rate is not related to the action of the medication.
    4. Electrolyte levels are not related to the action of the medication.

TEST-TAKING TIP: The medication is given to provide the baby with lung surfactant. The drug is given to treat respiratory distress syndrome (RDS). When preterm babies have RDS, they are having respiratory difficulty that leads to poor gas exchange. When there is poor gas exchange, the oxygen saturation drops. A normal O_2 saturation level, which is equal to or greater than 96%, therefore, indicates a positive outcome.

73. 1. A baby whose square window sign is 90° is preterm.
    2. A baby whose skin is cracked and leathery is exhibiting a sign of postmaturity.

3. A baby whose popliteal angle is 90° is full term.
4. A baby whose plantar creases are pronounced is full term.

TEST-TAKING TIP: A number of neonatal characteristics are assessed to determine the gestational age of a neonate. Four of those characteristics are square window sign, appearance of the skin, popliteal angle, and presence of plantar creases. The test taker should be familiar with the Ballard Scale and the many characteristics on which gestational age is measured.

74. 1. **Babies who have cardiac defects frequently feed poorly. And when they do feed, they frequently become cyanotic.**
    2. Sleeping is unlikely to trigger a cyanotic spell.
    3. Rocking is unlikely to trigger a cyanotic spell.
    4. Although the baby may be aroused when swaddled, it is unlikely to trigger a cyanotic spell.

TEST-TAKING TIP: Any activity that requires an increased oxygen demand can trigger a cyanotic spell in a neonate with a heart defect. The two activities that require the greatest amount of oxygen and energy are feeding and crying. In fact, because feeding demands that the baby be able to suck, swallow, and breathe rhythmically and without difficulty, many sick babies refuse to eat because it is such a demanding activity.

75. 1. It is not necessary to feed these babies via gastrostomy tubes.
    2. Blood-stained mucus is not associated with cleft lip or palate.
    3. It is not necessary to feed these babies via nasogastric tubes.
    4. **Cleft lip and palate babies require additional time to rest as well as to suck and swallow when being fed.**

TEST-TAKING TIP: Although cleft lips and palates do affect feeding, virtually all of the affected babies are able to feed orally and some are even able to breastfeed. But, feeding from a standard bottle and/or breastfeeding may prove to be impossible for some babies with cleft lips and/or palates. In those cases, there are a number of bottles that have been designed to facilitate their feeding so that neither gastrostomy tubes nor nasogastric tubes are needed. The Haberman feeder is one

example. Either expressed breast milk or formula can be put in the feeder.

76. 2 and 4 are correct.
    1. Vomiting is literally impossible.
    2. Babies with esophageal atresia would be expected to expel large amounts of mucus from the mouth.
    3. A ruddy complexion is related to polycythemia, not esophageal atresia.
    4. Abdominal distention can be seen with esophageal atresia as air enters the stomach via the trachea.
    5. Pigeon chest is not associated with esophageal atresia.

    TEST-TAKING TIP: With esophageal atresia, the esophagus ends in a blind pouch. In addition, there is usually a fistula connecting the stomach to the trachea. These babies are at high risk for respiratory compromise because they can aspirate the large quantity of oral mucus. The neonatologist should be notified whenever esophageal atresia is suspected.

77. 1. There is no need for Down syndrome children to undergo yearly glucose tolerance testing.
    2. Down syndrome babies are not at high risk for bleeding episodes.
    3. Down babies do not require special formulas. And although it can be a difficult beginning, many Down babies are successful breastfeeders.
    4. Because of the hypotonia of the respiratory accessory muscles, Down babies often need medical intervention when they have respiratory infections.

    TEST-TAKING TIP: Down syndrome babies not only have a characteristic appearance but also have physiological characteristics that the nurse must be familiar with. One of those characteristics is hypotonia. Because of this problem, Down babies are often difficult to feed during the neonatal period, have delayed growth and development, and have difficulty fighting upper respiratory illnesses.

78. 1. This baby has Down syndrome. The genetic disease is not associated with blood-tinged urine.
    2. Down babies are not at high risk for hemispheric paralysis.
    3. Cardiac anomalies occur much more frequently in Down babies than in other babies.

4. Down babies are no more at risk for hemolytic jaundice than are other babies.

TEST-TAKING TIP: Babies with Down syndrome have the following characteristic anomalies: low-set ears, simian creases, and slanted eyes. Because they are at high risk for internal anomalies as well, in particular cardiac defects, the nurse should carefully evaluate the babies for a heart murmur.

79. 1. Babies with TEF usually have the heads of their cribs elevated. The babies may be placed on one of their sides but should not be lain flat.
    2. Low nasogastric suction is usually maintained to minimize the amount of the baby's oral secretions.
    3. Babies that are born with TEF are kept NPO (nothing by mouth).
    4. There is no reason to place a TEF baby on a hypothermia blanket.

    TEST-TAKING TIP: Because the esophagus of a TEF baby ends in a blind pouch, he or she excretes large quantities of mucus from the mouth, placing the baby at high risk for aspiration. To decrease the potential for respiratory insult until surgery can take place, nasogastric suctioning is started and the baby's head is elevated.

80. 1. It is not painful for a baby with a cleft lip and palate to feed.
    2. It is likely that milk will be expelled from the baby's nose during feedings.
    3. Babies with clefts often take much longer to feed than do other babies.
    4. Babies with clefts usually consume the same milk, either breast milk or formula, that other babies consume.

    TEST-TAKING TIP: This question asks about the feeding of a baby with a cleft palate. Although the lip is intact, a cleft in the palate means that there is direct communication between the mouth and the sinuses. Because of the opening, milk is often expelled from the nose. Plus, the milk frequently enters the eustachian tubes. These babies, therefore, are at high risk for ear infections.

81. 1. Babies with 2-vessel cords are at high risk for renal defects.
    2. There is no relationship between a 2-vessel cord and a cardiac defect.

3. There is no relationship between a 2-vessel cord and glucose tolerance.
4. There is no relationship between a 2-vessel cord and the brain.

TEST-TAKING TIP: The umbilical cord is developed in fetal life at approximately the same time as is the renal system. Because of this fact, when a defect is seen in the umbilical cord, there may also be a defect in the renal system.

82. 1. It is not routinely necessary to perform nasogastric suctioning on a baby born with a meningomyelocele.
2. **The baby should be lain prone to prevent injury to the sac.**
3. It is not routinely necessary to administer oxygen to a baby born with a meningomyelocele.
4. A baby born with a meningomyelocele should not be swaddled.

TEST-TAKING TIP: The baby with meningomyelocele is born with an opening at the base of the spine through which a sac protrudes. The sac contains cerebral spinal fluid and nerve endings from the spinal cord. It is essential that the nurse not injure the sac; therefore, the baby should be placed in a prone position immediately after birth.

83. 1. **A diuretic will increase urinary output, which in turn will lead to weight loss.**
2. A drop in sodium is not a goal of diuretic therapy.
3. Rather than an increase in specific gravity, the nurse would expect to see a drop in specific gravity.
4. An increase in blood pressure is not a goal of diuretic therapy.

TEST-TAKING TIP: The heart is pumping inefficiently when a baby has congestive heart failure. Because of this pathology, the kidneys are poorly perfused, leading to fluid retention and weight gain. Diuretics are administered to improve the excretion of the fluid. When the urinary output is increased, the weight will drop and the urine will be less concentrated.

84. 1. Fatigue is an important nursing diagnosis for the baby with congestive heart failure, but it is not the priority diagnosis.
2. Activity intolerance is an important nursing diagnosis for the baby with congestive heart failure, but it is not the priority diagnosis.
3. Sleep pattern disturbance is an important nursing diagnosis for the baby with congestive heart failure, but it is not the priority diagnosis.
4. **Altered tissue perfusion is the priority diagnosis.**

TEST-TAKING TIP: Whenever the test taker is asked to identify the priority response, it is important to remember the hierarchy of needs. Respiratory issues almost always take precedence. Although the answer to this question does not refer to the respiratory system, it does relate to the oxygenation of the tissues. None of the other responses relates to critical physiological processes.

85. 1. The dose should not be readministered until it has been determined that the child's digoxin levels are within normal limits.
2. **The nurse should notify the physician that the baby has vomited the digoxin.**
3. This action is not needed. The apical pulse will have been assessed prior to the initial administration of the medication and assessing the two pulses together will provide no further information.
4. It is unlikely that the vomitus will be streaked with blood.

TEST-TAKING TIP: Vomiting is a sign of digoxin toxicity. This baby needs to have a digoxin level drawn. Because the nurse needs an order for the test, the nurse must notify the doctor of the problem.

86. 1. There should not be sensory loss in all four quadrants.
2. With a myelomeningocele (also known as meningomyelocele), there will be a sac at the base of the spine, not a tuft of hair.
3. **With a defect at L2, the nurse would expect to see paralysis of the legs.**
4. The Moro reflex will be asymmetrical because the enervation to the lower extremities is impaired.

TEST-TAKING TIP: If the test taker remembers that a sac with cerebral spinal fluid and nerves is seen at the base of the spine in a baby with myelomeningocele and that L2 innervates the motor nerves of the legs, the answer becomes obvious. This is an example of the importance of carefully studying normal anatomy and physiology and the pathophysiology of important diseases.

87. 1. Babinski and tonic neck reflexes are unrelated to the eye.
     2. Pseudostrabismus is normally seen in the neonate.
     3. Blood typing and Coombs' testing are unrelated to the eye.
     4. The baby should be assessed for signs of hydrocephalus, especially a disparity between the circumferences of the neonatal head and the neonatal chest.

TEST-TAKING TIP: Setting sun sign—when the sclera of the eye is visible above the iris of the eye—is one sign of hydrocephalus. An additional indication of hydrocephalus is finding that the head circumference of the baby is greater than 2 cm larger than the baby's chest circumference.

88. 1. The blood pressures in all four quadrants should be assessed.
     2. A bulging fontanel, not coarctation of the aorta, is indicative of hydrocephalus.
     3. At delivery, the hematocrit and hemoglobin will likely be the same as in a healthy baby.
     4. Harlequin coloration is a normal finding.

TEST-TAKING TIP: The pathophysiology of coarctation of the aorta provides the rationale for the assessment of the blood pressures. Because the narrowing of the aorta is usually distal to the ascending aorta, blood is able to pass unimpeded into the upper body but is unable to pass through the descending aorta toward the lower body. The blood pressures of the upper body, therefore, are much higher than the blood pressures in the lower extremities.

89. 1. Healthy babies should always be placed in the supine position for sleep and during unsupervised periods. For therapeutic reasons, however, sick babies may need to be placed in other positions.
     2. The prone position is not the appropriate position for a baby during a "tet" spell.
     3. Parents should place an infant during a "tet" spell into the knee-chest position.
     4. The Semi-Fowler's position is ordinarily a safe position for a baby with tetralogy of Fallot, but during a "tet" spell, the baby should be moved to the knee-chest position.

TEST-TAKING TIP: The four defects that are present in tetralogy of Fallot— ventricular septal defect, overriding aorta, pulmonary stenosis, and hypertrophied right ventricle—create a circulatory system in which much of the blood bypasses the lungs. As a result, a baby with tetralogy is predisposed to cyanotic, or "tet," spells. When a baby is placed in a squatting or knee-chest position, the femoral arteries are constricted, decreasing the amount of blood perfusing the lower body. This leads to improved perfusion to the upper body and the vital organs. With this action, the cyanotic spell will likely resolve.

90. 1. Cyanosis and clubbing are seen in children suffering from severe cyanotic defects and are not likely to develop with a small VSD.
     2. These symptoms will unlikely develop with a small VSD.
     3. This response is correct.
     4. Feeding difficulties and polycythemia are seen in children suffering from severe cyanotic defects.

TEST-TAKING TIP: The VSD—an opening between the ventricles of the heart—is the most common acyanotic heart defect seen. The defect leads to a left-to-right shunt as the left side of the heart is more powerful than the right side of the heart, causing a murmur. Small VSDs rarely result in severe symptoms and, in fact, often close over time without any treatment.

91. 1. Ventriculoperitoneal (VP) shunts are inserted for the treatment of hydrocephalus. A positive finding, therefore, would be decreasing head circumferences.
     2. VP shunts are not inserted for the treatment of cardiac arrhythmias or cardiac anomalies.
     3. VP shunts are not inserted for the treatment of hypertension.
     4. Setting sun sign is a sign of hydrocephalus. Appearance of setting sun sign would indicate that the shunt is functioning improperly.

TEST-TAKING TIP: One of the first signs of hydrocephalus in the neonate is increasing head circumferences because, as the fetal head is unfused, excess fluid in the brain forces the skull to expand. Once the diagnosis of hydrocephalus has been made, a VP shunt is usually inserted. The shunt is designed to remove excess cerebral spinal fluid from the ventricles of the brain. With the reduction in fluid, the size of the baby's head decreases.

92. 1. The baby is not suffering from a fluid volume deficit.
    2. If the fragile sac is injured, the baby is very high risk for infection.
    3. The defect is below the respiratory nerves. The baby is not at high risk for respiratory difficulties.
    4. Although babies with meningomyelocele must be fed in the prone position, they are able to eat without difficulty.

    TEST-TAKING TIP: **Babies with meningomyelocele, a form of spina bifida, are at very high risk for infection in the central nervous system until the defect is corrected. In addition, the vast majority of babies with myelomeningocele (also known as meningomyelocele), also have hydrocephalus for which they will receive a ventriculoperitoneal (VP) shunt. Plus, the most common problem associated with VP shunts is infection. Nurses, therefore, must care for these affected babies using strict aseptic technique.**

93. 1. Babies who have delayed meconium excretion may have Hirshsprung's disease.
    2. Tachycardia is not associated with Hirshsprung's disease.
    3. Rashes are not associated with Hirshsprung's disease
    4. Asymmetrical leg folds are related to developmental dysplasia of the hip, not to Hirshsprung's disease.

    TEST-TAKING TIP: **Hirshsprung's disease is defined as a congenital lack of parasympathetic innervation to the distal colon. Peristalsis, therefore, ceases at the end of the intestine. Because of the absence of peristalsis, the passage of meconium is delayed.**

94. 1. Excessive amounts of frothy saliva may indicate that the child has esophageal atresia.
    2. Blood-tinged vaginal discharge is a normal finding in female neonates.
    3. Milk-like secretion from the breast is a normal finding in neonates.
    4. It is normal for a baby's heart rate to speed slightly during inhalation and slow slightly during exhalation.

    TEST-TAKING TIP: **If the test taker is familiar with the characteristics of the normal neonate, the answer to this question is obvious. A baby whose esophagus ends in a blind pouch is unable to swallow his or her saliva. Instead, the mucus bubbles and drools from the mouth. Healthy babies, on the other hand, swallow without difficulty.**

95. 1. To treat developmental dysplasia of the hip, babies' legs are maintained in a state of abduction.
    2. DDH is not painful. Pain medication is not indicated.
    3. Casting is only done in cases where splinting is ineffective.
    4. There is no need to assess pedal pulses because they are unaffected in babies with DDH.

    TEST-TAKING TIP: **Because the pathology of DDH is related to the laxity of the hip joint, the rationale for the therapy is to maintain physiological positioning of the hip joint until the ligaments strengthen and mature. Keeping the legs in a state of abduction, the hip joint is maintained with the trochanter centered in the acetabulum.**

96. 1. With DDH there is reduced hip abduction.
    2. DDH is not associated with swelling at the site.
    3. The leg folds of the baby, both anteriorly and posteriorly, are frequently asymmetrical.
    4. Femoral pulses are unaffected by DDH.

    TEST-TAKING TIP: **Because of the subluxation of the hip, the gluteal and thigh folds of the baby usually appear asymmetrical. In addition to this finding, the nurse would expect to see reduced abduction of the hip and/or asymmetrical knee heights when the legs are flexed.**

97. 1. During the neonatal physical assessment, the nurse is unable to move a clubfoot into proper alignment.
    2. A positive Ortolani sign indicates the presence of developmental dysplasia of the hip.
    3. A shortened metatarsal arch is not diagnostic of clubfoot.
    4. The Babinski reflex is positive in all neonates.

    TEST-TAKING TIP: **The most common form of clubfoot is talipes equinovarus, when the baby's foot is in a state of inversion and plantar flexion. It is important for the nurse to distinguish between positional clubfoot that occurs from the baby's position in utero and resolves spontaneously, and pathology that requires orthopedic therapy.**

98. 1. The initial treatment plan for clubfoot usually includes a series of casts that slowly move the foot into proper alignment.
2. Harrington rod insertion has been used to treat scoliosis, not talipes equinovarus.
3. Pavlik harness is a therapy for a baby with developmental dysplasia of the hip.
4. Long-term bracing is not a common therapy for clubfoot.

TEST-TAKING TIP: This is an example of a question that may include a term that the test taker is unfamiliar with. If the test taker slowly breaks down the words into their component parts, the meaning of the term will become clear. The word "bilateral," of course, means that "both sides" of the body are affected. The word "talipes" is a word that contains two roots: "talis," meaning "ankle" and "pes," meaning "foot." The word, therefore, refers to a deformity of the foot and ankle—clubfoot. The term "equinovarus" specifically defines the type of clubfoot but, as the therapy is the same no matter which type of clubfoot the child suffers from, further analysis is not necessary to answer this question. (Talipes equinovarus clubfoot refers to a foot that is plantar flexed and turned inward.)

99. 2, 3, and 4 are correct.
1. Palpitations are not an early sign of congestive heart failure (CHF).
2. No matter whether a baby or an adult were developing CHF, the patient would be tachypneic.
3. No matter whether a baby or an adult were developing CHF, the patient would be tachycardic.
4. No matter whether a baby or an adult were developing CHF, the patient would be diaphoretic.
5. Irritability is not an early sign of CHF.

TEST-TAKING TIP: The term that is most descriptive in the phrase "congestive heart failure" is the word "failure." If the test taker remembers that, because of poor functioning, the heart is failing to oxygenate the body effectively, the test taker can remember the symptoms of the disease. When the body is being starved of oxygen, the body compensates by increasing respirations to take in more oxygen and the pulse rate speeds up to move the oxygenated blood more quickly through the body. Sweating is also a component of the early stages of the disease.

100. 1. Setting sun sign is a symptom of hydrocephalus. It is not a symptom of cardiac disease.
2. Anasarca refers to overall, systemic edema. It is seen is severe cardiovascular disease. A cardiac consult would be appropriate for this baby as would, perhaps, a renal consult.
3. A baby with flaccid extremities is exhibiting a neurological or musculoskeletal problem, not a cardiac problem.
4. A baby with polydactyly has more than 5 digits on the hands or feet. The finding has nothing to do with cardiac problems.

TEST-TAKING TIP: Although each of the answer options is abnormal, there is only one option that describes a symptom of a cardiac disease. The test taker must carefully discern what is being asked in each question to choose the one answer that relates specifically to the stem.

101. 1. A hole between the left and right ventricles is called a ventricular septal defect (VSD).
2. Unless the baby is decompensating, this defect rarely results in cyanosis. The blood is being oxygenated and, although there is mixed blood, the baby is sufficiently oxygenated.
3. There is a left to right shunt of blood with a PDA, resulting in oxygenated blood reentering the pulmonary system.
4. There is a left to right shunt rather than a right to left shunt.

TEST-TAKING TIP: The ductus arteriosus is a fetal circulatory duct that connects the pulmonary artery with the aorta. In utero, the blood is being oxygenated through the placenta, precluding the need for the blood to enter the lungs. In extrauterine life, however, the duct should close to create a one-way, intact system. When a ductus arteriosus stays open, a left to right shunt develops (because the left side of the heart is stronger than the right side of the heart) forcing the blood to reenter the lungs.

102. 3 and 5 are correct.
1. Transposition of the great vessels is a cyanotic defect that, if it stands alone, is incompatible with life.
2. Tetralogy of Fallot is a cyanotic defect characterized by four defects: VSD, pulmonic stenosis, overriding aorta, and right ventricular hypertrophy.

3. Ventricular septal defect (VSD) is the most common cardiac defect in neonates. It is an acyanotic defect with a left to right shunt. Already oxygenated blood reenters the pulmonary system.
4. Pulmonic stenosis is characterized by a narrowed pulmonic valve. The blood, therefore, is restricted from entering the pulmonary artery and the lungs to be oxygenated.
5. Patent ductus arteriosus (PDA) is a very common cardiac defect in preterm babies. It is an acyanotic defect with a left to right shunt. Already oxygenated blood reenters the pulmonary system.

TEST-TAKING TIP: The names of cardiac defects are very descriptive. Once the test taker remembers the pathophysiology of each of the defects, it becomes clear how the blood flow is affected. Of the choices in this question, the defects that are acyanotic defects, i.e., defects that allow blood to enter the lungs to be oxygenated, are the VSD and the PDA.

103. The term in column 1 is matched to the description in column 2.
1. Café au lait spot matches with D. A café au lait spot is a pale tan- to coffee-colored skin marking.
2. Hemangioma matches with A. A hemangioma is a raised blood vessel–filled lesion.
3. Mongolian spot matches with C. Mongolian spots are multiple grayish-blue, hyperpigmented skin areas.
4. Port wine stain matches with B. A port wine stain is a flat, sharply demarcated red-to-purple lesion.

TEST-TAKING TIP: This is simply a matching question. The test taker is asked to match the lesion that is seen in neonates with the description of the lesion. In the NCLEX-RN, this would be a drag-and-drop type of question. The test taker will be asked to drag the corresponding definition and drop it next to the name of the lesion.

104. 1. Galactosemia is one of the few diseases that is a contraindication for the intake of breast milk or any milk-based formula.
2. Galactosemia is a metabolic defect. There is no cardiovascular component.
3. Diarrhea and other malabsorption symptoms will be seen over time, but bloody stools would not be seen in the nursery.

4. Although vomiting and diarrhea do occur, the baby is unlikely to have abdominal pains.

TEST-TAKING TIP: There are many genetic metabolic diseases that may affect the neonate. Galactosemia, an autosomal recessive disease, is characterized by an inability to digest galactose, a by-product of lactose digestion. As breast milk and milk-based formulas are very high in lactose, affected babies must be switched to a soy-based formula.

105. 1. Because the head circumference is significantly larger than the chest circumference, the nurse should assess for another sign of hydrocephalus. A markedly enlarged or bulging fontanel is one of those signs.
2. Abdominal girth does not change when a child has hydrocephalus.
3. Hydrocephalus is not a cardiovascular problem.
4. Hydrocephalus is not a respiratory problem.

TEST-TAKING TIP: The test taker must remember that the head circumference should be approximately 2 cm larger than the chest circumference at birth. When the head circumference is markedly larger than expected, there is a possibility of hydrocephalus. The nurse should assess for other signs of the problem, such as enlarged fontanel size, setting sun sign, and bulging fontanels.

106. 1. Choanal atresia will affect the baby's ability to feed.
2. Digestion is unaffected by choanal atresia, a structural defect.
3. The immune response is unaffected by choanal atresia, a structural defect.
4. The renal system is unaffected by choanal atresia, a structural defect.

TEST-TAKING TIP: Choanal atresia, a congenital narrowing of the nasal passages, seriously affects babies' ability to feed. Babies are obligate nose breathers to enable them to suck-swallow-breathe in a rhythmic manner during feeding. If their nares are blocked, they are unable to breathe through their nose and, therefore, must stop feeding to breathe.

107. 1. A blockage in the gastrointestinal system may lead to polyhydramnios rather than oligohydramnios.

2. Oligohydramnios is not related to a defect in the hepatic system.
3. Oligohydramnios is not related to a defect in the endocrine system. Pregnancies of mothers with diabetes often are complicated by polyhydramnios.
4. Some defects of the renal system can lead to oligohydramnios.

TEST-TAKING TIP: The test taker must remember that most of the amniotic fluid produced during a pregnancy is produced by the fetal kidneys and is fetal urine. If there is a defect in the renal system, there may be a resulting decrease in the amount of fetal urine produced. Oligohydramnios would then result.

108. 1. Preeclampsia is not associated with esophageal atresia.
2. Idiopathic thrombocytopenia is not associated with esophageal atresia.
3. Polyhydramnios is often seen in pregnancies complicated by a fetus with a digestive blockage.
4. Severe anemia is not associated with esophageal atresia.

TEST-TAKING TIP: Babies swallow amniotic fluid in utero. When there is a blockage in the digestive system, they are unable to swallow the fluid. The fluid builds up in the uterus and polyhydramnios is noted.

109. 1. Digestive symptoms are not associated with a congenital diaphragmatic hernia.
2. High-pitched cries are associated with prematurity and some retardation syndromes.
3. The baby will develop respiratory distress very shortly after delivery.
4. Fecal incontinence is not associated with diaphragmatic hernia.

TEST-TAKING TIP: Abdominal organs are displaced into the thoracic cavity when a baby is born with a diaphragmatic hernia. Because of the defect, the respiratory tree does not develop completely. The newly delivered baby, therefore, is unable to breathe effectively.

110. 1. Oxytocin is administered to the mother, not to the baby.
2. Xylocaine is an anesthetic agent. It would not be administered in this situation.
3. Narcan is an opiate antagonist. It may be administered to a depressed baby at delivery.

4. Stadol is a synthetic opioid. It would not be administered in this situation.

TEST-TAKING TIP: It is important for the nurse to anticipate the needs of his or her clients. In this situation, because the mother has recently received an opioid analgesic, it is possible that the baby will experience central nervous system depression. In anticipation of this problem, the nurse, then, should have the opioid antagonist available for administration if the neonatologist should order it.

111. 1. Babies born via cesarean section usually have round, unmolded heads.
2. High forceps are not used in obstetrics today. High forceps, applied to babies' heads that are not well descended, are no longer used because of the high incidence of fetal damage that results. Instead, babies who fail to descend are now delivered via cesarean section.
3. Low forceps are applied when engagement is +2 or greater. The baby may develop forceps marks but would not develop a chignon.
4. Babies born via vacuum extraction often do develop chignons.

TEST-TAKING TIP: In common language, a chignon is a hairstyle that is characterized by a bun or knot of hair worn on the back of the head or nape of the neck. In obstetrics, a chignon is a round, bruised caput seen on the crown of the baby's head. It results from the pressure exerted on the scalp during a vacuum-assisted delivery.

112. 1. Vacuum-assisted deliveries result in injuries to the head and scalp, not to the feet.
2. The babies are at high risk for hyperbilirubinemia, not hypobilirubinemia.
3. Babies born via vacuum are not at high risk for hyperglycemia.
4. Babies born via vacuum are at high risk for cephalhematoma.

TEST-TAKING TIP: Babies born either via vacuum or via forceps are at high risk for cephalhematoma, as well as subdural hematoma. During mechanically assisted births, there often is trauma to the neonate's head and scalp. A cephalhematoma develops as a result of injury to superficial blood vessels. The blood loss accumulates in the subcutaneous space above the periosteum. The test taker should remember that babies born with **cephalhematomas are at high risk for hyperbilirubinemia.**

113. **1, 2, 3, and 4 are correct.**
1. The baby will complain of pain at the site.
2. If not in the immediate period after the injury, within a few days there will be a palpable lump on the bone at the site of the break.
3. Because of the break, the baby is likely to position the arm in an atypical posture.
4. Because of the injury to the bone, the baby is unable to respond with symmetrical arm movements.
5. It is very rare to see ecchymosis at the site of the break.

TEST-TAKING TIP: Clavicle breaks are a fairly common injury seen after a delivery. They usually result from a disproportion between the sizes of the maternal pelvis and the fetal body. Because shoulder dystocia is an obstetric emergency, threatening the life of the baby, obstetricians may purposefully break a baby's clavicle to enable the baby to be birthed as rapidly as possible.

114. 1. Clubfoot is a defect that usually develops from the positioning of the baby in utero.
2. Brachial palsy can result from either a traumatic vertex or breech delivery.
3. Gastroschisis, when skin does not cover the abdominal wall and the abdominal contents are exposed, develops during fetal development.
4. Congenital hydrocele, an accumulation of fluid in the testes of the male, develops when a membrane fails to develop between the peritoneal cavity and scrotal sac.

TEST-TAKING TIP: When babies are born with unexpected findings, the nurse must be familiar not only with the implications of the anomalies but also with an understanding of the etiology of the anomalies. If the anomaly were a result of birth trauma, the nurse must be able to clearly and accurately communicate to the parents the source of the birth injury without communicating an opinion on any potential blame for the problem.

115. 1. In twin-to-twin transfusion, the smaller twin has "donated" part of his or her blood supply to the larger twin.

2. The smaller twin is hypovolemic, so the likelihood of jaundice is small.
3. Opisthotonus is defined as a full-body spastic posture. This is unrelated to twin-to-twin transfusion.
4. Hydrocephalus is unrelated to twin-to-twin transfusion.

TEST-TAKING TIP: Twin-to-twin transfusion may occur in monochorionic twins because they share the same placenta. The blood from one twin, therefore, is able to be "transfused" into the cardiovascular system of the second twin. As a result, because of decreased oxygenation and nourishment, the donor develops intrauterine growth restriction and becomes anemic. Conversely, the recipient grows much larger and becomes hyperemic. Interestingly, the larger twin is the twin at highest risk for injury because of the potential for formation of thrombi and/or hyperbilirubinemia.

116. 1. The recipient twin's appearance is not characterized by the development of a rash.
2. The recipient is likely to be at least 20% larger than the donor twin.
3. The recipient, rather than the donor, will have an elevated hematocrit.
4. The recipient, rather than the donor, will be ruddy and plethoric.

TEST-TAKING TIP: The word "plethoric" refers to a red coloration. Because the recipient twin receives a "transfusion" from the donor, the recipient's skin color becomes dark pink, especially when crying. The donor, on the other hand, is pale and small.

117. 1. A baby who has lost 8% of his or her weight after only 24 hours of life is very high risk for altered growth.
2. Although a problem, the fact that the baby has yet to urinate does not indicate a risk for altered growth.
3. The average weight of a full-term neonate is between 2,500 and 4,000 grams. A baby weighing 3,000 grams, therefore, is well within norms.
4. Torticollis is a birth injury characterized by an abnormal positioning of the head. The head is deviated to one side.

TEST-TAKING TIP: The normal weight loss for newborn babies is between 5% and 10%. An 8% loss during the first 24 hours, therefore, places this baby at

high risk for altered growth. (The term "risk for" is very important. It does not mean that altered growth has already occurred, but rather that there is a strong possibility that altered growth will develop.) It is also important for the test taker to remember not to choose the option with an unfamiliar term, such as "torticollis," simply because it is unfamiliar.

118. 1. When a baby roots and sucks poorly, the baby is unable to transfer milk effectively. Because milk intake is the baby's source of fluid, the baby is high risk for fluid volume deficit.
2. Although a baby exhibiting fluid volume deficit may become activity intolerant, this is not the best answer.
3. Even when babies have poor rooting and sucking reflexes, they do not necessarily have poor gagging reflexes.
4. Babies are incapable of self-care.

TEST-TAKING TIP: The obvious nursing diagnosis related to poor rooting and sucking is "Deficient nutrition: less than body requirements." The test taker, however, is not given that choice. The test taker, therefore, must determine, which of the four available options is the best. Because dehydration is a consequence of altered fluid intake, that answer is the best response.

119. 14.16%
The formula for percentage of weight loss is: Original weight minus current weight divided by original weight. The value is then multiplied by 100 to convert the number into a percentage:
3199 − 2746 = 453
453/3199 = 0.1416 × 100 = 14.16%

TEST-TAKING TIP: Unless otherwise noted, the test taker should carry the math to the nearest hundredth place when performing calculations for infants and children. Because babies are very small, a fraction of a milligram (mg), kilogram (kg), and the like can make a significant difference.

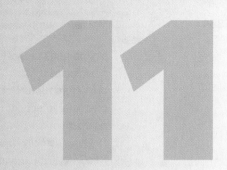

High-Risk Postpartum

As with the antepartum and intrapartum periods, there are several complications that can occur during the postpartum period. The questions in this chapter will enable the test taker to determine his or her preparedness for caring for complicated postpartum clients. The most common complications are related to infection, hypertensive illnesses, and excess blood loss. The nurse must be familiar with the precipitating factors that place a client at risk for these complications as well as the signs and symptoms of the problems and how to intervene effectively in each of the situations. Additional problems that the nurse may encounter are related to psychological responses of new mothers, breastfeeding problems, surgical complications, complications associated with chronic illnesses, and the like.

KEYWORDS

The following words include English vocabulary, nursing/medical terminology, concepts, principles, or information relevant to content specifically addressed in the chapter or associated with topics presented in it. English dictionaries, your nursing textbooks, and medical dictionaries such as *Taber's Cyclopedic Medical Dictionary* are resources that can be used to expand your knowledge and understanding of these words and related information.

Apresoline (hydralazine)
antidepressants (selective serotonin–reuptake inhibitors [SSRIs] such as Zoloft [sertraline] and Paxil [paroxetine])
Benadryl (diphenhydramine)
blocked milk duct
blood transfusion
breast abscess
breast enlargement
breast reduction
cesarean section
child abuse
child neglect
Compazine (prochlorperazine)
congenital defect
Coombs' test
Coumadin (warfarin)
cracked nipples
deep vein thrombosis (DVT)
dehiscence
eclampsia
engorgement
epidural anesthesia
fetal demise

forceps delivery
general anesthesia
gestational diabetes mellitus
grief and mourning
Hemabate (carboprost)
hematoma
heparin
HIV
infanticide
Lansinoh (lanolin breast cream)
macrosomia
magnesium sulfate
mastitis
Methergine (methylergonovine)
morphine sulfate
paralytic ileus
patient-controlled analgesia (PCA)
Phenergan (promethazine)
placental anomalies (accreta, battledore, circumvallate, succenturiate, velamentous cord insertion)
postpartum blues
postpartum depression
postpartum hemorrhage

postpartum psychosis
preeclampsia
premature rupture of the membranes
puerperal infection
puerperium
Reglan (metoclopramide)
RhoGAM (Rh [D] immune globulin)
rubella vaccine
Seconal (secobarbital)

self–breast milk expression
spinal anesthesia
substance abuse
titration
type 1 diabetes mellitus
type 2 diabetes mellitus
uterine atony
Zofran (ondansetron)

QUESTIONS

1. A gestational diabetic client, who delivered yesterday, is currently on the postpartum unit. Which of the following statements is appropriate for the nurse to make at this time?
   1. "Monitor your blood glucose five times a day until your 6-week checkup."
   2. "I will teach you how to inject insulin before you are discharged."
   3. "Daily exercise will help to prevent you from becoming diabetic in the future."
   4. "Your baby should be assessed every 6 months for signs of juvenile diabetes."

2. A client is receiving a blood transfusion after the delivery of a placenta accreta and hysterectomy. Which of the following complaints by the client would warrant immediately discontinuing the infusion?
   1. "My lower back hurts all of a sudden."
   2. "My hands feel so cold."
   3. "I feel like my heart is beating fast."
   4. "I feel like I need to have a bowel movement."

3. A client has just received Hemabate (carboprost) because of uterine atony not controlled by IV oxytocin. For which of the following side effects of the medication will the nurse monitor this patient? **Select all that apply.**
   1. Hyperthermia.
   2. Diarrhea.
   3. Hypotension.
   4. Palpitations.
   5. Anasarca.

4. A client, who is 2 weeks postpartum, calls her obstetrician's nurse and states that she has had a whitish discharge for 1 week but today she is "bleeding and saturating a pad about every ½ hour." Which of the following is an appropriate response by the nurse?
   1. "That is normal. You are starting to menstruate again."
   2. "You should stay on complete bed rest until the bleeding subsides."
   3. "Pushing during a bowel movement may have loosened your stitches."
   4. "The physician should see you. Please go to the emergency department."

5. The nurse is performing a postpartum assessment on a client who delivered 4 hours ago. The nurse notes a firm uterus at the umbilicus with heavy lochial flow. Which of the following nursing actions is appropriate?
   1. Massage the uterus.
   2. Notify the obstetrician.
   3. Administer an oxytocic as ordered.
   4. Assist the client to the bathroom.

6. A client has been receiving magnesium sulfate for severe preeclampsia for 12 hours. Her reflexes are 0 and her respiratory rate is 10. Which of the following situations could be a precipitating factor in these findings?
   1. Apical heart rate 104 bpm.
   2. Urinary output 240 mL/12 hr.
   3. Blood pressure 160/120.
   4. Temperature 100°F.

7. A client received general anesthesia during her cesarean section 4 hours ago. Which of the following postpartum nursing interventions is important for the nurse to make?
   1. Place the client flat in bed.
   2. Assess for dependent edema.
   3. Auscultate lung fields.
   4. Check patellar reflexes.

8. The nurse is developing a standard care plan for the post-cesarean client. Which of the following should the nurse plan to implement?
   1. Maintain client in left lateral recumbent position.
   2. Teach sitz bath use on second postoperative day.
   3. Perform active range-of-motion exercises until ambulating.
   4. Assess central venous pressure during first postoperative day.

9. The nurse has administered Benadryl (diphenhydramine) to a post-cesarean client who is experiencing side effects from the parenteral morphine sulfate that was administered 30 minutes earlier. Which of the following actions should the nurse perform following the administration of the drug?
   1. Monitor the urinary output hourly.
   2. Supervise while the woman holds her newborn.
   3. Position the woman slightly elevated on her left side.
   4. Ask any visitors to leave the room.

10. The nurse should suspect puerperal infection when a client exhibits which of the following?
    1. Temperature of 100.2°F.
    2. White blood cell count of 14,500 cells/mm³.
    3. Diaphoresis during the night.
    4. Malodorous lochial discharge.

11. A rubella nonimmune, breastfeeding client has just received the rubella vaccine. Which of the following side effects should the nurse warn the client about?
    1. The baby may develop a rash a week after the shot.
    2. The baby may temporarily reject the breast milk.
    3. The mother's milk supply may decrease precipitously.
    4. The mother's joints may become painful and stiff.

12. The nurse should expect to observe which behavior in a 3-week-multigravid postpartum client with postpartum depression?
    1. Feelings of infanticide.
    2. Difficulty with breastfeeding latch.
    3. Feelings of failure as a mother.
    4. Concerns about sibling jealousy.

13. Which symptom would the nurse expect to observe in a postpartum client with a vaginal hematoma?
    1. Pain.
    2. Bleeding.
    3. Warmth.
    4. Redness.

14. A breastfeeding woman calls the pediatric nurse with the following complaint: "I woke up this morning with a terrible cold. I don't want my baby to get sick. Which kind of formula should I have my husband feed the baby until I get better?" Which of the following replies by the nurse is appropriate at this time?
    1. "Any formula brand is satisfactory, but it is essential that it be mixed with water that has been boiled for at least 5 minutes."
    2. "Don't forget to pump your breasts every 3 hours while the baby is being fed the prescribed formula."
    3. "The best way to keep your baby from getting sick is for you to keep breastfeeding him rather than switching him to formula."
    4. "In addition to giving the baby formula, you should wear a surgical face mask when you are around him."

15. A woman who wishes to breastfeed advises the nurse that she had a breast reduction one year earlier. Which of the following responses by the nurse is appropriate?
    1. Advise the woman that unfortunately she will be unable to breastfeed.
    2. Examine the woman's breasts to see where the incision was placed.
    3. Monitor the baby's daily weights for excessive weight loss.
    4. Inform the woman that reduction surgery rarely affects milk transfer.

16. The nurse is caring for a postoperative cesarean client. The woman is obese and is an insulin-dependent diabetic. For which of the following complications should the nurse carefully monitor this client?
    1. Failed lactogenesis.
    2. Dysfunctional parenting.
    3. Wound dehiscence.
    4. Projectile vomiting.

17. A nurse who is called to a client's room notes that the client's cesarean incision has separated. Which of the following actions is the highest priority for the nurse to perform?
    1. Cover the wound with sterile wet dressings.
    2. Notify the surgeon.
    3. Elevate the head of the client's bed slightly.
    4. Flex the client's knees.

18. The nurse notes the following vital signs of a postoperative cesarean client during the immediate postpartum period: 100.0°F, P 68, R 12, BP 130/80. Which of the following is a correct interpretation of the findings?
    1. Temperature is elevated, a sign of infection.
    2. Pulse is too low, a sign of vagal pathology.
    3. Respirations are too low, a sign of medication toxicity.
    4. Blood pressure is elevated, a sign of preeclampsia.

19. The nurse is discharging five Rh-negative clients from the maternity unit. The nurse knows that the teaching was successful when the client who had which of the following deliveries asks why she must receive a RhoGAM injection? **Select all that apply.**
    1. Abortion at 10 weeks' gestation.
    2. Amniocentesis at 16 weeks' gestation.
    3. Fetal demise at 24 weeks' gestation.
    4. Birth of Rh-negative twins at 35 weeks' gestation.
    5. Delivery of a 40-week-gestation, Rh-positive baby.

20. In which of the following situations should a nurse report a possible deep vein thrombosis (DVT)?
    1. The woman complains of numbness in the toes and heel of one foot.
    2. The woman has cramping pain in a calf that is relieved when the foot is dorsiflexed.
    3. One of the woman's calves is swollen, red, and warm to the touch.
    4. The veins in the ankle of one of the woman's legs are spider-like and purple.

21. A woman, 26 weeks' gestation, has just delivered a fetal demise. Which of the following nursing actions is appropriate at this time?
    1. Remind the mother that she will be able to have another baby in the future.
    2. Dress the baby in a tee shirt and swaddle the baby in a receiving blanket.
    3. Ask the woman if she would like the doctor to prescribe a sedative for her.
    4. Remove the baby from the delivery room as quickly as possible.

22. A client, G1 P0000, is PP1 from a normal spontaneous delivery of a baby boy, Apgar 5/6. Because the client exhibited addictive behaviors, a toxicology assessment was performed; the results were positive for alcohol and cocaine. Which of the following interventions is appropriate for the nurse to perform for this postpartum client?
    1. Strongly advise the client to breastfeed her baby.
    2. Perform hourly incentive spirometer respiratory assessments.
    3. Suggest that the nursery nurse feed the baby in the nursery.
    4. Provide the client with supervised instruction on baby-care skills.

23. A client is 10 minutes postpartum from a forceps delivery of a 4,500-gram neonate with a cleft lip. The physician performed a right mediolateral episiotomy during the delivery. The client is at risk for each of the following nursing diagnoses. Which of the diagnoses is highest priority at this time?
    1. Ineffective breastfeeding.
    2. Fluid volume deficit.
    3. Infection.
    4. Pain.

24. A client is postpartum 24 hours from a spontaneous vaginal delivery with rupture of membranes for 42 hours. Which of the following signs/symptoms should the nurse report to the client's health care practitioner?
    1. Foul-smelling lochia.
    2. Engorged breasts.
    3. Cracked nipples.
    4. Cluster of hemorrhoids.

25. A client is 36 hours post–cesarean section. Which of the following assessments would indicate that the client may have a paralytic ileus?
    1. Abdominal striae.
    2. Oliguria.
    3. Omphalocele.
    4. Absent bowel sounds.

26. A client, 1 day postpartum (PP), is being monitored carefully after a significant postpartum hemorrhage. Which of the following should the nurse report to the obstetrician?
    1. Urine output 200 mL for the past 8 hours.
    2. Weight decrease of 2 pounds since delivery.
    3. Drop in hematocrit of 2% since admission.
    4. Pulse rate of 68 beats per minute.

27. A nurse is working on the postpartum unit. Which of the following patients should the nurse assess first?
    1. PP1 from vaginal delivery with complaints of burning on urination.
    2. PP2 from forceps delivery with blood loss of 500 mL at time of delivery.
    3. PP3 from vacuum delivery with hemoglobin of 7.2 g/dL.
    4. PO4 from cesarean delivery with complaints of firm and painful breasts.

28. A nurse has administered Methergine (methylergonovine) 0.2 mg po to a grand multipara who delivered vaginally 30 minutes earlier. Which of the following outcomes indicates that the medication is effective?
    1. Blood pressure 120/80.
    2. Pulse rate 80 bpm and regular.
    3. Fundus firm at umbilicus.
    4. Increase in prothrombin time.

29. A nurse on the postpartum unit is caring for two postoperative cesarean clients. One client had spinal anesthesia for the delivery and the other client had an epidural. Which of the following complications will the nurse monitor the spinal client for that the epidural client is much less high risk for?
    1. Pruritus.
    2. Nausea.
    3. Postural headache.
    4. Respiratory depression.

30. A postpartum woman has been diagnosed with postpartum psychosis. Which of the following signs/symptoms would the client exhibit?
    1. Hallucinations.
    2. Polyphagia.
    3. Induced vomiting.
    4. Weepy sadness.

31. The nurse is providing discharge counseling to a woman who is breastfeeding her baby. What should the nurse advise the woman to do if she should palpate tender, hard nodules in her breasts?
    1. Gently massage the areas toward the nipple, especially during feedings.
    2. Apply ice to the areas between feedings.
    3. Bottle feed for the next twenty-four hours.
    4. Apply lanolin ointment to the areas after each and every breastfeeding.

32. A woman states that all of a sudden her 4-day-old baby is having trouble feeding. On assessment, the nurse notes that the mother's breasts are firm, red, and warm to the touch. The nurse teaches the mother manually to express a small amount of breast milk from each breast. Which observation indicates that the nurse's intervention has been successful?
    1. The mother's nipples are soft to the touch.
    2. The baby swallows after every 5th suck.
    3. The baby's pre- and postfeed weight change is 20 milliliters.
    4. The mother squeezes her nipples during manual expression.

33. A client's vital signs and reflexes were normal throughout pregnancy, labor, and delivery. Four hours after delivery the client's vitals are 98.6°F, P 72, R 20, BP 150/100, and her reflexes are 4+. She has an intravenous infusion running with 20 units of Pitocin (oxytocin) added. Which of the following actions by the nurse is appropriate?
    1. Nothing, because the results are normal.
    2. Notify the obstetrician of the findings.
    3. Discontinue the intravenous immediately.
    4. Reassess the client after fifteen minutes.

34. A nurse is caring for a client, PP2, who is preparing to go home with her infant. The nurse notes that the client's blood type is O– (negative), the baby's type is A+ (positive), and the direct Coombs' test is negative. Which of the following actions by the nurse is appropriate?
    1. Advise the client to keep her physician appointment at the end of the week to receive her RhoGAM injection.
    2. Make sure that the client receives a RhoGAM injection before she is discharged from the hospital.
    3. Notify the client that because her baby's Coombs' test was negative she will not receive an injection of RhoGAM.
    4. Inform the client's physician that because the woman is being discharged on the second day, the RhoGAM could not be given.

35. The nurse is caring for a couple who are in the labor/delivery room immediately after the delivery of a dead baby who exhibited visible birth defects. Which of the following actions by the nurse is appropriate?
    1. Discourage the parents from naming the baby.
    2. Advise the parents that the baby's defects would be too upsetting for them to see.
    3. Transport the baby to the morgue as soon as possible.
    4. Give the parents a lock of the baby's hair and a copy of the footprint sheet.

36. The physician declares after delivering the placenta of a client during a cesarean section that it appears that the client has a placenta accreta. Which of the following maternal complications would be consistent with this diagnosis?
    1. Blood loss of 2,000 mL.
    2. Blood pressure of 160/110.
    3. Jaundiced skin color.
    4. Shortened prothrombin time.

37. Cloxacillin 500 mg by mouth four times per day for 10 days has been ordered for a client with a breast abscess. The client states that she is unable to swallow pills. The oral solution is available as 125 mg/5 mL. How many mL of medicine should the woman take per dose? **(Calculate to the nearest whole.)**
    _____ mL per dose.

38. A serum electrolyte report for a client, 1 day post–cesarean delivery for eclampsia, has just been received by the nurse. The client is receiving 5% dextrose in ½ normal saline IV at 125 mL/hr and magnesium sulfate 2 G/hr IV via infusion pump. Which of the following values should the nurse report to the surgeon?
    1. Magnesium 7 mg/dL.
    2. Sodium 136 mg/dL.
    3. Potassium 3.0 mg/dL.
    4. Calcium 9 mg/dL.

39. The home health nurse is visiting a client with HIV who is 6 weeks postdelivery. Which of the following findings would indicate that patient teaching by the nurse in the hospital was successful?
    1. The client is breastfeeding her baby every two hours.
    2. The client is using a diaphragm for family planning.
    3. The client is taking her temperature every morning.
    4. The client is seeking care for a recent weight loss.

40. A postpartum client has been diagnosed with deep vein thrombosis. For which of the following additional complications is this client high risk?
    1. Hemorrhage.
    2. Stroke.
    3. Endometritis.
    4. Hematoma.

41. A mother, G4 P4004, is 15 minutes postpartum. Her baby weighed 4,595 grams at birth. For which of the following complications should the nurse monitor this client?
    1. Seizures.
    2. Hemorrhage.
    3. Infection.
    4. Thrombosis.

42. A client who received a spinal for her cesarean delivery is complaining of pruritus and has a macular rash on her face and arms. Which of the following medications ordered by the anesthesiologist should the nurse administer at this time?
    1. Reglan (metoclopramide).
    2. Zofran (ondansetron).
    3. Compazine (prochlorperazine).
    4. Benadryl (diphenhydramine).

43. A woman with postpartum depression has been prescribed Zoloft (sertraline) 50 mg daily. Which of the following should the client be taught about the medication?
    1. Chamomile tea can potentiate the affect of the drug.
    2. Therapeutic effect may be delayed a week or more.
    3. The medication should only be taken whole.
    4. A weight gain of up to ten pounds is commonly seen.

44. A breastfeeding woman has been diagnosed with retained placental fragments 4 days postdelivery. Which of the following breastfeeding complications would the nurse expect to see?
    1. Engorgement.
    2. Mastitis.
    3. Blocked milk duct.
    4. Low milk supply.

45. The nurse assesses a 2-day postpartum, breastfeeding client. The nurse notes blood on the mother's breast pad and a crack on the mother's nipple. Which of the following actions should the nurse perform at this time?
    1. Advise the woman to wash the area with soap to prevent mastitis.
    2. Provide the woman with a tube of topical lanolin.
    3. Remind the woman that the baby can become sick if he drinks the blood.
    4. Get the woman an order for a topical anesthetic.

46. A client just delivered the placenta pictured below. The nurse will document that the woman delivered which of following placentas?

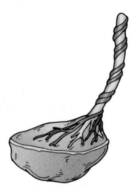

    1. Circumvallate placenta.
    2. Succenturiate placenta.
    3. Placenta with velamentous cord insertion.
    4. Battledore placenta.

47. The nurse administers RhoGAM to a postpartum client. Which of the following is the goal of the medication?
    1. Inhibit the mother's active immune response.
    2. Aggressively destroy the Rh antibodies produced by the mother.
    3. Prevent fetal cells from migrating throughout the mother's circulation.
    4. Change the maternal blood type to Rh-positive.

48. Which of the following comments suggest that a client whose baby was born with a congenital defect is in the bargaining phase of grief?
    1. "I hate myself. I caused my baby to be sick."
    2. "I'll take him to a specialist. Then he will get better."
    3. "I can't seem to stop crying."
    4. "This can't be happening."

49. A client is 1 day post–cesarean section with spinal anesthesia. Even though the nurse advised against it, the client has had the head of her bed in high Fowler's position since delivery. Which of the following complications would the nurse expect to see in relation to the client's action?
    1. Postpartum hemorrhage.
    2. Severe postural headache.
    3. Pruritic skin rash.
    4. Paralytic ileus.

50. A client is receiving IV heparin for deep vein thrombosis. Which of the following medications should the nurse obtain from the pharmacy to have on hand in case of heparin overdose?
    1. Vitamin K.
    2. Protamine.
    3. Vitamin E.
    4. Mannitol.

51. A client, who had no prenatal care, delivers a 10-lb 10-oz baby boy whose serum glucose result 1 hour after delivery was 20 mg/dL. Based on these data, which of the following tests should the mother have at her 6-week postpartum checkup?
    1. Glucose tolerance test.
    2. Indirect Coombs' test.
    3. Blood urea nitrogen (BUN).
    4. Complete blood count (CBC).

52. A client is to receive a blood transfusion after significant blood loss following a placenta previa delivery. Which of the following actions by the nurse is critical prior to starting the infusion? **Select all that apply.**
    1. Look up the client's blood type in the chart.
    2. Check the client's arm bracelet.
    3. Check the blood type on the infusion bag.
    4. Obtain an infusion bag of dextrose and water.
    5. Document the time the infusion begins.

53. A nurse is caring for the following four laboring patients. Which client should the nurse be prepared to monitor closely for signs of postpartum hemorrhage (PPH)? **Select all that apply.**
    1. G1 P0000, delivered a fetal demise at 29 weeks' gestation.
    2. G2 P1001, prolonged first stage of labor.
    3. G2 P0010, delivered by cesarean section for failure to progress.
    4. G3 P0200, delivered vaginally a 42-week, 2,200-gram neonate.
    5. G4 P3003, with a succenturiate placenta.

54. A client is 3 days post–cesarean delivery for eclampsia. The client is receiving hydralazine (Apresoline) 10 mg 4 times a day by mouth. Which of the following findings would indicate that the medication is effective?
    1. The client has had no seizures since delivery.
    2. The client's blood pressure has dropped from 160/120 to 130/90.
    3. The client's postoperative weight has dropped from 154 to 144 lb.
    4. The client states that her headache is gone.

55. A home care nurse is visiting a breastfeeding client who is 2 weeks postdelivery of a 7-lb baby girl over a midline episiotomy. Which of the following findings should take priority?
    1. Lochia is serosa.
    2. Client cries throughout the visit.
    3. Nipples are cracked.
    4. Client yells at the baby for crying.

56. A client who is post–cesarean section for severe preeclampsia is receiving magnesium sulfate via IV pump and morphine sulfate via patient-controlled anesthesia (PCA) pump. The nurse enters the room on rounds and notes that the client is not breathing. Which of the following actions should the nurse perform first?
    1. Give two breaths.
    2. Discontinue medications.
    3. Call a code.
    4. Check carotid pulse.

57. A breastfeeding client is being seen in the emergency department with a hard, red, warm nodule in the upper outer quadrant of her left breast. Her vital signs are: T 104.6°F, P 100, R 20, and BP 110/60. She has a recent history of mastitis and is crying in pain. Which of the following nursing diagnoses is highest priority?
    1. Ineffective breastfeeding.
    2. Infection.
    3. Ineffective individual coping.
    4. Pain.

58. A client is receiving an IV heparin drip at 16 mL/hr via an infusion pump for a diagnosis of deep vein thrombosis. The label on the ½ liter bag of D_5W indicates 25,000 units of heparin have been added. How many units of heparin is the client receiving per hour? (Calculate to the nearest whole.)
    _____ units per hour.

59. A nurse massages the atonic uterus of a woman who delivered 1 hour earlier. The nurse identifies the nursing diagnosis: Risk for injury related to uterine atony. Which of the following outcomes indicates that the client's condition has improved?
    1. Moderate lochia flow.
    2. Decreased pain level.
    3. Stable blood pressure.
    4. Fundus above the umbilicus.

60. Intermittent positive pressure boots have been ordered for a client who had an emergency cesarean section. Which of the following is the rationale for that order?
    1. Postpartum clients are at high risk for thrombus formation.
    2. Post-cesarean clients are at high risk for fluid volume deficit.
    3. Postpartum clients are at high risk for varicose vein development.
    4. Post-cesarean clients are at high risk for poor milk ejection reflex.

61. A client who received an epidural for her operative delivery has vomited twice since the surgery. Which of the following prn medications ordered by the anesthesiologist should the nurse administer at this time?
    1. Reglan (metoclopramide).
    2. Demerol (meperidine).
    3. Seconal (secobarbital).
    4. Benadryl (diphenhydramine).

62. A woman has just had a low forceps delivery. For which of the following should the nurse assess the woman during the immediate postpartum period?
    1. Infection.
    2. Bloody urine.
    3. Heavy lochia.
    4. Rectal abrasions.

63. A postpartum woman has been diagnosed with postpartum psychosis. Which of the following is essential to be included in the family teaching for this client?
    1. The woman should never be left alone with her infant.
    2. Symptoms rarely last more than one week.
    3. Clinical response to medications is usually poor.
    4. The woman must have her vitals assessed every two days.

64. A postoperative cesarean client, who was diagnosed with severe preeclampsia in labor and delivery, is transferred to the postpartum unit. The nurse is reviewing the client's doctor's orders. Which of the following medications that were ordered by the doctor should the nurse question?
    1. Methergine (methylergonovine).
    2. Magnesium sulfate.
    3. Advil (ibuprofen).
    4. Morphine sulfate.

65. A nurse administered RhoGAM to a client whose blood type is A+ (positive). Which of the following responses would the nurse expect to see? **Select all that apply.**
    1. Fever.
    2. Flank pain.
    3. Dark-colored urine.
    4. Swelling at the injection site.
    5. Polycythemia.

66. A couple, accompanied by their 5-year-old daughter, have been notified that their 32-week-gestation fetus is dead. The father is yelling at the staff. The mother is crying uncontrollably. The 5-year-old is banging the head of her doll on the floor. Which of the following nursing actions is appropriate at this time?
    1. Tell the father that his behavior is inappropriate.
    2. Sit with the family and quietly communicate sorrow at their loss.
    3. Help the couple to understand that their daughter is acting inappropriately.
    4. Encourage the couple to send their daughter to her grandparents.

67. The nurse is caring for a client, G3 P2002, whose infant has been diagnosed with a treatable birth defect. Which of the following is an appropriate statement for the nurse to make?
    1. "Thank goodness. It could have been untreatable."
    2. "I'm so happy that you have other children who are healthy."
    3. "These things happen. They are the will of God."
    4. "It is appropriate for you to cry at a time like this."

68. A client has given birth to a baby girl with a visible birth defect. Which of the following maternal responses would lead the nurse to suspect poor mother-infant bonding?
    1. The mother states, "I'm so tired. Please feed the baby in the nursery for me."
    2. The mother states, "Her eyes look like mine, but her chin is her Dad's."
    3. The mother says, "We have decided to name her Sarah after my mother."
    4. The mother says, "I breastfed her. I still need help swaddling her, though."

69. A client who has been diagnosed with deep vein thrombosis has been ordered to receive 12 units heparin/min. The nurse receives a 500-mL bag of D₅W with 20,000 units of heparin added from the pharmacy. At what rate in mL/hr should the nurse set the infusion pump? **(Calculate to the nearest whole.)**
    _____ mL/hr.

70. A client is being discharged on Coumadin (warfarin) post–pulmonary embolism after a cesarean delivery. Which of the following laboratory values indicates that the medication is effective?
    1. PT (prothrombin time): 12 sec (normal is 10–13 seconds).
    2. INR (international normalized ratio): 2.5 (normal is 1.0–1.4).
    3. Hematocrit 55%.
    4. Hemoglobin 10 g/dL.

71. The blood glucose of a client with type 1 diabetes 12 hours after delivery is 96 mg/dL. The client has received no insulin since delivery. The drop in serum levels of which of the following hormones of pregnancy is responsible for the glucose level?
    1. Estrogen.
    2. Progesterone.
    3. Human placental lactogen (hPL).
    4. Human chorionic gonadotropin (hCG).

72. A breastfeeding woman, 6 weeks postdelivery, must go into the hospital for a hemorrhoidectomy. Which of the following is the best intervention regarding infant feeding?
    1. Have the woman wean the baby to formula.
    2. Have the baby stay in the hospital room with the mother.
    3. Have the woman pump and dump her milk for two weeks.
    4. Have the baby bottle fed milk that the mother has stored.

73. A couple has delivered a 28-week fetal demise. Which of the following nursing actions are appropriate to take? **Select all that apply.**
    1. Swaddle the baby in a baby blanket.
    2. Discuss funeral options for the baby.
    3. Encourage the couple to try to get pregnant again in the near future.
    4. Ask the couple whether they would like to hold the baby.
    5. Advise the couple that the baby's death was probably for the best.

74. A client is being discharged on Coumadin (warfarin) post–pulmonary embolism after a cesarean delivery. Which of the following should be included in the patient teaching?
    1. Take only ibuprofen for pain.
    2. Avoid overeating dark green, leafy vegetables.
    3. Drink grapefruit juice daily.
    4. Report any decrease in urinary output.

75. A client just delivered the placenta pictured below. For which of the following complications should the nurse carefully observe the woman?

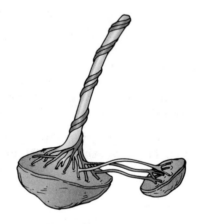

    1. Endometrial ischemia.
    2. Postpartum hemorrhage.
    3. Prolapsed uterus.
    4. Vaginal hematoma.

76. Which of the following is a priority nursing diagnosis for a woman, G10 P6226, who is PP1 from a spontaneous vaginal delivery with a significant postpartum hemorrhage?
    1. Alteration is comfort related to afterbirth pains.
    2. Risk for altered parenting related to grand multiparity.
    3. Fluid volume deficit related to blood loss.
    4. Risk for sleep deprivation related to mothering role.

77. A woman has just had a macrosomic baby after a 12-hour labor. For which of the following complications should the woman be carefully monitored?
    1. Uterine atony.
    2. Hypoprolactinemia.
    3. Infection.
    4. Mastitis.

78. On admission to the labor and delivery suite, the nurse assesses the discharge needs of a primipara who will be discharged home 4 days after a cesarean delivery. Which of the following questions should the nurse ask the client?
    1. "Have you ever had anesthesia before?"
    2. "Do you have any allergies?"
    3. "Do you scar easily?"
    4. "Are there many stairs in your home?"

79. A woman is receiving Paxil (paroxetine) for postpartum depression. To prevent a drug/food interaction, the client must be advised to refrain from consuming which of the following?
    1. Alcohol.
    2. Grapefruit.
    3. Milk.
    4. Cabbage.

80. A nurse is assessing a 1-day postpartum client who had a spontaneous vaginal delivery over an intact perineum. The fundus is firm at the umbilicus, lochia moderate, and perineum edematous. One hour after receiving ibuprofen 600 mg po, the client is complaining of perineal pain at level 9 on a 10-point scale. Based on this information, which of the following is an appropriate conclusion for the nurse to make about the client?
    1. She should be assessed by her doctor.
    2. She should have a sitz bath.
    3. She may have a hidden laceration.
    4. She needs a narcotic analgesic.

81. A breastfeeding mother calls the obstetrician's office with a complaint of pain in one breast. Upon inspection, a diagnosis of mastitis is made. Which of the following nursing interventions is appropriate?
    1. Advise the woman to apply ice packs to her breasts.
    2. Encourage the woman to breastfeed frequently.
    3. Inform the woman that she should wean immediately.
    4. Direct the woman to notify her pediatrician as soon as possible.

82. A woman who wishes to breastfeed advises the nurse that she has had breast augmentation surgery. Which of the following responses by the nurse is appropriate?
    1. Breast implants often contaminate the milk with toxins.
    2. The glandular tissue of women who need implants is often deficient.
    3. Babies often have difficulty latching to the nipples of women with breast implants.
    4. Women who have implants are often able exclusively to breastfeed.

83. A breastfeeding client calls her obstetrician stating that her baby was diagnosed with thrush and that her breasts have become infected as well. Which of the following organisms has caused the baby's and mother's infection?
    1. *Staphylococcus aureus.*
    2. *Streptococcus pneumoniae.*
    3. *Escherichia coli.*
    4. *Candida albicans.*

84. A client on the postpartum unit has been diagnosed with deep vein thrombosis. The following titration schedule is included in the client's orders:

    If INR is less than 1: administer 7,500 units heparin subcu
    If INR is 1.1 to 2: administer 5,000 units heparin subcu
    If INR is 2.1 to 3: administer 2,500 units heparin subcu
    If INR is greater than 3: administer 0 units heparin subcu

    The client's INR is 2.6. How many mL of heparin will the nurse administer if the available concentration of heparin is 5,000 units per 0.2 mL? (**Calculate to the nearest tenth.**)

    _____ mL.

85. A client is on magnesium sulfate via IV pump for severe preeclampsia. Other than patellar reflex assessments, which of the following noninvasive assessments should the nurse perform to monitor the client for early signs of magnesium sulfate toxicity?
    1. Serial grip strengths.
    2. Kernig assessments.
    3. Pupillary responses.
    4. Apical heart rate checks.

ANSWERS AND RATIONALES

The correct answer number and rationale for why it is the correct answer are given in boldface blue type. Rationales for why the other possible answer options are incorrect also are given, but they are not in boldface type.

1. 1. This is unnecessary. Gestational diabetic clients need not assess their blood glucose levels during the postpartum.
   2. This is unnecessary. Gestational diabetic clients need not inject insulin during the postpartum.
   3. **This is an appropriate statement to make.**
   4. This is not appropriate. Babies rarely develop diabetes before age 2. Plus, juvenile diabetes is now called type 1 diabetes.

   TEST-TAKING TIP: Women who develop gestational diabetes are high risk for developing type 2 diabetes. They should be encouraged to eat healthy foods and to exercise to prevent the onset of the chronic disease or, at the very least, to delay its onset.

2. 1. **Sudden lower back pain is a sign of a transfusion reaction.**
   2. This is not a sign of a transfusion reaction. The client may be nervous about receiving the blood.
   3. This is not a sign of a transfusion reaction. The client may be nervous about receiving the blood.
   4. This is not a sign of a transfusion reaction. The client is likely having a normal bowel movement.

   TEST-TAKING TIP: If the client is receiving the wrong type blood or is allergic to the blood, she will develop flank or kidney pain. Antibodies in the client's blood are likely destroying the donated blood. The transfusion should be stopped immediately and the reaction reported to the physician and to the blood bank.

3. **1 and 2 are correct.**
   1. **Hemabate can cause nausea, vomiting, diarrhea, and hyperthermia.**
   2. **Hemabate can cause nausea, vomiting, diarrhea, and hyperthermia.**
   3. Hypotension is not associated with Hemabate.
   4. Palpitations are not associated with Hemabate.
   5. Anasarca is not associated with Hemabate.

TEST-TAKING TIP: Hemabate is an oxytocic agent that acts on the myometrial tissue of the uterus. During the postpartum it acts directly at the site of placental separation to stop uncontrolled bleeding. Hemabate is a type of prostaglandin.

4. 1. This response is not appropriate. It is unlikely that this client is menstruating at 2 weeks postpartum.
   2. This response is not appropriate. This client needs to be evaluated.
   3. This response is not appropriate. This is an unlikely explanation for the bleeding.
   4. **This is the correct response. This client needs to be evaluated.**

   TEST-TAKING TIP: The quantity of lochia discharge is usually described as scant, moderate, or heavy. A heavy discharge is described as a discharge that saturates a pad in 1 hour or less. Because this client's lochia has already changed to alba (whitish), it is especially concerning that she is now experiencing a heavy lochia rubra (reddish) flow.

5. 1. The uterus is contracted. Massaging the uterus will not remedy the problem of heavy lochial flow.
   2. **It is important for the nurse to notify the physician. The client is bleeding more than she should after the delivery.**
   3. An oxytocic promotes contraction of the uterine muscle. The muscle is already contracted.
   4. The uterus is at the umbilicus. It is unlikely that it is displaced from a full bladder.

   TEST-TAKING TIP: The nurse must act as a detective to determine why he or she is seeing symptoms. In this scenario, the uterus is contracted and at the expected location—that is, firm at the umbilicus. The lochia flow, however, is heavy. The nurse must notify the practitioner for assistance because there is no additional action the nurse can take at this time.

6. 1. It is unlikely that an apical heart rate of 104 is responsible for the client's changes.
   2. **The urinary output is the likely cause of the client's changes.**
   3. It is unlikely that a blood pressure of 160/120 is responsible for the client's changes.

4. It is unlikely that a temperature of 100°F is responsible for the client's changes.

TEST-TAKING TIP: The hourly output for this client is 20 mL/hr. This is well below the minimum urinary output of 30 mL/hr. Because the medication is excreted via the kidneys, when a client's output is low, the concentration of the medication can increase to toxic levels in the bloodstream. This client is exhibiting signs of magnesium toxicity.

7. 1. The client should not be placed flat in bed. Her bed should be placed in the Sims position to enable her to aerate well.
   2. There is nothing in the scenario that suggests that this client is high risk for dependent edema.
   3. It is important for the nurse to auscultate the client's lung fields every 4 hours to assess for rales.
   4. There is nothing in the scenario that suggests that this client is high risk for an alteration in reflex response.

TEST-TAKING TIP: A cesarean section client is a postoperative client as well as a postpartum client. The nurse must perform needed physiological assessments. Because this client had general anesthesia during her surgery, she is high risk for pulmonary complications, including atelectasis and pneumonia.

8. 1. Postoperative cesarean clients should turn every 2 hours to prevent stasis of their lung fields.
   2. Sitz baths are rarely ordered for post-cesarean clients.
   3. Active range-of-motion exercises will help to prevent thrombus formation in post-cesarean patients.
   4. Central venous pressure is rarely assessed in post-cesarean clients.

TEST-TAKING TIP: Clients, whether they have intermittent positive pressure boots ordered or not, should be advised to move their legs actively at least a few times each hour. If the client exercises, she will be much less likely to develop deep vein thrombosis.

9. 1. It is unnecessary to monitor the client's hourly urinary output.
   2. This is an appropriate action.
   3. It is unnecessary for the client to be placed in this position.
   4. It is unnecessary for visitors to leave the client's room.

TEST-TAKING TIP: Benadryl is an antihistamine. One of the common side effects of Benadryl is sedation. It is very likely that this client will fall asleep while holding the baby. The nurse, therefore, should supervise the mother while she holds her baby.

10. 1. Puerperal infection is defined as a temperature of 100.4°F or higher after 24 hours postpartum.
    2. Although clients who develop endometritis will have significantly elevated white blood cell counts, a WBC count of 14,500 is normal for a postpartum client.
    3. Clients who develop infections may perspire profusely. However, diaphoresis is normally seen in postpartum clients, and is not in itself indicative of postpartum infection.
    4. A malodorous lochial flow is a common sign of a puerperal infection.

TEST-TAKING TIP: "Puerperium" is another word for "postpartum." Although a client may have a slight temperature elevation, an elevated white blood cell count, and/or be diaphoretic, all three symptoms are normally seen in the postpartum client. The only finding that would make a nurse suspect infection is the malodorous lochial flow. The other findings are well within normal range for a postpartum woman.

11. 1. The mother, not the baby, may develop a macular rash after receiving the injection. The baby will be unaffected.
    2. There is no evidence to suggest that babies whose mothers have received the rubella vaccine reject their mother's breast milk.
    3. There is no evidence to suggest that the mother's breast milk supply will drop.
    4. One out of 4 women complains of painful and stiff joints after receiving the injection.

TEST-TAKING TIP: Even though the benefits of receiving immunizations far outweigh the side effects of the medicines, anyone who receives a vaccine should be advised of the potential complications. It is especially important for mothers who are taking home newborn infants to receive anticipatory guidance regarding these changes and to be told that the baby's health will not be compromised.

12. 1. Feelings of infanticide are rare in clients diagnosed with postpartum depression.
    2. Difficulty latching babies to the breast is an independent problem from postpartum

depression. Some mothers with depression are successful breastfeeders, while some mothers who do not experience depression have difficulty latching their babies to the breast.

3. Mothers who experience postpartum depression often do feel like failures.
4. Concerns about sibling rivalry are not related to postpartum depression.

TEST-TAKING TIP: If a mother who is diagnosed with postpartum depression does have difficulty latching her baby to the breast, she may view this as yet another example of her poor parenting skills. The difficulty itself, however, is unrelated to the diagnosis.

13. 1. The client would be expected to complain of pain.
2. The nurse would not expect to see bleeding.
3. The nurse would not expect to note warmth.
4. The nurse would not expect to see redness.

TEST-TAKING TIP: A hematoma is a collection of blood under the skin. Although hematomas are usually simple bruises, large collections of blood can occur. Because the blood is trapped under the skin, the most common symptom is pain from the blood pressing on the pain sensors.

14. 1. This response is inappropriate. The client should not be advised to switch to formula.
2. This response is inappropriate. The client should not be advised to switch to formula.
3. This response by the nurse is appropriate.
4. This response is inappropriate. The client should not be advised to switch to formula.

TEST-TAKING TIP: First, the baby has already been exposed to the mother and will continue being exposed to her even if she switches to formula. More important, however, is the fact that the mother will produce antibodies that will be consumed by the baby in the breast milk. The baby will, therefore, be more protected by continuing to breastfeed because formula contains no protective properties.

15. 1. This may be true, but the mother may also be a successful breastfeeder.
2. This action can be helpful, but the placement of the incision will not necessarily determine the client's ability to breastfeed.

3. This action is very important.
4. This information is not accurate. Breast reduction surgery often does affect a woman's ability to breastfeed.

TEST-TAKING TIP: During breast reduction surgery, fat tissue is removed from the breast. Because the breast is much smaller, the nipple must be moved to a new location. During these procedures, the client's mammary ducts may be ligated. If the ducts are severed, the woman will not be able to transfer the milk produced in her glandular tissue to the baby. The most objective means of assessing milk transfer is by closely monitoring the baby's weights. Prefeed and postfeed weights as well as daily weights should be monitored.

16. 1. There is nothing in this client's history that would indicate that she could not produce breast milk.
2. There is nothing in this client's history that would indicate that she is at high risk for dysfunctional parenting.
3. This client is at high risk for wound dehiscence. Her wound healing may be impaired because of her diabetes and because of her obesity.
4. There is nothing in this client's history that would indicate that she is at high risk for projectile vomiting.

TEST-TAKING TIP: The fact that this client is postoperative cesarean section is irrelevant. This question could have been written by a surgical nursing professor rather than a parent-child nursing professor. The important pieces of information needed to answer this question correctly are that this client is obese and a type 1 diabetic and that she has had surgery.

17. 1. After the surgeon has been notified, the nurse should stay with the patient while another staff member gathers supplies, including a suture removal kit and personal protective equipment as well as sterile saline solution and a large syringe.
2. The highest priority action is to notify the surgeon.
3. After the surgeon has been notified, the nurse should elevate the client's bed slightly.
4. After the surgeon has been notified, the nurse should flex the client's knees slightly.

TEST-TAKING TIP: Positioning of the client is important, as the nurse wants to take as much stress off the incision as possible. If the surgeon is delayed, and the dehiscence is significant, the nurse must keep the intestines moist by placing sterile dressings that have been wetted with sterile saline, over the area (see Beattie, S. [2007]. Bedside emergency: Wound dehiscence. RN. Retrieved from: www.rnweb.com/rnweb/article/articleDetail.jsp?id(433110).

18. 1. This temperature elevation does not indicate infection.
    2. A low pulse rate is expected in the early postpartum period.
    3. The respiratory rate of 12 is well below normal. Peripartum clients' respiratory rates average 20 rpm.
    4. Although the systolic pressure is slightly elevated, a BP of 130/80 is within normal limits.

    TEST-TAKING TIP: Even though explanations are provided for each of the signs, the test taker must be able to determine which explanation is correct and which are erroneous. If the test taker consciously stops to think about each of the signs before looking at the explanations, he or she is less likely to be swayed by a wrong answer.

19. 1, 2, 3, and 5 are correct.
    1. The client should receive a RhoGAM injection after a spontaneous abortion.
    2. The client should receive a RhoGAM injection after an amniocentesis.
    3. The client should receive a RhoGAM injection after the delivery of a fetal demise.
    4. The client does not need a RhoGAM injection after the delivery of Rh-negative twins.
    5. The client should receive a RhoGAM injection after birth of an Rh-positive baby.

    TEST-TAKING TIP: RhoGAM, or Rh immune globulin, is administered to pregnant women at 28 weeks' gestation; after any invasive procedure, like an amniocentesis; after a preterm disruption of a pregnancy, like abortion or placental previa bleed; and after the delivery of an Rh+ infant. Because Rh-negative infants carry no Rh antigen, it is unnecessary to administer RhoGAM to their Rh-negative mothers.

20. 1. These findings are not consistent with a diagnosis of DVT. They may be due to a resolving epidural anesthesia.

2. These findings are normal. Many women complain of leg cramping.
3. These findings—swelling, redness, and warmth—indicate presence of a DVT.
4. These findings are normal. Many women develop spider veins during their pregnancies.

TEST-TAKING TIP: During the daily postpartum assessment, the nurse should assess for signs of thrombosis: pain, warmth, redness, and edema. The signs are usually unilateral. It is especially important for the nurse to refrain from palpating the calf too deeply because it is possible to dislodge a clot and cause a pulmonary embolism.

21. 1. This response is inappropriate. The client is not thinking about a future pregnancy at this time.
    2. This response is correct.
    3. This response is not appropriate. The nurse should ask the client if she would like to see or hold the baby.
    4. This response is not appropriate. The nurse should ask the client if she would like to see or hold the baby.

    TEST-TAKING TIP: The nurse should treat this baby with care and concern. Even though the baby has died he is still a valued child to the parents. The parents should be asked whether they would like to see or hold their baby. If they would, the nurse should help the parents to see the normalcy in their baby. Sedating a client only delays her inevitable grief.

22. 1. This action is inappropriate. Breastfeeding is contraindicated when the mother uses illicit drugs.
    2. This action is unnecessary. There is nothing in the scenario that implies that the client is having respiratory difficulties.
    3. This action is inappropriate. Rather, the nurse should encourage mother/baby interaction and provide the mother with parenting education.
    4. Providing instruction on baby-care skills is a very important action for the nurse to perform.

    TEST-TAKING TIP: Babies of mothers who are addicted to illicit drugs go through a withdrawal period and, because of the addiction, often have very disorganized behavior patterns. The nurse must provide guidance for the primipara regarding care of her difficult infant, especially because the client has already exhibited poor judgment. In addition, of course, the nurse must report the family to child protective services.

23. 1. Because the baby has a cleft lip, this is an appropriate nursing diagnosis, but it is not the highest priority diagnosis.
2. **This is the priority nursing diagnosis. Because the baby is macrosomic, the client is high risk for uterine atony that could lead to heavy vaginal bleeding possibly resulting in fluid volume deficit.**
3. Although the client is at high risk for infection, it is not highest priority. Infections take time to develop and this client is only 10 minutes postdelivery.
4. Although the client is at high risk for pain, especially from the episiotomy, this is not the highest priority nursing diagnosis.

TEST-TAKING TIP: **If the test taker remembers CAB as taught in CPR class—circulation, airway, breathing—he or she would realize that the client's fluid volume—that is, circulation—must take precedence.**

24. 1. **Foul-smelling lochia is a sign of endometritis.**
2. The nurse can assist the client with actions to relieve breast engorgement.
3. The nurse can assist the client with actions to relieve cracked nipples.
4. The nurse can assist the client with actions to relieve hemorrhoid pain.

TEST-TAKING TIP: **Some nursing actions are dependent functions. For example, nurses are able to administer antibiotics only after receiving a physician's order. Other actions, however, are independent actions. For example, assisting a client with engorged breasts to self-express breast milk, to apply warm soaks to the breasts, and to breastfeed effectively are independent actions. The nurse must report foul-smelling lochia to the physician so that the doctor can decide whether to order antibiotics for the client.**

25. 1. Abdominal striae are stretch marks. They are a normal side effect of pregnancy.
2. Oliguria is a complication that may develop after surgery, but it is not a symptom of paralytic ileus.
3. An omphalocele is a herniation of the intestines into the umbilical cord. It is sometimes seen in newborns.

4. **An absence of bowel sounds may indicate that a client has a paralytic ileus.**

TEST-TAKING TIP: **One of the complications of surgery and/or anesthesia is a paralytic ileus, the cessation of intestinal peristalsis. The client should be given nothing by mouth. Among other interventions, a nasogastric tube may be inserted to provide relief.**

26. 1. **This output is below the accepted minimum for 8 hours.**
2. This weight decrease following delivery is within normal limits.
3. A 2% drop in hematocrit is within normal limits.
4. This pulse rate is within normal limits.

TEST-TAKING TIP: **The nurse must divide the amount of urine output by the number of hours. The output in the scenario is equal to 25 mL/hr. This is well below the accepted output of 30 mL/hr. Plus, because this is a postpartum client, the nurse would expect high urinary outputs. Postpartum clients often have slowed heartbeats.**

27. 1. This client must be assessed—she likely has a urinary tract infection (UTI)—but another client should be checked first.
2. This client must be assessed—although her blood loss is within normal limits—but another client should be checked first.
3. **This client should be assessed first. The hemoglobin level is well below normal.**
4. This client must be assessed—she is likely engorged—but another client should be checked first.

TEST-TAKING TIP: **The nurse must recognize normal and abnormal findings. For example, 500 mL blood loss is an expected loss during a vaginal delivery. A hemoglobin of 7.2 g/dL, however, is well below the normal of 12 to 15 g/dL. This client is likely exhibiting signs of hypovolemia, including tachycardia, fatigue, and dizziness. She should be assessed first.**

28. 1. This blood pressure shows that no adverse side effects have resulted from the administration of the medication. One side effect of the medication is an elevation in blood pressure.
2. Pulse rate is unrelated to the administration of the medication.
3. **The fundal response indicates that the medication was effective in contracting the uterus.**

4. The prothrombin time is unrelated to the administration of the medication.

TEST-TAKING TIP: Methergine is an oxytocic agent. It is administered after delivery if the uterus is atonic or if the client is high risk for uterine atony. When the uterus is noted to be well contracted and at the appropriate position in the abdomen, the nurse can conclude that the medication action was successful.

29. 1. Both the spinal anesthesia and the epidural anesthesia clients are at high risk for developing pruritus.
2. Both the spinal anesthesia and the epidural anesthesia clients are at high risk for developing nausea.
3. **The client who has had the spinal anesthesia is much more likely to develop a postural headache than a client who had epidural anesthesia.**
4. Both the spinal anesthesia and the epidural anesthesia clients are at high risk for developing respiratory depression.

TEST-TAKING TIP: Both spinal anesthesia and epidural anesthesia are forms of regional anesthesia. The same medication is used and it is placed at the same vertebral level in both instances. Only spinal anesthesia is administered into the spinal space, leaving a wound through which spinal fluid can escape. When spinal fluid is lost from the spinal canal, clients are at high risk for developing postural headaches, also called spinal headaches, because of the change in pressure in the spinal canal.

30. 1. The client with postpartum psychosis will experience hallucinations.
2. Clients with diabetes mellitus, not postpartum psychosis, are polyphagic.
3. Clients with bulimia induce vomiting.
4. Clients with postpartum blues and/or postpartum depression are weepy and sad.

TEST-TAKING TIP: Clients who have been diagnosed with postpartum psychosis have a psychiatric disease. They experience hallucinations, usually auditory, including voices that may tell them to kill their babies.

31. 1. **This answer is correct. She should gently massage the area toward the nipple.**
2. The woman should apply warm soaks, not ice.

3. The woman should be advised to feed her baby frequently at the breast. She should not be advised to bottle feed.
4. The woman should apply lanolin (Lansinoh) to sore or cracked nipples, not for a problem of tender hard nodules.

TEST-TAKING TIP: A client who palpates a tender, hard nodule in her lactating breast is experiencing milk stasis. The stasis may be related to a blocked milk duct. It is very important that the woman gently massage the nodule while applying warm soaks and/or feeding her baby to prevent mastitis from developing.

32. 1. If the woman has manually removed milk from her breasts, her nipples will soften to the touch.
2. If the baby is latched well, he should swallow after every suck.
3. The nurse would expect the baby to transfer 60 mL or more at the feeding.
4. **The mother should not squeeze her nipple. The area behind the areola should be gently compressed.**

TEST-TAKING TIP: This client is complaining of engorgement. The baby is having difficulty latching because the breast is inflamed, making the nipple tense and short. When the woman manually removes a small amount of the foremilk, the nipple becomes easier for the baby to grasp.

33. 1. The results are not normal. This client's blood pressure is markedly elevated and the client is hyperreflexic.
2. **The nurse should notify the physician of the signs of preeclampsia.**
3. There is no need to discontinue the intravenous infusion.
4. The findings are consistent with signs of preeclampsia. It would be inappropriate to wait fifteen minutes to verify the results.

TEST-TAKING TIP: The hypertensive illnesses of pregnancy can develop at any time after 20 weeks' gestation through about 2 weeks postpartum. This client is exhibiting a late onset of preeclampsia—markedly elevated blood pressure and hyperreflexia. The physician should be notified of the changes.

34. 1. This response is incorrect. RhoGAM must be administered within 72 hours of delivery.
2. **This response is correct. The nurse should not finalize an Rh– (negative)**

client's discharge until the client has received her RhoGAM injection.

3. This response is incorrect. A negative direct Coombs' test means that no maternal antibodies were detected in the baby's circulatory system. The nurse would expect to detect a negative direct Coombs' test.

4. This response is unacceptable. Rh– (negative) clients should receive their RhoGAM injection before 72 hours postpartum or by discharge, whichever is earlier.

TEST-TAKING TIP: The administration of RhoGAM is the only way to prevent an Rh– (negative) client's body from mounting a full antibody response to the delivery of an Rh+ (positive) baby. It is malpractice for a nurse to discharge the client before she receives her injection or to delay the injection beyond the 72-hour deadline.

35. 1. This is inappropriate. Naming the baby is a means of acknowledging both the existence and the death of the baby.
2. This is inappropriate. Clients' imaginings of what the baby looks like are often much worse than the reality.
3. This is inappropriate. The couple should be provided time to be with their baby before transporting the baby to the morgue.
4. This is appropriate. The small mementos will provide the couple with something tangible to remember the pregnancy and baby by.

TEST-TAKING TIP: It is very difficult for parents who have delivered a fetal demise. The only contact they have had with the baby is through the pregnancy. Small mementos, such as a picture, lock of hair, or baby bracelet, provide the parents with tangible remembrances of the baby.

36. 1. The client with a placenta accreta is high risk for a large blood loss.
2. Placenta accreta is not related to a hypertensive state.
3. Placenta accreta is not related to the development of jaundice.
4. The nurse would not expect to detect a shortened prothrombin time when a client has a placenta accreta.

TEST-TAKING TIP: A placenta accreta's chorionic villi burrow through the endometrial lining into the myometrial lining. Separation of the placenta from the uterine wall is severely hampered. Clients often lose large quantities of blood, and it is not uncommon for the

physician to have to perform a hysterectomy to control the bleeding. Clients who have had multiple uterine scars are especially at high risk for this problem. If the test taker were unfamiliar with placenta accreta, he or she could deduce the answer, because the placenta is highly vascular and only one answer referred to a vascular issue. The average blood loss during a cesarean delivery is 1,000 mL.

37. 20 mL per dose
Formula:

$$\frac{\text{Known dosage}}{\text{Known volume}} = \frac{\text{Desired dosage}}{\text{Desired volume}}$$

$$\frac{125 \text{ mg}}{5 \text{ mL}} = \frac{500 \text{ mg}}{x \text{ mL}}$$

$$125\ x = 5 \times 500$$

$$125\ x = 2{,}500$$

$$x = 20 \text{ mL per dose}$$

TEST-TAKING TIP: The test taker must remember that a dose is defined as the quantity of medication that is administered to a client at one time. The client, then, is to receive 500 mg, or 20 mL, of the medication at each administration.

38. 1. A magnesium level of 7 mg/dL is therapeutic. This is an expected level.
2. The serum sodium level is normal.
3. The serum potassium is below normal. The nurse should report the finding to the physician.
4. The serum calcium is normal.

TEST-TAKING TIP: The test taker should be familiar with the normal values of commonly tested electrolytes. Although the normal magnesium level is 1.8 to 3.0 mg/dL, magnesium sulfate is being administered to raise the level in the client's bloodstream. The medication, which is an anticonvulsant, is being administered to prevent further seizures. The potassium level, however, is well below normal.

39. 1. Breastfeeding is contraindicated when a mother is HIV positive.
2. It is recommended that HIV-positive clients use condoms for family planning.
3. It is unnecessary to take her temperature every morning. If she should develop a fever, she should seek medical assistance as soon as possible, however.

4. The client should seek care for a recent weight loss. This may be a symptom of full-blown AIDS.

TEST-TAKING TIP: Although obstetric clients who enter the hospital are usually aware of their HIV status, the nurse must still review the actions that clients should take after discharge. These actions include taking all medications, bottle feeding rather than breastfeeding, and reporting any changes in health, like weight loss or the appearance of thrush.

40. 1. When a client has DVT she is clotting excessively. She is not at high risk for hemorrhage.
    2. The client is at high risk for stroke if a clot should travel to the brain through the vascular tree.
    3. The client is not at high risk for endometritis if she has DVT.
    4. The client is not at high risk for hematoma if she has DVT.

TEST-TAKING TIP: The test taker could deduce the answer to this question by determining the etiology of each of the problems. The only complication that is caused by a clot, which is the same etiology as the DVT, is a stroke.

41. 1. This client is not especially at high risk for seizures.
    2. The client should be monitored carefully for signs of postpartum hemorrhage.
    3. This client is not especially at high risk for infection.
    4. This client is not especially at high risk for thrombosis.

TEST-TAKING TIP: An average size baby weighs 2,500 to 4,000 grams. The baby in the scenario is macrosomic. As a result, the mother's uterus has been stretched beyond its expected capacity. The client is, therefore, at high risk for uterine atony, which could result in a postpartum hemorrhage.

42. 1. Reglan is an antiemetic. It is not the appropriate medication for this client.
    2. Zofran is an antiemetic. It is not the appropriate medication for this client.
    3. Compazine is an antiemetic. It is not the appropriate medication for this client.
    4. Benadryl is an antihistamine. It is the drug of choice for this client who has pruritus and a rash.

TEST-TAKING TIP: To answer this question, the test taker must first determine what the client's clinical problem is and then determine which medication will relieve that problem. The test taker, therefore, must be familiar with the actions of major medications. The client is exhibiting signs of an allergic response. Benadryl is the only choice that will inhibit the client's immune response.

43. 1. Chamomile tea has not been shown to potentiate the affect of Zoloft, but St. John's wort has.
    2. The therapeutic effect of selective serotonin receptor inhibitors (SSRIs) like Zoloft is delayed about 1 to 2 weeks from the time the medication is initiated.
    3. This response is incorrect. The medication can be crushed.
    4. A 10-lb weight gain is not associated with the medication.

TEST-TAKING TIP: Clients who receive medications for emotional problems as well as for physiological complaints expect to experience resolution of their symptoms in a timely fashion. If postpartum depression clients are not forewarned of the delay of the therapeutic effects, they may stop taking the medications prematurely, believing that the medicines are useless.

44. 1. The nurse would not expect to see engorgement.
    2. The nurse would not expect to see mastitis.
    3. The nurse would not expect to see a blocked milk duct.
    4. The nurse would expect that the woman would have a low milk supply.

TEST-TAKING TIP: The placenta produces the hormones of pregnancy, including estrogen and progesterone. When placental fragments are retained, those hormones are still being produced. Estrogen inhibits prolactin, which is the hormone of lactogenesis, or milk production. Women who have retained placental fragments, therefore, often complain of an insufficient milk supply for their babies.

45. 1. The woman should not wash with soap. Soaps destroy the natural lanolins produced by the body.
    2. A small amount of lanolin should be applied to the nipple after each feeding.

3. The baby will not become sick from the blood. The woman should be warned that he may spit up digested and/or undigested blood after the feeding, however.
4. Topical anesthetics are not used on the breasts. The woman could receive an oral analgesic, however.

TEST-TAKING TIP: Using lanolin on the breasts is a type of moist wound healing. The lanolin is soothing and allows the nipple to heal without a scab developing on the surface of the nipple. Mothers are often very concerned about their babies swallowing the blood. Ingesting the blood does not adversely affect the babies unless, of course, the mother is HIV positive or carries another bloodborne virus.

46. 1. A circumvallate placenta is a placenta with an inner ring created by a fold in the chorion and amnion. Clients with this type of placenta are at high risk for antepartal complications like preterm labor.
2. A succenturiate placenta is characterized by one primary placenta that is attached via blood vessels to satellite lobe(s). Clients with this type of placenta are at high risk for postpartum hemorrhage.
3. A placenta with a vellamentous insertion has an umbilical cord that is formed a distance from the placenta. Because the vessels are unsupported between the placenta and the cord, hemorrhage may result if one or more of the vessels tears.
4. **The battledore placenta is characterized by an umbilical cord that is inserted on the periphery of the placenta. Clients with this type of placenta are at high risk for preterm problems like preterm labor and hemorrhage.**

TEST-TAKING TIP: There are a number of placental variations. The test taker should be familiar with each of the variations and high-risk nature of each.

47. 1. The goal of the injection of RhoGAM is to inhibit the mother's immune response.
2. Immune globulin is composed of antibodies. When a client receives RhoGAM, she receives passive antibodies to inhibit her immune response.
3. Passive antibodies cannot prevent the migration of fetal cells throughout the mother's bloodstream.
4. A client's blood type is determined by her DNA. RhoGAM cannot change a client's DNA.

TEST-TAKING TIP: When a client receives RhoGAM, she receives passive Rh antibodies. If any Rh antigen is circulating in the mother's bloodstream, the antibodies will destroy it. As a result, there will be no antigen in the mother's body to stimulate her mast cells to have an active antibody response. In essence, therefore, RhoGAM is injected to inhibit the client's immune response.

48. 1. This client is voicing anger at herself.
2. **This client is exhibiting the bargaining stage of grief.**
3. This client is exhibiting signs of depression.
4. This client is exhibiting denial.

TEST-TAKING TIP: Although clients do not go through the stages of grief linearly, they do express the many stages of grief while they mourn the loss of their child of fantasy. Bargaining is a particularly vulnerable time for parents. Unscrupulous practitioners can make a great deal of money from couples who believe that their child can be cured from "special medicines" or "procedures."

49. 1. This client in high-Fowler's position is no more at high risk for postpartum hemorrhage than a spinal anesthesia client who has been kept flat after surgery.
2. **The nurse would expect the client to complain of a severe postural headache.**
3. This client is no more at high risk for a pruritic rash than a spinal anesthesia client who has been kept flat after surgery.
4. This client is no more at high risk for paralytic ileus than a spinal anesthesia client who has been kept flat after surgery.

TEST-TAKING TIP: Postpartum hemorrhage, pruritic rash, and paralytic ileus are complications seen in post-cesarean clients, whether they received general anesthesia, epidural anesthesia, or spinal anesthesia. Only spinal clients, most notably those who elevate soon after surgery, are at high risk for postural headaches.

50. 1. Vitamin K is the antidote for Coumadin (warfarin) overdose, not for heparin overdose.
2. **Protamine is the antidote for heparin overdose.**
3. Vitamin E is not correct.
4. Mannitol is not correct.

TEST-TAKING TIP: When heparin is administered, clients must be monitored carefully for signs of hemorrhage. Protamine is the antidote for heparin overdose. Conversely, the antidote for Coumadin, another medication often administered to clients with DVT, is vitamin K.

51. 1. The client should have a glucose tolerance test done at about 6 weeks postpartum. Women who give birth to hypoglycemic and/or macrosomic babies are at increased risk of developing type 2 diabetes.
2. There is no indication in the scenario of Rh incompatibility that would require that an indirect Coombs' test be done.
3. There is no indication in the scenario that this client has impaired kidney function and should have a BUN done.
4. There is no indication in the scenario that this client should have a CBC done. There is no indication of anemia or infection.

TEST-TAKING TIP: The baby born to this mother is hypoglycemic and is macrosomic. The most common cause of these two neonatal complications is maternal diabetes. It is recommended that mothers who are diabetic during pregnancy—that is, gestational diabetics—be assessed for type 2 diabetes at about 6 weeks postpartum.

52. 1, 2, 3, and 5 are correct.
1. The nurse must check the client's blood type.
2. The nurse must check the client's name by checking the bracelet and asking the client her name.
3. The nurse must compare the client's blood type with the blood type on the infusion bag.
4. The nurse must obtain an infusion of normal saline, not dextrose and water.
5. The time the infusion begins and ends must be documented.

TEST-TAKING TIP: The potential for blood transfusion incompatibility is very real. It is essential, therefore, that two health care practitioners check simultaneously to make sure that the client is receiving the correct blood. If any sign of a reaction should develop, the transfusion should be stopped immediately. Only normal saline solution is used as a solution immediately before or after blood administration. Dextrose in water will hemolyze the red

blood cells. In addition, a special filtered infusion set must be used.

53. 2 and 5 are correct.
1. Preterm labor clients are not especially at high risk for postpartum hemorrhage.
2. Clients who have had a prolonged first stage of labor are at high risk for postpartum hemorrhage (PPH).
3. Cesarean section clients are not especially at high risk for PPH.
4. Postdates clients who deliver small babies are not especially at high risk for PPH.
5. Clients with a succenturiate placenta are at high risk for PPH.

TEST-TAKING TIP: The muscles of the uterus of a client who has experienced a prolonged first stage of labor are fatigued. In the postpartum period, therefore, they may fail to contract fully enough to control bleeding at the site of placental separation. A succenturiate placenta is characterized by one primary placenta that is attached via blood vessels to satellite lobe(s). These clients must be monitored carefully for postpartum hemorrhage.

54. 1. Hydralazine is administered as an antihypertensive, not specifically as an anti-seizure medication. Magnesium sulfate is the drug administered as an anticonvulsant to women with eclampsia.
2. Hydralazine is an antihypertensive. The change in blood pressure indicates that the medication is effective.
3. The weight loss is secondary to fluid loss.
4. The hydralazine is not administered to treat a headache.

TEST-TAKING TIP: Hydralazine is an antihypertensive medication. The goal, therefore, is for the blood pressure to drop. A change in BP from 160/120 to 130/90 is evidence of a therapeutic effect.

55. 1. Lochia serosa at 2 weeks postpartum is unusual, but it does not put the client or her baby in imminent danger.
2. This client is exhibiting signs of postpartum depression. This is a problem that must be remedied, but it does not put the client or her baby in imminent danger.
3. The client's cracked nipples do need intervention, but they do not put the client or her baby in imminent danger.
4. The client is exhibiting inappropriate behavior when she yells at the baby for crying. The nurse must make additional

assessments to determine whether there is any other evidence of abuse or neglect.

TEST-TAKING TIP: The baby is the most vulnerable member of the mother-infant dyad. Because the baby is completely dependent on the care of the mother, if the nurse discovers any behavior or other evidence that makes him or her suspicious of child abuse or neglect, he or she is obligated both morally and legally to report the situation. Clients who are experiencing postpartum depression usually perform baby care competently.

56. 1. The nurse should call a code before beginning rescue breathing.
2. The nurse should call a code first and then discontinue the medication.
3. The nurse should call a code first.
4. The nurse should call a code before checking the carotid pulse.

TEST-TAKING TIP: The nurse should call a code as soon as he or she discovers a client who is nonresponsive. Immediately after calling the code, the nurse should stop the medications, begin rescue breathing, and provide chest compressions, if necessary, until the code team arrives. Only after receiving an order to do so should the nurse administer calcium gluconate, the antidote to magnesium sulfate.

57. 1. Infection, not ineffective breastfeeding, is the priority nursing diagnosis.
2. Infection is the priority nursing diagnosis. A temperature of 104.6°F, as well as the client's other signs/symptoms, should immediately suggest the presence of infection.
3. Infection, not ineffective individual coping, is the priority nursing diagnosis.
4. Infection, not pain, is the priority nursing diagnosis.

TEST-TAKING TIP: This client has a breast abscess. Although all of the nursing diagnoses are important, the most important diagnosis is infection. It is the only one of the four diagnoses that is related to the acute problem. Ineffective breastfeeding contributed to the development of the infection. Because of the infection, the client is in pain and is coping poorly. Once the abscess is drained and the antibiotics have been administered, the

other three diagnoses will be on the road to being resolved.

58. **800 units/hour**
The formula to determine the number of units that the client is receiving per hour is:

total number of units : mL of IV solution = x units : flow rate

$$25{,}000 \text{ units} : 500 \text{ mL} = x : 16 \text{ mL/hr}$$

$$500\,x = 25{,}000 \times 16$$

$$x = \frac{25{,}000 \times 16}{500}$$

$$x = 800 \text{ units/hr}$$

TEST-TAKING TIP: To make sure that he or she is calculating the amount correctly, the test taker can label each number and cancel to make sure that the result is in the units requested. As can be seen above, the mL's drop out and the values that are left are units/hr.

59. 1. A moderate lochia flow would indicate that the action was successful.
2. Decreased pain is not an expected outcome of uterine massage for uterine atony.
3. A stable postpartum blood pressure is not directly related to the action of uterine massage.
4. The expected outcome would be that the uterus is contracted at or below the umbilicus.

TEST-TAKING TIP: Expected outcomes relate to specific nursing diagnoses that are developed after making an assessment. This client's uterine muscle was boggy. The nursing action taken—massage—related directly to the nursing assessment—atonic uterus—and the outcome—normal lochia—indicated that the action was successful.

60. 1. This rationale is correct. Because of an elevation in clotting factors, all postpartum clients are at high risk for thrombus formation.
2. The positive pressure boots improve blood return to the heart by preventing pooling of blood in the extremities. They are not applied to treat hypovolemia.
3. The rationale for the use of positive pressure boots is not related to varicose vein development. Varicose veins would, however, increase a client's potential for developing deep vein thrombosis.

4. The rationale for the use of positive pressure boots has nothing to do with a client's milk ejection reflex.

TEST-TAKING TIP: The client in the scenario is post–cesarean section. The surgeon has ordered intermittent positive pressure boots for her because she is at high risk for thrombus formation and because she is on bed rest. Clients who deliver vaginally do not need the boots because they are able to ambulate immediately after delivery and, therefore, rarely experience pooling of blood in their extremities.

61. 1. Reglan is an antiemetic. It is one drug that may be administered to a client who is vomiting after surgery.
2. Demerol is a narcotic analgesic. It is not the appropriate medication for this client.
3. Seconal is a sedative. It is not the appropriate medication for this client.
4. Benadryl is an antihistamine. It is not the appropriate medication for this client.

TEST-TAKING TIP: This client is exhibiting a common side effect of regional anesthesia: nausea and vomiting. Antiemetics are the medications of choice for this problem. Many prn medications are ordered for postsurgical clients. The test taker must become familiar with the actions and the uses of each of them.

62. 1. The nurse should monitor the client for signs of infection after the first 24 hours have passed.
2. The client is not at high risk for bloody urine.
3. The client should be monitored carefully for heavy lochia.
4. The client is not at high risk for rectal abrasions.

TEST-TAKING TIP: The key to answering this question is the time frame stipulated in the stem of the question—"the immediate postpartum period." There are two main maternal complications associated with forceps use—hemorrhage and infection. Hemorrhage usually occurs early, secondary to cervical, vaginal, or perineal lacerations. Infection usually develops later in the postpartum period secondary to contamination of the uterine cavity during the application of the forceps.

63. 1. It is essential that the client never be left alone with her baby.

2. The statement is untrue. There is no set time frame for the resolution of the symptoms of postpartum psychosis.
3. Clinical response to medications is usually quite good.
4. The client's vital signs need not be assessed frequently.

TEST-TAKING TIP: Clients who have been diagnosed with postpartum psychosis have been known to have homicidal and suicidal ideations. Because the baby and other children are vulnerable, the mother should always be supervised when in their presence. In addition, if she exhibits suicidal behaviors, she should be supervised at all times.

64. 1. Methergine is contraindicated for this client.
2. Magnesium sulfate is the drug of choice for the treatment of severe preeclampsia.
3. Ibuprofen is a nonsteroidal anti-inflammatory drug (NSAID). It is an appropriate medication for the treatment of postpartum cramping. It is not contraindicated for this client.
4. Morphine sulfate is a narcotic analgesic. It is an appropriate medication for the treatment of postsurgical pain. It is not contraindicated for this client.

TEST-TAKING TIP: Methergine is an oxytocic agent. It acts directly on the myofibrils of the uterus. Secondarily, it also contracts the muscles of the vascular tree. As a result, clients' blood pressure tends to elevate when they receive this medication. Methergine should not be administered to a client whose blood pressure is 130/90 or higher.

65. 1, 2, and 3 are correct.
1. The nurse would expect to see fever, flank pain, and dark-colored urine.
2. The nurse would expect to see fever, flank pain, and dark-colored urine.
3. The nurse would expect to see fever, flank pain, and dark-colored urine.
4. Rh– (negative) clients often complain of swelling at the injection site. This is an expected finding.
5. The nurse would expect to see a hemolytic response, not polycythemia.

TEST-TAKING TIP: When RhoGAM is administered to an Rh+ (positive) client, antibodies against the client's red blood cells are being injected into her body. A hemolytic response similar to one seen

when a client receives the wrong type of blood may develop.

66. 1. This father is grieving. His anger is appropriate at this time.
 2. This action is appropriate. The nurse is acknowledging that every member of the family is grieving the loss.
 3. Five-year-old children do not understand death. They do respond to their parents' unusual behaviors.
 4. Even though it is very difficult for the parents to deal with their own grief while caring for their daughter, the young girl may feel abandoned if sent unexpectedly to her grandparents.

TEST-TAKING TIP: Each member of a family will grieve differently. One of the important actions for the nurse is to help the members of the family to communicate with one another. Children do not understand the finality of death until about age 9, but pre–schoolage children often feel guilty when bad things happen. It is important for the nurse to communicate clearly that the child was not responsible for the death of the fetus.

67. 1. This statement is inappropriate. Any defect is devastating for the parents to accept.
 2. This statement is inappropriate. This child is affected. That is all that matters.
 3. This statement is inappropriate. The nurse must not impose his or her beliefs on the couple.
 4. This statement is appropriate. Clients may need help or permission to express their grief.

TEST-TAKING TIP: Nurses must be very careful how they speak with and care for clients who have had a baby that is less than perfect. Couples expect to birth perfect babies. When a baby who has a problem is born, the couple must grieve their "baby of fantasy," while they bond with and accept their "baby of reality."

68. 1. This statement by the mother may be a true statement, but it may communicate the mother's difficulty with accepting her baby.
 2. This statement is an example of positive maternal bonding.
 3. This statement is an example of positive maternal bonding.
 4. This statement is an example of positive maternal bonding.

TEST-TAKING TIP: Babies with defects are more likely to be victims of child abuse and neglect than are healthy, normal babies. Nurses must evaluate the bonding between the mother and her baby. If the nurse is concerned about the bonding relationship, he or she must monitor the mother's care and, if necessary, refer the family for a home-care nurse evaluation and/or to child protective services.

69. 18 mL/hour.
 The formula for determining the flow rate is:

 Total number of units : mL of IV solution

 $$= \text{Units/min} : x \text{ flow rate}$$

 20,000 units : 500 mL = 12 units/min : x mL/hr

 Because the order is written in units/min, the test taker must determine how many units the client is receiving per hour:
 (12 units/min × 60 min/hr = 720 units/hr)

 20,000 units : 500 mL = 720 units/hr : x

 20,000 x units = 500 mL × 720 units/hr

 $$x = \frac{500 \text{ mL} \times 720 \text{ units/hr}}{20,000 \text{ units}}$$

 $$x = 18 \text{ mL/hr}$$

TEST-TAKING TIP: The test taker must remember that pumps are always programmed in mL/hr. Because the question included a rate of units/min, to calculate the pump rate, units/min had to be converted to units/hr. In addition, it must be remembered that per a Joint Commission on Accreditation of Hospitals directive, "units" must always be written out fully— that is, not abbreviated as "U."

70. 1. The PT is normal. For someone taking warfarin, the PT time should be prolonged 1.5 to 2.0 times normal.
 2. The INR should be between 2 and 3.
 3. The hematocrit is elevated. It should be within normal limits.
 4. The hemoglobin is below normal. It should be within normal limits.

TEST-TAKING TIP: Coumadin interferes with the clotting of blood. The PT and/or INR will be monitored to determine whether the medication is effective. If the PT is more than 2 times normal or the INR is over 3, the client is at high risk for hemorrhage.

71. 1. The drop in estrogen is not related to the glucose level.
2. The drop in progesterone is not related to the glucose level.
3. The drop in human placental lactogen (hPL) is related to the glucose level.
4. The drop in human chorionic gonadotropin is not related to the glucose level.

TEST-TAKING TIP: The hormone hPL is an insulin antagonist. Throughout pregnancy, the insulin needs of type 1 diabetics rise incrementally as the levels of hPL in the bloodstream rise. Once the placenta is birthed, however, the levels drop precipitously. As a result, it is not uncommon for the glucose levels of type 1 diabetics to be within normal limits for a day or so after delivery—as seen in this client.

72. 1. It is unnecessary to wean the baby to formula.
2. Optimally, the baby should stay in the hospital room with the mother.
3. It is unnecessary for the mother to pump and dump for 2 weeks.
4. Although the baby could drink milk stored by the mother, this is not the best solution.

TEST-TAKING TIP: Other than the period of time that the mother is in the surgical suite, there is unlikely to be anything that would warrant separating the mother from her baby. The surgeon and anesthesiologist should be able to prescribe medicines that are compatible with breastfeeding. Plus, the client could easily feed her baby while lying in a comfortable position. The client should be admitted to a hospital room that would be safe for a 6-week-old baby.

73. 1, 2, and 4 are correct.
1. This is an appropriate action. The baby should be handled with respect.
2. This is an appropriate action. Funerals help clients to achieve closure and to provide others with a means of acknowledging the baby's death.
3. This is inappropriate. The couple must grieve the loss of this child.
4. This is an appropriate action. Although there are some clients who will decline to hold their babies, the action is very important for those who accept the opportunity.
5. This action is inappropriate. Stating that the loss of a baby is for the best is very demeaning and unfeeling.

TEST-TAKING TIP: Clients must be encouraged and assisted through the process of grieving and mourning their babies. In addition, as most women will remain on the obstetric unit, there must be a mechanism, like a specific picture placed on the woman's door, for communicating to every department in the hospital, from nursing to housekeeping to dietary, that the client has had a fetal death.

74. 1. Ibuprofen is an NSAID. It can exacerbate the action of Coumadin. The client should be encouraged to take acetaminophen, if needed, for pain.
2. This action is correct. Dark green, leafy vegetables contain vitamin K. The vitamin would decrease the anticoagulant affect of Coumadin.
3. The client should be advised to avoid drinking grapefruit juice. It may increase the action of Coumadin.
4. The client should be advised to report signs of internal bleeding, such as hematuria. Decreased urinary output would not be expected in a client taking Coumadin.

TEST-TAKING TIP: Patient education is essential when clients are discharged on powerful medications like Coumadin. The nurse must consider all aspects of the client's daily life, including diet (see above regarding dark green, leafy vegetables); herbs taken (some, such as ginkgo biloba, and ginger, can increase the action of the medication); activities (clients should avoid playing contact sports, using razors); and the like.

75. 1. Endometrial ischemia is not a complication of a succenturiate placenta.
2. The nurse should carefully monitor this client for signs of postpartum hemorrhage.
3. The client is not especially at high risk for a prolapsed uterus.
4. The client is not at high risk for a vaginal hematoma.

TEST-TAKING TIP: Because a succenturiate placenta has extra lobe(s), the client is at high risk for hemorrhage from one or more of the lobes. The professional who performed the delivery may have noted one lobe but may not have realized that an additional lobe is still in utero.

76. 1. This is an important nursing diagnosis, but it is not the priority diagnosis.

2. This is an important nursing diagnosis, but it is not the priority diagnosis.
3. Fluid volume deficit related to blood loss is the priority nursing diagnosis.
4. This is an important nursing diagnosis, but it is not the priority diagnosis.

TEST-TAKING TIP: It is likely that most clients will have multiple nursing diagnoses. The nurse must then determine which is (are) the priority diagnosis(ses). It is essential that the nurse remember Maslow's Hierarchy of Needs. Although psychosocial needs are very important, the physiological needs, especially those related to the respiratory and the cardiovascular systems, must take precedence.

77. 1. This client is high risk for uterine atony.
2. The client is not at high risk for hypoprolactinemia.
3. The client is not at high risk for infection.
4. The client is not at high risk for mastitis.

TEST-TAKING TIP: The uterus of a woman who delivers a macrosomic baby has been stretched beyond the usual pregnancy size. The muscle fibers of the myometrium, therefore, are stretched. After delivery the muscles are unable to contract effectively to stop the bleeding at the placental separation site.

78. 1. This is an important question to ask the client but it is unrelated to her discharge needs.
2. This is an important question to ask the client but it is unrelated to her discharge needs.
3. This is an important question to ask the client but it is unrelated to her discharge needs.
4. The client has had major surgery. The client will need some assistance when she returns home, especially if she has a number of stairs to climb.

TEST-TAKING TIP: Discharge care must begin on admission to the hospital. Cesarean section clients will need some assistance after discharge, especially if they must climb up and down stairs.

79. 1. Clients should be warned about consuming alcohol when taking Paxil.
2. Grapefruit is not contraindicated for clients who have been prescribed Paxil.
3. Milk is not contraindicated for clients who have been prescribed Paxil.
4. Cabbage is not contraindicated for clients who have been prescribed Paxil.

TEST-TAKING TIP: Paxil is an antidepressant. Although the concurrent use of alcohol and Paxil has not been shown to adversely affect clients' abilities, it is advised that alcohol not be consumed while taking the medication. Some clients have actually reported that they experienced a craving for alcohol while taking the medication.

80. 1. The client should be assessed by her health care practitioner.
2. The client may need a sitz bath, but should be assessed first.
3. It is unlikely that this client has a hidden laceration as her lochial flow is normal.
4. The client may benefit from a narcotic, but should be assessed first.

TEST-TAKING TIP: This client is complaining of an excessive amount of pain after having received a relatively large dose of ibuprofen. Because the perineum is edematous, the lochial flow is normal, and the pain level is well above that expected, the nurse should suspect that the client has developed a hematoma. The client should be assessed by her health care provider.

81. 1. This action is inappropriate. The woman should apply warm soaks to the breast.
2. The action is appropriate. The woman should breastfeed frequently.
3. The woman should be discouraged from weaning.
4. It is unnecessary for the client to notify the pediatrician. The baby's health is not in jeopardy.

TEST-TAKING TIP: Mastitis is a breast infection. Usually only one duct system is affected by the bacteria. If the mother were to wean abruptly, milk stasis would occur, the bacteria would proliferate, and a breast abscess is likely to develop. The mother should feed her baby frequently, use warm soaks to promote milk flow, and notify her obstetrician. Antibiotics are usually prescribed to eradicate the bacteria.

82. 1. This response is incorrect. The implants usually do not leach toxins into the surrounding tissue.
2. The glandular tissue of most women who choose to have breast augmentation surgery is normal.
3. This information is incorrect. Implants usually do not affect a baby's ability to latch.

4. This information is true. Women who have had augmentation surgery usually are able to breastfeed exclusively.

TEST-TAKING TIP: Because breast implants are usually inserted behind the breast tissue, the mammary ducts are rarely affected. Daily weights of babies whose mothers have had breast enlargements should be monitored as a precaution, but most of these mothers do produce sufficient quantities of breast milk.

83. 1. *Staphylococcus aureus* is the most common bacteria to cause mastitis.
    2. *Streptococcus pneumoniae* is a major cause of pneumonia.
    3. Certain strains of *Escherichia coli* cause severe gastritis.
    4. The baby and mother are infected with *Candida albicans*.

TEST-TAKING TIP: When breastfeeding babies develop thrush, the mothers are at high risk for developing a yeast infection of the breast. Because they are both infected, it is critical that they be treated simultaneously for a minimum of 2 weeks. If they are not treated aggressively, they will continue to reinfect each other.

84. 0.1 mL
    Because the INR is between 2.1 and 3, the nurse must administer 2,500 units of heparin subcu. To determine the quantity of heparin that the nurse must administer, a ratio and proportion equation should be set up:

$$\frac{\text{Known dose}}{\text{Known volume}} = \frac{\text{Desired dose}}{\text{Desired volume}}$$

$$\frac{5{,}000 \text{ units}}{0.2} = \frac{2{,}500 \text{ units}}{x \text{ mL}}$$

$$5{,}000\, x = 2{,}500 \times 0.2$$

$$x = \frac{2{,}500 \times 0.2}{5{,}000}$$

$$x = 0.1 \text{ mL}$$

TEST-TAKING TIP: The test taker should not let the titration protocol confuse him or her. The test taker simply must choose the dosage that meets the given criteria. Because the INR in the scenario is 2.6, the test taker can quickly see that the dosage that must be administered is 2,500 units: 2.1 < 2.6 < 3.

85. 1. Serial grip strengths can be performed to monitor a client for magnesium sulfate toxicity.
    2. Kernig's assessment is performed when checking for nuchal rigidity in a client with meningitis.
    3. Pupillary responses are performed when a client has had a head injury or is not responsive.
    4. Apical heart rate checks are performed when a client has a cardiac disease or is receiving digoxin.

TEST-TAKING TIP: The only accurate way to assess for magnesium toxicity is to do a serum magnesium level. Normal magnesium levels are 1.8 to 3.0 mg/dL. Therapeutic levels are 4 to 8 mg/dL. Reflex depression begins to appear when the levels reach 8 to 12 mg/dL. When levels rise to 15 mg/dL or higher, respiratory depression and, eventually, cardiac arrest occur. Hourly grip strengths performed with reflex assessments are excellent noninvasive assessments to monitor for neuromuscular blockage. If changes are noted, the nurse can notify the health care provider, who can order a stat magnesium level.

Comprehensive Examination

1. The nurse is caring for a client, 37 weeks' gestation, who was just told that she is group B strep + (positive). The client states, "How could that happen? I only have sex with my husband. Will my baby be OK?" Based on this information, which of the following should the nurse communicate to the client?
   1. The client's partner must have acquired the bacteria during a sexual encounter.
   2. The bacteria do not injure babies, but they could cause the client to have a bad sore throat.
   3. The client is high risk for developing pelvic inflammatory disease from the bacteria.
   4. Antibiotics will be administered during labor to prevent vertical transmission of the bacteria.

2. The nurse is caring for a client in labor and delivery with the following history: G2 P1000, 39 weeks' gestation in transition phase, FH 135 with early decelerations. The client states, "I'm so scared. Please make sure the baby is OK!" Which of the following responses by the nurse is appropriate?
   1. "There is absolutely nothing to worry about."
   2. "The fetal heart rate is within normal limits."
   3. "How did your first baby die?"
   4. "Was your first baby preterm?"

3. A certified nursing assistant (CNA) is working with a registered nurse (RN) in the neonatal nursery. It would be appropriate for the nurse to delegate which of the following actions to the assistant?
   1. Admission assessment on a newly delivered baby.
   2. Patient teaching of a neonatal sponge bath.
   3. Placement of a bag on a baby for urine collection.
   4. Hourly neonatal blood glucose assessments.

4. A fetus is in the LOA position in utero. Which of the following findings would the nurse observe when doing Leopold's maneuvers?
   1. Hard, round object in the fundal region.
   2. Flat object above the symphysis pubis.
   3. Soft, round object on the left side of the uterus.
   4. Small objects on the right side of the uterus.

5. A woman is being interviewed by a triage nurse at a medical doctor's office. Which of the following signs/symptoms by the client would warrant the nurse to suggest that a pregnancy test be done? **Select all that apply.**
   1. Amenorrhea.
   2. Fever.
   3. Fatigue.
   4. Nausea.
   5. Dysuria.

6. A woman is seeking counseling regarding tubal ligation. Which of the following should the nurse include in her discussion?
   1. The woman will no longer menstruate.
   2. The surgery should be done when the woman is ovulating.
   3. The surgery is easily reversible.
   4. The woman will be under anesthesia during the procedure.

7. A woman is admitted to the labor and delivery unit with active tuberculosis. She has not been under a physician's care and is not on medication. Which of the following actions should the nursery nurse perform when the neonate is delivered?
   1. Isolate the baby from the other babies in a special care nursery.
   2. Keep the baby in the regular care nursery but separated from the mother.
   3. Isolate the baby with the mother in the mother's room.
   4. Obtain an order from the doctor for antituberculosis medications for the baby.

8. A client has just received synthetic prostaglandins for the induction of labor. The nurse plans to monitor the client for which of the following side effects?
   1. Nausea and uterine tetany.
   2. Hypertension and vaginal bleeding.
   3. Urinary retention and severe headache.
   4. Bradycardia and hypothermia.

9. The triage nurse in an obstetric clinic received the following four messages during the lunch hour. Which of the women should the nurse telephone first?
   1. "My section incision from last week is leaking a whitish yellow discharge and I have a fever. What should I do?"
   2. "I am 39 weeks pregnant with my first baby. I am having contractions about every ten minutes."
   3. "My boyfriend and I had intercourse this morning and our condom broke. What should we do?"
   4. "I started my period yesterday. I need some medicine for these terrible menstrual cramps."

10. A patient is placed on bed rest at home for mild preeclampsia at 38 weeks' gestation. Which of the following must the nurse teach the patient regarding her condition?
    1. Eat a sodium-restricted diet.
    2. Check her temperature 4 times daily.
    3. Report swollen hands and face.
    4. Limit fluids to 1 liter per day.

11. The health care practitioner caring for a pregnant client diagnosed with gonorrhea writes the following order: ceftriaxone 250 mg IM × one dose. The medication is available in 1-gram vials. The nurse adds 8 mL of normal saline to the vial. How many mL of the medication should the nurse administer? **Calculate to the nearest whole.**

    _____ mL.

12. A 42-week-gestation neonate is being assessed. Which of the following findings would the nurse expect to see?
    1. Folded and flat pinnae.
    2. Smooth plantar surfaces.
    3. Loose and peeling skin.
    4. Short pliable fingernails.

13. A 39-week-gestation client is admitted to the labor and delivery unit for a scheduled cesarean delivery. The nurse should inform the surgeon regarding which of the following admission laboratory findings?
    1. Potassium 4.9 mEq/L.
    2. Sodium 136 mEq/L.
    3. Platelet count 75,000 cells/mm^3.
    4. White blood cell count 15,000 cells/mm^3.

14. A mother questions the nurse about when the newborn screening tests for inborn diseases will be performed. Which of the following is an appropriate response by the nurse?
   1. The doctor took blood from the baby's umbilical cord at birth.
   2. A sample of the baby's first urine and first stool were sent for testing.
   3. A vial of blood was drawn and sent when the baby was admitted to the nursery.
   4. Blood from the baby's heel was sent after the baby had been fed a few times.

15. On vaginal exam it is noted that the fetus is in the LSA position and −2 station. Place an "X" on the diagram in the quadrant where the fetal heart would best be assessed.

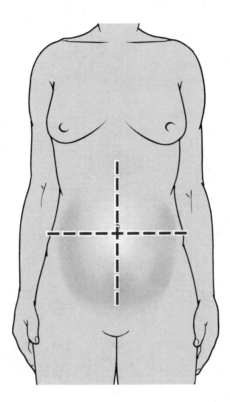

16. The nurse would be concerned that a 26-week-gravid client is carrying an unwanted pregnancy when the client makes which of the following statements?
   1. "The baby hasn't started to move yet."
   2. "My back aches every night when I get home from work."
   3. "I am finding it very hard always to eat the right things."
   4. "I am no longer able to wear my old clothes."

17. A young man is planning to use the condom as a contraceptive device. The nurse should teach him that which of the following actions is needed to maximize the condom's effectiveness?
   1. Use only water-soluble lubricants.
   2. Use only natural lambskin condoms.
   3. Apply the condom to a flaccid penis.
   4. Apply it tightly to the tip of the penis.

18. In 2000, the perinatal mortality rate in one county was 16. The nurse interprets that information as which of the following?
   1. 16 babies died between 28 and 40 weeks' gestation per 1,000 full-term pregnancies.
   2. 16 babies died between 28 weeks' gestation and 28 days of age per 1,000 live births.
   3. 16 babies died between birth and 1 month of life per 1,000 full-term pregnancies.
   4. 16 babies died between 1 month of life and 1 year of life per 1,000 live births.

19. Which of the electronic fetal monitor tracings shown below would the nurse interpret as indicating umbilical cord compression?

1.

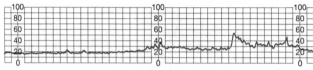

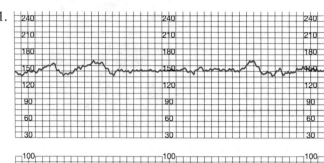

2.

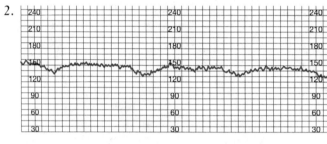

3.

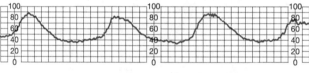

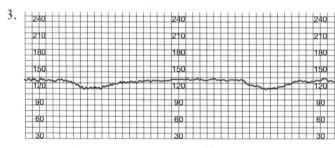

4.

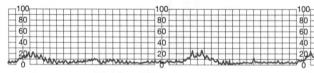

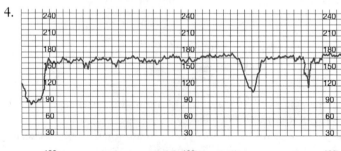

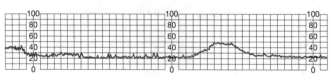

20. A client has been admitted with a diagnosis of threatened abortion. She is wearing a pad that weighed 15 grams when it was clean. It now weighs 30 grams. How many mL of blood can the nurse estimate that the client has lost? **Calculate to the nearest whole.**
    _____ mL.

21. A school nurse is discussing the male reproductive system with the students in a high school health class. Which of the following information about the hormone testosterone should be included in the discussion?
    1. "Testosterone is what makes boys more muscular than girls."
    2. "The level of testosterone in boys changes every month like female hormones do."
    3. "Testosterone is produced by the male prostate gland."
    4. "The production of testosterone usually stops by the time a man is fifty years old."

22. A woman is in the "taking-hold phase" of the postpartum period. Which of the following behaviors would the nurse expect to see?
    1. The woman is on the telephone relating her experiences to family and friends.
    2. The woman asks for a meal tray and eats a variety of foods brought from home.
    3. The woman is interested in learning baby-care skills from the nurse.
    4. The woman takes a nap after each breastfeeding and each meal.

23. A client's amniocentesis results are reported as 45, X. How should the nurse interpret these findings?
    1. The fetus is nonviable.
    2. The fetus is a normal female.
    3. The baby will be a hermaphrodite.
    4. The girl will be short and sterile.

24. The nurse is teaching a new mother about the physical characteristics and needs of her baby. Which of the following statements should the nurse include in her discussion?
    1. "The anterior fontanelle will close by the time the baby is 18 months of age."
    2. "The grasp reflex will last until the baby is about 10 months old."
    3. "Your baby can see shapes but will not be able to see colors clearly for about 6 months."
    4. "Your baby will likely be started on solid foods when he is 2 to 3 months of age."

25. A laboring woman, G4 P3003, who was 6 cm dilated 1 hour ago cries, "Hurry. I have to go to the bathroom to have a bowel movement." The nurse notes that there is an increase in bloody show. Which of the following actions by the nurse is appropriate?
    1. Assess cervical dilation.
    2. Help the woman to the bathroom.
    3. Ask the woman if she needs pain medicine.
    4. Check the fetal heart rate.

26. A birth plan is being developed by a pregnant couple. Which of the following items should be included in the plan?
    1. The method of infant feeding the mother plans on using.
    2. The name and address of her health care insurance company.
    3. The couple's baby name preferences.
    4. The couple's cell phone numbers.

27. When providing contraceptive counseling to a woman, which of the following factors should the nurse consider? **Select all that apply.**
    1. Age.
    2. Obstetric history.
    3. Religious beliefs.
    4. Employment.
    5. Body structure.

28. A baby is born addicted to crack cocaine. Which of the following signs/symptoms would the nurse expect to see?
    1. Hyperreflexia.
    2. Anorexia.
    3. Constipation.
    4. Hypokalemia.

29. A woman, contracting every 3 min × 60 seconds, suddenly develops an amniotic fluid embolism. Which of the following signs/symptoms would the nurse observe?
    1. Sudden gush of fluid from the vagina.
    2. Intense and unrelenting uterine pain.
    3. Precipitous dilation and expulsion of the fetus.
    4. Chest pain with dyspnea and cyanosis.

30. A client complaining of frequency, urgency, and burning on urination is seen by her health care practitioner. Which of the following factors in the client's history places her at risk for these complaints?
    1. The client urinates immediately after every sexual encounter.
    2. The client uses the diaphragm as a family planning method.
    3. The client wipes from front to back after every toileting.
    4. The client changes her peripads every two hours during her menses.

31. On the third postpartum day a client tells the nurse that she feels sad and that she cries easily. The nurse should explain about which of the following?
    1. These feelings are normal and should diminish when the baby is a week or so old.
    2. The physician will likely order an antidepressant for the client to take at home.
    3. If the client focuses on the fact that she has a healthy baby, the feelings will cease.
    4. When the client is home with her family and friends, her sad feelings will disappear.

32. A nurse is reading a research study that states, "There is a strong negative correlation between the independent and dependent variables ($r = -0.85$)." The nurse interprets the statement as which of the following?
    1. The dependent variable caused a change in the independent variable.
    2. The independent and dependent variables are significantly different.
    3. As values of the independent variable go up, values of the dependent variable go down.
    4. When the confidence interval is computed, the negative value will change to positive.

33. A nurse notes that a baby is lying in a crib in the tonic neck position. In which of the following positions is the baby lying?
    1. One of the baby's arms and one of its legs are extended to the same side the baby's head is facing.
    2. When the baby faces straight ahead, the baby's head tilts toward one side.
    3. Both the baby's back and head are sharply arched backward and resist being moved to midline.
    4. When the baby lies prone, the baby's body arches to one side.

34. A doula is working with a laboring woman who is 6 cm dilated and is contracting every 3 min × 60 sec on an oxytocin drip. Which of the following interventions should the nurse suggest the doula perform?
    1. Regulate the oxytocin drip rate.
    2. Check the vaginal dilation of the client.
    3. Encourage the woman to use breathing techniques.
    4. Monitor the client for uterine hyperstimulation.

35. A pregnant woman is complaining of ptyalism. The nurse should teach the woman to try which of the following self-care measures?
    1. Use an astringent mouthwash.
    2. Elevate her legs frequently.
    3. Eat high-fiber foods.
    4. Void when the urge is felt.

36. The nurse is counseling a woman who has been diagnosed with mild osteoporosis. Which of the following should be included in the counseling session?
    1. Begin a regimen of walking each day.
    2. Refrain from drinking chocolate milk.
    3. Increase her daily intake of red meat.
    4. Only wear shoes with rubber soles.

37. It is noted that a baby admitted to the nursery has translucent skin with visible veins. Because of this finding, the nurse should monitor this baby carefully for which of the following?
    1. Polycythemia.
    2. Hypothermia.
    3. Hyperglycemia.
    4. Polyuria.

38. A 32-week-gravid client presents in the emergency department with severe abdominal pain, rigid abdomen, and scant dark red bleeding. The nurse should assess this client for which of the following?
    1. Signs of pulmonary edema.
    2. Enlarging abdominal girth measurements.
    3. Hyporeflexia and confusion.
    4. Signs of diabetic coma and ketosis.

39. The doctor has ordered a contraction stress test. The nurse should interpret which of the following as a negative test?
    1. The fetal heart remains stable in relation to 3 contractions.
    2. The uterine contractions last longer than 90 seconds.
    3. The mother reports a pain level that is less than 5 on a 10-point scale.
    4. The baby moves spontaneously 3 times in 20 minutes.

40. A nurse who is creating a pedigree of a woman's family tree includes the following symbols. The symbols represent which of the following relationships?

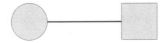

    1. A healthy sister and brother.
    2. A couple who have mated.
    3. A grandmother and her grandson.
    4. A father and his daughter.

41. A woman, who is in pain from a diagnosis of mastitis, has abruptly weaned her baby to a bottle. Her actions place the woman at high risk for which of the following?
    1. Mammary rupture.
    2. Postpartum psychosis.
    3. Supernumerary nipples.
    4. Breast abscess.

42. The triage nurse is interviewing a client, 19 years old, unmarried, who states, "I felt a hard thing on the lip of my vagina this morning. It doesn't hurt." Which of the following questions is most important for the nurse to ask at this time?
    1. "Have any of your partners ever hurt you?"
    2. "Do you ever have unprotected intercourse?"
    3. "Have you ever had a baby?"
    4. "Do you think you may be pregnant?"

43. A breastfeeding mother and her baby are being discharged home after delivery. The nurse is providing anticipatory guidance about what signs to expect the baby to exhibit every 24 hours by the end of the first week. Which of the following should the nurse include in his/her instructions?
    1. The baby will have at least 6 wet diapers.
    2. The baby will have at least 6 pasty stools.
    3. The baby will breastfeed at least 6 times.
    4. The baby will gain at least 6 ounces.

44. Please indicate the frequency and duration of the contraction pattern shown below.

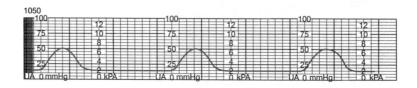

_____ min × _____ sec

45. The nurse documents a woman's gravidity and parity as G6 P3214. Which of the following obstetric histories is consistent with this notation?
    1. The woman is currently pregnant, has 3 living children.
    2. The woman is currently pregnant, had 2 full-term pregnancies.
    3. The woman is not currently pregnant, had 4 preterm babies.
    4. The woman is not currently pregnant, had 1 abortion.

46. The nurse is teaching a woman how to do the pelvic tilt exercise. In the teaching session, which of the following should the nurse tell the woman to do?
    1. Stand with the back of her heels and shoulders touching a wall.
    2. Bend laterally back and forth from one side to the other.
    3. Move so that her back alternately is concave and convex.
    4. Lie flat on her back and move her hips from side to side.

47. A 6-month-old child has been diagnosed with a significant hearing loss. Which of the following complications that occurred immediately after delivery could have resulted in this condition?
    1. Necrotizing enterocolitis.
    2. Hypoglycemia.
    3. Bronchopulmonary dysplasia.
    4. Kernicterus.

48. During a vaginal delivery of a macrosomic baby, the nurse midwife requests nursing assistance. Which of the following actions by the nurse would be appropriate?
    1. Estimate fetal length and weight.
    2. Assess intensity of contractions.
    3. Provide suprapubic pressure.
    4. Assist woman with breathing.

49. A 1-week-postpartum client calls her obstetrician's office and states, "I am a breastfeeding mother and my nipples are cracked and bleeding." Which of the following comments by the nurse is appropriate at this time?
    1. "You will need to be seen by the doctor today."
    2. "The blood will make the baby very sick. You should pump and dump your milk for at least 1 week."
    3. "You are very high risk for infection. You should cleanse your nipples with dilute hydrogen peroxide twice every day."
    4. "Lanolin cream applied after each feeding will help you to heal."

50. A postpartum client, who delivered her baby vaginally 2 hours earlier, just voided 100 mL in the bathroom. After returning to bed, the nurse makes the following assessment: fundus 4 cm above the umbilicus and deviated to the right with moderate lochia rubra. Which of the following nursing diagnoses is appropriate at this time?
    1. Impaired skin integrity.
    2. Fluid volume deficit.
    3. Impaired urinary elimination.
    4. Toileting self-care deficit.

51. A nurse should monitor a client who is postpartum from a forceps delivery for which of the following complications?
    1. Placental abruption.
    2. Seizure.
    3. Idiopathic thrombocytopenia.
    4. Infection.

52. A fetal fibronectin assessment of the cervicovaginal fluids of a 28-week gravida is positive. Based on the results, which of the following complaints should the nurse advise the client to report immediately to the health care provider?
    1. Headache.
    2. Visual disturbances.
    3. Uterine cramping.
    4. Oliguria.

53. A breastfeeding client asks the nurse to make sure that her newborn is positioned and latched well at the breast. Which of the following assessments would indicate that the baby is poorly latched?
    1. The baby swallows after every suckle.
    2. The baby's body is facing the mother's body.
    3. The baby's lower lip is curled under.
    4. The baby is lying at the level of the mother's breasts.

54. A fetus, descending through the birth canal, is going through the cardinal moves of labor. Please place the following moves in chronological order.
    1. External rotation.
    2. Flexion.
    3. Extension.
    4. Internal rotation.
    5. Expulsion.

55. The nurse is working with a pregnant woman who states that she is a vegan. Which of the following actions by the nurse is appropriate?
    1. Advise the mother that she must eat some animal protein during her pregnancy.
    2. Refer the woman to a nutritionist for diet counseling.
    3. Remind the mother that cashews and coconut are excellent sources of calcium.
    4. Congratulate the woman on agreeing to eat eggs and milk.

56. When caring for a woman whom a nurse suspects is being abused by her partner, the nurse should do which of the following?
    1. Ask the client directly about how she sustained her injuries.
    2. Counsel the client on how her behavior probably provoked the attack.
    3. Inform the client that the police must arrest her partner.
    4. Give the client a pamphlet with the names of matrimonial attorneys.

57. The nurse is caring for a baby whose blood type is A+ (positive) and direct Coombs' test is + (positive), and whose mother's blood type is O+ (positive). Which of the following nursing diagnoses is appropriate for this baby?
    1. Risk for injury to the central nervous system.
    2. Risk for fluid volume deficit.
    3. Risk for interrupted family processes.
    4. Risk for impaired parent-infant attachment.

58. Which of the following complications of labor and delivery may develop when a baby enters the pelvis in the LMP position?
   1. Cephalopelvic disproportion.
   2. Placental abruption.
   3. Breech presentation.
   4. Acute fetal distress.

59. A 36-week-gestation client is having an amniocentesis. For which of the following reasons is the test likely being conducted?
   1. Genetic evaluation.
   2. Assessment of intrauterine growth restriction.
   3. Assessment of fetal lung maturation.
   4. Hormonal studies.

60. A client on the obstetric unit is receiving IV medications per physician's orders. On rounds the nurse notes that the client's IV has infiltrated. Which of the following actions should the nurse perform first?
   1. Determine whether the infusion is a vesicant.
   2. Stop the infusion and remove the catheter.
   3. Document the occurrence in the medical record.
   4. Elevate the extremity and monitor the site.

61. A client asks the nurse to explain what luteinizing hormone (LH) does in the body. The nurse explains which of the following?
   1. "It accelerates the growth and maturation of an egg in your ovary."
   2. "It enhances the potential for the sperm to fertilize the mature egg."
   3. "It promotes the movement of the egg through the fallopian tube."
   4. "It stimulates the monthly release of a mature egg from your ovary."

62. The nurse is obtaining the first postpartum meal for a client who has stated that she practices Mormonism (the Church of Jesus Christ of Latter-Day Saints). Which of the following items should the nurse remove from the clients' food tray?
   1. Caffeinated coffee.
   2. Cheeseburger.
   3. Fried fish.
   4. Pork sausage.

63. A couple has decided not to circumcise their son. Based on this decision, which of the following instructions should the nurse include in the parent teaching?
   1. The couple should check their son's temperature every evening because he will be high risk for urinary tract infections.
   2. The couple should fully retract the foreskin to assess for the presence of exudate every morning.
   3. The pediatrician will observe the baby void during each well-baby examination to assess for a phimosis.
   4. The prepuce should be cleansed with soap and water every day during the baby's sponge bath.

64. A client, 6 cm and 80% effaced, has just received Demerol (meperidine) 50 mg IV for pain. Which of the following fetal heart changes would the nurse expect to observe on the internal fetal monitor tracing?
   1. Drop in baseline heart rate.
   2. Increase in number of variable decelerations.
   3. Decrease in variability.
   4. Rise in number of early decelerations.

65. Which of the following features would the nurse expect to be absent in an 8-week-gestation embryo?
   1. Four-chambered heart.
   2. Fingers and toes.
   3. Fully formed genitalia.
   4. Facial features.

66. A client, who is 6 hours post–vaginal delivery, has a BP of 150/110. Her last 4 BP readings were: 114/88, 120/80, 134/86, 140/90. Which of the following questions should the nurse ask the client at this time?
    1. "Have you had a bowel movement since delivery?"
    2. "Is there anything that is making you anxious about the baby?"
    3. "When you last went to the bathroom were you bleeding heavily?"
    4. "Do you have a headache or blurring of your vision?"

67. A baby is exhibiting signs of neonatal abstinence syndrome. Which action would be appropriate for the nursery nurse to make?
    1. Cover the baby with at least two blankets.
    2. Stimulate the baby with rattles.
    3. Play soft classical music in the nursery.
    4. Attach a mobile to the crib.

68. A mother, 39 weeks' gestation, is admitted to the labor suite with rupture of membranes 15 minutes earlier and contractions q 8 minutes × 30 seconds. On vaginal exam, the cervix is 4 cm dilated and 80% effaced, and the station is –2. The baby is found to be in the LSP position. The fetal heart rate is 144 with average variability and variable decelerations. Which of the following complications of labor must the nurse assess this client for at this time?
    1. Precipitous delivery.
    2. Chorioamnionitis.
    3. Uteroplacental insufficiency.
    4. Prolapsed cord.

69. Young pregnant adolescents have increased nutritional needs as compared with pregnant adults. Which of the following foods would meet those needs?
    1. Banana.
    2. Cheeseburger.
    3. Strawberries.
    4. Rice.

70. The nurse is caring for a client and her partner who just birthed a 33-week fetal demise. Which of the following actions by the nurse is appropriate at this time?
    1. Recommend that the woman be moved to a medical unit.
    2. Refrain from discussing the loss with the couple.
    3. Ask the couple if they would like to hold their baby.
    4. Obtain an order for a milk suppressant for the mother.

71. A woman asks the nurse to recommend the best douche for use after menstruation. Which of the following responses by the nurse is appropriate?
    1. "Tap water with white vinegar is most refreshing and least allergenic."
    2. "It is really best for women not to douche."
    3. "Any of the over-the-counter douches is satisfactory."
    4. "It is best to douche during menstruation rather than after it is over."

72. During a postpartum examination, the nurse notes that a client's left calf is warm and swollen. Which of the following actions by the nurse is appropriate at this time?
    1. Notify the client's physician.
    2. Teach the client to massage her leg.
    3. Apply ice packs to the client's leg.
    4. Encourage the client to ambulate.

73. A nurse sees an overweight woman looking at the babies through the nursery window. The woman asks the nurse when the babies go to their mothers for feedings and about the location of the nearest stairwell. Which of the following replies by the nurse is most appropriate at this time?
    1. "The babies go to their mothers whenever they seem hungry."
    2. "Please let me escort you to the mother's room you are here to visit."
    3. "The babies are in the mothers' rooms for the majority of the day."
    4. "Most of our visitors prefer to use the elevator to return to the lobby."

74. Without doing a vaginal examination, a nurse concludes that a primigravida, who has received no medications during her labor, is in transition. Which of the following signs/symptoms would lead a nurse to that conclusion?
    1. The woman fell asleep during a contraction.
    2. The woman yelled at her partner and vomited.
    3. The woman laughed at something on the television.
    4. The woman began pushing with each contraction.

75. A male baby is born with scant amounts of vernix caseosa in his axillae and groin, scant amounts of lanugo on his shoulders, testes in his scrotum, and a strong suck. The nurse would estimate that the baby is which of the following gestational ages?
    1. 22 weeks.
    2. 28 weeks.
    3. 32 weeks.
    4. 38 weeks.

76. The mother of a neonate with Down syndrome wishes to breastfeed. Which of the following considerations should the nurse make in relation to the mother's wishes?
    1. The mother should be encouraged to feed expressed breast milk via a bottle.
    2. Down syndrome babies consume more calories than unaffected neonates.
    3. Because of the weight of the neonatal head, the side-lying position must be used.
    4. The baby will likely have a weak suck due to congenitally poor muscle tone.

77. A neonate in the nursery, whose mother had no prenatal care, has been diagnosed with macrosomia. For which of the following signs/symptoms should the nurse carefully monitor this baby?
    1. Jaundice.
    2. Jitters.
    3. Blepharitis.
    4. Strabismus.

78. The nurse in the obstetrician's office is caring for four 25-week-gestation prenatal clients who are carrying singleton pregnancies. With which of the following clients should the nurse carefully review the signs and symptoms of preterm labor?
    1. African American, 15 years old, with newly diagnosed gestational diabetes.
    2. Asian American, 23 years old, with five-year-old twins who were born at term.
    3. Jewish, 25 years old, working as a certified public accountant.
    4. Mormon, 33 years old, who recently moved into a new apartment.

79. A woman has been diagnosed with chlamydia. The nurse would expect the client to complain of which of the following signs/symptoms?
    1. No signs or symptoms.
    2. Painful lesions on the labia.
    3. Foul-smelling discharge.
    4. Severe lower abdominal pain.

80. A woman and man have the following genotypes for an autosomal dominant disease: Aa and Aa. If asked, which of the following should the nurse say is the probability of their child having the disease?
    1. 25% probability.
    2. 50% probability.
    3. 75% probability.
    4. 100% probability.

81. The nurse is providing patient teaching to a client who plans to bottle feed her newborn infant. Which of the following information should be included in the education session?
    1. The baby should be burped after every 3 ounces of formula.
    2. If the bottle nipple is not filled throughout the feeding, the baby may take in a large amount of air.
    3. The best way to heat formula for the baby is in the microwave.
    4. If the mother is busy with her other children, she can prop the baby bottle up on a blanket or towel.

82. The nurse has received change of shift report on the following four clients. Which of the clients should the nurse assess first?
    1. G1 P0000, 9 weeks' gestation, hyperemesis gravidarum, vomited twice during the last shift.
    2. G2 P0101, 24 weeks' gestation, receiving terbutaline po q 2 h for preterm labor, no complaints of cramping during last shift.
    3. G1 P0000, 1 day postpartum, vacuum extraction, for bilateral tubal ligation during this shift.
    4. G2 P0101, 2 days postpartum, spontaneous delivery, had asthma attack during last shift.

83. Using the graph below, of the following weights, how many grams would a 34-week neonate need to weigh to be labeled appropriate-for-gestational age?
    1. 500 grams.
    2. 1,700 grams.
    3. 2,900 grams.
    4. 4,100 grams.

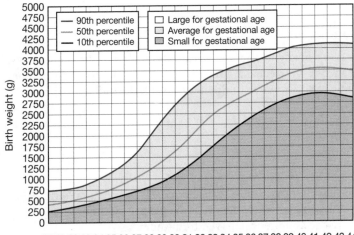

84. A client is receiving terbutaline (Brethine) IV for preterm labor. Which of the following maternal findings would warrant stopping the infusion?
    1. Cardiac arrhythmias.
    2. Respiratory rate 24 rpm.
    3. Blood pressure 90/60.
    4. Hypocalcemia.

85. A breastfeeding client, 6 days postdelivery, calls the postpartum unit stating, "I think I am engorged. My breasts are very hard and hot and they really hurt." Which of the following questions should the nurse ask at this time?
    1. "Have you taken a warm shower this morning?"
    2. "Do you have an electric breast pump?"
    3. "How much did you have to drink yesterday?"
    4. "When was the last time you fed the baby?"

86. A client's vital signs during labor and delivery were: BP 100/58–110/66, T 98.6°F–98.8°F, P 72–80 bpm, R 20–24 rpm. The client's vitals 2 hours postpartum are BP 100/56, TPR 99.4°F, P 70 bpm, R 20 rpm. Which of the following actions should the nurse perform at this time?
    1. Check the client's lochia flow.
    2. Ask the client if she is having chills.
    3. Encourage the client to drink fluids.
    4. Assess the client's lung fields.

87. A G1 P0000 gravida, whose labor was uneventful, delivered 1 minute ago. The baby's Apgar score at this time is 3. Which of the following actions is appropriate for the nurse to make?
    1. Administer ophthalmic prophylaxis.
    2. Place the baby on the abdomen of the mother.
    3. Obtain assistance for neonatal resuscitation.
    4. Repeat the score to confirm its accuracy.

88. The nurse has identified the following nursing diagnosis for a postpartum (PP) client: Potential for fluid volume deficit. Which of the following goals for the mother is appropriate?
    1. Minimal perineal pain.
    2. Normal lochial flow.
    3. Normal temperature.
    4. Weight reduction.

89. An infant of a diabetic mother, 40 weeks' gestation, weight 4,500 grams, has just been admitted to the neonatal nursery. The neonatal intensive care nurse will monitor this baby for which of the following? **Select all that apply.**
    1. Hyperreflexia.
    2. Hypoglycemia.
    3. Respiratory distress.
    4. Opisthotonus.
    5. Nuchal rigidity.

90. A nurse has just inserted an orogastric gavage tube into a preterm baby. When would the nurse determine that the tube is in the proper location?
    1. When gastric aspirate is removed from the tube.
    2. When the baby suckles on the tubing.
    3. When respirations are unlabored during tube insertion.
    4. When the tubing can be inserted no farther.

91. A client asks the nurse, "Could you explain how the baby's blood and my blood separate at delivery?" Which of the following responses is appropriate for the nurse to make?
    1. "When the placenta is born, the circulatory systems separate."
    2. "When the doctor clamps the cord, the blood stops mixing."
    3. "The separation happens after the baby takes the first breath. The baby's oxygen no longer has to come from you."
    4. "The blood actually never mixes. Your blood supply and the baby's blood supply are completely separate."

92. A 4-day-old breastfeeding neonate, whose birth weight was 2,678 grams, has lost 286 grams since its cesarean birth. Which of the following actions should the nurse take?
1. Nothing, because this is an acceptable weight loss.
2. Advise the mother to stop breastfeeding and give formula.
3. Notify the neonatologist of the excessive weight loss.
4. Give the baby dextrose water between breast feedings.

93. A nurse has provided a young woman with preconception counseling. Which of the statements by the woman indicates that the teaching was successful? **Select all that apply.**
1. "As soon as I think I may be pregnant, I should stop drinking alcohol."
2. "It is important for me to see my medical doctor for a complete physical."
3. "I should make sure that my daily multivitamin contains folic acid."
4. "When I go to my dentist for a checkup I should state that I may be pregnant."
5. "From now until I deliver I should refrain from eating sushi and rare meat."

94. A client who had a vaginal delivery 2 hours earlier has just been transferred to the postpartum unit from labor and delivery. Which of the following nursing care goals is of highest priority?
1. The client will breastfeed her baby every 2 hours.
2. The client will consume a nutritious diet.
3. The client will have a moderate lochial flow.
4. The client will ambulate in the hallways every shift.

95. The nurse who has just performed a vaginal examination notes that the fetus is in the LOP position. Which of the following clinical assessments would the nurse expect to note at this time?
1. Complaints of severe back pain.
2. Rapid descent and effacement.
3. Irregular and hypotonic contractions.
4. Rectal pressure with bloody show.

96. A client with type 1 diabetes mellitus is 6 weeks pregnant. Her fasting glucose and hemoglobin A_{1C} are noted to be 168 mg/dL and 12%, respectively. Which of the following nursing diagnoses is appropriate for the nurse to make at this time?
1. Altered maternal skin integrity.
2. Deficient maternal fluid volume.
3. Risk for fetal injury.
4. Fetal urinary retention.

97. A client who is 18 weeks' gestation has been diagnosed with a hydatiform mole (gestational trophoblastic disease). In addition to vaginal loss, which of the following signs/symptoms would the nurse expect to see?
1. Hyperemesis and hypertension.
2. Diarrhea and hyperthermia.
3. Polycythemia.
4. Polydipsia.

98. A woman who states that she smokes 2 packs of cigarettes each day is admitted to the labor and delivery suite in labor. The nurse should monitor this labor for which of the following?
1. Delayed placental separation.
2. Late decelerations.
3. Shoulder dystocia.
4. Precipitous fetal descent.

99. A nurse has just received report on 4 neonates in the newborn nursery. Which of the babies should the nurse assess first?
    1. Neonate whose mother is HIV positive.
    2. Neonate whose mother is group B streptococcus positive.
    3. Neonate whose mother's labor was 12 hours long.
    4. Neonate whose mother gained 45 pounds during her pregnancy.

100. The umbilical cord is being clamped by the obstetrician. Which of the following physiological changes is taking place at this time?
    1. The baby's blood bypasses its pulmonary system.
    2. The baby's oxygen level begins to drop.
    3. Bacteria begin to invade the baby's bowel.
    4. Bilirubin rises in the baby's bloodstream.

The correct answer number and rationale for why it is the correct answer are given in **boldface blue type**. Rationales for why the other possible answer options are incorrect also are given, but they are not in boldface type.

1. 1. This statement is incorrect. Approximately ⅕ of all women carry group B strep as normal flora. This is not a sexually transmitted infection.
   2. This statement is incorrect. Group B strep can seriously injure babies. Group A beta hemolytic strep causes strep throat.
   3. This statement is incorrect. The bacteria rarely cause illness in the mother.
   4. **This statement is accurate. Antibiotics will be administered to the mother during labor and delivery to prevent vertical transmission.**

   TEST-TAKING TIP: Vertical transmission refers to the transmission of disease from the mother to the baby. Group B strep is called the "baby killer." If a mother is colonized with the bacteria, the baby may be exposed if the membranes rupture or when the baby passes through the birth canal.

2. 1. This is an inappropriate response. Even though it is very likely that the baby will be fine, the nurse does not know for certain that the baby will be well.
   2. **This is the best response for the nurse to make. The nurse is providing the client with accurate, reassuring information without guaranteeing that there will definitely be a positive outcome.**
   3. This response is inappropriate. The client is in the transition phase of labor. She is not in a position to discuss the circumstances of her first baby's death.
   4. This response is inappropriate. The parity cited indicates that the baby was full-term.

   TEST-TAKING TIP: Clients who have experienced fetal loss or the loss of a newborn are often very anxious during pregnancy, labor and delivery, and the early newborn period. The nurse must accept the client's concern and acknowledge the client's grief. It is also important for the nurse to keep the client well informed of all assessments and interventions related to the baby.

3. 1. An admission assessment should be performed by the nurse.
   2. Patient teaching should be performed by the nurse.
   3. **A urinary drainage bag may be put in place by the CNA.**
   4. The nurse should perform the hourly blood glucose assessments.

   TEST-TAKING TIP: Nursing assistants do not have the education to perform sophisticated client care skills. An initial assessment, patient teaching, and invasive neonatal procedures all should be performed by a skilled professional. The placement of a drainage bag is a task that the CNA could be taught to perform.

4. 1. If the nurse had noted a hard, round object—the fetal head—in the fundal region, he or she would have concluded that the fetus was in the sacral presentation.
   2. If the nurse had noted a flat object—the fetal back—above the symphysis, he or she would have concluded that the fetus was in a horizontal lie.
   3. If the nurse had noted a soft, round object—the fetal buttocks—on the left side of the uterus, he or she would have concluded that the fetus was in a horizontal lie.
   4. **A nurse could conclude that a fetus is in the LOA when feeling small objects—the fetal arms and legs—on the right side of the uterus.**

   TEST-TAKING TIP: This is a difficult question. The test taker must clearly understand that in the LOA position the occiput of a fetus is presenting. The back of the baby would be felt on the left side of the uterus and the small parts of the baby would be felt on the right side of the uterus.

5. **1, 3, and 4 are correct.**
   1. **Pregnancy is the most common cause of amenorrhea.**
   2. Although a client's temperature is slightly elevated (about 0.2°C above normal) during pregnancy, a nurse would not associate a fever with pregnancy.
   3. **A common complaint of women in early pregnancy is fatigue.**
   4. **A common complaint of women in early pregnancy is nausea.**
   5. Although gravidas complain of urinary frequency early in pregnancy, they should not complain of dysuria.

   TEST-TAKING TIP: This question is easily answered if the test taker is familiar with the presumptive signs of pregnancy—that is, the subjective complaints of pregnancy.

6. 1. This response is incorrect. Women who have bilateral tubal ligations (BTLs) do still menstruate until they reach menopause.
   2. The surgery can be performed at any time except between 2 days and 6 weeks postpartum.
   3. Although BTLs have been reversed, the success rate of the reversals is very low.
   4. This response is correct. BTL surgery, usually performed laparoscopically, is done under general anesthesia.

   TEST-TAKING TIP: Because scar tissue forms at the site of the BTL, it is very difficult to have a successful reversal of the procedure. Even though a sperm may be able to traverse the tube after reconstructive surgery has taken place, the fertilized egg is often too large to migrate through the tube to the uterus for implantation. Women are at high risk for ectopic pregnancies after tubal reconstructive surgery.

7. 1. It is unnecessary to isolate the baby in a special care nursery.
   2. This response is accurate. The baby can be cared for in the well-baby nursery, but must be kept separated from its mother.
   3. This is an unsafe practice. The baby could develop TB if kept in a room with the mother.
   4. This is unnecessary. The baby does not have TB. The mother has TB.

   TEST-TAKING TIP: Tuberculosis is transmitted via respiratory droplets. Because the mother has not been given medication, she is communicable. This is one of the few instances when mothers and babies must be kept apart. Only after it has been determined that the mother has been on medication a sufficient period of time should she and the baby have physical contact.

8. 1. Two side effects of prostaglandin administration are nausea and uterine tetany.
   2. Hypertension and vaginal bleeding are not associated with prostaglandin administration.
   3. Urinary retention and severe headache are not associated with prostaglandin administration.
   4. Bradycardia and hypothermia are not associated with prostaglandin administration.

   TEST-TAKING TIP: The test taker must be familiar with the side effects of commonly administered medications. Prostaglandins are frequently administered to women who are to be induced but who have low Bishop scores.

9. 1. The nurse should call the postoperative cesarean client back first. It sounds, from her description, that she has a wound infection.
   2. This client is a primigravida and, if she is in labor, is in the early phase of the first stage. Her call must be returned, but it can wait.
   3. This client needs emergency contraception. Although the medicine must be taken within 72 hours of intercourse, the nurse can wait to return her call.
   4. This client is complaining of menstrual pain. Although she needs pain medicine, the nurse can wait to return her call.

   TEST-TAKING TIP: To answer this question, the test taker must prioritize care. The woman who is most vulnerable at this time is the woman with a wound infection. If she truly does have a wound infection, she will need to be seen by the health care practitioner, have a culture of the wound taken, and be put on antibiotics.

10. 1. The client should be encouraged to have a normal sodium intake.
    2. It is unnecessary for the client to assess her temperature.
    3. The client should call her primary caregiver to report swollen hands and face.
    4. The client should not limit her intake of fluids.

    TEST-TAKING TIP: Clients with mild preeclampsia who progress to severe preeclampsia usually develop swollen hands and face. The symptoms occur as a result of the third spacing of fluid, which, in turn, occurs as a result of the reduced colloidal pressure in the vascular tree.

11. 2 mL
    The formula for ratio and proportion is:
    $$\frac{\text{Known dose}}{\text{Known volume}} = \frac{\text{Desired dose}}{\text{Desired volume}}$$
    1 gram/8 mL = 250 mg/x mL
    1,000 mg/8 mL = 250 mg/x mL
    1,000 x = 2,000
    x = 2 mL

    TEST-TAKING TIP: If the test taker always uses the formula, inserting the correct values into the respective locations, he or she will be unlikely to make any calculation errors. The known dose and volume are given—that is, 1 gram in 8 mL. The test taker must convert grams to mg, cross multiply, and solve for x.

12. 1. Folded and flat pinnae are seen in preterm newborns, not postmature babies.
2. Smooth plantar surfaces are seen in preterm newborns, not postmature babies.
3. **The skin of the post-term baby is loose because the baby has depleted most of the subcutaneous fat stores and is peeling because of the dehydration and advanced age of the baby.**
4. The nurse would expect to see long fingernails that may be tinged green from exposure to meconium.

TEST-TAKING TIP: If the test taker were unsure of the answer to this question, an educated response could have been made. Post-term babies are in utero beyond the normal life of the placenta. They are deprived of nourishment, hydration, and oxygenation because of this. Loose skin often connotes a loss of weight, and peeling skin is seen in poorly nourished and hydrated individuals. The test taker could deduce that choice 3 is the correct response.

13. 1. The client's potassium level is normal.
2. The client's sodium level is normal.
3. **The platelet count is well below normal.**
4. The white blood cell count is normal for a 38-week-gestation woman.

TEST-TAKING TIP: The normal platelet count is 150,000 to 400,000 cells/mm³. This client's cell count is well below normal. Clients with low platelet counts are high risk for bleeding spontaneously. Although the white blood cell count is elevated for a nonpregnant woman, it is normal for a perinatal client.

14. 1. A sample of cord blood is taken but it is not used to check for inborn diseases. Rather, the baby's blood type and Coombs' test are assessed from the cord blood sample.
2. Inborn diseases are not detected from urine or stool samples.
3. This answer is incorrect. Admission blood is not used to check for inborn diseases.
4. **This answer is correct. Because many of the inborn diseases are related to metabolism of foods, the baby must be fed a few times before the blood can be drawn.**

TEST-TAKING TIP: The genetic disease phenylketonuria (PKU) is one of the many metabolic illnesses that babies are

assessed for. Babies with PKU lack the enzyme needed for fully metabolizing phenylalanine, an essential amino acid. To accurately assess whether the baby lacks the enzyme or not, the baby must have consumed the proteins that are present in breast milk or formula before the blood test is performed.

15. The test taker should place an "X" in the diagram's left upper quadrant.

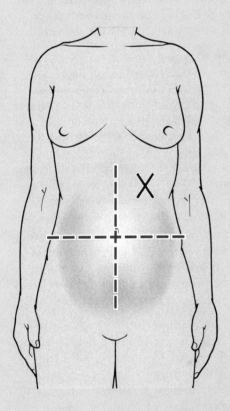

TEST-TAKING TIP: The best way for the test taker to remember the placement of the fetal heart electrode is to remember that the heartbeat is best heard through the fetal back. Because the baby is in the breech position and is not yet engaged, the heart would be located in an upper quadrant and because the baby is in the LSA position, the electrode should be placed in the left upper quadrant.

16. 1. Quickening should be felt by 20 weeks' gestation at the latest. The nurse, therefore, should be concerned that this pregnancy is unwanted.
2. Backaches are normal, expected complaints of pregnancy.
3. This comment shows the frustration that the mother is feeling about maintaining a

nutritious diet for her child. It does not indicate a rejection of the pregnancy.
4. This comment shows the frustration that the mother is feeling about her changing body image.

TEST-TAKING TIP: When women whose pregnancies are beyond 20 weeks' gestation state that they have yet to feel the baby move, the nurse must consider the possibility that the woman is rejecting her pregnancy. The nurse should attempt to intervene during the pregnancy rather than waiting until the baby is delivered.

17. 1. This response is correct. Only water-based lubricants should be used with the condom.
2. Natural lambskin condoms do not protect the wearer from viral sexually transmitted illnesses. Latex condoms do protect the wearer.
3. The condom should be applied to an erect penis.
4. A small reservoir should be left in the condom at the tip of the penis.

TEST-TAKING TIP: The condom is an excellent birth control and infection control device if it is used properly. The nurse must be prepared to educate clients, both male and female, in its correct use.

18. 1. This statement is incorrect. A perinatal mortality rate of 16 means that 16 babies died between 28 weeks' gestation and 28 days of age per 1000 live births.
2. **This statement is correct. A perinatal mortality rate of 16 means that 16 babies died between 28 weeks' gestation and 28 days of age per 1,000 live births.**
3. This statement is incorrect. A perinatal mortality rate of 16 means that 16 babies died between 28 weeks' gestation and 28 days of age per 1,000 live births.
4. This statement is incorrect. A perinatal mortality rate of 16 means that 16 babies died between 28 weeks' gestation and 28 days of age per 1,000 live births.

TEST-TAKING TIP: The perinatal period is defined as the time period between 28 weeks' gestation and 4 weeks (or 28 days) after delivery. The best way to remember that definition is to remember that the prefix "peri" means "around" and the word "natal" refers to "birth." The perinatal period, therefore, is the time period around the birth.

19. 1. This fetal heart tracing shows a healthy fetus with good variability and accelerations.
2. This fetal heart tracing indicates that the fetus is experiencing head compression—early decelerations.
3. This fetal heart tracing indicates the presence of uteroplacental insufficiency—late decelerations.
4. **This fetal heart tracing indicates the presence of cord compression—variable decelerations.**

TEST-TAKING TIP: One way to remember why variable decelerations indicate cord compression is the fact that the cord is a free-flowing object in the uterine cavity. It can be compressed, therefore, at a variety of times. For example, if the baby moves a certain way, the cord can be compressed. Or when the mother moves to a new position, the cord can be compressed. The decelerations seen, therefore, occur at times independent of timing of the contractions.

20. 15 mL
   30 grams − 15 grams = 15 grams
   The client has lost approximately 15 mL of blood.

TEST-TAKING TIP: The test taker must remember that 1 mL of fluid = 1 gram of fluid. This is true of blood, water, breast milk, or any other natural fluid.

21. 1. **This response is true. Testosterone is responsible for the development of the male secondary sex characteristics.**
2. This response is incorrect. Unlike the monthly hormonal fluctuations seen in the female, testosterone levels are relatively constant at all times.
3. This response is incorrect. Testosterone is produced by the testes.
4. Although the level of testosterone does drop slightly with age, the testes will produce the hormone throughout life.

TEST-TAKING TIP: Even though the female carries the fetus, the male reproductive system is also essential to procreation. It is important, therefore, for the test taker to be familiar with the anatomy and physiology of both the male and the female reproductive systems.

22. 1. Mothers who discuss their labor and delivery experiences are exhibiting a characteristic of the "taking-in" postpartum phase.

2. Mothers who eat quantities of food are exhibiting a characteristic of the "taking-in" postpartum phase.

3. When mothers are interested in learning baby-care skills from the nurse, they are exhibiting signs of the "taking-hold" postpartum phase.

4. Mothers who express intense fatigue and take naps throughout the day are exhibiting a characteristic of the "taking-in" postpartum phase.

TEST-TAKING TIP: The "taking-hold" phase is the postpartum period when mothers regain their independence and express interest in caring for their neonate. Prior to that time, mothers express the need to be cared for while they internalize their labor and delivery experience.

23. 1. The amniocentesis results indicate Turner's syndrome—45, X, a genetic anomaly—but the fetus is viable.

2. This is not a normal female, although the child will be phenotypically female.

3. The child will be phenotypically female.

4. Turner's syndrome girls are characterized by short stature, broad chests, and the inability to conceive.

TEST-TAKING TIP: The genetic anomaly 45, X is the only monosomy that is viable. No child can survive missing a complete autosome or with only a single Y sex chromosome. There is no mental retardation associated with Turner's syndrome.

24. 1. The anterior fontanel will close by the time the baby is about 18 months of age.

2. The grasp reflex will disappear when the baby is about 3 months of age.

3. Babies see colors at birth. And they see quite well when they are about 12 to 18 inches away from an object.

4. Babies are usually started on solids at 4 to 6 months of age.

TEST-TAKING TIP: The obstetric nurse must be familiar with normal growth and development. It is essential that nurses provide parents with anticipatory guidance regarding their child's normal growth and development milestones.

25. 1. This action is appropriate. It is very likely that this client is fully dilated because she is complaining of the urge to push.

2. This action is appropriate only if the nurse, after examining the woman, determines that she is not fully dilated.

3. This action is inappropriate. Not only has the client not complained of pain, she is likely fully dilated and ready to push.

4. There is nothing in the scenario that indicates that the fetus is in danger at this time.

TEST-TAKING TIP: This client is a multipara. Even though her last vaginal examination indicated that she was in active labor 1 hour ago, the test taker must remember that the transition phase of labor, on average, lasts only 10 minutes in multiparas. It is very likely that this client has experienced very rapid cervical change and is now in the second stage of labor. The urge to push, a classic sign of the second stage of labor, feels very similar to the urge to have a large bowel movement.

26. 1. The couple should include in the birth plan whether the mother plans to breastfeed or bottle feed the baby.

2. It is unnecessary to include in the birth plan the name and address of the woman's health insurance company.

3. It is unnecessary to include in the birth plan the couple's baby name preferences.

4. It is unnecessary to include in the birth plan the couple's cell phone numbers.

TEST-TAKING TIP: If the test taker remembers the rationale for the birth plan, he or she will easily be able to choose the correct response to this question. The birth plan is a document that a couple creates to facilitate communication between themselves and health care professionals in relation to the couple's wishes for the birth.

27. 1, 2, and 3 are correct.
1. The client's age should be considered by the nurse.

2. The client's obstetric history should be considered by the nurse.

3. The client's religious beliefs should be considered by the nurse.

4. The client's employment is not usually relevant in relation to her choice of family planning method.

5. The client's body structure is not usually relevant in relation to her choice of family planning method.

TEST-TAKING TIP: Many issues will determine a client's willingness and ability to

use family planning methods. For example, if a client is a devout Catholic, she may refuse to use any method other than a natural family planning method. If a client states that she feels she has completed her family, she may be interested in a permanent family planning method. A woman over 35 who smokes should be advised not to use a hormonally based method for health considerations.

28. 1. The nurse would expect that the baby would be hyperreflexic.
    2. Babies who are showing signs of addiction often repeatedly mouth for food rather than showing signs of anorexia.
    3. Babies who are showing signs of addiction often have diarrhea, not constipation.
    4. Hypokalemia is not related to neonatal cocaine addiction.

    TEST-TAKING TIP: Babies who are withdrawing from crack cocaine exhibit agitated behaviors, including hyperreflexia, high-pitched crying, and disorganized behavioral states.

29. 1. These signs are evident when the amniotic sac ruptures, not when a client experiences an amniotic fluid embolism.
    2. Intense, unrelenting uterine pain is seen with placental abruption and uterine rupture, not with amniotic fluid embolism.
    3. Precipitous dilation and expulsion of the fetus describes a precipitous delivery.
    4. **Chest pain with dyspnea and cyanosis are the classic signs of amniotic fluid embolism.**

    TEST-TAKING TIP: When amniotic fluid enters the vascular tree, it acts like any foreign body. When it reaches the lung fields, gas exchange is adversely affected. The woman experiences the same symptoms as if a thrombus had migrated to her lungs.

30. 1. Voiding after each sexual encounter decreases women's chances of developing a urinary tract infection.
    2. Clients who use the diaphragm as a family planning device are at high risk for urinary tract infections.
    3. To prevent the introduction of rectal flora into the urinary tract, it is important for women to wipe from front to back after toileting.

    4. Because blood is an ideal medium for bacterial growth, it is recommended that women change their peripads frequently.

    TEST-TAKING TIP: Women are much more at high risk for UTI than are men because of the close proximity of the urethra to the vagina and rectum. Women should be counseled on ways to prevent UTI and women who are prone to UTI should consider changing their family planning method from the diaphragm to another method.

31. 1. This statement is true. The client's feelings are normal.
    2. Because the postpartum blues usually last less than 2 weeks, it is unlikely that the physician will order antidepressants for the client.
    3. This statement is incorrect. It is not possible to change one's feelings by merely "thinking" positive thoughts.
    4. This statement is inappropriate. The blues may continue for up to 10 days, well after the client returns home.

    TEST-TAKING TIP: Postpartum blues are considered normal. About 80% of women experience them. They are related to the hormonal shifts that occur after delivery as well as fatigue and the emotional stress of having full responsibility for the care and well-being of a neonate.

32. 1. Correlational statistics never indicate cause and effect relationships.
    2. There is no indication of a significant relationship—designated by a *P* value—in the scenario.
    3. This statement is accurate. In a negative correlation, as the values of one variable rise, the values of the other variable drop.
    4. This statement is meaningless.

    TEST-TAKING TIP: The test taker must be very careful when interpreting correlational statistics. Correlations merely communicate whether variables covary. Correlations should never be interpreted as cause and effect relationships.

33. 1. This is an accurate description of the tonic neck position.
    2. This is a description of a child with torticollis.
    3. This is a description of a child with opisthotonus.

4. This is a description of a baby exhibiting the trunk incurvation reflex.

TEST-TAKING TIP: Tonic neck position is one of the neonatal reflexes. The reflex usually disappears between 3 and 4 months. It has been suggested that the reflex developed to prevent babies from rolling over onto their bellies, a high-risk position that predisposes babies to SIDS.

34. 1. It is not appropriate for the nurse to delegate the regulation of the oxytocin drip rate to the doula.
    2. It is not appropriate for the nurse to delegate the monitoring of the client's vaginal dilation to the doula.
    3. **The doula is an expert in assisting laboring clients to work with their labors.**
    4. It is not appropriate for the nurse to delegate the monitoring for hyperstimulation to the doula.

TEST-TAKING TIP: The role of the doula is as a labor support. Doulas intervene to help clients to relax and work with their labors. It is inappropriate for doulas to perform any professional nursing care such as evaluating electronic monitor tracings, administering medications, performing physical assessments, and the like.

35. 1. **This response is correct. Women who complain of ptyalism should be advised to use an astringent mouthwash.**
    2. Elevating one's legs will not alleviate a woman's complaint of ptyalism.
    3. Eating high-fiber foods will not alleviate a woman's complaint of ptyalism.
    4. Voiding when the urge is felt will not alleviate a woman's complaint of ptyalism.

TEST-TAKING TIP: Some women complain of ptyalism during pregnancy. The excessive salivation is caused by the increase in vascularity of the mucous membranes as a result of elevated estrogen levels in the bloodstream.

36. 1. **Walking is an excellent preventive exercise for women who are at high risk for osteoporosis.**
    2. **Chocolate milk contains calcium and vitamin D. The intake of both substances is important in the prevention of osteoporosis.**
    3. Red meat is not high in calcium or vitamin D.

4. The type of shoe worn by a woman will not affect her bone density.

TEST-TAKING TIP: A woman's bone health is positively affected by her participation in exercise. Weight-bearing exercises, like walking, jogging, running, and weight lifting, provide the most benefit for women who are at high risk for osteoporosis.

37. 1. The nurse would not expect the baby to be polycythemic.
    2. **The nurse should watch the baby who has transparent skin with visible veins for hypothermia.**
    3. The nurse would expect the baby to be hypoglycemic rather than hyperglycemic.
    4. The nurse would not expect the baby to have polyuria.

TEST-TAKING TIP: Translucent skin with visible veins, a sign of prematurity, indicates that the subcutaneous fat has yet to be deposited. Because subcutaneous fat is an insulating substance, the baby is at high risk for hypothermia.

38. 1. The symptoms in the scenario are related to placental abruption, not pulmonary edema.
    2. **The nurse should observe for enlarging abdominal girth measurements.**
    3. Hyporeflexia and confusion are not symptoms of placental abruption.
    4. The symptoms in the scenario are related to placental abruption, not diabetic coma and ketosis.

TEST-TAKING TIP: When a nurse suspects placental abruption, he or she should monitor the gravida for enlarging abdominal girth, a board-like abdomen, and unrelenting pain. The nurse should also monitor the fetal heart rate for dysrhythmias. Placental abruption is an obstetric emergency.

39. 1. **A negative contraction stress test is defined as a stable fetal heart rate during 3 consecutive contractions.**
    2. The length of contractions is not considered when a contraction stress test is performed.
    3. The mother's pain level is not considered when a contraction stress test is performed.
    4. Fetal movement is not considered when a contraction stress test is performed.

TEST-TAKING TIP: A contraction stress test is performed to determine the ability of the fetus to withstand the stress of labor. If the heart rate remains stable during

3 consecutive contractions—a negative test—the fetus is assumed to be healthy. A compromised fetus's heart rate would decelerate during contractions. This is defined as a positive test.

40. 1. The symbol represents a couple who have mated, not a healthy sister and brother.
    2. The symbol represents a couple who have mated.
    3. The symbol represents a couple who have mated, not a grandmother and her grandson.
    4. The symbol represents a couple who have mated, not a father and his daughter.

TEST-TAKING TIP: When a female (circle) and a male (square) are connected with a single line on a pedigree, a couple who have mated is represented. A circle and square connected by a double line indicates a consanguineous couple (blood relatives) who have mated.

41. 1. She is not high risk for mammary rupture.
    2. She is not high risk for postpartum psychosis.
    3. She is not high risk for supernumerary nipples.
    4. The client is high risk for the development of a breast abscess.

TEST-TAKING TIP: When clients wean abruptly, the breasts become engorged with milk. Mastitis is a breast infection usually caused by *Staphylococcus aureus*. When the milk is not removed from the breast, an abscess, or collection of pus, can develop in the breast.

42. 1. Although this question is important, it is not the best question to ask at this time. In addition, an injury would be painful.
    2. This is the best question to ask at this time.
    3. Although this question is important, it is not the best question to ask at this time.
    4. Although this question is important, it is not the best question to ask at this time.

TEST-TAKING TIP: This is an unmarried woman who may be having intercourse with men or women who are intimate with others. The young woman may be feeling a lesion caused by a sexually transmitted infection (STI), such as a syphilis chancre or a perineal wart.

43. 1. The baby should have a minimum of 6 wet diapers during each 24-hour period.
    2. The baby should have 3 to 4 loose, bright yellow stools during each 24-hour period.

Babies who consume formula often have pasty, brownish-colored stools.
    3. The baby should breastfeed a minimum of 8 times in a 24-hour period.
    4. Neonates gain, on average, about 5 oz per week, not 6 oz in a 24-hour period.

TEST-TAKING TIP: Breastfeeding mothers often worry whether their babies are receiving enough to eat. It is important, therefore, to provide the mothers with objective assessments that inform them that their babies are receiving enough fluids and nutrition: at least 6 wet diapers per day and 3 to 4 loose, bright yellow stools per day. In addition, the mother can take the baby to the pediatrician's office for periodic weight evaluations.

44. Q 3 min × 60 sec

TEST-TAKING TIP: Frequency (always measured in minutes [min]) is defined as the time period from the beginning of one contraction to the beginning of the next contraction. Duration (always measured in seconds [sec]) is defined as the time period from the beginning of one contraction to the end of the same contraction.

45. 1. The client is not currently pregnant and has 4 living children.
    2. The client is not currently pregnant and has had 3 full-term pregnancies.
    3. The client is not currently pregnant and has had 2 preterm deliveries.
    4. The client is not currently pregnant and has had 1 abortion.

TEST-TAKING TIP: Gravidity (G) is defined as the total number of pregnancies a woman has had, including a current pregnancy. Parity (P) refers to deliveries. The four numbers following the P refer to the following: full-term pregnancies, preterm pregnancies, abortions, living children. The client in the scenario, therefore, has been pregnant 6 times, had 3 full-term deliveries, 2 preterm deliveries, 1 abortion, and has 4 living children. Since 3 + 2 + 1 = 6, the client has delivered all of her pregnancies.

46. 1. A woman should be encouraged to stand erect to improve her posture but this action is not related to the pelvic tilt.
    2. This can be a valuable exercise but it is not the pelvic tilt.
    3. The woman successively changes her back from a concave to a convex posture when doing the pelvic tilt.

4. It is recommended that pregnant women not lie flat on their back.

TEST-TAKING TIP: The pelvic tilt is an excellent exercise for pregnant women. It helps to strengthen as well as to relax the muscles of the lower back. The test taker should be familiar not only with the name of exercises or other procedures but also with the precise way each is performed.

47. 1. NEC does not result in hearing loss.
2. Hypoglycemia does not result in hearing loss.
3. Bronchopulmonary dysplasia does not result in hearing loss.
4. A baby who has had kernicterus can develop hearing loss.

TEST-TAKING TIP: Kernicterus occurs when bilirubin in the bloodstream reaches toxic levels. Bilirubin is neurotoxic. Early signs of kernicterus are lethargy, sleepiness, and poor feeding. Severe kernicterus, when babies develop seizures and opisthotonus, can result in a number of neurological problems, including cerebral palsy, sensory deficits, and behavioral disorders.

48. 1. This action will not assist the midwife with the delivery of the baby.
2. This action will not assist the midwife with the delivery of the baby.
3. Suprapubic pressure can help to dislodge the shoulders of a macrosomic baby and facilitate the delivery.
4. This action will not assist the midwife with the delivery of the baby.

TEST-TAKING TIP: Macrosomia can lead to shoulder dystocia during a delivery. Suprapubic pressure helps to dislodge the shoulders and enable the baby to be delivered. Nurses must not apply fundal pressure in this situation. Rather than facilitating delivery of the shoulders, fundal pressure can actually worsen the dystocia.

49. 1. It is unnecessary for the woman to be seen by the obstetrician for cracked nipples.
2. There is no need to pump and dump. The blood will not injure the baby.
3. Hydrogen peroxide should not be applied to the nipples.
4. Lanolin cream applied after each feeding is an excellent therapy for cracked nipples.

TEST-TAKING TIP: The nurse should also ask the client about the baby's latch, making sure that the baby's mouth is wide, lips are flanged, and tongue is below the breast and lying on the baby's gums.

50. 1. There is nothing in the scenario that indicates that the client's skin integrity is impaired.
2. Although the woman's bladder is full, at this time the client is not bleeding heavily.
3. This answer is correct. The client has not emptied her bladder.
4. The client is able to walk back and forth to the toilet on her own. Her problem is related to an inability to empty her bladder.

TEST-TAKING TIP: The test taker must remember that postpartum clients eliminate large quantities of fluids through their kidneys. When only 100 mL is voided and the uterus is displaced, the nurse must conclude that the client has not emptied her bladder.

51. 1. Placental abruption occurs before the delivery of the baby.
2. Clients who have had forceps deliveries are no more at high risk for seizures than other postpartum clients.
3. Clients who have had forceps deliveries are no more at high risk for idiopathic thrombocytopenia than other postpartum clients.
4. Clients who have had forceps deliveries are at high risk for infection.

TEST-TAKING TIP: The vagina is not a sterile space. Because the forceps are applied through the vagina into the sterile uterine cavity, there is a possibility of bacteria ascending into the upper gynecological system.

52. 1. Headache is associated with preeclampsia, not preterm labor.
2. Visual disturbances are associated with preeclampsia, not preterm labor.
3. The nurse should advise the client immediately to report any uterine cramping.
4. Oliguria is associated with preeclampsia, not preterm labor.

TEST-TAKING TIP: A positive fetal fibronectin assessment between 22 and 37 weeks' gestation puts a client at high risk for preterm labor. All of the other symptoms— headache, visual disturbance, and oliguria— are associated with preeclampsia. The test taker could have made an educated guess regarding the correct response to the question had he or she noted the relationship among the three other options.

53. 1. Babies who swallow after every suck usually are latched well.
    2. To latch well, babies should face their mother's body.
    3. When babies' lips are curled under, they are unable to create a satisfactory suck. In addition, it is usually painful for the mother.
    4. Neonates should be placed at the level of their mother's breasts to breastfeed.

    TEST-TAKING TIP: To create a good latch, babies should have a large quantity of breast tissue in their mouth, lips should be well flanged at the breast, and their tongue should cup around their mother's breast.

54. 2, 4, 3, 1, 5 is the correct order.

    TEST-TAKING TIP: For the fetus to traverse the birth canal, the baby must flex its head so that the chin is on the chest and then must rotate through the pelvis. When the baby's head is flexed, the smallest diameter of the fetal head will present to the pelvis. As the baby proceeds through the moves—descent, internal rotation, extension, external rotation, and expulsion—it will progress from the intrauterine environment to the external environment.

55. 1. Although it is not easy, it is possible to consume enough protein to sustain a pregnancy on a vegan diet.
    2. This action is essential. Women's protein demands increase during pregnancy. Nutrition counselors are qualified to evaluate a pregnant woman's total protein and essential amino acid intake.
    3. This response is incorrect. Cashews and coconut are not excellent sources of calcium.
    4. This response is incorrect. Vegans eat no animal protein.

    TEST-TAKING TIP: Nurses do receive nutrition education during their nursing programs. They are not, however, experts in the field. It is very important for nurses to know the limits of their knowledge. Because protein, as well as calcium intake, is essential for a healthy pregnancy, it is important for the nurse to refer the client to the expert in the field.

56. 1. This action is appropriate. The client must be asked about her injuries.
    2. This is inappropriate. No one deserves to be abused.
    3. This is inappropriate. The police may not have enough evidence to make an arrest.
    4. This is inappropriate.

    TEST-TAKING TIP: Clients rarely discuss domestic violence issues unless they are asked directly about them. Even if the nurse does not see evidence of injury, he or she should inquire about the client's relationship during each nurse-patient encounter.

57. 1. This is an appropriate nursing diagnosis because this child is at high risk for developing hyperbilirubinemia.
    2. This baby is not at high risk for fluid volume deficit.
    3. This baby is not at high risk for interrupted family processes.
    4. This baby is not at high risk for impaired parent-infant attachment.

    TEST-TAKING TIP: The baby in the scenario is exhibiting signs of ABO incompatibility. The mother's blood type is O+ while the baby's type is A+. Because the baby's direct Coombs' test is positive, the nurse should conclude that the baby has anti-A antibodies in the bloodstream against the A antigen. If the baby's blood should start to hemolyze, high levels of bilirubin will be released into the baby's bloodstream. High levels of bilirubin can damage the baby's central nervous system.

58. 1. Because a larger diameter of the fetal head is presenting to the pelvis in the LMP position, cephalopelvic disproportion is possible.
    2. Placental abruption is not higher risk for the delivery of a baby in LMP position than it is for a baby in any other position.
    3. LMP is a vertex, not a breech, position.
    4. Acute fetal distress is not higher risk for the delivery of a baby in LMP position than it is for a baby in any other position.

    TEST-TAKING TIP: When a baby's mentum is presenting to the birth canal, the baby's head has failed to flex during descent. As a result, rather than the smallest diameter of the fetal head presenting to the pelvis, a larger diameter is presenting. Cephalopelvic disproportion is a possible consequence.

59. 1. A genetic amniocentesis is performed between 12 and 16 weeks' gestation.
    2. Intrauterine growth restriction is detected via ultrasound.
    3. A lecithin/sphingomyelin ratio and/or a shake test can be performed on amniotic fluid to determine whether the fetal

lung fields are mature. These tests are performed during the third trimester.

4. Hormonal studies would not be conducted on the amniotic fluid.

TEST-TAKING TIP: To answer this question correctly, the test taker must attend carefully to the gestational age when the test is being conducted. Even though amniocenteses are performed to obtain fetal cells for genetic analysis, those tests are not performed during the third trimester.

60. 1. Although this action is very important, the infusion should first be discontinued. If the fluid is a vesicant, the physician should then be notified.
    2. The first thing the nurse should do is to discontinue the infusion.
    3. The nurse should document the occurrence after the important interventions have been performed.
    4. After discontinuing the infusion, the arm should be elevated and, if appropriate, warm soaks applied.

TEST-TAKING TIP: Although most IV fluids administered in the obstetric area do not harm the tissues if they should extravasate, some, like antibiotics, can adversely affect the vessels and surrounding tissues. The nurse must be knowledgeable about the actions he or she should take if an infiltration should occur.

61. 1. Follicle-stimulating hormone (FSH), not LH, accelerates the growth and maturation of an egg in the ovary.
    2. This response is untrue. LH does not enhance the potential of the sperm to fertilize an egg.
    3. This response is untrue. LH does not facilitate the egg's movement through the fallopian tube.
    4. This response is correct. LH stimulates the release of a mature egg from the ovary each month.

TEST-TAKING TIP: FSH stimulates the growth and maturation of the egg, while LH stimulates its release from the ovary. The woman's temperature will drop slightly when she experiences the LH surge.

62. 1. The nurse should remove the caffeinated coffee from the food tray.
    2. The nurse need not remove the cheeseburger from the food tray.
    3. The nurse need not remove the fried fish from the food tray.

4. The nurse need not remove the pork sausage from the food tray.

TEST-TAKING TIP: Mormons are forbidden from drinking caffeinated beverages, like coffee and colas, and are forbidden from smoking and from drinking alcohol. To show respect, the nurse should remove the offending beverage from the woman's food tray.

63. 1. The incidence of UTIs is slightly higher in boys who have not been circumcised, but there is no need to check the baby's daily temperature.
    2. The prepuce should not be fully drawn back during the newborn period because of the potential for inducing pain and scarring.
    3. The pediatrician will not have to evaluate the baby. Phimosis, or a tightened prepuce, may be present at birth or may develop subsequent to an infection. The mother, therefore, should be advised to watch that the baby's urine flows freely when he voids.
    4. This response is correct. The baby's prepuce should be cleansed with soap and water during the daily bath. The mother should not force the foreskin to retract, but if it does naturally loosen from the glans, she should gently clean underneath.

TEST-TAKING TIP: Whether or not to circumcise a male child is a decision for the parents to make. There is some evidence that males are much less at risk of developing sexually transmitted infections if they are circumcised and the incidence of UTI is slightly higher in boys who have not been circumcised. The American Academy of Pediatrics, however, does not recommend that all males be circumcised.

64. 1. The nurse would not expect to see a drop in the baseline fetal heart rate.
    2. The nurse would not expect to see an increase in variable decelerations.
    3. The nurse would expect to see a decrease in the baseline variability.
    4. The nurse would not expect to see an increase in early decelerations.

TEST-TAKING TIP: Demerol is a narcotic analgesic. Narcotics are central nervous system (CNS) depressants. The baseline variability is an expression of the interaction between the parasympathetic

and sympathetic nervous systems of the fetus. Because the narcotic enters the fetal vascular system through the placenta, the fetal CNS is depressed. As a result, the variability drops.

65. 1. The four-chambered heart is present by 8 weeks' gestation.
2. Although webbed and short, fingers and toes are visible by 8 weeks' gestation.
3. The genitalia are not fully formed until about 12 weeks' gestation.
4. The facial features are all present by 8 weeks' gestation.

TEST-TAKING TIP: By the time the embryo reaches 8 weeks' gestation virtually all organ systems are present. Male genitalia will be differentiated by 12 weeks if testosterone is produced. If no testosterone is produced, female genitalia develop. Maturation continues in all organ systems through the remainder of the pregnancy.

66. 1. This question is not appropriate in relation to the clinical findings.
2. This question is not appropriate in relation to the clinical findings.
3. This question is not appropriate in relation to the clinical findings.
4. This question is important for the nurse to ask at this time.

TEST-TAKING TIP: Even though the client is postdelivery, her blood pressures are rising. It is likely that she is developing preeclampsia. Among the symptoms that clients with severe preeclampsia experience are headache, blurred vision, and epigastric pain.

67. 1. Neonates who are exhibiting signs of neonatal abstinence syndrome are not at high risk of becoming hypothermic. In addition, neonates should be swaddled rather than covered with blankets. When a baby is covered, the blankets may inadvertently cover the baby's face, obstructing the baby's nasal passages.
2. Neonates who are exhibiting signs of neonatal abstinence syndrome should be kept in a low-stimulation environment.
3. Neonates who are exhibiting signs of neonatal abstinence are often soothed by the playing of soft classical music.
4. Neonates who are exhibiting signs of neonatal abstinence syndrome should be kept in a low-stimulation environment.

TEST-TAKING TIP: Neonatal abstinence syndrome is the title given to the signs and symptoms exhibited by babies during the drug withdrawal period. The babies are hyperreflexic and agitated during this period; therefore, keeping them in a soothing, low-stimulation environment is optimal.

68. 1. The baby is not yet engaged. It is very unlikely that the client will experience a precipitous delivery.
2. The membranes have been ruptured a very short time. The client is not at high risk for infection at this time.
3. The fetal heart rate is showing variable decelerations, the baby is not postdates, and there is no evidence of other placental issues. The client is not at high risk for uteroplacental insufficiency.
4. The membranes are ruptured, the baby is not engaged, the baby is in the sacral position, and the fetal heart rate is showing variable decelerations. The nurse should assess this client carefully for prolapsed cord.

TEST-TAKING TIP: The test taker must methodically consider the many factors in the scenario before determining the correct answer to this question. The key items that must be considered are fetal heart rate, time since rupture of membranes, fetal position, fetal station, and gestational age.

69. 1. A banana is an excellent fruit choice, but it does not meet the young woman's iron or calcium needs.
2. Cheeseburgers meet both iron and calcium needs.
3. Strawberries are an excellent fruit choice, but they do not meet the young woman's iron or calcium needs.
4. Rice is high in protein and does contain some calcium, but it is not a good iron source.

TEST-TAKING TIP: The best way to remember the special nutritional needs of young pregnant adolescents is to remember that they are still growing themselves. As a result, they need the minerals, calcium and iron, as well as protein for their own growth and development as well as to meet the needs of the growing fetus. Of the choices, only cheeseburgers meet all those needs.

70. 1. This action is not advisable unless the woman requests the move.
2. This action is inappropriate. The nurse must acknowledge the loss of the baby.

3. This action is appropriate. The nurse should offer the couple the opportunity to hold their baby.
4. This action is inappropriate. The administration of milk suppressants is not recommended because of the adverse side effects of the medications.

TEST-TAKING TIP: Unless the couple view and hold their baby, they will have no tangible person to mourn. If they should decide not to see their baby, nurses should take pictures of the baby. In the future, the couple can look at the pictures to remember their loss. In addition, clients who have had a fetal loss should be forewarned that they may lactate. This can be very stressful for a grieving woman if she is unprepared.

71. 1. It is recommended that women not douche.
    2. It is recommended that women not douche.
    3. It is recommended that women not douche.
    4. It is recommended that women not douche.

TEST-TAKING TIP: Douching not only adversely affects the vaginal environment, it also can force endometrial tissue into the tubes and onto the ovaries, resulting in endometriosis, especially during the menses.

72. 1. The client's physician should be notified.
    2. It is inappropriate to massage the client's leg.
    3. It is inappropriate to apply ice packs to the leg.
    4. It is inappropriate to encourage the client to walk.

TEST-TAKING TIP: Clients who exhibit any or all of the following symptoms— erythema, warmth, edema, pain—in one or both calves may have a deep vein thrombosis. The physician should be notified so that diagnostic tests can be ordered. If the woman were to ambulate or if she were to massage her leg, the thrombus could become dislodged.

73. 1. The nurse should refrain from giving any information to the woman regarding the babies' schedules.
    2. The nurse should politely escort the woman to a postpartum room, if appropriate, or off the unit if she is not visiting a patient.

3. The nurse should refrain from giving any information to the woman regarding the babies' schedules.
4. The nurse should politely escort the woman to a postpartum room, if appropriate, or off the unit if she is not visiting a patient.

TEST-TAKING TIP: The physical characteristics and actions of the woman in the scenario are consistent with those of women who abduct neonates. By asking the client which patient the woman wishes to visit, the nurse will be able to determine whether the woman is a legitimate visitor.

74. 1. It is very unlikely that a woman in transition would fall asleep during contractions.
    2. These are characteristic actions of laboring women who are in transition.
    3. It is very unlikely that a woman in transition would be watching television.
    4. Pushing is characteristic of stage 2 of labor.

TEST-TAKING TIP: Transition is the most forceful phase of the first stage of labor. The contractions are strong and frequent and mothers, especially primigravidas, are usually fatigued and very uncomfortable during the phase. Vomiting is commonly seen during this phase.

75. 1. At 22 weeks, testes are not yet descended, the suck is weak, and lanugo and vernix are present.
    2. At 28 weeks, testes may begin to descend, the suck is weak, and lanugo and vernix are abundant.
    3. At 32 weeks, testes may have descended, the suck is improving but still poor, and lanugo and vernix are abundant.
    4. At 38 weeks, testes are fully descended, the suck is strong, and the amount of lanugo and vernix is minimal.

TEST-TAKING TIP: The test taker should be familiar with major fetal development milestones. Preterm babies are born covered in lanugo and vernix, have weak sucks, and, if male, have not developed sufficiently to have their testes present in their scrotal sacs.

76. 1. If a mother wishes to breastfeed, the nurse should assist her to do so.
    2. Down syndrome babies require the same number of calories as do other babies.
    3. The mother can breastfeed the Down baby in any position—side-lying, cradle, cross-cradle, or football—as long as she provides the jaw support that the baby

needs. Mothers of Down babies often find that the football hold works best.

4. Down syndrome babies are hypotonic. They often have a weak suck at birth.

TEST-TAKING TIP: Simply because a baby has a congenital defect does not mean that the baby will be unable to breastfeed. The nurse should assess each situation individually and provide assistance when needed. If additional help is required, a lactation consultant should be requested.

77. 1. Macrosomic babies are no more at high risk for jaundice than are babies of average weight.
2. Macrosomic babies are at high risk for jitters.
3. Macrosomic babies are no more at high risk for blepharitis, inflammation of the eyelash follicles, than are babies of average weight.
4. All babies are born with a pseudostrabismus. The muscles of the eyes usually mature by 6 months when the strabismus ceases.

TEST-TAKING TIP: To answer this question correctly, the test taker must fully understand the physiology of pregnancy and the pathophysiology of a major cause of macrosomia—namely, maternal gestational diabetes. The high glucose levels in the maternal bloodstream easily cross the placenta, resulting in high glucose levels in the fetus. The babies metabolize the glucose, resulting in a proportionate increase in body weight. When the babies deliver, their bodies continue to excrete high levels of insulin but the high levels of glucose are no longer available. Hypoglycemia and jitters (a symptom of hypoglycemia) result. Because the mother in this scenario had had no prenatal care, it is very possible that she had undiagnosed gestational diabetes.

78. 1. This client is high risk for preterm labor because she is African American, under 17 years of age, and has been diagnosed with gestational diabetes, a vascular disease.
2. Although twin pregnancies are at high risk for preterm labor, this client currently is carrying a single fetus. Plus, Asian American women are not at high risk for preterm labor.

3. Neither Jewish clients nor clients who work as CPAs are at high risk for preterm labor.
4. Clients who follow the Mormon religion are not at high risk for preterm labor. Simply because a client has had a recent move does not place her at high risk for preterm labor.

TEST-TAKING TIP: It has been shown that there are many risk factors for preterm labor, including non-white race, age over 35 or under 17, and maternal medical disease.

79. 1. Most women have no complaints.
2. Most women have no complaints.
3. Most women have no complaints.
4. Most women have no complaints.

TEST-TAKING TIP: Chlamydia is known as a "silent" disease because about 75% of infected women and about 50% of infected men have no symptoms. If symptoms do occur, they usually appear within a few weeks of the exposure (see http://www. cdc.gov/std/chlamydia/STDFact-Chlamydia.htm).

80. 1. There is a 75% probability that their child will have the disease.
2. There is a 75% probability that their child will have the disease.
3. There is a 75% probability that their child will have the disease.
4. There is a 75% probability that their child will have the disease.

TEST-TAKING TIP: The test taker should create and analyze a Punnett square:

Father:	A	a
Mother: A	AA	Aa
a	Aa	aa

Because only 1 dominant gene need be present for a dominant disease to be exhibited, each child has a $\frac{3}{4}$ or 75% probability of having the disease.

81. 1. Newborn babies should be burped after consuming every 1/2 to 1 ounce of formula.
2. This statement is true. To prevent ingestion of air, the bottle nipple should be filled with formula throughout the feeding.
3. Formula should never be heated in the microwave.

4. Because of the potential for aspiration, baby bottles should never be propped.

TEST-TAKING TIP: Mothers who decide to bottle feed their babies must be educated regarding safe bottle-feeding practices. Not only is propping unsafe but it also decreases the amount of quality time the mother has with her baby.

82. 1. This client did vomit twice last shift, but she is not the highest risk of the nurse's patients.
    2. This client is at high risk for preterm labor, but she is not the highest risk of the nurse's patients.
    3. This client does need to be given preoperative teaching and prepared for surgery, but she is not the highest risk of the nurse's patients.
    4. This client should be seen first. Although obstetrically she is not at high risk, her care must take priority because she had a pulmonary episode during the prior shift.

TEST-TAKING TIP: When taking a comprehensive examination, the test taker should be prepared to answer complex questions. This question requires the test taker to consider a variety of issues including antepartum clients versus postpartum clients, obstetric complications versus medical complications, and preoperative issues versus standard care issues.

83. 1. A 34-week baby weighing 500 grams would be classified as small-for-gestational age.
    2. A 34-week baby weighing 1,700 grams would be classified as small-for-gestational age.
    3. A 34-week baby weighing 2,900 grams would be classified as appropriate-for-gestational age.
    4. A 34-week baby weighing 4,100 grams would be classified as large-for-gestational age.

TEST-TAKING TIP: The test taker must be prepared to interpret simple graphs. Appropriate-for-gestational age babies are babies who weigh between the 10th and 90th percentile for a specific gestational age.

84. 1. The presence of cardiac arrhythmias warrants termination of the medication.
    2. A respiratory rate of 24 does not warrant termination of the medication.
    3. The blood pressure may rise. A blood

pressure of 90/60 does not warrant termination of the medication.
    4. Hypocalcemia does not warrant termination of the medication.

TEST-TAKING TIP: Terbutaline is a beta agonist used to treat preterm labor. Tachycardia is an expected side effect of the medication, but its use is contraindicated in clients with dysrhythmias or with a heart rate over 140 bpm.

85. 1. A warm shower may help to promote the milk ejection reflex, but this is not the question the nurse should ask at this time.
    2. The client may need to pump her breasts to soften them enough for the baby to latch well, but this is not the question the nurse should ask at this time.
    3. Unless a client has a very low intake, the quantity of fluids that the client consumes is not related to the quantity of milk she will produce.
    4. The nurse should ask the client when she fed the baby last.

TEST-TAKING TIP: Engorgement rarely develops if a mother breastfeeds frequently. Breastfeeding mothers should be encouraged to feed every 2 to 3 hours. Plus, it is especially important to encourage them never to skip a feeding. If they must give the baby a bottle in place of a breastfeeding, they should pump their breasts at the same time as the missed feeding.

86. 1. The vital signs are normal. There is no indication that the client may be bleeding heavily at this time.
    2. The client's temperature, although higher than during labor, is not elevated significantly. This is not the appropriate action to take at this time.
    3. The only significant change in vitals is a rise in temperature to 99.4°F. Because the client has recently delivered, it is likely that the elevation is related to dehydration. The nurse should encourage the client to drink fluids.
    4. There is nothing in the scenario that indicates that the client may have a pulmonary problem. This is not the appropriate action to take at this time.

TEST-TAKING TIP: The only significant change in the client's vital signs from the intrapartum period to the postpartum

period is the elevation in the temperature. Since the temperature is not high enough to signal an infection, it is likely related to dehydration. She should drink fluids. If the client were becoming hypovolemic from blood loss, the nurse would have noted a marked elevation in pulse rate but likely no change in blood pressure. Because the blood volume of women rises dramatically during pregnancy, their bodies are able to compensate for an extended period of time before hypotension is noted.

87. 1. It is inappropriate to insert eye prophylaxis when the baby needs resuscitation.
2. This action is inappropriate. The baby needs to be resuscitated.
3. An Apgar score of 3 is an indication for neonatal resuscitation.
4. There is no need to repeat the score until 5 minutes after birth. The score of 3 at 1 minute is enough evidence to warrant resuscitation.

TEST-TAKING TIP: An Apgar score of 8 or above indicates that the baby is making a smooth transition into extrauterine life. A score of 3 indicates a baby that is severely compromised. Resuscitation should be instituted as quickly as possible.

88. 1. Although minimal perineal pain is a goal for the PP client, it is not related to the nursing diagnosis of potential for fluid volume deficit.
2. Normal lochial flow is a goal related to the nursing diagnosis of potential for fluid volume deficit.
3. Although a normal temperature is a goal for the PP client, it is not related to the nursing diagnosis of potential for fluid volume deficit.
4. The PP client is expected to have some weight reduction, but that goal is not related to the nursing diagnosis of potential for fluid volume deficit.

TEST-TAKING TIP: The nursing process is an important tool used by nurses to provide care. To provide needed care, the nurse must determine goals for his or her clients. The goals are related to the nursing diagnoses. When fluid volume deficit is of concern, the nurse must consider loss of fluids through bleeding, excessive voiding, or other means. The nursing goal is that the client not bleed heavily.

89. 2 and 3 are correct.
1. The baby is no more at high risk for hyperreflexia than are other neonates.
2. The nurse should monitor the baby for respiratory distress and hypoglycemia.
3. The nurse should monitor the baby for respiratory distress and hypoglycemia.
4. The baby is no more at high risk for opisthotonus than are other neonates.
5. The baby is no more at high risk for nuchal rigidity than are other neonates.

TEST-TAKING TIP: Babies of diabetic mothers are at high risk for respiratory distress because their lung fields develop more slowly than the lung fields of babies of normoglycemic mothers. Even full-term infants of diabetic mothers sometimes have respiratory difficulties.

90. 1. The tube is placed through the mouth into the baby's stomach. When gastric juices are aspirated, the nurse knows that the tubing is in the stomach.
2. Babies will often suckle on items in their mouths. This does not mean, however, that the tubing is in place.
3. Even if the tubing is inserted correctly into the stomach, the baby may exhibit some respiratory difficulties.
4. Even though the nurse meets resistance when inserting the tube, this does not mean that it has been inserted into the stomach.

TEST-TAKING TIP: When a tube is inserted into a baby for a gavage feeding, the nurse must be certain that the tube has entered the stomach and not the lung fields. There are a number of actions the nurse can take to ensure the tube's placement, including injecting air into the tubing and listening with a stethoscope for the "rush" as it enters the stomach as well as aspirating the stomach contents.

91. 1. This response is incorrect. The maternal and fetal circulatory systems are independent throughout pregnancy.
2. This response is incorrect. The maternal and fetal circulatory systems are independent throughout pregnancy.
3. This response is incorrect. The maternal and fetal circulatory systems are independent throughout pregnancy.
4. This response is correct. The maternal and fetal circulatory systems are independent throughout pregnancy.

TEST-TAKING TIP: The fetal circulation and maternal circulation are independent of each other. Oxygen and nutrients enter into the fetal system across cell membranes in the placenta. Similarly, waste products from the fetus are eliminated through the maternal system across the same cell membranes.

92. 1. The weight loss is excessive. This response is not acceptable.
    2. It is inappropriate to recommend that the woman stop breastfeeding. It may be appropriate to add supplementation, however.
    3. The nurse should notify the neonatologist of the excessive weight loss.
    4. It is inappropriate for the baby to receive dextrose water between feedings.

    TEST-TAKING TIP: Babies can safely lose between 5% and 10% of their birth weights in the first few days of life. Instead of calculating the exact weight loss for this baby, however, the test taker can determine what a 10% weight loss would be for the baby and compare that figure to the child's actual weight loss: $2678 \times 0.1 = 267.8$. Because the baby has lost more than 10% of its birth weight (286 > 267.8), it is easy to determine that the weight loss is excessive.

93. 2, 3, 4, and 5 are correct.
    1. Because the majority of fetal development occurs during the embryonic period, and many women are unaware that they are pregnant until well into that period, it is too late to stop drinking alcohol when the woman "thinks" that she may be pregnant.
    2. To make sure that a woman is not suffering from a disease that could adversely affect a pregnancy, or that pregnancy would adversely affect a woman's health, it is important for a woman to have a complete medical checkup prior to becoming pregnant.
    3. Because folic acid supplementation has been found to reduce the incidence of some birth defects, women should take a daily multivitamin that includes folic acid when they are trying to become pregnant.
    4. Because dental x-rays could injure the developing embryo, a woman should tell her dentist that she is trying to become pregnant so that the dentist can shield her abdomen during the x-ray.
    5. Pregnant women are especially high risk for contracting listeriosis. The offending organism, *Listeria*

monocytogenes, is found in sushi and rare meat, as well as in a number of other foods.

TEST-TAKING TIP: Embryogenesis often occurs before a woman is aware that she is pregnant. Because teratogenic insults can injure the developing embryo, it is essential that women plan their pregnancies and avoid teratogens when attempting to become pregnant.

94. 1. Breastfeeding every 2 hours is an important nursing care goal for a postpartum client, but it is not highest priority.
    2. A nutritious diet is an important nursing care goal for a postpartum client, but it is not highest priority.
    3. The nursing care goal of a moderate lochial flow for a postpartum client is of highest priority.
    4. Walking in the hallways every shift is an important nursing care goal for a postpartum client, but it is not highest priority.

    TEST-TAKING TIP: The test taker should consider the acronym CAB (circulation, airway, breathing) to determine which nursing care goal is of highest priority. The care goal related to lochial flow is directly related to circulation (C). If the client were to bleed heavily, her circulation would be compromised.

95. 1. The nurse would expect the client to complain of severe back pain.
    2. Descent is often slowed when the baby is in a posterior position.
    3. The nurse would not expect to see hypotonic or irregular contractions.
    4. The nurse would not expect rectal pressure or an increase in bloody show.

    TEST-TAKING TIP: When the fetus is in a posterior position, the occiput of the baby's head presses against the coccyx during every contraction. This action is very painful. None of the other responses is directly linked to a posterior fetal position.

96. 1. A nursing diagnosis of altered skin integrity (maternal) is not related to the clinical scenario.
    2. A nursing diagnosis of maternal deficient fluid volume is not related to the clinical scenario.
    3. A nursing diagnosis of risk for fetal injury is an appropriate nursing diagnosis.

4. A nursing diagnosis of fetal urinary retention is not related to the clinical scenario.

TEST-TAKING TIP:: The client in the scenario has an elevated fasting blood glucose level as well as an elevated glycohemoglobin level. The nurse knows, therefore, that the client is currently hyperglycemic and has been hyperglycemic over the past 3 months. Because hyperglycemia is teratogenic, the fetus is at high risk for injury or, in other words, at high risk for birth defects.

97. 1. Hyperemesis and hypertension are often seen in clients with hydatiform mole.
    2. Neither diarrhea nor hyperthermia is associated with hydatiform mole.
    3. Polycythemia is not associated with hydatiform mole.
    4. Polydipsia is not associated with hydatiform mole.

TEST-TAKING TIP: Because the levels of human chorionic gonadotropin (hCG) are markedly elevated with hydatiform mole, women often experience persistent vomiting into the second trimester. In addition, signs of preeclampsia, such as hypertension, appear before 20 weeks' gestation in clients with molar pregnancies.

98. 1. Delayed placental separation is not associated with maternal cigarette smoking.
    2. The nurse should carefully monitor the labor for late decelerations.
    3. Shoulder dystocia is not associated with maternal cigarette smoking.
    4. Precipitous fetal descent is not associated with maternal cigarette smoking.

TEST-TAKING TIP: Smoking affects the oxygenation ability of the placenta. Indeed, the placentas of women who smoke are often small, infarcted, and/or calcified. During labor, therefore, there is a strong likelihood that uteroplacental insufficiency will be evident. Late decelerations are indicative of uteroplacental insufficiency.

99. 1. Babies whose mothers are HIV positive are not at high risk during the immediate neonatal period.
    2. This is the correct response. Babies who are born to mothers who are GBS positive are at high risk for sepsis. The incidence of sepsis is reduced, however, when the mother receives IV antibiotics during labor.
    3. Twelve hours is not an abnormal length for a patient's labor.
    4. Although 45 pounds higher than the recommended weight gain for pregnancy, this baby is not highest priority.

TEST-TAKING TIP: Each of the responses includes either a number or a disease process. To answer the question, the nurse must determine which of the answer options is a high-risk state during the immediate neonatal period. Even though babies born to women who are HIV positive may acquire the infection, the baby will not be adversely affected by the virus immediately after birth. (In fact, if the babies are treated, transmission rates are very low.) Babies born to mothers who are GBS positive, however, may develop sepsis while in the neonatal nursery.

100. 1. This is an incorrect answer. The blood bypasses the pulmonary system during fetal circulation.
     2. This is a correct answer. When the cord is clamped, the blood is no longer being oxygenated through the placenta. The baby's oxygen levels, therefore, begin to drop.
     3. Bacteria will not colonize the bowel until the baby has been in the extrauterine environment and has eaten.
     4. Bilirubin levels usually begin to rise on day 2.

TEST-TAKING TIP: If the test taker remembers the role of the umbilical cord, the answer becomes very clear. The change in the blood gasses—drop in oxygen levels with a concomitant rise in carbon dioxide levels—is one of the important triggers that stimulates babies to breathe.

References

American Cancer Society. (2012). Retrieved from http://cancer.org/index

American College of Obstetricians and Gynecologists. (2012). Retrieved from http://acog.org/

American Society for Reproductive Medicine. (2012). Retrieved from http://asrm.org/ASRM_homepage/

Beattie, S. (2007). Bedside emergency: Wound dehiscence. *RN*. Retrieved from http://rnweb.com/rnweb/article/articleDetail.jsp?id=433110

Bishop, E.H. (1964). Pelvic scoring for elective induction. *Obstetrics & Gynecology, 24*, 266.

Centers for Disease Control and Prevention. (n.d.) Retrieved from http://cdc.gov/

Dietary guidelines for Americans. (2010). Retrieved from http://health.gov/dietaryguidelines/dga2010/DietaryGuidelines2010.pdf

Guidelines for Catholics on the evaluation and treatment of infertility. (n.d.). Catholic infertility. Retrieved from http://catholicinfertility.org/guidelines.html

Infertility: An overview. (2003). Birmingham, AL: American Society for ReproductiveMedicine. Retrieved from http://asrm.org/uploadedFiles/ASRM_Content/Resources/Patient_Resources/Fact_Sheets and_Info_Booklets/infertility_overview.pdf

IOM (Institute of Medicine). (2011b). *Dietary reference intakes for energy, carbohydrate, fiber, fat, fatty acids, cholesterol, protein, and amino acids.* Washington, DC: The National Academies Press.

Marron, R.L., Lanphear, B.P., Kouides, R., et al. (1998). Efficacy of informational letters on hepatitis immunization rates in university students. *Journal of American College Health, 47*(3), 123–127.

My Sister's Place, Inc. (2009). Retrieved from http://mysistersplacedc.org/.

2010 NCLEX-RN® detailed test plan. (2010). Chicago, IL: National Council of State Boards of Nursing.

Office of Dietary Supplements (NIH). (2011). Retrieved from http://ods.od.nih.gov/

Planned Parenthood. (2012). Retrieved from http://plannedparenthood.org.

Preimplantation Genetic Diagnosis International Society. (2012). Retrieved from http://pgdis.org/

RAINN: Rape, Abuse and Incest National Network. (2009). Retrieved from http://rainn.org/

Rasmussen, K.M., Abrams, B., Bodnar, L.M., et al. (2009). *Weight gain during pregnancy: Reexamining the guidelines.* Washington, DC: National Academy of Sciences. Retrieved from http://iom.edu/~/media/Files/Report%20Files/2009/Weight-Gain-During-Pregnancy-Reexamining-the-Guidelines/Report%20Brief%20-%20Weight%20Gain%20During%20Pregnancy.pdf

Ross, A.C., Taylor, C.L., Yaktine, A.L., et al. (2011). *Dietary reference intakes for calcium and vitamin D.* Institute of Medicine. Retrieved from http://nationalacademyofsciencescalvitD.pdf

Stanford, J.B., White, G.L., & Hatasaka, H. (2002). Timing intercourse to achieve pregnancy: Current evidence. *Obstetrics & Gynecology, 100*(6), 1333–1341.

Tool kit for teen care: Suggested responses to common adolescent-related telephone questions (2nd ed). (2009). Washington, DC: The American College of Obstetricians and Gynecologists. Retrieved from http://acog.org/~/media/Departments/Adolescent%20Health%20Care/Teen%20Care%20Tool%20Kit/SuggestedResponsesLT2.pdf?dmc=1&ts=20120227T1605503280

USDA. (n.d.). *Choose my plate*. Retrieved from http://choosemyplate.gov/foodgroups/dairy_counts.html

U.S. Department of Health and Human Services. (2012). *Health information privacy*. Retrieved from http://hhs.gov/ocr/privacy/hipaa/understanding/index.html

U.S. eligibility criteria for contraceptive use. (2010). *MMWR, 59* (RR-4), 1–88. Retrieved from http://cdc.gov/mmwr/pdf/rr/rr5904.pdf

U.S. Food and Drug Administration. (2012). Retrieved from http://fda.gov/default.htm

Workowski, K.A., & Berman, S.M. (2010). Sexually transmitted diseases treatment guidelines, 2010. *MMWR, 59* (RR-12), 1–112. Retrieved from http://cdc.gov/std/treatment/2010/STD-Treatment-2010-RR5912.pdf

World Alliance for Breastfeeding Action. (n.d.). Retrieved from http://waba.org.my/index.htm

World Health Organization. (2012). Retrieved from http://who.int/en/

Index

A

Abdominal pain
  afterbirth pains, 216, 232
  incisions, cesarean section clients, 210, 225
  in pregnancy, 98, 117, 239–240, 256–257
  when ovulation occurs, 12, 30, 32
Abduction of newborns, 179, 203, 404, 421
ABO incompatibility, 321, 339–340, 401, 418
  Coombs' test, 321, 340
Abortion
  discussing with client, 59, 76
  spontaneous
    incomplete, 240, 258
      RhoGAM injection following, 249, 271
      showing concern for client, 240, 257
Abruptio placentae, 287, 305
  from auto accident, 240, 257–258
  cocaine use and, 287, 305–306
  differentiating from placenta previa, 287, 306
  enlarging abdominal girth measurements and, 399, 415
  fundal height and, 287, 305
Abstinence syndrome, neonatal, 322, 341, 403, 420
  hypoglycemia, ruling out, 323, 342
  soothing newborns with classical music, 403, 420
  swaddling, 322, 341
Abuse
  denial of, 64, 82
  giving client options and safety plan, 64, 82–83
  "honeymoon phase," 64, 83
  postpartum, of infant, 371, 386–387
  during pregnancy, 252, 275
  questioning about, 63–64, 82–83, 401, 418
  signs of, 63–64, 82–84
Accelerations (fetal heart) during fetal movement, 137, 137f, 154
Acetaminophen, liquid, 169, 190
Achondroplasia, 21, 41
Acidosis, 245–246, 266–267
Acquired immune deficiency syndrome (AIDS). *See* HIV (human immunodeficiency syndrome)/AIDS (acquired immune deficiency syndrome)
Acrocyanosis, 163, 182
Active alert period (newborn), 165, 184–185
Active phase of labor, 143
Acupressure, in labor, 141, 159
Addicted mother
  instruction on baby-care skills, 367, 380–381
  reporting to child protective services, 367, 381
Adolescents
  access to birth control methods, 46, 76
    state-specific methods not on NCLEX-RN, 76
  childbirth education, 130, 147
  date rape, protecting from, 64, 84
  female condoms, 58, 75

pregnancy, 250–251, 273–274
  diet, 403, 420
Adoption, 16, 35
African culture, expressing breast milk into babies' eyes to prevent infections, 176, 198–199
Afterbirth pains, 216, 232
AIDS (acquired immune deficiency syndrome). *See* HIV (human immunodeficiency syndrome)/AIDS (acquired immune deficiency syndrome)
Alcohol consumption, breastfeeding and, 174, 196
Alendronate (Fosamax), for osteoporosis, 62, 80
Ambulation, postpartum, 212, 214, 226, 229–230
Amenorrhea
  anorexia nervosa, 63, 82
  excessive exercise and, 13, 33, 63, 82
  lactational amenorrhea method (LAM), 59, 77
  presumptive sign of pregnancy, 88, 104
Amniocentesis, 22, 26, 28, 43, 46
Amnioinfusion, 289, 308
Amniotic fluid, 101, 121
  embolism, 286–287, 304–305, 398, 414
  meconium-stained fluid, 289, 307–308
  nitrazine paper, assessing fluid with, 282, 300
  smell of, 282, 300–301
Amniotomy, 132, 149, 283, 301
  prolapsed cord, 295, 317
Anasarca, 334, 358
Anemia
  pregnant client, 95, 111–112
    diet, 240, 257
  sickle cell anemia, 27, 47, 247, 268
    screening, 162, 180
Anesthesia
  epidural
    hypotension following, 140, 157–158
    spinal versus epidural anesthesia in cesarean section clients, 291, 310, 368, 382, 385
  general
    antacids presurgically, 291, 310
    cricoid pressure, applying, 291, 291f, 311, 311f
    history of scoliosis surgery, 292, 312
  spinal
    epidural versus spinal anesthesia in cesarean section clients, 291, 310, 368, 382, 385
    positioning clients postanesthesia, 210, 224
    post-cesarean section, postural headaches and, 371, 382, 385
Anorexia nervosa
  amenorrhea, 63, 82
  excessive exercise, 63, 82
  significant weight loss, 63, 82
Answers and rationales
  antepartum, 104–125
    high-risk, 254–277
  comprehensive examination, 409–426

D